W9-BAF-436

Drugs, Society, and Human Behavior

Drugs, Society, and Human Behavior Twelfth Edition

Charles Ksir
University of Wyoming

Carl L. Hart
Columbia University

Oakley Ray
Vanderbilt University

Boston   Burr Ridge, IL   Dubuque, IA   Madison, WI   New York
San Francisco   St. Louis   Bangkok   Bogotá   Caracas   Kuala Lumpur
Lisbon   London   Madrid   Mexico City   Milan   Montreal   New Delhi
Santiago   Seoul   Singapore   Sydney   Taipei   Toronto

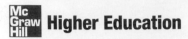

Higher Education

DRUGS, SOCIETY, AND HUMAN BEHAVIOR
Published by McGraw-Hill, a business unit of The McGraw-Hill Companies, Inc., 1221 Avenue of the Americas, New York, NY, 10020. Copyright © 2008, 2006, 2004, 2002, 1999, 1996, 1993, 1987, 1983, 1978, 1972 by The McGraw-Hill Companies, Inc. All rights reserved. No part of this publication may be reproduced or distributed in any form or by any means, or stored in a database or retrieval system, without the prior written consent of The McGraw-Hill Companies, Inc., including, but not limited to, in any network or other electronic storage or transmission, or broadcast for distance learning. Some ancillaries, including electronic and print components, may not be available to customers outside the United States.

This book is printed on acid-free paper.

3 4 5 6 7 8 9 0 DOC/DOC 0 9 8 7

ISBN: 978-0-07-352961-5
MHID: 0-07-352961-3

Vice President and Editor-in-Chief: *Emily Barrosse*
Publisher: *William R. Glass*
Sponsoring Editor: *Joseph Diggins*
Director of Development: *Kathleen Engelberg*
Senior Developmental Editor: *Kirstan Price*
Editorial Coordinator: *Sarah Hill*
Executive Marketing Manager: *Nick Agnew*
Managing Editor: *Jean Dal Porto*
Project Manager: *Jean R. Starr*
Art Director: *Jeanne Schreiber*
Art Editor: *Ayelet Arbel*
Illustrators: *Lotus Art*
Designer: *Marianna Kinigakis*
Cover and interior design: *Pam Verros*
Cover photo: © *Marie Bertrand/images.com/Veer*
Manager, photo research: *Brian J. Pecko*
Developmental Editor for Technology: *Julia D. Akpan*
Media Producer: *Michele Borrelli*
Production Supervisor: *Jason I. Huls*
Composition: *by Techbooks*
Printing: *45# New Era Matte, R. R. Donnelley & Sons*

Credits: The credits section for this book begins on page C1 and is considered an extension of the copyright page.

Library of Congress Cataloging-in-Publication Data
Ksir, Charles
    Drugs, society, and human behavior / Charles Ksir, Carl L. Hart, Oakley Ray.—12th ed.
        p. cm.
    Includes bibliographical references and index.
    ISBN-13: 978-0-07-352961-5 (softcover : alk. paper)
    ISBN-10: 0-07-352961-3 (softcover : alk. paper)
        1. Psychotropic drugs. 2. Drug abuse. 3. Drug abuse—Social aspects. 4. Neuropsychopharmacology. I. Ray, Oakley Stern. II. Hart, Carl L. III, Title.
    RM315.R372008
    362.29—dc22   2006048144

The Internet addresses listed in the text were accurate at the time of publication. The inclusion of a Web site does not indicate an endorsement by the authors of McGraw-Hill, and McGraw-Hill does not guarantee the accuracy of the information presented at these sites.

www.mhhe.com

Brief Contents

Contents

List of Boxes

Drugs in the Media

Drugs in Depth

Taking Sides

Mind/Body Connection

Targeting Prevention

DSM-IV-TR

Preface

Today's media-oriented college students are aware of many issues relating to drug use. Nearly every day we hear new concerns about methamphetamine, club drugs, legal pharmaceuticals, and the effects of tobacco and alcohol, and most of us have had some personal experience with these issues through family, friends, or coworkers. This course is one of the most exciting students will take because it will help them relate the latest information on drugs to their effects on society and human behavior. Students will not only be in a better position to make decisions to enhance their own health and well-being, but they will also have a deeper understanding of the individual problems and social conflicts that arise when others misuse and abuse psychoactive substances.

Much has changed in the 35 years since *Drugs, Society, and Human Behavior* was first published. The 1970s were a period of widespread experimentation with marijuana and hallucinogens, while the 1980s brought increased concern about illegal drugs and conservatism, along with decreased use of alcohol and all illicit drugs. Not only did drug-using behavior change, but so did attitudes and knowledge. And, of course, in each decade the particular drugs of immediate social concern have changed: LSD gave way to angel dust, then to heroin, then to cocaine and crack. In the 1990s, we saw increased use of LSD and marijuana, but not to the levels of the 1970s.

Recent Trends

The most alarming trend in recent years has been the increased misuse of prescription opioid pain relievers such as Oxycontin and Vicodin. These pharmaceuticals have now replaced cocaine as the leading cause of drug overdose deaths in the United States (not counting alcohol overdoses), and they have joined methamphetamine and Ecstasy as leading causes of concern about drug misuse and abuse. Methamphetamine, Esctasy, GHB, and the misuse of prescription painkillers are the big news items in the new century.

Meanwhile, our old standbys, alcohol and tobacco, remain with us and continue to create serious health and social problems. Regulations undergo frequent changes, new scientific information becomes available, and new approaches to prevention and treatment are being tested, but the reality of substance use and abuse always seems to be with us.

This text approaches drugs and drug use from a variety of perspectives—behavioral, pharmacological, historical, social, legal, and clinical—which will help students connect the content to their own interests.

Special Features

Updated Content in the Twelfth Edition

Throughout each chapter, we have included the very latest information and statistics, and the Drugs in the Media feature has allowed us to comment on breaking news right up to press time. In addition, we have introduced many timely topics and issues that are sure to pique students' interest and stimulate class discussion.

The following are just some of the new and updated topics in the twelfth edition:

- Statistics on drug use in various populations (Chapter 1), on drug-related toxicity from the new DAWN system (Chapter 2), and on Americans in prison (Chapter 3)
- Fear and decision making (Chapter 2)
- Treatments for ADHD (Chapter 6), sleep disorders (Chapter 7), and bipolar disorder (Chapter 8)
- Alcohol sales and consumption, alcohol effects on traffic accidents, and new alcohol inhaling devices (Chapter 9)

- Tobacco consumption and tobacco-related mortality (Chapter 10)
- Consumption of coffee and other beverages containing caffeine (Chapter 11)
- Heroin usage rates (Chapter 13)
- Medical marijuana, including recent U.S. Supreme Court decisions (Chapter 15)
- Nutritional ergogenic aids (Chapter 16)
- Effective prevention programs (Chapter 17)
- New medical approaches to the treatment of dependence (Chapter 18)

Focus Boxes

Boxes are used in *Drugs, Society, and Human Behavior* to explore a wide range of current topics in greater detail than is possible in the text itself. The boxes are organized around key themes.

Drugs in the Media Our world revolves around media of all types—TV, films, radio, print media, and the Web. To meet students on familiar ground, we have included Drugs in the Media boxes, which take an informative and critical look at these media sources of drug information. Students can build their critical thinking skills while reading about such topics as alcohol advertising, media coverage of prescription drugs, and the presentation of cigarette smoking in films.

Taking Sides These boxes discuss a particular drug-related issue or problem and ask students to take a side in the debate. This thought-provoking material will help students apply what they learned in the chapter to real-world situations. Taking Sides topics include potential medical uses of marijuana and heroin, current laws relating to drug use, and the use of animals in drug testing.

Mind/Body Connections The Mind/Body Connection boxes highlight the interface between the psychological and the physiological aspects of substance use, abuse, and dependence. These boxes help students consider influences on their own attitudes toward drug use. Topics include religion and drug use, the social and emotional costs of smoking, and the nature of dependence.

Targeting Prevention The Targeting Prevention boxes offer perspective and provoke thought regarding which drug-related behaviors we, as a society, want to reduce or prevent. Topics include syringe exchange programs, criminal penalties for use of date rape drugs, and non-drug techniques for overcoming insomnia. These boxes help students better evaluate prevention strategies and messages.

Drugs in Depth These boxes examine specific, often controversial, drug-related issues such as crack babies, nutritional supplements for improving sports performance, and the growing number of people in prison for drug-related offenses. Drugs in Depth boxes are a perfect starting point for class or group discussion.

Online Learning Center Resources These boxes, found at the opening of each chapter, direct students toward the useful resources available on the Online Learning Center for *Drugs, Society, and Human Behavior.* These resources include learning objectives, glossary flashcards, Web activities, chapter quizzes, audio chapter summaries, and links. Students can use Online Learning Center resources to improve their grades and get the most out of this course.

Check Yourself! Activities

These self-assessments, found at the end of most chapters, help students put health concepts into practice. Each Check Yourself! activity asks students to answer questions and analyze their own attitudes, habits, and behaviors. Self-assessments are included in such areas as sleep habits, daily mood changes, alcohol use, caffeine consumption, and consideration of consequences.

Attractive Design and Illustration Package

The inviting look, bold colors, and exciting graphics in *Drugs, Society, and Human Behavior* draw the reader in with every turn of the page. Sharp and appealing photographs, attractive illustrations, and informative tables support and clarify the chapter material. The twelfth edition features more than 100 new photos.

Pedagogical Aids

Although all the features of *Drugs, Society, and Human Behavior* are designed to facilitate and improve learning, several specific learning aids have been incorporated into the text:

- **Chapter Objectives:** Chapters begin with a list of objectives that identify the major concepts and help guide students in their reading and review of the text.

- **Definitions of Key Terms:** Key terms are set in boldface type and are defined on the same page in corresponding boxes. Other important terms in the text are set in italics for emphasis. Both approaches facilitate vocabulary comprehension.

- **Chapter Summaries:** Each chapter concludes with a bulleted summary of key concepts. Students can use the chapter summaries to guide their reading and review of the chapters.

- **Review Questions:** A set of questions appears at the end of each chapter to aid students in their review and analysis of chapter content.

- **Appendices:** The appendices include handy references on brand and generic names of drugs and on drug resources and organizations.

- **Summary Drugs Chart:** A helpful chart of drug categories, uses, and effects appears on the back inside cover of the text.

Supplements

A comprehensive package of supplementary materials designed to enhance teaching and learning is available with *Drugs, Society, and Human Behavior*.

Instructor Teaching Tools from the Online Learning Center www.mhhe.com/ksir12e

The following instructor resources are available for download from the Online Learning Center; to obtain a password to download these teaching tools, please contact your local sales representative.

- **Instructor's Manual:** Organized by chapter, the Instructor's Manual includes chapter objectives, key terms, chapter outlines, key points, suggested class discussion questions and activities, and video suggestions.

- **Test Bank:** Revised and expanded for the twelfth edition, the test bank now includes more questions for each chapter. The questions are available as Word files and with **the EZ Test computerized testing software.** EZ Test provides a powerful, easy-to-use test maker to create printed quizzes and exams. For secure online testing, exams created in EZ Test can be exported to WebCT, Blackboard, PageOut, and EZ Test Online. EZ Test comes with a Quick Start Guide, user's manual, and Flash tutorials. Additional help is available online at www.mhhe.com/eztest.

- **PowerPoint Slides:** Updated and expanded for the twelfth edition, the PowerPoint slides include key lecture points and images from the text and other sources.

- **Image Bank:** Expanded for the twelfth edition, the image bank contains over 200 images from the text and other sources.

Student Resources Available with *Drugs, Society, and Human Behavior*

- **Online Learning Center (www.mhhe.com/ ksir12e):** Student study and learning tools on the **free** Online Learning Center include chapter objectives, glossary flashcards, self-correcting quizzes, Web activities, audio chapter summaries, and links.

- **HealthQuest 4.2:** An optional CD-ROM that can be packaged with the text, HealthQuest includes tutorials, assessments, and behavior change guidance. Sample HealthQuest Activities for *Drugs, Society, and Human Behavior* are included on the Online Learning Center.

Classroom Performance System (CPS)

CPS, a wireless response system, brings interactivity into the classroom or lecture hall. Each student uses a wireless response pad similar to a television remote to instantly respond to polling or quiz questions. Results can be posted for immediate viewing by the instructor and entire class. Contact your local sales representative for more information about using CPS with *Drugs, Society, and Human Behavior.*

PageOut
www.pageout.net

PageOut is a free, easy-to-use program that enables instructors to quickly develop websites for their courses. PageOut can be used to create a course home page, an instructor home page, an interactive syllabus that can be linked to elements in the Online Learning Center, weblinks, online discussion areas, an online grade book, and much more. Contact your McGraw-Hill sales representative to obtain a password for PageOut.

Course Management Systems

The Online Learning Center can also be customized to work with popular course-management systems such as WebCT and Blackboard. The McGraw-Hill Instructor Advantage program offers access to a complete online teaching website called the Knowledge Gateway, toll-free phone support, and unlimited e-mail support directly from WebCT and Blackboard. Instructors who use 500 or more copies of a text can enroll in the Instructor Advantage Plus program, which provides on-campus, hands-on training from a certified platform specialist.

Primis Online
www.mhhe.com/primis

Primis Online is a database-driven publishing system that allows instructors to create customized textbooks, lab manuals, or readers for their courses directly from the Primis website. The custom text can be delivered in print or electronic (eBook) form. A Primis eBook is a digital version of the customized text sold directly to students as a file downloadable to their computer or accessed online by password. *Drugs, Society, and Human Behavior* can be customized using Primis Online.

Acknowledgments

We would like to express our appreciation to the following instructors who reviewed the previous edition and helped lay the groundwork for the improvements and changes needed in the twelfth edition:

M. J. Basti, *Cuesta Community College*
M. Harry Daniels, *University of Florida*
Julie David, *Normandale Community College*
Jay Elliott, *Medical University of South Carolina*
Jeanne Freeman, *California State University, Chico*
Anne Garcia, *Washtenaw Community College*
Jamie Johnson, *Western Illinois University*
Richard Larkin, *Harper College*
Steven Strazza, *The College of Saint Rose*
Bob Walsh, *Utah Valley State College*

Charles Ksir
Carl L. Hart
Oakley Ray

Drug Use in Modern Society

The interaction between drugs and behavior can be approached from two general perspectives. Certain drugs, the ones we call psychoactive, have profound effects on behavior. Part of what a book on this topic should do is describe the effects of these drugs *on behavior,* and later chapters do that in some detail. Another perspective, however, views drug taking as *behavior.* The psychologist sees drug-taking behaviors as interesting examples of human behavior that are influenced by many psychological, social, and cultural variables. In the first section of this text, we focus on drug taking as behavior that can be studied in the same way that other behaviors, such as aggression, learning, and human sexuality, can be studied.

1 **Drug Use: An Overview**
Which drugs are being used and why?

2 **Drug Use as a Social Problem**
Why does our society want to regulate drug use?

3 **Drug Products and Their Regulations**
What are the regulations, and what is their effect?

1

Drug Use: An Overview

Objectives

When you have finished this chapter, you should be able to:

- **Develop an analytical framework for understanding any specific drug-use issue.**

- **Apply four general principles of psychoactive drug use to any specific drug-use issue.**

- **Explain the differences between misuse, abuse, and dependence.**

- **Describe how four revolutions in pharmacology have helped to shape attitudes about drugs.**

- **Describe the general trends of increases and decreases in drug use in the U.S. since 1975.**

- **Remember several correlates and antecedents of adolescent drug use.**

- **Describe correlates and antecedents of drug use in the terminology of risk factors and protective factors.**

- **Discuss motives that people may have for illicit and/or dangerous drug-using behavior.**

"The Drug Problem"

Talking About Drug Use

"Drug use on the rise" is a headline that has been seen quite regularly over the years. It gets our attention. At any given time the unwanted use of some kind of drug can be found to be increasing, at least in some group of people. How big a problem does the current headline represent?

Before you can meaningfully evaluate the extent of such a problem or propose possible solutions, it helps to define what you're talking about. In other words, it helps to be more specific about just what the problem is. Most of us don't really view the problem as drug use, if that includes your Aunt Margie's taking two aspirins when she has a headache. What we really mean is that some drugs being used by some people or in some situations constitute problems with which our society must deal.

Journalism students are told that an informative news story must answer the questions *who, what, when, where, why,* and *how.* Let's see how answering the same questions plus one more question—*how much*—can help us analyze problem drug use.

- *Who* is taking the drug? We are more concerned about a 15-year-old girl drinking a beer than we are about a 21-year-old woman doing the same thing. We worry more about a 10-year-old boy chewing tobacco than we do about a 40-year-old man chewing it (unless we happen to be riding right behind him when he spits out the window). And, although we don't like anyone taking heroin, we undoubtedly get

Online Learning Center Resources

www.mhhe.com/ksir12e

Visit our Online Learning Center (OLC) for access to these study aids and additional resources.

- Learning objectives
- Glossary flashcards
- Web activities and links
- Self-scoring chapter quiz
- Audio chapter summaries

more upset when we hear about the girl next door becoming a user.

- *What* drug are they taking? This question should be obvious, but often it is overlooked. A simple claim that a high percentage of students are "drug users" doesn't tell us if there has been an epidemic of methamphetamine use or if the drug referred to is alcohol (more likely). If someone begins to talk about a serious "drug problem" at the local high school, the first question should be "what drug or drugs?"

- *When* and *where* is the drug being used? The situation in which the drug use occurs often makes all the difference. The clearest example is the drinking of alcohol; if it is confined to appropriate times and places, most people accept drinking as normal be-

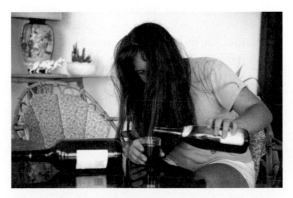

Our concern about the use of a substance often depends on who is using it.

havior. When an individual begins to drink on the job, at school, or in the morning, that behavior is evidence of a drinking problem. Even subcultures that accept the use of illegal drugs might distinguish between acceptable and unacceptable situations; some college-age groups might accept marijuana smoking at a party but not just before going to a calculus class!

- *Why* a person takes a drug or does anything else is a tough question to answer. Nevertheless, it is important in some cases. If a person takes Vicodin because her doctor prescribed it for the knee injury she got while skiing, most of us would not be concerned. If, on the other hand, she takes that drug on her own, just because she likes the way it makes her feel, then we should begin to worry about possible abuse of the drug. The motives for drug use, as with motives for other behaviors, can be complex. Even the person taking the drug might not be aware of all the motives involved. One way a psychologist can try to answer *why* questions is to look for consistency in the situations in which the behavior occurs (when and where). If a person drinks only with other people who are drinking, we may suspect social motives; if a person often drinks alone, we may suspect that the person is trying to deal with personal problems by drinking.

- *How* the drug is taken can often be critical. South American Indians who chew coca leaves absorb cocaine slowly over a long period. The same total amount of cocaine "snorted" into the nose produces a more rapid, more intense effect of shorter duration and probably leads to much stronger dependence. Smoking cocaine in the form of "crack" produces an even more rapid, intense, and brief effect, and dependence occurs very quickly.

- *How much* of the drug is being used? This isn't one of the standard journalism questions, but it is important when describing drug use. Often the difference between

Drugs in the Media

Reporting on the "Drug du Jour"

At the beginning of this millennium, newspaper and television stories about drugs are dominated by the so-called **club drugs,** such as Ecstasy and GHB. Before that there was a wave of media reports about crystal meth and other forms of methamphetamine. In the mid-1980s, it was crack cocaine. Of course these waves of media focus are associated with waves of drug use, but the news media all seem to jump on the latest "drug du jour" (drug of the day) at the same time. For example, the U.S. Drug Enforcement Administration (DEA) announced in 2000 that the club drugs were its highest priority, and this means more news stories about arrests of distributors for these types of drugs.

One question that doesn't get asked much is this: What role does such media attention play in popularizing the current drug fad, perhaps making it spread farther and faster than would happen without the publicity? About 30 years ago, in a chapter titled "How to Create a Nationwide Drug Epidemic," journalist

E. M. Brecher described a sequence of news stories that he believed were the key factor in spreading the practice of sniffing the glues sold to kids for assembling plastic models of cars and airplanes (see *volatile solvents* in Chapter 7). He argued that, without the well-meant attempts to warn people of the dangers of this practice, it would probably have remained isolated to a small group of youngsters in Pueblo, Colorado. Instead, sales of model glue skyrocketed across America, leading to widespread restrictions on sales to minors.

Thinking about the kinds of things such articles often say about the latest drug problem, are there components of those articles that you would include if you were writing an advertisement to promote use of the drug? Do you think such articles actually do more harm than good, as Brecher suggested? If so, does the important principle of a free press mean there is no way to reduce the impact of such journalism?

what one considers normal use and what one considers abuse of, for example, alcohol or a prescription drug comes down to how much a person takes.

Four Principles of Psychoactive Drugs

Now that we've seen how helpful it can be to be specific when talking about drug use, let's look for some organizing principles.

Are there any general statements that can be made about **psychoactive** drugs—those compounds that alter consciousness and affect mood? Four basic principles seem to apply to all of these drugs.

1. *Drugs, per se, are not good or bad.* There are no "bad drugs." When drug abuse, drug dependence, and deviant drug use are talked about, it is the behavior, the way the drug is being used, that is being referred to. This statement sounds controversial and has angered some prominent political fig-

ures and drug educators. It therefore requires some defense. For a pharmacologist, it is difficult to view the drug, the chemical substance itself, as somehow possessing evil intent. It sits there in its bottle and does nothing until we put it into a living system. From the perspective of a psychologist who treats drug users, it is difficult to imagine what good there might be in heroin or cocaine. However, heroin is a perfectly good painkiller, at least as effective as morphine, and it is used medically in many countries. Cocaine is a good local anesthetic and is still used for medical procedures, even in the United States. Each of these drugs can also produce bad effects when people abuse them. In the cases of heroin and cocaine, our society has weighed its perception of the risks of bad consequences against the potential benefits and decided that we should severely restrict the availability of these substances. It is wrong, though, to place all of the blame for these bad consequences on the drugs themselves and to conclude that they are simply "bad" drugs. Many people tend to view some of these substances as possessing an almost magical power to produce evil. When we blame the substance itself, our efforts to correct drug-related problems tend to focus exclusively on eliminating the substance, perhaps ignoring all of the factors that led to the abuse of the drug.

2. *Every drug has multiple effects.* Although a user might focus on a single aspect of a drug's effect, we do not yet have compounds that alter only one aspect of consciousness. All psychoactive drugs act on more than one place in the brain, so we might expect them to produce complex psychological effects. Also, virtually every drug that acts in the brain also has effects on the rest of the body, influencing blood pressure, intestinal activity, or other functions.

3. *Both the size and the quality of a drug's effect depend on the amount the individual has taken.* The relationship between dose and effect works in two ways. By increasing the dose, there is usually an increase in the same effects noticed at lower drug levels. Also, at different dose levels there is often a change in the kind of effect, an alteration in the character of the experience.

4. *The effect of any psychoactive drug depends on the individual's history and expectations.* Because these drugs alter consciousness and thought processes, the effect they have on an individual depends on what was there initially. An individual's attitude can have a major effect on his or her perception of the drug experience. The fact that relatively inexperienced users can experience a high when smoking oregano and dry oak tree leaves—thinking it's good **marijuana**—should come as no surprise to anyone

who has arrived late at a party and felt a "buzz" after one drink rather than the usual two or three. It is not possible, then, to talk about many of the effects of these drugs independent of the user's history and attitude and the setting.

How Did We Get Here?

Have Things Really Changed?

Drug use is not new. Humans have been using alcohol and plant-derived drugs for thousands of years—as far as we know, since *Homo sapiens* first appeared on the planet. Recorded history indicates that some of these drugs were used not just for their presumed therapeutic effects but also for recreational purposes. In some of the highly developed ancient cultures, psychoactive plants played important economic and religious roles. There is also evidence that some people have always overused, misused, or abused these substances.

Drugs play a much different role in modern society than they did even 100 years ago. Major events have occurred in pharmacology and medicine that have produced revolutionary changes in the way in which we view drugs. In addition, recent cultural revolutions have influenced our attitudes and behavior regarding drugs and drug use.

club drugs: drugs associated with use at all-night dance parties, known as "raves," held in dance clubs, abandoned warehouses, and increasingly in more traditional nightclubs as the rave-party generation moves into its 20s. The drugs most commonly included in this group include the hallucinogen MDMA ("Ecstasy"; Chapter 14) and the depressants GHB and Rohypnol ("roofies"; Chapter 7).

psychoactive: having effects on thoughts, emotions, or behavior.

marijuana (mare i *wan* ah): also spelled "marihuana." Dried leaves of the *Cannabis* plant.

Drugs in Depth

Important Definitions—and a Caution!

Some terms that are commonly used in discussing drugs and drug use are difficult to define with precision, partly because they are so widely used for many different purposes. Therefore, any definition we offer should be viewed with caution because each represents a compromise between leaving out something important versus including so much that the defined term is watered down.

The word **drug** will be defined as "any substance, natural or artificial, other than food, that by its chemical nature alters structure or function in the living organism." One obvious difficulty is that we haven't defined *food,* and how we draw that line can sometimes be arbitrary. Alcoholic beverages, such as wine and beer, may be seen as either drug, food, or both. Are we discussing how much sherry wine to include in beef Stroganoff, or are we discussing how many ounces of wine can be consumed before becoming intoxicated? Since this is not a cookbook but, rather, a book on the use of psychoactive chemicals, we will view all alcoholic beverages as drugs.

Illicit drug is a term used to refer to a drug that is unlawful to possess or use. Many of these drugs are available by prescription, but when they are manufactured or sold illegally they are illicit. Traditionally, alcohol and tobacco have not been considered illicit substances even when used by minors, probably because of their widespread legal availability to adults. Common household chemicals, such as glues and paints, take on some characteristics of illicit substances when people inhale them to get "high."

Deviant drug use is drug use that is not common within a social group *and* that is disapproved of by the majority, causing members of the group to take corrective action when it occurs. The corrective action may be informal (making fun of the behavior, criticizing the behavior) or formal (incarceration, treatment). Some examples of drug use might be deviant in the society at large but accepted or even expected in particular subcultures. We still consider this behavior to be deviant, since it makes more sense to apply the perspective of the larger society.

Drug misuse generally refers to the use of prescribed drugs in greater amounts than, or for purposes other than, those prescribed by a physician or dentist. For nonprescription drugs or chemicals such as paints, glues, or solvents, misuse might mean any use other than the use intended by the manufacturer.

Abuse consists of the use of a substance in a manner, amounts, or situations such that the drug use causes problems or greatly increases the chances of problems occurring. The problems may be social (including legal), occupational, psychological, or physical. Once again, this definition gives us a good idea of what we're talking about, but it isn't precise. For example, some would consider any use of an illicit drug to be abuse because of the possibility of legal problems, but many people who have tried marijuana would argue that they had no problems and therefore didn't abuse it. Also, the use of almost any drug, even under the orders of a physician, has at least some potential for causing problems. The question might come down to how great the risk is and whether the user is recklessly disregarding the risk. How does cigarette smoking fit this definition? Should all cigarette smoking be considered drug abuse? For someone to receive a diagnosis of having a *substance abuse disorder* (see DSM-IV-TR feature in Chapter 2), the use must be recurrent, and the problems must lead to significant impairment or distress.

Addiction is a controversial and complex term that has different meanings for different people. Because the term is so widely used in everyday conversation, it is risky for us to try to give it a precise, scientific definition, and then have our readers use their own long-held perspectives whenever we use the term. Therefore, we have avoided using this term where possible, instead relying on more precisely defined terms such as *dependence*.

Drug **dependence** refers to a state in which the individual uses the drug so frequently and consistently that it appears that it would be difficult for the person to get along *without* using the drug. For some drugs and some users, there are clear withdrawal signs when the drug is not taken, implying a *physiological dependence*. Dependence can take other forms, as shown in the DSM-IV-TR feature in Chapter 2. If a great deal of the individual's time and effort is devoted to getting and using the drug, if the person often winds up taking more of the substance than he or she intended, and if the person has tried several times without success to cut down or control the use, then the person meets the criteria for dependence.

Taking Sides

Can We Predict or Control Trends in Drug Use?

Looking at the overall trends in drug use, it is clear that significant changes have occurred in the number of people using marijuana, cocaine, alcohol, and tobacco. However, while it's easy to describe the changes once they have happened, it's much tougher to predict what will come next. Maybe even harder than predicting trends in drug use is knowing what social policies are effective in controlling these trends. The two main kinds of activities that we usually look to as methods to prevent or reduce drug use are legal controls and education (including advertising campaigns). How effective do you think laws have been in helping prevent or reduce drug use? Be sure to consider laws regulating sales of alcohol and tobacco to minors in your analysis. What about the public advertising campaigns you are familiar with? How about school-based prevention programs? As you go through the remainder of this book, these questions will come up again, along with more information about specific laws, drugs, and prevention programs. For now, choose which side you would rather take in a debate on the following proposition: broad changes in drug use reflect shifts in society and are not greatly influenced by drug-control laws, antidrug advertising, or drug-prevention programs in schools.

Four Pharmacological Revolutions

One hundred years ago, most Americans had a very different view of medicines than we have today. Only a few drugs had powerful effects, and these were used to treat a wide variety of ailments. The idea that a drug could be a specific treatment for a specific disease was only a dream. As a consequence, most people had limited faith in the power of drugs and were cautious about using them. Our modern attitudes about drugs are based to a great extent on several important advances in pharmacology.

The first revolution brought some major communicable diseases well under control. The use of *vaccines,* which began with Pasteur, Jenner, and Koch in the 19th century, has had a major impact on our society. The deadly disease smallpox was almost entirely eliminated, and other serious diseases are virtually a thing of the past; diphtheria, polio, and whooping cough are nearly unheard of, except when we refer to the vaccines for them. Measles, mumps, and tetanus also are preventable now through the development of specific vaccines. *Vaccines helped convince the public that medicine is capable of produc-* *ing drugs with very powerful and very selective beneficial effects.*

The second pharmacological revolution resulted from the introduction of *antibiotics:* "sulfa" drugs, penicillin, and then others. First proven effective during World War II, they continue to save lives daily. These drugs not only cure such previously dreaded diseases as syphilis and pneumonia but can also prevent or treat infections resulting from injury or surgery, thus saving both lives and limbs. *Antibiotics helped give us faith in drugs as effective cures for serious illnesses.* We now expect that when we get sick we will go to a physician who will prescribe a drug that will make us better.

The first two revolutions might be too pervasive and too close to home for most of us to appreciate their importance. This is not the case with the third pharmacological revolution—the development of **psychopharmacology** that began in the 1950s (see Chapter 8). The most

psychopharmacology: the study of the behavioral effects of drugs.

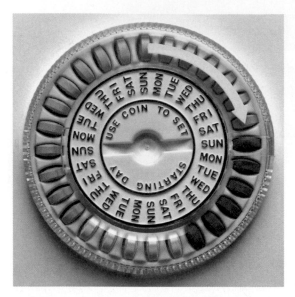

Oral contraceptives were one of the first drugs to be widely used by healthy people to exert chemical control over the functioning of their bodies.

important single event was the introduction of the antipsychotic drugs for the treatment of schizophrenia and other major psychotic disorders. These drugs have freed thousands of patients from long-term hospitalization and have helped restructure our society's approach to mental illness on several levels. One important, but little-studied, effect on our culture came about because these drugs have their primary effect on mental processes. *Because of advances in psychopharmacology, we came to accept the notion that drugs can have powerful effects on our emotions and our perceptions.* Perhaps the psychopharmacological revolution of the 1950s helped set the stage for the "psychedelic" experimentation of the 1960s.

The fourth pharmacological revolution, the development of the *oral contraceptive,* contributed to the sexual revolution, which was beginning to occur in the 1950s and has not yet stabilized. It is probably true that the opportunity for unmarried couples to engage in sex without fear of pregnancy contributed to a greater sexual freedom in the 1960s and 1970s.

That a married woman could be relatively certain for the first time of having several years of her life uninterrupted by pregnancy made it possible for her to commit to attaining more education and to developing her career. Perhaps those social changes were ready to happen without "the pill," but we all began to think in terms of *planning* for pregnancy and childbirth. This control factor might be one of the most pervasive and subtle influences of the oral contraceptive on our society's view of drugs. *With oral contraceptives, powerful chemicals clearly labeled as drugs were not being used to prevent or treat disease but were being used by healthy people to gain chemical control over their own bodies.* This may have helped pave the way for attempts to control emotions and thoughts by using chemistry.

Recent Cultural Change

After World War II, Americans enjoyed a period of growth and prosperity. Concerns about substance abuse were not a major cultural feature of the era that is immortalized in reruns of "Leave it to Beaver." There was some worry about alcohol use being such an accepted part of business and social life, as seen in the 1962 film *Days of Wine and Roses,* and there was a little fascination with the world of jazz music and heroin use, revealed in the 1955 film *The Man With the Golden Arm.* Still, it is revealing that in the early days of rock and roll music the older generation was concerned about the music's possible influence on sexuality, and there was no implied association with drug use. The phrase, "sex, drugs, and rock and roll" wasn't heard before the 1960s.

The mid-1960s was an era of rapid cultural change all over the world, especially in the United States. The Beatles, the civil rights movement, and the Vietnam war were all part of the mix, as was a newfound interest in marijuana and other drugs. Lysergic acid diethylamide (LSD) became a household word, and "psychedelic" referred not only to the experiences of drug users, but also to flamboyant styles of music, art, and clothing. At colleges and universities, parties that had previously featured beer kegs now often included pills and passing around a marijuana joint. Drug use became a common theme on television and in the movies, from *Yellow Submarine* (1968) and *Easy Rider* (1969) through 1978's *Up in Smoke.*

Of course, those who were older or more conservative reacted. Richard Nixon appealed to the "silent majority" in a 1969 speech on Vietnam, and in 1971 was the first to declare a "War on Drugs." However, the 1970s continued to be an era of greater tolerance for drug use, as indicated by the lowering of drinking ages in many states, as well as the lowering of penalties for possession of marijuana (see Chapter 15).

American society in the 1980s became less tolerant of differences, foreigners, pornography, experimental drug use, and young people questioning America's traditional ideals. Congress debated a constitutional amendment to ban the burning of the American flag. Penalties for violating drug laws, which had been loosened in the 1970s, were increased and broadened. The drinking age, which most states had lowered during the 1970s, was increased to 21 again. Authority was back, along with conformity and materialism. College students were being criticized for their focus on the dollar value of their degree rather than on the experience of learning.

The 1990s seemed largely to be a continuation of the 1980s, with a little softening of attitudes toward drugs. Marijuana use increased somewhat among high school students, but the dominant culture remained socially and politically conservative and focused on the wealth that was being generated by the stock market in general and Internet industries in particular.

Not long after the new century opened, the American economy began to slow and people began to question whether the stock market was really the answer to all our important social questions. Then the World Trade Center attack inspired a stronger sense of patriotism and "pulling together" than America had known in decades. But the broadening gap between rich and poor, continuing racial issues, and an increasingly obvious generational rift indicate

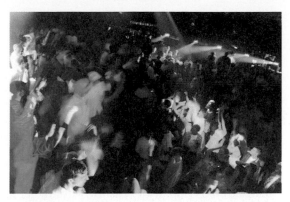

Raves are representative of youth culture and have been associated with so-called club drugs.

the potential for future cultural clashes that will have drugs and drug policy at the forefront. One issue that will help define the next cultural trend is the medicinal marijuana movement (Chapter 15). The federal government stands solidly opposed to increased availability of marijuana for medical purposes, while states are acting to allow such availability. Another issue has been that of the "rave" dance culture among youth and its association with club drugs. Federal lawmakers express horror and outrage while proposing more restrictive measures. The conflict does not appear to be only over drugs, but includes hip-hop, trance, and techno music and other aspects of youth culture that upset the mostly older people representing the dominant culture in America.

Drugs and Drug Use Today

Extent of Drug Use

In trying to get an overall picture of drug use in today's society, we quickly discover that it's not easy to get accurate information. It's not possible to measure with great accuracy the use of, let's say, cocaine in the United States. We don't really know how much is imported and sold, because most of it is illegal. We don't really know how many cocaine users there are in the country, because we have no good way of counting them. For some things, such as prescription drugs, tobacco, and alcohol, we have a wealth of sales information and can make much better estimates of rates of use. Even there, however, our information might not be complete (home-brewed beer would not be counted, for example, and prescription drugs might be bought and then left unused in the medicine cabinet).

Let us look at some of the kinds of information we do have. A large number of survey questionnaire studies have been conducted in junior highs, high schools, and colleges, partly because this is one of the easiest ways to get a lot of information with a minimum of fuss. Researchers have always been most interested in drug use by adolescents and young adults, because this age is when drug use usually begins and reaches its highest levels.

This type of research has a couple of drawbacks. The first is that we can use this technique only on the students who are in classrooms. We can't get this information from high school dropouts. That causes a bias, because those who skip school or have dropped out are more likely to use drugs.

A second limitation is that we must assume that most of the self-reports are done honestly. In most cases, we have no way of checking to see if Johnny really did smoke marijuana last week, as he claimed on the questionnaire. Nevertheless, if every effort is made to encourage honesty (including assurances of anonymity), we expect that this factor is minimized. To the extent that tendencies to overreport or underreport drug use are relatively constant from one year to the next, we can use such results to reflect trends in drug use over time and to compare relative reported use of various drugs.

Let's look first at the drugs most commonly reported by young college students in a recent nationwide sample. Table 1.1 presents data from

Table 1.1
Percentage of College Students One to Four Years beyond High School Reporting Use of Seven Types of Drugs (2004)

Drug	Ever Used	Used in Past 30 Days	Used Daily for Past 30 Days
Alcohol	85	68	3.7
Cigarettes	NA	24	13.8
Marijuana/hashish	49	19	4.5
Inhalants	8	0.4	0.0
Amphetamines	13	3.2	0.2
Hallucinogens	12	1.3	0.0
Cocaine (all)	10	2.4	0.0
Crack	2.0	0.4	0.0

Source: Monitoring the Future Project, University of Michigan and Substance Abuse and Mental Health Services Administration.

Drugs in Depth

Methamphetamine Use in Your Community

Assume that you have just been appointed to a community-based committee that is looking into drug problems. A high school student on the committee has just returned from a residential treatment program and reports that methamphetamine use has become "very common" in local high schools. Some members of the committee want to call in some experts immediately to give school-wide assemblies describing the dangers of methamphetamine. You have asked for a little time to check out the student's story to find out what you can about the actual extent of use in the community and report back to the group in a month. Make a list of potential information sources and the type of information each might provide. How close do you think you could come to making an estimate of how many current methamphetamine users there are in your community? Do you think it would be above or below the national average?

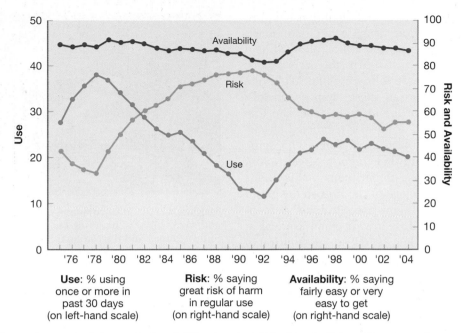

Use: % using
once or more in
past 30 days
(on left-hand scale)

Risk: % saying
great risk of harm
in regular use
(on right-hand scale)

Availability: % saying
fairly easy or very
easy to get
(on right-hand scale)

Figure 1.1   Marijuana: Trends in Perceived Availability, Perceived Risk of Regular Use, and Prevalence of Use in the Past 30 Days for 12th Graders

SOURCE: Johnston, et al. *Monitoring the Future National Survey Results on Drug Use, 1975–2004. Volume I: Secondary School Students* (NIH Publication No. 05-5727). Bethesda, MD.: National Institute on Drug Abuse, 2005.

one of the best and most complete research programs of this type, the Monitoring the Future Project at the University of Michigan. Data are collected each year from more than 15,000 high school seniors in schools across the United States, so that nationwide trends can be assessed. Data are also gathered from 8th- and 10th-graders and from college students. Three numbers are presented for each drug: the percentage of college students (one to four years beyond high school) who have *ever* used the drug, the smaller percentage who report having used it within the past *30 days,* and the still smaller percentage who report *daily* use for the past 30 days.[1] Note that most of these college students have tried alcohol at some time in their lives. Half have tried marijuana, and most students report never having tried the rest of the drugs listed. Also note that daily use of any of these drugs other than cigarettes can be considered rare.

Trends in Drug Use

The high school senior survey, conducted annually for almost 30 years, demonstrates long-term trends. One of the most interesting graphs from this study looks at the prevalence of reported marijuana use in the past 30 days, and relates this to a couple of beliefs about marijuana.[2] Figure 1.1 shows that marijuana use among high school seniors increased from 1975 through 1978 and then declined fairly dramatically throughout the 1980s. This represents a large change in drug-using behavior, from a high of 37 percent of seniors reporting recent marijuana use in 1978, to a low of 12 percent in 1992. The decline then reversed itself, climbing back to 24 percent reporting recent use in 1997, and then slowly declining to just under 20 percent in 2004.

Marijuana is important because it is by far the most frequently used illicit drug, but the same study found a similar, if less dramatic, pattern for trends in recent alcohol use and in recent use of illicit drugs other than marijuana: peak usage around 1980, followed by a decline to the lowest use in the early 1990s, and a small increase following that. We'd like to know what caused these changes, so let's start by looking at the attitude data. The line on the graph in Figure 1.1 labeled "risk" shows the percentage of students who agree with the statement that there is "great risk of harm in regular use of marijuana." This line is almost a mirror image of the line on the graph representing marijuana use. Students' perception of risk was at its lowest when use was at its highest in the late 1970s, and perception of risk reached a peak in the early 1990s when use was at its lowest. We'd like to be able to say that when more students are afraid to use marijuana this causes fewer of them to use it, and that's probably the correct way of looking at this. But we cannot rule out the possibility that the cause works the other way around: When more students are using marijuana and it is more familiar, fewer students are afraid of the risks.

The third line on the graph is also important. Notice that from 1975 through 2004, almost 90 percent of the 12th-graders said it would be fairly easy or very easy for them to get marijuana if they wanted it. In the context of the other two lines, it is surprising how stable this perception is over time. This line represents *perceived* availability—90 percent of the students believe they could get marijuana, but most of them haven't actually bought any. This graph seems to support the idea that if we want to reduce marijuana use among high school students, trying to make marijuana less available might not have much impact, whereas changing the students' attitudes about the risks of using marijuana might be more effective. In other words, the marijuana is always there, but the students will decide whether they are going to use it based on their attitudes.

In addition to the surveys of students, broad-based self-report information is also gathered through house-to-house surveys. With

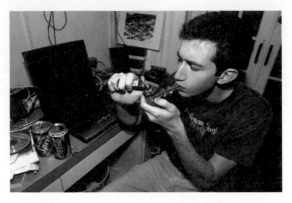

Marijuana is the most commonly used illicit drug, and major surveys including the Monitoring the Future Project and the National Survey on Drug Use and Health track trends in its usage.

proper sampling techniques, these studies can estimate the drug use in most of the population, not just among students. This technique is much more time consuming and expensive, it has a greater rate of refusal to participate, and we must suspect that individuals engaged in illegal drug use would be reluctant to reveal that fact to a stranger on their doorstep. Table 1.2 presents data from the National Survey on Drug Use and Health (formerly called the National Household Survey) obtained from face-to-face, computer-assisted interviews done with more than 68,000 individuals in carefully sampled households across the United States. Because rates of use for most substances are highest in the 18–25 age group, we are presenting data for different demographic groups using only that age group (except for alcohol, where the grouping is all adults over 21). The table shows males typically are more likely to use these substances than females, and those with college degrees are less likely to use tobacco or marijuana than those with high school diplomas. Among the racial/ethnic comparisons, more whites report using these substances than blacks, Hispanics, or Asians.

Some of the results from the National Survey can be compared with similar household surveys conducted as far back as 1965; Figure 1.2 displays the trends in reported past

Table 1.2
Drug Use among 18 to 25-year-olds: Percentage Reporting Use in the Past 30 Days

Drug	Male	Female	White	African American	Hispanic	Native American	Asian	High School Graduate	College Graduate
Alcohol (Age 21+)	65	56	68	48	48	56	47	56	78
Tobacco (all types)	52	37	51	35	35	55	28	46	34
Marijuana	20	12	18	17	10	24	6	16	12
Cocaine	3	2	3	1	2	3	0.2	2	2

Source: Substance Abuse and Mental Health Services Administration. (2005). *Overview of Findings from the 2004 National Survey on Drug Use and Health* (Office of Applied Studies, NSDUH Series H-27, DHHS Publication No. SMA 05-4061). Rockville, MD.

month use of marijuana for two different age groups. This study shows the same pattern as the Monitoring the Future study of 12th-graders: Marijuana use apparently grew throughout the 1970s, reaching a peak in about 1980, and then declining until the early 1990s, when it increased again.

Figure 1.3 shows trends in the *30-day* figures for the 18 to 25 age group for alcohol, marijuana, and cocaine since 1974. Again, we see that the peak of reported use of all these substances was in 1980.

Finding such a similar pattern in two different studies using different sampling

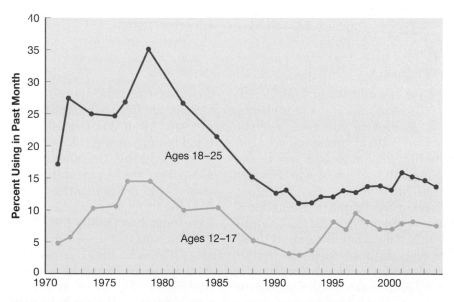

Figure 1.2   Marijuana Use among Persons Ages 12–25, by Age Group: 1971–2004

SOURCE: Substance Abuse and Mental Health Services Administration. (2005). *Overview of Findings from the 2004 National Survey on Drug Use and Health* (Office of Applied Studies, NSDUH Series H-27, DHHS Publication No. SMA 05-4061). Rockville, MD.

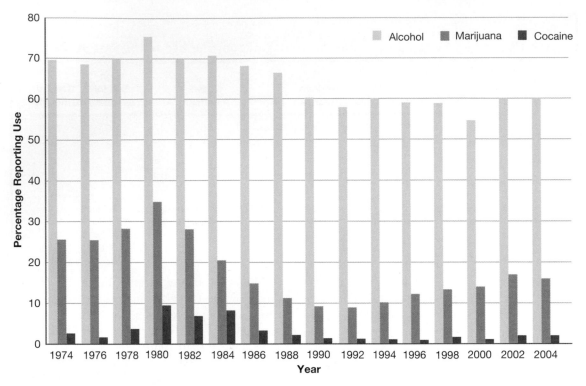

Figure 1.3   Trends in Reported Drug Use within the Past 30 Days for Young Adults Ages 18 to 25

SOURCE: Substance Abuse and Mental Health Services Administration. (2005). *Overview of Findings from the 2004 National Survey on Drug Use and Health* (Office of Applied Studies, NSDUH Series H-27, DHHS Publication No. SMA 05-4061). Rockville, MD.

techniques gives us additional confidence that these trends have been real and probably reflect broad changes in American society over this time. Political observers will be quick to note that Ronald Reagan was president during most of the 1980s, when use of marijuana and other drugs was declining, while Bill Clinton was in office during most of the 1990s, when these rates rose. Were these changes in drug use the result of more conservative drug-control policies under the Reagan administration and more liberal policies under the Clinton administration? There are two reasons to think that is not the answer. First, the timing is not quite right. President Reagan was elected in 1980, took office in 1981, and didn't begin focusing on the

"Just Say No" antidrug messages until 1983. Most of the important legislation was passed in 1986. All of this was after the downward trend in drug use had already begun. It seems more likely that the Reagan administration recognized the opportunity provided by an underlying change in attitude among the general public. The government's policies might have helped to amplify the effects of this underlying social change, but they did not create it. The same timing problem is associated with trying to link drug use to the Clinton presidency: The election was in 1992, and increased use was already beginning in 1993, during the first year of the Clinton administration. Also, the Clinton administration can hardly be accused of having liberal drug-control policies—drug-control budgets and arrests for drug violations were both higher than in any previous administration. We don't have a good explanation for the generational differences in the use of illicit drugs, but the differences are obviously fairly large.

Correlates of Drug Use

Once we know that a drug is used by some percentage of a group of people, the next logical step is to ask about the characteristics of those who use the drug, as compared with those who don't. Often the same questionnaires that ask each person which drugs they have used also include several questions about the persons completing the questionnaires. The researchers might then send their computers "prospecting" through the data to see if certain personal characteristics can be correlated with drug use. But these studies rarely reveal much about either very unusual or very common types or amounts of drug use. For example, if we send a computer combing through the data from 1,000 questionnaires, looking for characteristics correlated with heroin use, only one or two people in that sample might report heroin use, and you can't correlate much based on one or two people. Likewise, it would be difficult to identify the distinguishing characteristics of the people who have "ever tried" alcohol, because that group usually represents more than 90 percent of the sample.

Much of the research on **correlates** of drug use has used marijuana smoking as an indicator, partly because marijuana use has been a matter of some concern and partly because enough people have tried it so that meaningful correlations can be done. Other studies focus on early drinking or early cigarette smoking. We have already seen that age, gender, racial/ethnic grouping, and education level are all related to rates of drug use.

You may be surprised at some of the factors that generally do *not* correlate well with alcohol or drug use. One of these is the *socioeconomic status (SES)* of the family.

Whether reporting on illicit drug use or level of drinking, most studies find little correlation to family income level. These results surprise people who think it's the kids with all the money who use drugs, as well as other people who believe that it's the poor kids who use drugs. In fact, those families living in poverty do have somewhat higher levels of illicit drug use. So very low SES does play a role in drug and alcohol use, but, for the vast majority of the population, SES is not a significant factor. Another surprise for most people is the consistent finding that *personality problems* are poor predictors of drug use. Even though many theories of drug use assume that people use alcohol or drugs because of low self-esteem, depression, or anxiety, many studies have found that measures of these characteristics are only weakly correlated with drug use. People often report that they drink or use drugs when they're depressed or anxious, but they are probably referring to a temporary *state* of depression or anxiety, as opposed to a long-term personality *trait*. Self-esteem apparently has complicated relationships to drug use because there is evidence that young people sometimes enhance their self-esteem by becoming involved with a drug- or alcohol-using group. Also, please remember that these surveys are examining the overall range of drug or alcohol use as found in the population at large, as opposed to looking selectively at that small fraction of people who have substance-use disorders.

Increasingly, researchers are analyzing the correlates of drug use in terms of *risk factors* and *protective factors*. Risk factors are those correlates that lead to an increased risk for drug use, while protective factors are those correlates that are associated with lower rates of drug use. A recent study, based on data obtained from the National Survey on Drug Use

correlate (*core a let*): a variable that is statistically related to some other variable, such as drug use.

Table 1.3
Risk and Protective Factors Associated with Adolescent Marijuana Use in the Past Year

Domain	Factors	Odds Ratio	Domain	Factors	Odds Ratio
COMMUNITY			**PEER/INDIVIDUAL**		
	Risk			**Risk**	
	Community norms toward substance use			Friends' substance use	
	Multiple substances	5.09		Multiple substances	8.05
	Marijuana (try once or twice)	4.14		Marijuana	6.25
	Availability of marijuana	2.72		Antisocial behavior	7.10
	Community attitudes toward substance use			Individual attitudes toward marijuana use	4.47
	Multiple substances	2.23		Friends' attitudes toward substance use	
	Marijuana (try once or twice)	1.95		Multiple substances	4.19
	Community disorganization and crime	1.43		Marijuana (try once or twice)	4.37
				Perceived risk of substance use	
	Protective			Multiple substances	3.76
	Exposed to prevention messages in media	0.70		Marijuana	3.48
	Neighborhood cohesiveness	0.79		Risk-taking proclivity	3.27
				Protective	
FAMILY				Religiosity	0.47
	Risk			Participated in two or more extracurricular activities	0.52
	Parental attitudes toward substance use		**SCHOOL**		
	Multiple substances	2.84		**Risk**	
	Marijuana (try once or twice)	2.47		Perceived prevalence of substance use	
	Parental monitoring	2.60		Multiple substances	6.05
				Marijuana	4.78
	Protective			Low academic performance	1.81
	Parents are source of social support	0.40		**Protective**	
	Parental encouragement	0.59		Sanctions against substance use at school	
	Parents communicate about substance use	0.97		Multiple substances	0.28
				Marijuana	0.52
				Commitment to school	0.45
				Exposed to prevention messages in school	0.63

continued

and Health, examined risk and protective factors regarding use of marijuana among adolescents (ages 12–17).[3] This large-scale study provides some of the best information we have about the correlates of marijuana use among American adolescents. As shown in Table 1.3, the factors were organized into several areas: community, family, peer/individual, and school. The most significant factors are reported in Table 1.3.

> **Table 1.3**
> *continued*
>
> ---
>
> Notes:
>
> The odds ratio indicates the increase or decrease in the odds of a respondent reporting past-year use of marijuana with higher scores on each scale. For example, people who report that they engaged in frequent fighting, stealing, or other antisocial behaviors during the past year were 7.10 times more likely to say they used marijuana than people who scored low on this "antisocial" scale. An odds ratio of 1.0 means there is no change in the odds of using marijuana with different scores on that scale. Risk factors have odds ratios higher than 1.0. Protective factors have odds ratios lower than 1.0. For example, those who report that their parents are a source of social support (they can talk to them about problems, etc.) are less than half as likely (0.40) to report marijuana use.
>
> *Community Norms Toward Substance Use* is based on questions such as, "How many adults that you know personally would you say use marijuana or hashish?" (or other substances for the "multiple substances" scale).
>
> *Community Attitudes Toward Substance Use* is based on questions such as, "How do you think that most adults in your neighborhood would feel about you trying marijuana or hashish once or twice?"
>
> *Community Disorganization and Crime* is based on questions such as, "How much do you agree or disagree that there is a lot of crime in your neighborhood (street fights, graffiti, abandoned buildings)?
>
> *Neighborhood Cohesiveness* asks questions about how often people in your neighborhood help each other out and visit each other's homes.
>
> *Parental Monitoring* asks questions about how often parents check on your homework, limit TV watching, require chores, etc.
>
> *Parental Encouragement* asks how often parents tell you they are proud of you, or let you know that you have done a good job.
>
> *Antisocial Behavior* asks how often during the past year you have gotten into a serious fight, carried a gun, sold drugs, stolen, or attacked someone.
>
> *Risk-Taking Proclivity* asks whether you get a kick out of doing dangerous things, and how often you wear a seat belt.
>
> *Religiosity* asks about attendance at religious services and the importance of religious beliefs.
>
> *Low Academic Performance* asks about your recent grade point average.
>
> *Commitment to School* asks how much you like going to school, and whether the classes are important and interesting.

In some ways, the results confirm what most people probably assume: the kids who live in rough neighborhoods, whose parents don't seem to care what they do, who have drug-using friends, who steal and get into fights, who aren't involved in religious activities, and who don't do well in school are the most likely to smoke marijuana. The same study analyzed cigarette smoking and alcohol use, with overall similar results. The study also reveals how strong each of these relationships is, and it also shows that some of the variables analyzed did not correlate with drug use. For example, Table 1.3 includes one non-significant factor for comparison purposes: Parents Communicate about Substance Use. This scale asked how often during the past year the adolescent had talked to at least one parent about the dangers of drug use. In Table 1.3, the odds ratio for this scale was very close to 1.0,

no correlation at all. How can this be? Don't those TV commercials encourage parents to do this, and claim that parents are the "anti-drug"? This result points out the problem with a correlational study: Some adolescents smoked marijuana and also had a discussion with a parent about the dangers of drug use. In many cases, the parent might have had this conversation *because* the adolescent was caught or admitted using marijuana. In other cases, the parent might have had the conversation and prevented the adolescent from smoking marijuana. We might have two different causal relationships producing opposite effects on this scale, resulting in no overall correlation.

Another example of the limitation of correlational studies is the link between marijuana smoking and poor academic performance. Does smoking marijuana cause the user to get lower

Mind/Body Connection

Religion and Drug Use

More than three-fourths of American adolescents report that religion plays an important part in their lives. In study after study, those young people who report more involvement with religion (they attend services regularly and say their religion influences how they make decisions) are less likely to smoke cigarettes, drink alcohol, or use any type of illicit drug.

Consider your own feelings about religion and about drug use. Why do you think this relationship between "religiosity" and lower rates of drug use is such a consistent finding? If you have friends from different religious backgrounds, discuss this relationship with them. Some religions have specific teachings against any alcohol use or tobacco use, but the general relationship seems to hold even for those religions that do not forbid these behaviors (at least for adults). What other factors related to religious involvement in general might serve as protective factors against the use of these substances?

behavior—what some researchers refer to as *problem* behaviors. We all can think of individual exceptions to this rule, but correlational studies over many years all come to the same conclusion: If you want to find the greatest number of young people who use illicit drugs, look among the same people who are getting in trouble in other ways.

Antecedents of Drug Use

Finding characteristics that tend to be associated with drug use doesn't help us understand causal relationships very well. For example, do adolescents first become involved with a deviant peer group and then use drugs, or do they first use drugs and then begin to hang around with others who do the same? Does drug use cause them to become poor students and to fight and steal? To answer such questions, we might interview the same individuals at different times and look for **antecedents,** characteristics that predict later initiation of drug use. One such study conducted in Finland found that future initiation of substance use or heavy alcohol use can be predicted by several of the same risk factors we have already discussed: aggressiveness, conduct problems, poor academic performance, "attachment to bad company," and parent and community norms more supportive of drug use.[4] Because these factors were measured *before* the increase in substance use, we are more likely to conclude that they may be *causing* substance use. But some other, unmeasured, variables might be causing both the antecedent risk factors and the subsequent substance use to emerge in these adolescents' lives.

A few scientists have been able to follow the same group of people at annual intervals for several years in what is known as a **longitudinal study.** One such study has tracked more than 1,200 participants from a predominantly African-American community in Chicago from ages 6 through 32.[5] Males who had shown a high "readiness to learn" in

grades? Or is it the kids who are getting low grades anyway who are more likely to smoke marijuana? One indication comes from the analysis of risk and protective factors for cigarette smoking in this same study. The association between low academic performance and cigarette smoking was even stronger than the association between low academic performance and marijuana smoking. This leads most people to conclude that it's the kids who are getting low grades anyway who are more likely to be cigarette smokers, and the same conclusion can probably be reached about marijuana smoking.

The overall picture that emerges from studies of risk and protective factors is that the same adolescents who are likely to smoke cigarettes, drink heavily, and smoke marijuana are also likely to engage in other deviant behaviors, such as vandalism, stealing, fighting, and early sexual

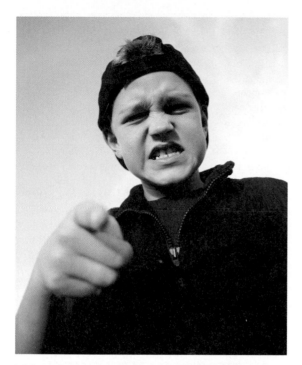

Males who are aggressive in early elementary school are more likely to be drug users as adults.

first grade were less likely to be cocaine users as adults, but females with poor academic performance in first grade had lower rates of cocaine use than females with higher first-grade scores. Males who were either "shy" or "aggressive" in first grade were more likely to be adult drug users compared to the students who had been considered neither shy nor aggressive 26 years earlier. It is much more difficult to obtain this type of data, and it is somewhat surprising that any variables measured at age six could reliably predict adult drug use.

Gateway Substances One very important study from the 1970s pointed out a typical sequence of involvement with drugs.[6] Most of the high school students in that group started their drug involvement with beer or wine. The second stage involved hard liquor, cigarettes, or both; the third stage was marijuana use; and only after going through those stages did they try

other illicit substances. Not everyone followed the same pattern, but only 1 percent of the students began their substance use with marijuana or another illicit drug. It is as though they first had to go through the **gateway** of using alcohol and, in many cases, cigarettes. The students who had not used beer or wine at the beginning of the study were much less likely to be marijuana smokers at the end of the study than the students who had used these substances. The cigarette smokers were about twice as likely as the nonsmokers to move on to smoking marijuana.

If the gateway theory can explain something about later drug use, then perhaps looking at those people who followed the traditional order of substance use (alcohol/cigarettes, followed by marijuana, followed by other illicit drugs) and comparing them to people who followed different orders of use might tell us something useful about the importance of particular orders of initiation. One recent study examined 375 homeless "street" youth, ages 13–21, in Seattle.[7] They were asked at what age they first started using various substances, and then grouped into categories depending on whether they followed the traditional gateway order or some other order of initiation. The order of use did not predict current levels or types of drug use in this population, leading the study's authors to conclude that knowing which substances people use first might not be very important in helping to prevent future escalation of drug use.

One possible interpretation of the gateway phenomenon is that young people are exposed to alcohol and tobacco and that these substances

antecedent (ant eh *see* dent): a variable that occurs before some event such as the initiation of drug use.
longitudinal study (lon jeh *too* di nul): a study done over a period of time (months or years).
gateway: one of the first drugs (e.g., alcohol or tobacco) used by a typical drug user.

Targeting Prevention

Preventing What?

Chapter 1 provides an overview of psychoactive drug use, primarily based on data from the United States. As we look forward to the topic of prevention, it's appropriate to think about what aspects of psychoactive drug use we would most like to reduce. Following are some perspectives:

- We should work to prevent any use of tobacco or alcohol by those under age 21, as well as any use of drugs such as marijuana, cocaine, and LSD. These drugs are all illegal, and we know that early use of tobacco and alcohol is associated with a greatly increased risk of illicit drug use in the future.
- Focusing only on drug use ignores the fact that illicit drug use is usually part of a larger pattern of deviant or antisocial behavior. Therefore, our efforts would be more effective if we were to target younger people and work to prevent poor

academic performance, fighting, shoplifting, and other early indicators of this lifestyle, in addition to early experimentation with tobacco and alcohol.

- Wait a minute! We're confusing what might be desirable with what might be possible. We can't prevent everyone from doing things we don't like. For example, as adults most people will drink alcohol at least once in a while, yet perhaps only 10 percent of drinkers have most of the problems. Trying to prevent all drug use and other undesirable behavior is just too big a job, and it violates our sense of individual freedom. We need to focus our efforts on preventing abuse and the crime that goes with it. That's a much smaller problem, and we have a better chance of success.

With which of these perspectives do you most agree at this point? Are there other perspectives not represented by these three?

---

somehow make the person more likely to go on to use other drugs. Because most people who use these gateway substances do not go on to become cocaine users, we should be cautious about jumping to that conclusion. More likely is that early alcohol use and cigarette smoking are common indicators of the general deviance-prone pattern of behavior that also includes an increased likelihood of smoking marijuana or trying cocaine.

Because beer and cigarettes are more widely available to a deviance-prone young person than marijuana or cocaine, it is logical that beer and cigarettes would most often be tried first. The socially conforming students are less likely to try even these relatively available substances until they are older, and they are less likely ever to try the illicit substances. Let's ask the question another way: If we developed a prevention program that stopped all young people from smoking cigarettes, would that cut down on marijuana smoking? Most of us think it might, because people who don't want to suck tobacco smoke into their lungs

probably won't want to inhale marijuana smoke either. Would such a program keep people from getting *D* averages or getting into other kinds of trouble? Probably not. In other words, we think of the use of gateway substances not as the *cause* of later illicit drug use but, instead, as an early indicator of the basic pattern of deviant behavior resulting from a variety of psychosocial risk factors.

Motives for Drug Use

To most of us, it doesn't seem necessary to find explanations for normative behavior; we don't often ask why someone takes a pain reliever when she has a headache. Our task is to try to explain the drug-taking behavior that frightens and infuriates—the deviant drug use. We should keep one fact about human conduct in mind throughout this book: Despite good, logical evidence telling us we "should" avoid certain things, we all do some of them anyway. We know that we shouldn't eat that second piece of pie or have that third drink on an empty

stomach. Cool-headed logic tells us so. We
would be hard pressed to find good, sensible
reasons why we should smoke cigarettes, drive
faster than the speed limit, go skydiving, sleep
late when we have work to do, flirt with someone and risk an established relationship, or use
cocaine. Whether one labels these behaviors
sinful or just stupid, they don't seem to be designed to maximize our health or longevity.

But humans do not live by logic alone; we
are social animals who like to impress each
other, and we are pleasure-seeking animals.
These factors help explain why people do
some of the things they shouldn't, including
using drugs.

The research on correlates and antecedents
points to a variety of personal and social variables that influence our drug taking, and many
psychological and sociological theorists have
proposed models for explaining illegal or excessive drug use. We have seen evidence for
one common reason that some people begin to
take certain illegal drugs: usually young, and
somewhat more often male than female, they
have chosen to identify with a deviant subculture. These groups frequently engage in a variety of behaviors not condoned by the larger
society. Within that group, the use of a particular drug might not be deviant at all but might,
in fact, be expected. Occasionally the use of a
particular drug becomes such a fad among a
large number of youth groups that it seems to
be a nationwide problem. However, within any
given community there will still be people of
the same age who don't use the drug.

Rebellious behavior, especially among
young people, serves important functions not
only for the developing individual but also for
the evolving society. Adolescents often try very
hard to impress other people and may find it
especially difficult to impress their parents. An
adolescent who is unable to gain respect from
people or who is frustrated in efforts to "go his
or her own way" might engage in a particularly
dangerous or disgusting behavior as a way of
demanding that people be impressed or at least
pay attention.

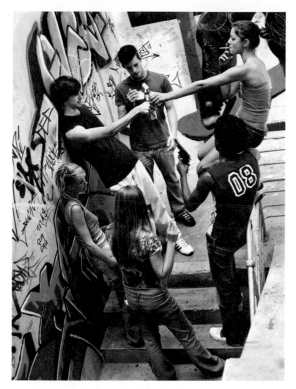

People who use drugs and who identify with a
deviant subculture are more likely to engage in a
variety of behaviors not condoned by society.

One source of excessive drug use may be
found within the drugs themselves. Many of
these drugs are capable of *reinforcing* the behavior that gets the drug into the system.
Reinforcement means that, everything else
being equal, each time you take the drug you
increase slightly the probability that you will
take it again. Thus, with many psychoactive
drugs there is a constant tendency to increase
the frequency or amount of use. Some drugs

reinforcement: a procedure in which a behavioral
event is followed by a consequent event such that
the behavior is then more likely to be repeated. The
behavior of taking a drug may be reinforced by the
effect of the drug.

(such as intravenous heroin or cocaine) appear to be so reinforcing that this process occurs relatively rapidly in a large percentage of those who use them. For other drugs, such as alcohol, the process seems to be slower. In many people, social factors, other reinforcers, or other activities prevent an increase. For some, however, the drug-taking behavior does increase and consumes an increasing share of their lives.

Most drug users are seeking an altered state of consciousness, a different perception of the world than is provided by normal, day-to-day activities. Many of the high school students in the nationwide surveys report that they take drugs "to see what it's like," or "to get high," or "because of boredom." In other words, they are looking for a change, for something new and different in their lives. This aspect of drug use was particularly clear during

the 1960s and 1970s, when LSD and other perception-altering drugs were popular. We don't always recognize the altered states produced by other substances, but they do exist. A man drinking alcohol might have just a bit more of a perception that he's a tough guy, that he's influential, that he's well liked. A cocaine user might get the seductive feeling that everything is great and that she's doing a great job (even if she isn't). Many drug-abuse prevention programs have focused on efforts to show young people how to feel good about themselves and how to look for excitement in their lives without using drugs.

Another thing seems clear: Although societal, community, and family factors (the outer areas of Figure 1.4) play an important role in determining whether an individual will first *try* a drug, with increasing use the individual's own experiences with the drug become in-

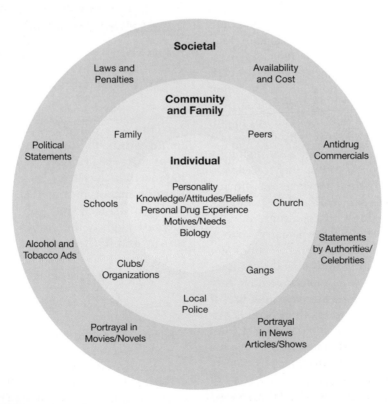

Figure 1.4   Influences on Drug Use

creasingly important. For those who become seriously dependent, the drug and its actions on that individual become central, and social influences, availability, cost, and penalties play a less important role in the continuation of drug use.

Summary

- In discussing a drug-use issue, you must consider who is using the drug, what drug is being used, when and where the drug use is occurring, why the person is using the drug, how the person is taking the drug, and how much drug is being used.

- No drug is either entirely good or bad, and every drug has multiple effects. The size and type of effect depends on the dose of the drug and the user's history and expectations.

- Deviant drug use includes those forms of drug use not considered either normal or acceptable by the society at large. Drug misuse is using a drug in a way that was not intended by its manufacturer. Drug abuse is drug use that causes problems. (If frequent and serious, then a diagnosis of substance abuse disorder is applied.) Drug dependence involves using the substance more often or in greater amounts than the user intended, and having difficulty stopping or cutting down on its use.

- The introduction of vaccines, antibiotics, psychotherapeutic drugs, and oral contraceptives has influenced our current views of drugs and drug use.

- Among American college students, about 70 percent can be considered current (within the past 30 days) users of alcohol, about 25 percent current smokers of tobacco cigarettes, about 20 percent current marijuana users, and less than 2 percent current users of cocaine.

- Both alcohol and illicit drug use reached an apparent peak around 1980, then decreased until the early 1990s, with a slower increase after that. Current rates of use are lower than at the peak.

- Adolescents who use illicit drugs (mostly marijuana) are more likely to know adults who use drugs, less likely to believe that their parents would object to their drug use, less likely to see their parents as a source of social support, more likely to have friends who use drugs, less likely to be religious, and more likely to have academic problems. Neither personality nor socioeconomic status appears to be important in predicting drug use.

- A typical progression of drug use starts with cigarettes and alcohol, then marijuana, then other drugs such as amphetamines, cocaine, or heroin. However, there is no evidence that using one of the "gateway" substances causes one to escalate to more deviant forms of drug use.

- People may use illicit or dangerous drugs for a variety of reasons: They may be part of a deviant subculture, they may be signaling their rebellion, they may find the effects of the drugs to be reinforcing, or they may be seeking an altered state of consciousness. The specific types of drugs and the ways they are used will be influenced by the user's social and physical environment. If dependence develops, then these environmental factors may begin to have less influence.

Review Questions

1. Besides asking a person the question directly, what is one way a psychologist can try to determine why a person is taking a drug?
2. What two characteristics of a drug's effect might change when the dose is increased?
3. In what way might the development of oral contraceptives have changed people's views of drugs to make experimenting with psychoactive drugs more likely?

4. In about what year did drug use in the United States peak?

5. What are the two types of large drug-use surveys sponsored by the federal government on a regular basis?

6. About what percentage of college students use marijuana?

7. What is the relationship between socioeconomic status and illicit drug use or heavy drinking?

8. Name one risk factor and one protective factor related to the family/parents.

References

1. Johnston, L. D., P. M. O'Malley, J. G. Bachman, and J. E. Schulenberg. *Monitoring the Future National Survey Results on Drug Use, 1975–2004. Volume II: College Students and Adults Ages 19–45* (NIH Publication No. 05-5728). Bethesda, MD: National Institute on Drug Abuse, 2005.

2. Johnston, L. D., P. M. O'Malley, J. G. Bachman, and J. E. Schulenberg. *Monitoring the Future National Survey Results on Drug Use, 1975–2004. Volume I: Secondary School Students* (NIH Publication No. 05-5727). Bethesda, MD: National Institute on Drug Abuse, 2005.

3. Wright, D., & M. Pemberton. *Risk and Protective Factors for Adolescent Drug Use: Findings from the 1999 National Household Survey on Drug Abuse* (DHHS Publication No. SMA 04-3874, Analytic Series A-19). Rockville, MD: Substance Abuse and Mental Health Services Administration, Office of Applied Studies, 2004.

4. Poikolainen, Kari. "Antecedents of Substance Use in Adolescence." *Current Opinion in Psychiatry* 15 (2002), pp. 241–45.

5. Ensminger, M. E., H. S. Juon, and K. E. Fothergill. "Childhood and Adolescent Antecedents of Substance Use in Adulthood." *Addiction* 97 (2002), pp. 833–44.

6. Kandel, D., & R. Faust. "Sequence and Stages in Patterns of Adolescent Drug Use." *Archives of General Psychiatry* 32 (1975), pp. 923–32.

7. Ginzler, J. A., and others. "Sequential Progression of Substance Use among Homeless Youth: An Empirical Investigation of the Gateway Theory." *Substance Use & Misuse* 38 (2003), pp. 725–58.

Check Yourself

Do Your Goals and Behaviors Match?

One interesting thing about young people who get into trouble with drugs or other types of deviant behavior is that they often express fairly conventional long-term goals for themselves. In other words, they want or perhaps even expect to be successful in life, but then do things that interfere with that success. One way to look at this is that their long-term goals don't match up with their short-term behavior. Everyone does this sort of thing to some extent—you want to get a good grade on the first exam, but then someone talks you into going out instead of studying for the next one. Or perhaps you hope to lose five pounds but just can't pass up that extra slice of pizza.

Make yourself a chart that lists your long-term goals down one side and has a space for short-term behaviors down the other side, like the one that follows:

Write in your goal under each category as best you can. Then think about some things you do occasionally that tend to interfere with your achieving that goal and put a minus sign next to each of those behaviors. After you have gone through all the goals, write down some short-term behaviors that you could practice to assist you in achieving each goal, and put a plus sign beside each of those behaviors.

How does it stack up? Are there some important goals for which you have too many minuses and not enough plusses? If study skills and habits, relationship problems, or substance abuse appear to be serious roadblocks for your success, consider visiting a counselor or therapist to get help in overcoming them.

	Goals (Long-Term)	Behaviors (Short-Term)
Educational		
Physical health and fitness		
Occupational		
Spiritual		
Personal relationships		

2

Drug Use as a Social Problem

Objectives

When you have finished this chapter, you should be able to:

- **Distinguish between the federal government's regulatory approach before the early 1900s and now.**

- **Distinguish between acute and chronic toxicity and between physiological and behavioral toxicity.**

- **Describe the two types of data collected in the DAWN system and know the top four drug classes for emergency room visits and for mortality.**

- **Understand why the risks of HIV/AIDS and hepatitis are higher among injection drug users.**

- **Define tolerance, physical dependence, and behavioral dependence.**

- **Understand that the scientific perspective on substance dependence has changed in recent years.**

- **Differentiate between abuse disorder and substance dependence disorder using diagnostic criteria.**

- **Debate the various theories on the cause of dependence.**

- **Describe four ways it has been proposed that drug use might cause an increase in crime.**

As we look into the problems experienced by society as a result of the use of psychoactive drugs, we need to consider two broad categories. Tho first category is the problems directly related to actually taking the drug, such as the risk of developing dependence or of overdosing. Second, because the use of certain drugs is considered a deviant act, the continued use of those drugs by some individuals represents a different set of social problems, apart from the direct dangers of the drugs themselves. These problems include arrests, fines, jailing, and the expenses associated with efforts to prevent misuse and to treat abuse and dependence. We begin by examining the direct drug-related problems that first raised concerns about cocaine, opium, and other drugs. Problems related to law enforcement, prevention, and treatment will be examined more thoroughly in Chapters 3, 17, and 18.

Laissez-Faire

In the 1800s, the U.S. government, like the majority of countries around the world, had virtually no laws governing the sale or use of most drugs. The idea seemed to be that, if the seller wanted to sell it and the buyer wanted to buy

Online Learning Center Resources

www.mhhe.com/ksir12e

Visit our Online Learning Center (OLC) for access to these study aids and additional resources.

- Learning objectives
- Glossary flashcards
- Web activities and links
- Self-scoring chapter quiz
- Audio chapter summaries

it, let them do it—**laissez-faire,** in French. This term has been used to characterize the general nature of the U.S. government of that era. In the 21st century, hundreds of drugs are listed as federally controlled substances, the U.S. government spends more than 12 billion dollars each year trying to control their sale and use, and 1.5 million arrests are made each year for violating controlled substance laws. What happened to cause the leaders of the "land of the free" to believe it was necessary to create especially restrictive regulations for some drugs?

Three main concerns aroused public interest: (1) *toxicity:* some drug sellers were considered to be endangering the public health and victimizing individuals because they were selling dangerous, toxic chemicals, often without labeling them or putting appropriate warnings on them; (2) *dependence:* some sellers were seen as victimizing individuals and endangering their health by selling them habit-forming drugs, again often without appropriate labels or warnings; and (3) *crime:* the drug user came to be seen as a threat to public safety—the attitude became widespread that drug-crazed individuals would often commit horrible, violent crimes. In Chapter 3, we will look at the roots of these concerns and how our current legal structures grew from them. For now, let's look at each issue and develop ground rules for the discussion of toxicity, dependence, and drug-induced criminality.

Toxicity

Categories of Toxicity

The word **toxic** means "poisonous, deadly, or dangerous." All the drugs we discuss in this text can be toxic if misused or abused. We will use the term to refer to those effects of drugs that interfere with normal functioning in such a way as to produce dangerous or potentially dangerous consequences. Seen in this way, for example, alcohol can be toxic in high doses because it suppresses respiration—this can be dangerous if breathing stops long enough to induce brain damage or death. But we can also consider alcohol to be toxic if it causes a person to be so disoriented that, for them, otherwise normal behaviors, such as driving a car or swimming, become dangerous. This is an example of something we refer to as **behavioral toxicity.** We make a somewhat arbitrary distinction, then, between behavioral toxicity and "physiological" toxicity—perhaps taking advantage of the widely assumed mind-body distinction, which is more convenient than real. The only reason for making this distinction is that it helps remind us of some important kinds of toxicity that are special to psychoactive drugs and that are sometimes overlooked.

Why do we consider physiological toxicity to be a "social" problem? One view might be that if an individual chooses to take a risk and harms his or her own body, that's the individual's business. But impacts on hospital emergency rooms, increased health insurance rates, lost productivity, and other consequences of physiological toxicity mean that social systems also are affected when an individual's health is put at risk, whether by drug use or failure to wear seat belts.

Another distinction we make for the purpose of discussion is **acute** versus **chronic.** Most of the time when people use the word *acute,* they mean "sharp" or "intense." In medicine an acute condition is one that comes on suddenly, as opposed to a chronic or long-lasting condition. When talking about drug effects, we can think of the acute effects as those that result from a single administration of a drug or are a

Drugs in the Media

Counting Crack Babies

One toxicity issue that received national media attention was the effect of crack cocaine use on the unborn child during pregnancy. The image of the "crack baby" is a powerful one: born to a mother who was smoking crack during her pregnancy and up until the time of delivery, the infant is cocaine-dependent at birth, suffers withdrawal agonies, and continues to suffer developmental abnormalities. In the early 1990s, politicians and news media attracted our attention by describing the plight of these innocent victims of drug abuse and by suggesting that large numbers of children were affected. While even one of these tragedies is too high a rate, just how many really occur? How can we find out?

The Partnership for a Drug-Free America in 1992 began running an ad showing crack in a baby bottle, claiming that "a crack baby is born every 5 minutes." This works out to about 100,000 infants a year. Were there that many crack babies?

The 1991 Household Survey data estimated that 280,000 women of all ages may have used crack at some time during the year. Perhaps most of these were of childbearing age, but most were not using the drug frequently and most were not pregnant, so 100,000 crack babies would seem high. A call to the Partnership office revealed they had gotten the 100,000 figure from the 1989 National Drug Control Strategy published by the White House. The estimated 100,000 "cocaine babies" referred to in this document seems to be an estimate of the number of babies whose mothers used any form of cocaine, even once, at some time during their pregnancy.

Media reports used numbers ranging from 60,000 to more than 300,000 per year in referring to crack babies. If we mean only those babies who are born dependent because of recent heavy crack smoking by the mother, then all these numbers are probably too high. (Crack babies are discussed further in Chapter 6.) Why do you think politicians and the media tend to oversell the latest drug problem to the public?

---

direct result of the actual presence of the drug in the system at the time. For example, taking an overdose of heroin can lead to acute toxicity. By contrast, the chronic effects of a drug are those that result from long-term exposure and can be present whether or not the substance is actually in the system at a given point. For example, smoking cigarettes can eventually lead to various types of lung disorders. If you have emphysema from years of smoking, that condition is there when you wake up in the morning and when you go to bed at night, and whether your most recent cigarette was five minutes ago or five days ago doesn't make much difference.

Using these definitions, Table 2.1 (p. 30) can help give us an overall picture of the possible toxic consequences of a given type of drug. However, knowing what is *possible* is different from knowing what is *likely*. How can we get an idea of which drugs are most likely to produce adverse drug reactions?

Drug Abuse Warning Network

In an effort to monitor the toxicity of drugs other than alcohol, the U.S. government set up the Drug Abuse Warning Network (**DAWN**). This system collects data on drug-related emergency room visits from hospital emergency

laissez-faire (lay say fair): a hands-off approach to government.

toxic: poisonous, dangerous.

behavioral toxicity: toxicity resulting from behavioral effects of a drug.

acute: referring to drugs, the short-term effects of a single dose.

chronic: referring to drugs, the long-term effects from repeated use.

DAWN: Drug Abuse Warning Network. System for collecting data on drug-related deaths or emergency room visits.

Table 2.1
Examples of Four Types of Drug-Induced Toxicity

Acute (Immediate)

Behavioral	"Intoxication" from alcohol, marijuana, or other drugs that impair behavior and increase danger to the individual
Physiological	Overdose of heroin or alcohol causing the user to stop breathing

Chronic (Long-term)

Behavioral	Personality changes reported to occur in alcoholics and suspected by some to occur in marijuana users (a motivational syndrome)
Physiological	Heart disease, lung cancer, and other effects related to smoking; liver damage resulting from chronic alcohol exposure

departments in major metropolitan areas around the country. When an individual goes to an emergency room with any sort of problem related to drug misuse or abuse, each drug involved (up to six) is recorded. For each drug or drug type, staff members can add up the number of visits associated with that particular drug. The visit could be for a wide variety of reasons, such as injury due to an accident, accidental overdose, a suicide attempt, or a distressing panic reaction that is not life-threatening to the patient. The emergency room personnel who record these incidents do not need to determine that the drug actually *caused* the visit, only that some type of drug misuse or abuse was involved. This avoids many of the subjective judgments that would vary from place to place and from day to day, especially when (as is often the case) more than one drug is involved. If someone is in an automobile accident after drinking alcohol,

smoking marijuana, and using some cocaine, rather than trying to say which one of these substances was responsible for the accident, each of them is counted as being involved in that emergency room visit.

Because not every emergency room in the U.S. participates in the DAWN system, for many years the sampled data were used to estimate the overall number of emergency room visits for the entire country. Because of concerns about the accuracy of those estimates, the 2003 results were not used in that way. The numbers for emergency room visits for 2003 shown on the left side of Table 2.2 (p. 31) are the totals from the sampled hospitals, so they are about two-thirds the magnitude of the numbers found in previous reports (and in previous editions of this text).[1]

The DAWN system collects another set of data on drug-related deaths, with the reports being completed by medical examiners (coroners) in the same metropolitan areas around the U.S. The agency responsible for the DAWN data (the Office of Applied Studies from the Substance Abuse and Mental Health Services Administration) became so concerned about the accuracy of national estimates that they have stopped providing overall national totals and rankings by drug type. The numbers on the right side of Table 2.2 were derived by adding up the reported number of deaths in 2003 related to each drug type from each of the 32 major metropolitan areas.[2]

Alcohol is treated somewhat differently than other drugs in the sample. Whenever an emergency room visit or a death is related only to alcohol use by an adult, the DAWN system does not keep track of that. Alcohol-related problems are counted when alcohol and some other drug are involved (alcohol-in-combination); in the latest report alcohol alone is recorded if the individual is under 21 years of age. Notice that alcohol-in-combination is near the top ranking in both types of data, a place it has held for many years. In fact, if alcohol were counted alone its numbers would be large enough to make the other drugs seem much less important beside it. This seems to

Table 2.2
Toxicity Data from the Drug Abuse Warning Network (DAWN) for 2003

DRUG-RELATED EMERGENCY ROOM VISITS			DRUG-RELATED DEATHS		
Rank	**Drug**	**Number**	**Rank**	**Drug**	**Number**
1.	Cocaine	125,921	1.	Opioids (not heroin)	3,667
2.	Alcohol-in-combination	118,724	2.	Cocaine	3,142
3.	Opioids (not heroin)	87,319	3.	Alcohol-in-combination	2,482
4.	Marijuana	79,663	4.	Benzodiazepeines	1,611
5.	Benzodiazepines	75,481	5.	Antidepressants	1,566
6.	Heroin	47,604	6.	Methadone	1,171
7.	Stimulants (includes methamphetamine)	42,538	7.	Sedative-Hypnotics (non-benzodiazepeine)	882
8.	PCP	4,581	8.	Heroin	792
9.	MDMA (Ecstasy)	2,221	9.	Stimulants (includes methamphetamine)	584
10.	Inhalants	1,681	10.	Marijuana	304

indicate that alcohol is a fairly toxic substance. It can be, but let us also remember that about half of all adult Americans drink alcohol at least once a month, whereas only a small percentage of the adult population uses cocaine, a drug that is also at the top of both lists. The DAWN system does not correct for differences in rates of use, but rather gives us an idea of the relative impact of a substance on medical emergencies and drug-related deaths. Cocaine has vied with alcohol-in-combination for the top spot on these lists since the mid-1980s. Legal drugs are found on both lists, with prescription opioids now at the top of the mortality data. Including the widely prescribed hydrocodone (Vicodin) and oxycodone (Oxycontin), these drugs are increasingly marketed through Internet pharmacies that might be contributing to the increased number of toxic reactions. Other groups of prescription drugs, such as benzodiazepine sedatives (e.g., Xanax) and sleeping pills (e.g., Halcion) and the antidepressants, are relatively important, especially in the category of drug-related deaths.

The importance of drug combinations, particularly combinations with alcohol, in contributing to these numbers cannot be overstressed. Typically about half of the emergency room visits involve more than one substance, and about three-fourths of the drug-related deaths include multiple drugs. By far the most common "other" drug is alcohol. The most dramatic case is for the benzodiazepines. In 2003, only 16 of the 1,611 benzodiazepine-related

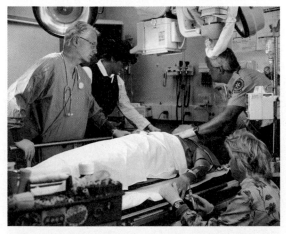

The Drug Abuse Warning Network (DAWN) uses data from hospital emergency rooms to monitor drug toxicity.

deaths were reported as single-drug deaths, implying that the real danger lies in combining sedatives or sleeping pills with alcohol.

How Dangerous Is the Drug?

Now that we have some idea of the drugs contributing to the largest numbers of toxic reactions in these two sets of data, let's see if we can use that information to ask some questions about the relative danger to a person taking one drug versus another. We mentioned that the DAWN data do not correct for frequency of use. However, in Chapter 1 we reviewed other sets of data that provide information on the relative rates of use of different drugs, such as the National Survey on Drug Use and Health discussed on pages 12–14. The populations and sampling methods are different, so we're not going to be able to make fine distinctions with any degree of accuracy. But we know, for example, that roughly eight times as many people report current use of marijuana as report current use of cocaine. The 2003 DAWN mortality report shows roughly six times as many cocaine-related deaths as marijuana-related deaths. If one-eighth as many users experience six times as many deaths, can we say that the risk of death to an individual cocaine user is 48 times the risk of death to an individual marijuana user? That's too precise an answer, but is seems pretty clear that cocaine is relatively much more toxic than marijuana.

We should point out an important difference in the latest DAWN report for 2003 regarding heroin. In past DAWN reports, if a blood sample was positive for morphine, this was recorded under the heroin/morphine category, because it is not possible to distinguish heroin from morphine with the standard toxicology screens. However, morphine is also fairly widely used as a legal prescription pain reliever, so previous reports probably overestimated the number of toxic reactions to heroin itself. In the 2003 data, for the first time heroin is counted separately only if there is specific information that the person actually used heroin. Since that information is not always available, especially after someone has died, the new reports probably underestimate the total number of toxic reactions to heroin. As a result, heroin appears to have dropped from third place in drug-related deaths to eighth place. This change is likely due to changes in the way the records are kept rather than to changes in heroin itself or in its use.

We cannot tell precisely from the DAWN data how many total deaths are related to the use of cocaine or heroin, because not all coroners are included in the system. Data are gathered from metropolitan areas that include about a third of the U.S. population, but they are areas that have higher than average use of illicit drugs. A very rough estimate of the total annual number of deaths related to cocaine, for example, might be three times the reported DAWN figure, or about 9,000 per year. The total for all illicit drugs, including cocaine, heroin, marijuana, and methamphetamine, might be approximately 15,000. Using the same proportions, estimated annual deaths associated with the use of the prescription narcotic analgesics, antidepressants, benzodiazepines, and over-the-counter pain relievers would be roughly 20,000. For comparison, alcohol is estimated to be responsible for 100,000 deaths annually (see Chapter 9), and more than 400,000 annual deaths are attributed to cigarette smoking (see Chapter 10). Of course, many more people use those substances, and in terms of *relative* danger of toxicity, heroin and cocaine are undoubtedly more dangerous than prescription drugs,

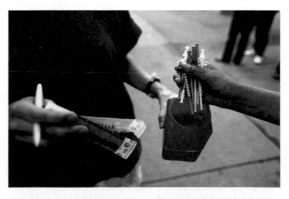

Needles are collected through an exchange program in an effort to prevent the spread of HIV among needle-using users.

Mind / Body Connection

Fear and Decision Making

Fear is a useful emotion. Being afraid of something that threatens you helps you to avoid the real dangers that do exist in our world. But, of course, fear also can be irrational, far out of proportion to any real threat. When that happens, as individuals we might be hampered by being unable to use elevators or ride in airliners, or fear of contamination might seriously interfere with our social lives. Fear is also a favorite tool of many politicians. If they can convince us that there is a real threat of some kind and they offer to protect us from it, we are likely to elect them and to give them the power or funding they seek to provide that protection. Again, this is a rational and perfectly appropriate governmental response to the extent that the threat is both real and likely to harm us, but sometimes it is difficult to get it right. Maybe the U.S. government underestimated the threat of Hurricane Katrina. Maybe because of the horrible televised images of the World Trade Center attack we overestimate the threat of Al Quaeda. Raising fears about specific types of drugs has been a staple of politics and government in the U.S.

for more than 100 years, from the age of Demon Rum through heroin, marijuana, LSD, PCP, cocaine, MDMA (Ecstasy) and methamphetamine. How do we get it right?

On an individual level, most of us are sufficiently afraid of the possible consequences of using illicit drugs that we avoid using them at all. If those fears are overblown, so what? As long as we avoid using dangerous drugs we can see those fears as being useful. But a politician can easily amplify fears about a drug and use that fear to help get elected, and to pass laws that go too far, compared to the actual magnitude of the threat. Think about frightening things you have heard about specific drugs. For example, there has been a lot of talk about "meth" labs exploding and about the toxic effects of exposure to the harsh chemicals used in making methamphetamine. How can you evaluate such stories other than to go look up statistics on the actual occurrences of such events? Remember to use your common sense. If a story seems to be outrageous, there's a pretty good chance that someone is overstating the actual risk.

---

alcohol, or cigarettes. However, in looking at the *total* impact of these drug-related deaths on American society, you might conclude that politicians and the news media have been paying a disproportionate amount of attention to cocaine, heroin, and methamphetamine.

Blood-Borne Diseases

One specific toxicity concern for users who inject drugs is the potential for spreading blood-borne diseases, such as **HIV, AIDS,** and the life-threatening liver infections hepatitis B and hepatitis C. These viral diseases can all be transmitted through the sharing of needles. In a recent study of injecting drug users in six U.S. cities, rates of HIV infection ranged from a low of 3 percent to a high of almost 30 percent, representing a serious public health hazard. Rates of hepatitis B infection among injecting drug users were higher, ranging from 50 percent to 80 percent, and rates were even higher for hepa-

titis C (66 percent to 93 percent). Since rates increased with age, the authors stressed the need for prevention programs targeting younger people who have recently begun injecting drugs.[3]

This type of drug-associated toxicity is not due to the action of the drug itself, but is incidental to the sharing of needles, no matter which drug is injected or whether the injection is intravenous or intramuscular. An individual drug user may inject 1,000 times a year, and that represents a lot of needles. In several states and cities, drug paraphernalia laws make it illegal to obtain syringes or needles without a prescription, and the resulting shortage of new, clean syringes increases the likelihood that drug users will share needles. One response to this has been the development of syringe exchange programs, in

HIV: human immunodeficiency virus.
AIDS: acquired immunodeficiency syndrome.

Targeting Prevention

Clean Needles?

The spread of the human immunodeficiency virus (HIV) among drug users is associated primarily with the sharing of the needles used for injecting heroin and other drugs. Evidence from several studies indicates that HIV transmission can be reduced if clean syringes and needles are made readily available to injecting drug users. Do you know whether a user of illicit drugs in your community can get access to clean syringes and needles?

You might start learning about this by asking a local pharmacist to see what the rules are for purchasing these items, as well as how expensive they are. It will also be interesting to see how the pharmacist reacts to your questions about this topic. How do you react to the idea of possibly being

looked at as a user of illegal drugs? You might take this book along to show that you do have an academic reason for asking!

Once you find out what the situation is with direct purchasing, see if you can discover if there is a needle exchange program in your community. This will be a little harder, but you can start by looking up "public health" in the phone book and calling that office.

Are there steps your community could take to make clean needles more readily available to users of illicit drugs? Do you believe that such programs encourage or condone drug use? Would the program help prevent the spread of HIV in your community? Visit the Online Learning Center for links to more information on needle exchange programs.

which new, clean syringes are traded for used syringes. Although the U.S. Congress has prohibited the use of federal funds to support these programs, based on the theory that they provide moral encouragement for illegal drug use, exchange programs have been funded by state and local governments, and many other countries support such programs. Evidence shows that given the opportunity, drug injectors increase their use of clean syringes, rates of infection are lowered, and the programs more than pay for themselves in the long run.[4] Despite political opposition, syringe exchange currently represents one of the most practical ways to prevent the spread of these blood-borne diseases among drug users and from them to the non-drug-using population.

Substance Dependence: What Is It?

All our lives we have heard people talk about "alcoholics" and "users," and we're sure we know what we're talking about when one of these terms is used. Years ago when people first

became concerned about some people being frequent, heavy users of cocaine or morphine, the term *habituation* was often used. If we try to develop scientific definitions, terms such as *alcoholic* or *user* are actually hard to pin down. For example, not everyone who is considered an alcoholic drinks every day—some drink in binges, with brief periods of sobriety in between. Not everyone who drinks every day is considered an alcoholic—a glass of wine with dinner every night doesn't match most people's idea of alcoholism. The most extreme examples are easy to spot: the homeless man dressed in rags, drinking from a bottle of cheap wine, or the heroin user who needs a fix three or four times a day to avoid withdrawal symptoms. No hard-and-fast rule for quantity or frequency of use can help us draw a clear line between what we want to think of as a "normal drinker" or a "recreational user" and someone who has developed a dependence on the substance, who is compelled to use it, or who has lost control over use of the substance. It would be nice if we could separate substance use into two distinct categories: In one case, the individual controls the use of the substance; in the other case, the substance seems to take control of the individual. However, the real world of substance use, misuse, abuse, and dependence does not come wrapped in such convenient packages.

Three Basic Processes

The extreme examples mentioned above, of the homeless wine drinker or the frequent heroin user, typically exhibit three characteristics of their substance use that distinguish them from first-time or occasional users. These appear to represent three processes that may occur with repeated drug use, and each of these processes can be defined and studied by researchers interested in understanding drug dependence.

Tolerance Tolerance refers to a phenomenon seen with many drugs, in which repeated exposure to the same dose of the drug results in a lesser effect. There are many ways this diminished effect can occur, and some examples are given in Chapter 5. For now, it is enough for us to think of the body as developing ways to compensate for the chemical imbalance caused by introducing a drug into the system. As the individual experiences less and less of the desired effect, often the tolerance can be overcome by increasing the dose of the drug. Some regular drug users might eventually build up to taking much more of the drug than it would take to kill a nontolerant individual.

Physical Dependence Physical dependence is defined by the occurrence of a **withdrawal syndrome.** Suppose a person has begun to take a drug and a tolerance has developed. The person increases the amount of drug and continues to take these higher doses so regularly that the body is continuously exposed to the drug for days or weeks. With some drugs, when the person stops taking the drug abruptly, a set of symptoms begins to appear as the drug level in the system drops. For example, as the level of heroin drops in a regular user, that person's nose might run and he or she might begin to experience chills and fever, diarrhea, and other symptoms. When we have a drug that produces a consistent set of these symptoms in different

individuals, we refer to the collection of symptoms as a withdrawal syndrome. These withdrawal syndromes vary from one class of drugs to another. Our model for why withdrawal symptoms appear is that the drug initially disrupts the body's normal physiological balances. These imbalances are detected by the nervous system, and over a period of repeated drug use the body's normal regulatory mechanisms compensate for the presence of the drug. When the drug is suddenly removed, these compensating mechanisms produce an imbalance. Tolerance typically precedes physical dependence. To continue with the heroin example, when it is first used it slows intestinal movement and produces constipation. After several days of constant heroin use, other mechanisms in the body counteract this effect and get the intestines moving again (tolerance). If the heroin use is suddenly stopped, the compensating mechanisms produce too much intestinal motility. Diarrhea is one of the most reliable and dramatic heroin withdrawal symptoms.

Because of the presumed involvement of these compensating mechanisms, the presence of a withdrawal syndrome is said to reflect **physical** (or physiological) **dependence** on the drug. In other words, the individual has come to depend on the presence of some amount of that drug to function normally; removing the drug leads to an imbalance, which is slowly corrected over a few days.

Psychological Dependence Psychological dependence (also called *behavioral dependence*) can be defined in terms of observable behavior. It is

---

tolerance: reduced effect of a drug after repeated use.
withdrawal syndrome: a consistent set of symptoms that appears after discontinuing use of a drug.
physical dependence: drug dependence defined by the presence of a withdrawal syndrome, implying that the body has become adapted to the drug's presence.
psychological dependence: behavioral dependence; indicated by high rate of drug use, craving for the drug, and a tendency to relapse after stopping use.

indicated by the frequency of using a drug or by the amount of time or effort an individual spends in drug-seeking behavior. Often it is accompanied by reports of *craving* the drug or its effects. A major contribution of behavioral psychology has been to point out the scientific value of the concept of **reinforcement** for understanding psychological dependence.

The term *reinforcement* is used in psychology to describe a process: A behavioral act is followed by a consequence, resulting in an increased tendency to repeat that behavioral act. The consequence may be described as pleasurable or as a "reward" in some cases (e.g., providing a tasty piece of food to someone who has not eaten for a while). In other cases, the consequence may be described in terms of escape from pain or discomfort. The behavior itself is said to be strengthened, or *reinforced,* by its consequences. The administration of certain drugs can reinforce the behaviors that led to the drug's administration. Laboratory rats and monkeys have been trained to press levers when the only consequence of lever pressing is a small intravenous injection of heroin, cocaine, or another drug. Because some drugs but not others are capable of serving this function, it is possible to refer to some drugs as having

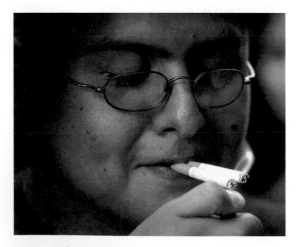

Frequent drug use, craving for the drug, and a high rate of relapse after quitting indicate psychological dependence.

"reinforcing properties" and to note that there is a general correlation between those drugs and the ones to which people often develop psychological dependence.

Changing Views of Dependence

Until the 20th century, the most common view was probably that dependent individuals were weak-willed, lazy, or immoral (the "moral model"). Then medical and scientific studies began of users of alcohol and opioids. It seemed as if something more powerful than mere self-indulgence was at work, and the predominant view began to be that dependence is a drug-induced illness.

Early Medical Models If heroin dependence is induced by heroin, or alcohol dependence by alcohol, then why do some users develop dependence and others not? An early guess was simply that some people, for whatever reasons, were exposed to large amounts of the substance for a long time. This could happen through medical treatment or self-indulgence. The most obvious changes resulting from long exposure to large doses are the withdrawal symptoms that occur when the drug is stopped. Both alcohol and the opioids can produce rather dramatic withdrawal syndromes. Thus, the problem came to be associated with the presence of physical dependence (a withdrawal syndrome), and enlightened medically oriented researchers went looking for treatments based on reducing or eliminating withdrawal symptoms. According to the most narrow interpretation of this model, the dependence itself was cured when the person had successfully completed withdrawal and the symptoms disappeared, although, of course, there was concern that people often reacquired the pattern of frequent, heavy use.

Pharmacologists and medical authorities continued into the 1970s to define *dependence* as occurring only when physical dependence was seen. Based on this view, public policy decisions, medical treatment, and individual drug-use decisions could be influenced by the question "Is this an addicting drug?" If some drugs produce dependence but others do not, then legal restrictions on specific drugs, care in the medical use of those drugs, and education in avoiding the recreational use of those drugs are appropriate. The determination of whether a drug is or is not "addicting" was therefore crucial.

In the 1960s, some drugs, particularly marijuana and amphetamines, were not considered to have well-defined, dramatic, physical withdrawal syndromes. The growing group of interested scientists began to refer to drugs such as marijuana, amphetamines, and cocaine as "merely" producing psychological dependence, whereas heroin produced a "true addiction," which includes physical dependence. The idea seemed to be that psychological dependence was "all in the head," whereas with physical dependence actual bodily processes were involved, subject to physiological and biochemical analysis and possibly to improved medical treatments. This was the view held by most drug-abuse experts in the 1960s.

Positive Reinforcement Model In the 1960s, a remarkable series of experiments began to appear in the scientific literature—experiments in which laboratory monkeys and rats were given intravenous **catheters** connected to motorized syringes and controlling equipment so that pressing a lever would produce a single brief injection of morphine, an opioid very similar to heroin. In the initial experiments, monkeys were exposed for several days to large doses of morphine, allowed to experience the initial stages of withdrawal, and then connected to the apparatus to see if they would learn to press the lever, thereby avoiding the withdrawal symptoms. These experiments were based on the predominant view of drug use as being driven by physical dependence. The monkeys did learn to press the levers.

As these scientists began to publish their results and as more experiments like this were done, interesting facts became apparent. First, monkeys would begin pressing and maintain pressing without first being made physically dependent. Second, monkeys who had given themselves only fairly small doses and who had never experienced withdrawal symptoms could be trained to work very hard for their morphine. A history of physical dependence and withdrawal didn't seem to have much influence on response rates in the long run. Clearly, the small drug injections themselves were working as positive reinforcers of the lever-pressing behavior, just as food can be a positive reinforcer to a hungry rat or monkey. Thus, the idea spread that drugs can act as reinforcers of behavior and that this might be the basis of what had been called psychological dependence. Drugs such as amphetamines and cocaine could easily be used as reinforcers in these experiments, and they were known to produce strong psychological dependence in humans. Animal experiments using drug self-administration are now of central importance in determining which drugs are likely to be used repeatedly by people, as well as in exploring the basic behavioral and biological features associated with drug dependence.[5]

Which Is More Important, Physical Dependence or Psychological Dependence?

The animal research that led to the positive reinforcement model implies that psychological dependence is more important than physical dependence in explaining repeated drug use, and this has led people to examine the lives of heroin users from a different perspective. Stories were told of users who occasionally stopped

---

reinforcement: a procedure in which a behavioral event is followed by a consequent event such that the behavior is then more likely to be repeated. The behavior of taking a drug may be reinforced by the effect of the drug.

catheters (*cath* a ters): plastic or other tubing implanted into the body.

DSM-IV-TR

Psychiatric Diagnosis of Substance Use Disorders

Diagnostic Criteria for Substance Dependence

A maladaptive pattern of substance use, leading to clinically significant impairment or distress, as manifested by three (or more) of the following, occurring at any time in the same 12-month period:

1. Tolerance, as defined by either of the following:
   a. A need for markedly increased amounts of the substance to achieve intoxication or desired effect
   b. Markedly diminished effect with continued use of the same amount of the substance
2. Withdrawal, as manifested by either of the following:
   a. The characteristic withdrawal syndrome for the substance
   b. The same (or a closely related) substance is taken to relieve or avoid withdrawal symptoms
3. The substance is often taken in larger amounts or over a longer period than was intended.
4. There is a persistent desire or unsuccessful efforts to cut down or control substance use.
5. A great deal of time is spent in activities necessary to obtain the substance.
6. Important social, occupational, or recreational activities are given up or reduced because of substance use.
7. The substance use is continued despite knowledge of having a persistent or recurrent physical or psychological problem that is likely to have been caused or exacerbated by the substance.

- With physiological dependence: evidence of tolerance or withdrawal (i.e., either Item 1 or 2 is present)
- Without physiological dependence: no evidence of tolerance or withdrawal (i.e., neither Item 1 nor 2 is present)

Diagnostic Criteria for Substance Abuse

A. A maladaptive pattern of substance use leading to clinically significant impairment or distress, as manifested by one (or more) of the following, occurring within a 12-month period:
   1. Recurrent substance use resulting in failure to fulfill major role obligations at work, school, or home
   2. Recurrent substance use in situations in which it is physically hazardous
   3. Recurrent substance-related legal problems
   4. Continued substance use despite having persistent or recurrent social or interpersonal problems caused or exacerbated by the effects of the substance
B. The symptoms have never met the criteria for substance dependence for this class of substance.

taking heroin, voluntarily going through withdrawal so as to reduce their tolerance level and get back to the lower doses of drug they could more easily afford. When we examine the total daily heroin intake of many users, we see that they do not need a large amount and that the agonies of withdrawal they experience are probably more like a prolonged case of intestinal flu. We have known for a long time that heroin users who have already gone through withdrawal in treatment programs or in jail have a high probability of returning to active heroin use. In other words, if all we had to worry about was users' avoiding withdrawal symptoms, the problem would be much smaller than it actually is.

Psychological dependence, based on *reinforcement,* is increasingly accepted as the real driving force behind repeated drug use, and tolerance and physical dependence are now seen as related phenomena that sometimes occur but probably are not critical to the development of frequent patterns of drug-using behavior.

Researchers and treatment providers rely heavily on the definitions of *substance dependence* and *substance abuse* developed by the American Psychiatric Association and presented in their *Diagnostic and Statistical Manual* (DSM-IV-TR).[6] These are presented in outline form above. Notice that both substance dependence and substance abuse are complex behavioral definitions, and the exact set of behaviors seen may vary from person to person. Also, substance dependence may occur either with or without physiological dependence, as defined by the appearance of tolerance or withdrawal. Thus, physiological dependence is a secondary issue and is not the key to a diagnosis of substance dependence.

Broad Views of Substance Dependence

If we define drug dependence not in terms of withdrawal but in more behavioral or psychological terms, as an overwhelming involvement with getting and using the drug, then might this model also be used to describe other kinds of behavior? What about a man who visits prostitutes several times a day, someone who eats large amounts of food throughout the day, or someone who places bets on every football and basketball game, every horse race or automobile race, and who spends hours each day planning these bets and finding money to bet again? Shouldn't these also be considered examples of dependence? Do the experiences of overeating, gambling, sex, and drugs have something in common—a common change in physiology or brain chemistry or a common personality trait that leads to any or many of these compulsive behaviors? Are all of these filling an unmet social or spiritual need? More and more, researchers are looking for these common threads and discussing "dependencies" as a varied set of behavioral manifestations of a common dependence process or disorder.

Is Dependence Caused by the Substance?

Especially with chemical dependence, many people speak as though the substance itself is the cause of the dependence. Certainly some drugs are more likely than others to result in dependence. For example, it is widely believed that heroin and crack cocaine are both extremely likely to lead to compulsive use. In contrast, most users of marijuana report occasional

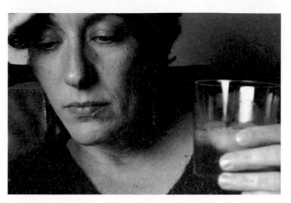

Alcohol causes serious dependence in perhaps 1 of 10 drinkers.

use and little difficulty in deciding when to use it and when not to. We also know that some methods of taking a drug (e.g., intravenous injection) are more likely to result in repeated use than other methods of taking the same drug (by mouth, for instance). We can determine which drugs, or which methods of using those drugs, pose the greatest risk for dependence. One major study reviewed 350 published articles to come up with relative ratings, then had the preliminary tables reviewed by a panel of psychopharmacologists for suggested changes.[7] Based on that report, we can classify psychoactive drugs into seven categories of "dependence potential." Smoked or injected methamphetamine would probably be in one of the top two categories in such a ranking (see Table 2.3). The range of risk of dependence depends to some extent upon the drug itself, but also depends upon its method of use (as well as a variety of other biological, psychological, and social factors). Thus, the substance itself cannot be seen as the entire cause of the problem, even though some people would like to put all the blame on "demon rum" or on heroin or crack cocaine.

When we extend the concept of dependence to other activities, such as gambling, sex, or overeating, it seems harder to place the entire blame on the activity, again because many people do not exhibit compulsive patterns of such behaviors. Some activities might be more of a problem than others—few people become dependent on filling out income tax forms,

Table 2.3
Dependence Potential of Psychoactive Drugs

Very high:	Heroin (IV)
	Crack cocaine
High:	Morphine (injected)
	Opium (smoked)
Moderate/high:	Cocaine powder (snorted)
	Tobacco cigarettes
	PCP (smoked)
Moderate:	Diazepam (Valium)
	Alcohol
	Amphetamines (oral)
Moderate/low:	Caffeine
	MDMA* (Ecstasy)
	Marijuana
Low:	Ketamine (see Chapter 14)
Very low:	LSD†
	Mescaline
	Psilocybin

*MDMA, methylenedioxy methamphetamine

†LSD, lysergic acid diethylamide

whereas a higher proportion of all those who gamble become overwhelmingly involved. Still, it is wrong to conclude that any activity is by its nature always "habit forming."

When a chemical is seen as causing the dependence, there is a tendency to give that substance a personality and to ascribe motives to it. When we listen either to a practicing user's loving description of his interaction with the drug or to a recovering alcoholic describe her struggle against the bottle's attempts to destroy her, the substance seems to take on almost human characteristics. We all realize that is going too far, yet the analogy is so powerful that it pervades our thinking. **Alcoholics Anonymous (AA)** members often describe alcohol as being "cunning, baffling, and powerful" and admit that they are powerless against such a foe. And those seeking the prohibition of alcohol, cocaine, marijuana, heroin, and other drugs have over the years tended to demonize those substances, making

them into powerful forces of evil. The concept of a "war on drugs" reflects in part such a perspective—that some drugs are evil and war must be waged against the substances themselves.

Is Dependence Biological?

In recent years, interest has increased in the possibility that all compulsive behaviors might have some common physiological or biochemical action in the brain. For example, many theorists have recently focused on dopamine, one of the brain's important neurotransmitters, which some believe to play a large role in positive reinforcement. The idea is that any drug use or other activity that has pleasurable or rewarding properties spurs dopamine activity in a particular part of the brain. This idea is discussed more fully in Chapter 4. Although this theory has been widely tested in animal models and much evidence is consistent with it, considerable evidence also shows that this model is too simple and that other neurotransmitters and other brain regions are also important. A great deal of attention has been given to reports from various brain-scanning experiments done on drug users. For example, cues that stimulate craving for cocaine activate many areas that are widely separated in the brain, including some that are known to be dopamine-rich areas and some that are not.[8] Although these studies show some of the physiological *consequences* produced by cocaine or by even thinking about cocaine, they have not yet been useful in examining the possible biological *causes* of dependence. One important question that remains is whether the brains of people who have used cocaine intermittently show different responses, compared with the brains of dependent cocaine users. Ultimately, the strongest demonstration of the power of such techniques would be if it were possible to know, based on looking at a brain scan, whether a person had developed dependence. Many previous biological theories of dependence have failed this test: so far, no genetic, physiological or biochemical marker has been found that strongly predicts drug dependence.

Is There an "Addictive Personality"?

Perhaps the explanation for why some people become dependent but others do not lies in the personality—that complex set of attributes and attitudes that develops over time, partly as a result of particular experiences. Is there a common personality factor that is seen in compulsive drug users but not in others? This type of research has been conducted for decades, and its value is still controversial. The problem with many studies on practicing or recovering users is that it is not possible to know whether the alcohol or other drug use has changed the person's personality. In retrospective studies of personality tests given to college students who later became dependent on alcohol, the prealcoholic students showed what would be considered a "normal" overall personality profile. However, they also tended to be more independent, nonconformist, gregarious, and impulsive. One personality characteristic that has frequently been associated with early substance use and abuse is called sensation-seeking.[9] Once again, although there is a statistical relationship, many other factors also play a role, and we have yet to discover a particular personality type that seems destined to develop compulsive patterns of substance use.

Is Dependence a Family Disorder?

Although few scientific studies have been done, examination of the lives of alcohol-dependent individuals reveals some typical patterns of family adaptation to the problem. A common example in a home with an alcohol-dependent father is that the mother enables this behavior, by calling her husband's boss to say he is ill or by making excuses to family and friends for failures to appear at dinners or parties and generally by caring for her incapacitated husband. The children might also compensate in various ways, and all conspire to keep the family secret. Thus, it is said that alcohol dependence often exists within a dysfunctional family—the functions of individual members adjust to the needs created by the presence of excessive drinking. This new arrangement can make it difficult for the drinker alone to change his or her behav-

ior, because doing so would disrupt the family system. Some people suspect that certain family structures actually enhance the likelihood of alcohol abuse or dependence developing. For example, the "codependent" needs of other family members to take care of someone who is dependent on them might facilitate drunkenness.

Much has been written about the effects on children who grow up in an "alcoholic family," and there is some indication that even as adults these individuals tend to exhibit certain personality characteristics. The "adult children of alcoholics" are then perhaps more likely to become involved in dysfunctional relationships that increase the likelihood of alcohol abuse, either in themselves or in another family member. Again, the evidence indicates that such influences are statistical tendencies and are not all-powerful. It is perhaps unfortunate that some people with alcoholic parents have adopted the role of "adult children" and try to explain their entire personalities and all their difficulties in terms of that status.

Is Substance Dependence a Disease?

The most important reason for adopting a disease model for dependence is based on the experiences of the founders of AA and is discussed in Chapter 9. Psychiatrists had commonly assumed that alcohol dependence was secondary to another disorder, such as anxiety or depression, and often attempted to treat the presumed underlying disorder while encouraging the drinker to try to "cut down." The founders of AA believed that alcohol dependence itself was the primary problem and needed to be recognized as such and treated directly. This is the reason for the continued insistence that alcohol dependence is a disease—

Alcoholics Anonymous (AA): a worldwide organization of self-help groups based on alcoholics helping each other achieve and maintain sobriety.

that it is often the primary disturbance and deserves to stand in its own right as a recognized disorder requiring treatment.

On the other hand, Peele[10] and others have argued that substance dependence does not have many of the characteristics of some classic medical diseases, such as tuberculosis or syphilis: We can't use an X-ray or blood test to reveal the underlying cause, and we don't have a way to treat the underlying cause and cure the symptoms—we don't really know that there is an underlying cause, because all we have are the symptoms of excessive involvement. Furthermore, if substance dependence itself is a disease, then gambling, excessive sexual involvement, and overeating should also be seen as diseases. This in turn weakens our normal understanding of the concept of disease. The disease model is perhaps best seen as an analogy—substance dependence is *like* a disease in many ways, but that is different from insisting that it *is* a disease. One reason for the conflict over the disease model of dependence may be differences in how we think of the term *disease*. For example, many would agree that high blood pressure is considered a disease—it's certainly viewed as a medical disorder. We know that high blood pressure can be produced by genetic factors, cigarette smoking, diet, lack of exercise, or by other medical conditions. In that context, the idea that alcohol or drug dependence is like a disease doesn't seem so far-fetched. This is taking a broad, **biopsychosocial** perspective that dependence might be related to dysfunctions of biology, personality, social interactions, or a combination of these factors.

Crime and Violence: Does Drug Use Cause Crime?

It might seem obvious to a reader of today's newspapers or to a viewer of today's television that drugs and crime are linked. There are frequent reports of killings attributed to warring gangs of drug dealers. Our prisons house a large population of people convicted of drug-

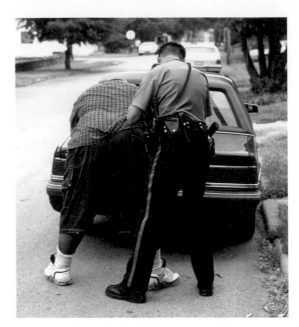

There are more than 1.5 million drug arrests every year.

related crimes, and several reports have revealed that a large fraction of arrestees for non-drug felonies have positive results from urine tests for illicit substances.

The belief that there is a causal relationship between many forms of drug use and criminality probably forms the basis for many of our laws concerning drug use and drug users. The relationship between crime and illegal drug use is complex, and only recently have data-based statements become possible. Facts are necessary because laws are enacted on the basis of what we believe to be true.

The basis for concern was the belief that drug use *causes* crime. The fact that drug users engage in robberies or that car thieves are likely to also use illicit drugs does not say anything about causality. Both criminal activity and drug use could well be caused by other factors, producing both types of deviant behavior in the same individuals. There are several senses in which it might be said that drugs cause crime, but the most frightening possibility is that drug use somehow *changes the individual's personality in a lasting way,* making him or her into a "criminal type." For example, during the 1924 debate that led to prohibition of heroin sales in the United States, a testifying physician asserted, regarding users, that heroin "dethrones their moral responsibility." Another physician testified that some types of individuals will have their mental equipment "permanently injured by the use of heroin, and those are the ones who will go out and commit crimes." Similar beliefs are reflected in the introductory message in the 1937 film *Reefer Madness,* which referred to marijuana as "The Real Public Enemy Number One!" and described its "soul-destroying" effects as follows:

> emotional disturbances, the total inability to direct thought, the loss of all power to resist physical emotions, leading finally to acts of shocking violence . . . ending often in incurable insanity.

Such verbal excesses seem quaint and comical these days, but the underlying belief that drug use changes people into criminals still can be detected in much current political rhetoric. You should remember from Chapter 1 that longitudinal research on children and adolescents has led to the conclusion that indicators of criminal or antisocial behavior usually occur before the first use of an illicit drug. The interaction over time between developing drug-use "careers" and criminal careers is complex and interactive, but it is incorrect to conclude that using any particular drug will turn a person into a criminal.[11]

A second sense in which drug use might *cause* criminal behavior is when the person is *under the influence* of the drug. Do the acute effects of a drug make a person *temporarily* more likely to engage in criminal behavior? There is little good evidence for this with most illicit substances. In most individuals, marijuana produces a state more akin to lethargy than to crazed violence (see Chapter 15), and heroin tends to make its users more passive and perhaps sexually impotent (see Chapter 13). Stimulants such as amphetamine and cocaine

can make people paranoid and "jumpy," and this can contribute to violent behavior in some cases (see Chapter 6). The hallucinogen PCP causes disorientation and blocks pain, so users are sometimes hard to restrain (see Chapter 14). This has led to a considerable amount of folklore about the dangerousness of PCP users, although actual documented cases of excessive violence are either rare or nonexistent. A study of U.S. homicide cases found that every year about 5 percent are considered to be drug-related. However, most of these are murders that occur in the context of drug trafficking, so it cannot be said that increased violence results from the pharmacological actions of the drugs.[12]

While there is some question as to whether the direct influence of illicit drugs produces a person more likely to engage in criminal or violent behavior, there has been less doubt about one commonly used substance: alcohol. Many studies indicate that alcohol is clearly linked with violent crime. In many assaults and sexual assaults, alcohol is present in both assailant and victim. Most homicides are among people who know each other—and alcohol use is associated with half or more of all murders. Drinking at the time of the offense was reported in about 25 percent of assaults and more than one-third of all rapes and sexual assaults, with drinking rates closer to two-thirds for cases of domestic violence.[13] Victims of violent crime report that they believe the offender had been using alcohol in 25 percent of the cases, compared to about 5 percent of the cases in which they believe the offender had been using drugs other than alcohol.[11] Even with such strong correlational evidence linking alcohol use with crime and violence, there is still debate about how much of the effect is related to the "disinhibitory" pharmacological action of alcohol, and how much is related to other factors. For example, several

> **biopsychosocial:** a theory or perspective that relies on the interaction of biological, individual psychological, and social variables.

studies that have controlled for age, sex, and a generalized tendency to engage in problem behaviors have concluded that both drinking and criminal violence are associated with young males who exhibit a range of antisocial behaviors, and that the immediate contribution of being intoxicated might be small.[12]

A third sense in which drug use may be said to cause crime refers to *crimes carried out for the purpose of obtaining money* to purchase illicit drugs. Among jail inmates who had been convicted of property crimes, about one-fourth reported that they had committed the crime to get money for drugs. Also, about one-fourth of those convicted of drug crimes reported that they had sold drugs to get money for their own drug use.[12]

From 1987 through 2003, the U.S. Justice Department collected data on drug use from people arrested and booked into jails for serious crimes. The interviewers tried not to sample too many people who were arrested for drug sale or possession, so that usually fewer than 20 percent of those in the study had been arrested on drug charges. All interviews and urine tests were anonymous; about 90 percent of arrestees who were asked agreed to an interview, and about 90 percent of those agreed to provide urine specimens. In 2003, in 39 sites around the country, a median figure of 67 percent of the adult male arrestees tested positive for the presence of at least one of the five drugs of interest (cocaine, marijuana, methamphetamine, opiates, and PCP). Marijuana was the drug most frequently detected (44 percent), followed by cocaine (30 percent).[14] This level of drug use among those arrested for nondrug crimes is quite high; how can we account for it? First, those who adopt a deviant lifestyle might engage in both crime and drug use. Second, because most of these arrests were for crimes in which profit was the motive, the arrestees might have been burglarizing a house or stealing a car to get money to purchase drugs.

The commission of crimes to obtain money for expensive illicit drugs is due to the artifi-

Taking Sides

Are Current Laws Fair?

People do things all the time that are potentially dangerous for themselves and potentially messy and expensive for others. Driving faster than the speed limit, driving without a seat belt, and riding a motorcycle without a helmet are examples, some of which may not be illegal where you live. In what ways are these behaviors similar to a person snorting cocaine or injecting heroin into his or her veins? In what ways are they different? Do you feel that the laws as they currently exist in your area are appropriate and fair in dealing with these behaviors? If it were up to you, would you outlaw some things that are now legal, legalize some things that are now controlled, or some of each?

cially high cost of the drugs, not primarily to a pharmacological effect of the drug. The inflated cost results from drug controls and enforcement. Both heroin and cocaine are inexpensive substances when obtained legally from a licensed manufacturer, and it has been estimated that if heroin were freely available it would cost no more to be a regular heroin user than to be a regular drinker of alcohol. The black-market cost of these substances makes the use of cocaine or heroin consume so much money.

The fourth and final sense in which drug use causes crime is that *illicit drug use is a crime.* At first that may seem trivial, but there are two senses in which it is not. First, we are now making more than 1.5 million arrests for drug-law violations each year, and more than half of all federal prisoners are convicted on drug charges. Thus, drug-law violations are one of the major types of crime in the United States. Second, it is likely that the relationship between drug use and other forms of deviant behavior is strengthened by the fact that drug use is a crime. A person willing to commit one type of crime might be more willing than the average person to commit another type of crime. Some of the people who are actively trying to impress others by living dangerously and committing criminal acts might be drawn to illicit drug use as an obvious way to demonstrate their alienation from society. To better understand this relationship, imagine what might happen if the use of marijuana were legalized. Presumably, a greater number of otherwise law-abiding citizens might try using the drug, thus reducing the correlation between marijuana use and other forms of criminal activity. The concern over possibly increased drug use is, of course, one major argument in favor of maintaining legal controls on the illicit drugs.

Why We Try to Regulate Drugs

We can see that there are reasonable concerns about the potential toxicity and habit-forming nature of some drugs and even the criminality of some drug users. But the drugs that have been singled out for special controls, such as heroin, cocaine, and marijuana, are not unique in their association with toxicity, dependence, or criminal behavior. Tobacco, alcohol, and many legally available prescription drugs are also linked to these same social ills. At the beginning of the chapter we mentioned another important source of social conflict over drug use. Once a substance is regulated in any way, those regulations will be broken by some. This produces enormous social conflict and results in many problems for society. From underage drinking to injecting heroin, from Internet sales of prescription narcotics to "date-rape" drugs, the conflicts resulting from particular kinds of drug use lead to additional costs to American society (police, courts, prisons, treatment, etc.) beyond the direct drug effects of toxicity, dependence, and links to other kinds of criminal behavior. Our current laws do not represent a rationally devised plan to counteract the most realistic of these concerns in the most effective manner. In fact, most legislation is passed in an atmosphere of emotionality, in response to a specific set of concerns. Often the problems have been there for a long time, but public attention and concern have been recently aroused and Congress must respond. Sometimes

members of Congress or government officials play a major role in calling public attention to the problem for which they offer the solution: a new law, more restrictions, and a bigger budget for some agency. This is what is known in political circles as "starting a prairie fire." As we will see in Chapter 3, often the prairie fires include a lot of emotion-arousing rhetoric that borders on the irrational, and sometimes the results of the prairie fire and the ensuing legislation are unexpected and undesirable.

Summary

- American society has changed from being one that tolerated a wide variety of individual drug use to being one that attempts strict control over some types of drugs. This has occurred in response to social concerns about drug toxicity, dependence potential, and drug-related crime and violence.

- *Toxicity* can refer either to physiological poisoning or to dangerous disruption of behavior. Also, we can distinguish acute toxicity, resulting from the presence of too much of a drug, from chronic toxicity, which results from long-term exposure to a drug.

- Heroin and cocaine have high risks of toxicity per user, but their overall public health impact is low compared to tobacco and alcohol.

- Prescription drugs are also important contributors to overall drug toxicity figures.

- Drug dependence does not depend solely on the drug itself, but the use of some drugs is more likely to result in dependence than is the use of other drugs.

- The idea that opioid drugs or marijuana can produce violent criminality in their users is an old and largely discredited idea. Opioid users seem to engage in crimes mainly to obtain money, not because they are made more criminal by the drugs they take. One drug that is widely accepted as contributing to crimes and violence is alcohol.

- There are more than 1.5 million arrests each year in the United States for drug-law violations.

- Laws that have been developed to control drug use have a legitimate social purpose, which is to protect society from the dangers caused by some types of drug use. Whether these dangers have always been viewed rationally, and whether the laws have had their intended results, can be better judged after we have learned more about the drugs and the history of their regulation.

Review Questions

1. The French term *laissez-faire* is used to describe what type of relationship between a government and its people?
2. What three major concerns about drugs led to the initial passage of laws controlling their availability?
3. Long-term, heavy drinking can lead to permanent impairment of memory. What type of toxicity is this (acute or chronic; physiological or behavioral)?
4. What two kinds of data are recorded by the DAWN system?
5. What drug other than alcohol is mentioned most often in both parts of the DAWN system?
6. Why has AIDS been of particular concern for users of illicit drugs?
7. What drugs and methods of using them are considered to have very high dependence potential?
8. What is the apparent dependence potential of hallucinogenic drugs, such as LSD and mescaline?
9. What are four ways in which drug use might theoretically cause crime?
10. About how many arrests are made each year in the United States for violations of drug laws?

References

1. Substance Abuse and Mental Health Services Administration, Office of Applied Studies. Drug Abuse Warning Network, 2003: Interim National Estimates of Drug-Related Emergency Department Visits. DAWN Series D-26, DHHS Publication No. (SMA) 04-3972. Rockville, MD, 2004.
2. Drug Abuse Warning Network, 2003: Area Profiles of Drug-Related Mortality. DAWN Series D-27, DHHS Publication No. (SMA) 05-4023. Rockville, MD, 2005.
3. Murrill, C. S., and others. "Age-Specific Seroprevalence of HIV, Hepatitis B Virus, and Hepatitis C Virus Infection Among Injection Drug Users Admitted to Drug Treatment in 6 US Cities." *American Journal of Public Health* 92 (2002), pp. 385–87.
4. Ksobiech, K. "A Meta-Analysis of Needle Sharing, Lending, and Borrowing Behaviors of Needle Exchange Program Attenders." *AIDS Education and Prevention* 15 (2003), pp. 257–68.
5. Katz, J. L., & S. T. Higgins. What Is Represented by Vertical Shifts in Self-Administration Dose-Effect Curves?" *Psychopharmacology* 17 (2004), pp. 360–61.
6. American Psychiatric Association. *Diagnostic and Statistical Manual of Mental Disorders,* 4th ed. Washington, DC: American Psychological Association, 2000.
7. Gable, R. S. "Toward a Comparative Overview of Dependence Potential and Acute Toxicity of Psychoactive Substances Used Nonmedically." *American Journal of Drug and Alcohol Abuse* 19 (1993), pp. 263–81.
8. Kilts, C. D., and others. "The Neural Correlates of Cue-Induced Craving in Cocaine-Dependent Women." *American Journal of Psychiatry* 161 (2004), pp. 233–41.
9. Crawford, A. M., and others. "Parallel Developmental Trajectories of Sensation Seeking and Regular Substance Use in Adolescents." *Psychology of Addictive Behaviors* 17 (2003), pp. 179–92.
10. Peele, S. "What Addiction Is and Is Not: The Impact of Mistaken Notions of Addiction." *Addictive Behaviors* 8 (2000), pp. 599–607.
11. Simpson, M. "The Relationship Between Drug Use and Crime. A Puzzle Inside an Enigma." *International Journal of Drug Policy* 14 (2003), pp. 307–19.
12. Bureau of Justice Statistics. *Drugs and Crime Facts.* (Pub. No. NCJ 165148). Washington, DC: U.S. Department of Justice, 2004.
13. National Institute on Alcohol Abuse and Alcoholism. *Tenth Special Report to the U.S. Congress on Alcohol and Health.* (Pub. No. 00-1583). Bethesda, MD: National Institutes of Health, 2000.
14. National Opinion Research Center. *Drug and Alcohol Use and Related Matters Among Arrestees, 2003.* Washington, DC: U.S. Department of Justice, 2004.

Check Yourself

Are You Hooked On an Activity?

Think of an activity other than substance use that you either really enjoy or find yourself doing a lot. This can be a hobby, such as playing video games or watching movies; something more energetic, such as skiing or mountain biking; or something that involves spending money, such as buying books, CDs, or clothing or shopping on the Internet or TV shopping channels. It can be sexual behavior or gambling, or it can even be working longer hours than most people. Now, with the most "addictive" of those activities in mind, go through the *DSM-IV-TR* diagnostic criteria one by one and ask whether your nondrug "habit" meets each criterion, obviously substituting the behavior in question for the words *the substance* and *substance use*. Probably the most informative questions in this context are the following (note the words in italics):

- Have you *often* done more of the behavior or for a longer period than you intended?
- Have you *persistently* tried to cut down or control the behavior?
- Have you given up *important* social, occupational, or recreational activities because of this behavior?
- Is the behavior continuing despite recurrent physical or psychological problems *caused or made worse* by the behavior?

If you answered yes to all four questions, then whether or not you agree that you meet abuse or dependence criteria, you should consider talking to a behavioral health professional to obtain some assistance in reducing the impact of this behavior on your life.

Check Yourself

Any drug that has the ability to affect you in any way also has the potential to be toxic if used in too great a quantity or in the wrong combination with other drugs. If you use alcohol or other drugs, use the following assessment to estimate the risk of toxicity to which your drug use exposes you.

1. When you take over-the-counter medications, including headache remedies, do you read the instructions carefully and make sure not to exceed the recommended dose?
2. If you are already taking some sort of medication on a regular basis, do you always check with your doctor or pharmacist about the safety of taking any additional drug along with your regular medication?
3. Do you check the expiration dates of drugs in your medicine cabinet before using them?
4. If you drink alcohol, do you drink only in moderation and check to make sure the alcohol won't interact with a drug you are also taking?
5. Do you avoid taking drugs prescribed for someone else and avoid the use of street drugs of unknown strength and purity?

If you answered yes to all these questions, you are probably a responsible consumer of alcohol, prescription, and over-the-counter drugs, and it is unlikely that you will suffer from drug toxicity.

Drug Products and Their Regulations

Objectives

When you have finished this chapter, you should be able to:

- Discuss the role of reformist attitudes and social concerns in moving the U.S. government toward drug regulations.

- Understand the major purposes and influence of the 1906 Pure Food and Drugs Act.

- Understand the evolution, major purposes, and influence of the 1914 Harrison Act.

- Describe the process of approval for new pharmaceuticals.

- Describe drugs and dietary supplements as defined by the FDA.

- Describe the historical sequence of controls on opioids, cocaine, marijuana, and other controlled substances.

- Understand controlled substance schedules (I-V).

- Explain the impact of mandatory minimum sentencing.

- Explain what makes particular drug paraphernalia illegal.

- Compare and contrast the major types of drug testing.

- Explain how drug control efforts affect the federal budget, international relations, and the criminal justice systems.

Once upon a time in the United States, there weren't any federal regulations about drug use. That lasted for about two years. In 1791, Congress passed an excise tax on whiskey, which resulted in a disagreement that historians call the Whiskey Rebellion. West of the Appalachian Mountains, where most whiskey was made, the farmers refused to pay the tax and tarred and feathered revenue officers who tried to collect it. In 1794, President George Washington called in the militia, which occupied counties in western Pennsylvania and sent prisoners to Philadelphia for trial. The militia and the federal government carried the day. The Whiskey Rebellion was an important test for the new government because it clearly established that the federal government had the power to enforce federal laws within the states.

In Chapter 2, we saw that drug regulations are passed mainly for what is perceived to be the public good. As the story of the laws and regulations about drugs unfolds, it will become clear that most of the debate centers on the question "What is the public good?" Issues of fact, morality, health, personal choice, and social order are intertwined—and sometimes confused. Our laws concerning drug use resemble a patchwork quilt reflecting the many social changes that have occurred in this country. If we want to understand our current drug laws, we must see how they have evolved over the years in response to one social crisis after another.

Online Learning Center Resources

www.mhhe.com/ksir12e

Visit our Online Learning Center (OLC) for access to these study aids and additional resources.

- Learning objectives
- Glossary flashcards
- Web activities and links
- Self-scoring chapter quiz
- Audio chapter summaries

The Beginnings

Reformism

The current federal approaches to drug regulation can be traced to two pieces of legislation passed in 1906 and 1914. The nation was moving out of the gilded age of *laissez-faire* capitalism into the reform area, in which legislation was passed regulating business and labor practices, meatpacking, and food production. This general movement toward improvement of our nation's moral character led in 1919 to a constitutional amendment prohibiting the sale of alcoholic beverages. America's "Noble Experiment" with federal alcohol prohibition during the 1920s played a very important role in how the nation approached other substances associated with the social problems described in Chapter 2.

Also, the period between 1890 and 1920 has been called the "nadir of race relations" in the United States. During the Civil War, many Northerners had favored the integration of blacks into society. After the Civil War, blacks moved north to take jobs in factories, the U.S. Army battled Native Americans in the West, Chinese immigrants came in large numbers to build the intercontinental railroads and to work in mines, Mexican laborers came to the South and Southwest to work in the fields, and immigrants from Italy, Ireland, and other parts of Europe also came to contribute labor to all these efforts. For some, this was just too much

social change in too short a time period. Racism became more widespread and open across the entire country, and was targeted against all these groups. Many of the first labor unions were openly racist, trying to protect jobs for "real" Americans. For many Americans, concerns about drunkenness, crime, drug misuse, and other forms of deviant behavior came to be associated with minority racial groups, adding fuel not only to beliefs about the immorality of members of those races, but also to the desire to pass tough laws regulating these undesirable behaviors. The legacy of those beliefs and those laws remains with us today.

Issues Leading to Legislation

The trend toward reform was given direction and energy by the public discussion of several drug-related problems, and those first federal drug laws reflected the specific problems that fueled their passage. In the early 1800s, opium (see Chapter 13) was the medical doctor's most reliable and effective medicine, used for a variety of conditions but most notably as a pain reliever. Physicians prescribed various forms of opium liberally and with only limited concern about patients developing dependence. Commercial production of pure **morphine** from opium in the 1830s was followed by the introduction of the hypodermic syringe in the 1850s, and this more potent delivery method led to increasing medical recognition of the negative aspects of "morphinism," an analogy with the term *alcoholism*. By the start of the 20th century, most physicians were aware of the dangers of morphine overuse, but many patients had developed morphine dependence under their doctor's care and relied upon their physicians and pharmacists for a regular supply. Physicians debated whether their morphine-dependent patients had developed a unique disorder requiring continued treatment (a medical view of dependence), or whether they were merely weak-willed or simply seeking pleasure in the drug's effects (a moral model of dependence).

Drugs in the Media

Is Media Coverage of New Prescription Drugs Too Rosy?

Until fairly recently, U.S. pharmaceutical companies weren't allowed to advertise prescription drugs directly to consumers, so the companies placed their advertising in medical journals. After all, these drugs cannot be obtained by the consumer unless prescribed by a physician. A few years ago, however, some companies began running ads that did not mention a drug but referred to certain medical conditions, such as baldness or erectile dysfunction, and suggested that consumers talk to their doctors. In 1997, the Food and Drug Administration began to allow commercials on radio and television to mention drugs by name. The ads must also mention the most important warnings and possible side effects associated with the drug. While such brief messages cannot provide complete information about the risks, costs, and benefits of new drugs, they may sway consumers' and physicians' demand for a drug.

In many ways, news coverage of new drugs has the same deficiencies as advertising. A *New England Journal of Medicine* study published in May 2000 found that most news stories do not fully convey the risks and cost of drugs. When a medical breakthrough is announced, fame for investigators and their institutions, future research grants, and corporate profits are often at stake, so reporters are barraged with daily news releases, expert testimonials, and public relations phone calls, which can cloud news judgment. Enthusiastic reporters may not be skeptical about what they read and may not put the benefits of a drug in context. For example, they may paint a drug as providing a big breakthrough when in reality it decreases a disease's mortality rate by only a few percentage points. Overstating drug benefits can create demand among consumers, with the possible effect of physicians writing prescriptions for expensive drugs with potentially harmful side effects.

Watch for drug advertisements and news stories for several days, and check for answers to these questions: Does the ad make it clear what disease or condition the drug treats? What kinds of conditions seem to be most common among advertised prescription drugs? Does the ad's list of side effects and warnings sound potentially worse than the disorder being treated? In a news story, do you think the reporter gave a balanced picture of the benefits and risks of the medication covered? How do you think your physician would react to your suggesting that he or she prescribe a specific drug?

During the reform era, the moral model became increasingly popular.

Patent Medicines The broadest impact on drug use in this country came from the widespread legal distribution of **patent medicines.** Patent medicines were dispensed by traveling peddlers and were readily available at local stores for self-medication. Sales of patent medicines increased from $3.5 million in 1859 to $74 million in 1904.

Within the United States, conflict increased between the steady progress of medical science and the therapeutic claims of the patent medicine hucksters. The alcohol and other habit-forming drug content of the patent medicines was also a matter of concern. One medicine, Hostetter's Bitters, was 44 percent alcohol, and another, Birney's Catarrh Cure, was 4 percent cocaine. In October 1905, *Collier's* magazine culminated a prolonged attack on patent medicines with a well-documented, aggressive series titled "Great American Fraud."[1]

Opium and the Chinese The roots of Chinese opium smoking and the history of the Opium Wars are discussed in Chapter 13. In the mid-1800s,

> **morphine:** a narcotic, the primary active chemical in opium. Heroin is made from morphine.
> **patent medicines:** medicines sold directly to the public.

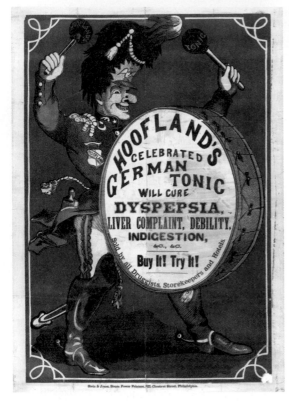

Many patent medicines contained habit-forming drugs. This tonic from the 1860s was about 30 percent alcohol.

many British and some American merchants were engaged in the lucrative sale of opium to the Chinese, and many reformers and world leaders disapproved. In 1833, the United States signed its first treaty agreeing to control international trade in opium, and a regulatory tax on crude opium imported into this country was legislated in 1842.

The United States imported Chinese workers after the Civil War, mainly to help build the rapidly expanding railroads, and some of these people brought with them the habit of smoking opium. As always happens when a new pleasure is introduced into a society, the practice of opium smoking spread rapidly. Also, as always happens, the new practice upset the status quo and caused society to react. A contemporary report in 1882 described both the spread of opium smoking in San Francisco and the reactions it elicited:

> The practice spread rapidly and quietly among this class of gamblers and prostitutes until the latter part of 1875, at which time the authorities became cognizant of the fact, and finding . . . that many women and young girls, as also young men of respectable family, were being induced to visit the dens, where they were ruined morally and otherwise, a city ordinance was passed forbidding the practice under the penalty of a heavy fine or imprisonment, or both. Many arrests were made, and the punishment was prompt and thorough.[2]

This 1875 San Francisco ordinance was the first U.S. law forbidding opium smoking. In 1882, New York State passed a similar law aimed at opium use in New York City's expanding Chinatown. An 1890 federal act permitted only American citizens to import opium or to manufacture smoking opium in the United States. Although this law is sometimes viewed as a racist policy, it was partly in response to an 1887 agreement with China, which also forbade American citizens from engaging in the Chinese opium trade.

As more states and municipalities outlawed opium dens, the cost of black-market

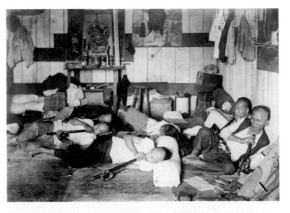

Opium smoking spread widely following its introduction in the nineteenth century.

opium increased, and many of the lower-class opium users took up morphine or heroin, which were readily available and inexpensive.

Cocaine Pure **cocaine** (see Chapter 6) became available in the mid-1800s, and its use increased over time. By 1900, its presence in many patent medicines and tonics (including the original Coca-Cola), and its ready availability by mail order and in pharmacies led medical experts to be increasingly concerned about the effects of overuse. In the early 1900s, drug reformers repeatedly raised this public issue: Cocaine sniffing had become widespread among Southern "negroes," and it was responsible for an increase in violent crimes perpetrated by those among the "lower class" of blacks in the South. The widespread distribution of this largely unsubstantiated fear was especially important in building support for federal drug control laws among Southern senators and congressmen despite their typical "states' rights" opposition to increasing federalism.[3]

1906 Pure Food and Drugs Act

President Theodore Roosevelt recommended in 1905 "that a law be enacted to regulate interstate commerce in misbranded and adulterated foods, drinks, and drugs."[4] The 1906 publication of Upton Sinclair's *The Jungle,* exposing the horribly unsanitary conditions in the meatpacking industry, shocked Congress and America. Five months later, the Pure Food and Drugs Act was passed. This 1906 act prohibited interstate commerce in adulterated or misbranded foods and drugs, bringing the federal government full force into the drug marketplace. Subsequent modifications have built on it. A drug was defined as "any substance or mixture of substances intended to be used for the cure, mitigation, or prevention of disease." Of particular importance was the phrasing of the law with respect to misbranding. Misbranding referred *only to the label, not to general advertising,* and covered "any

statement, design, or device regarding . . . a drug, or the ingredients or substances contained therein, which shall be false or misleading in any particular."

The act specifically referred to alcohol, morphine, opium, cocaine, heroin, *Cannabis indica* (marijuana), and several other agents. Each package was required to state how much (or what proportion) of these drugs was included in the preparation. This meant, for example, that the widely sold "cures" for alcohol or morphine dependence had to indicate that they contained another habit-forming drug. However, as long as the ingredients were clearly listed on the label, any drug could be sold and bought with no federal restrictions. The goal was to protect people from unscrupulous merchants, not from themselves. The 1906 Pure Food and Drugs Act provided the rootstock on which all our modern laws regulating pharmaceuticals have been grafted.

Harrison Act of 1914

In the early 1900s, Dr. Hamilton Wright, the father of American narcotics laws, decided the United States could gain favored trading status with China by leading international efforts to aid the Chinese in their efforts to reduce opium importation. At the request of the United States, an international conference met in 1912 to discuss controls on the opium trade. Great Britain, which was giving up a very lucrative business, wanted morphine, heroin, and cocaine included as well, because, as opium was being controlled, these German products were replacing it.[5] Eventually, several nations agreed to control both international trade and domestic sale and use of these substances. In response, Dr. Wright drafted a bill, which was submitted by Senator Harrison of New York, titled "An Act to provide for the registration

cocaine: a stimulant; the primary active chemical in coca.

of, with collectors of internal revenue, and to impose a special tax upon all persons who produce, import, manufacture, compound, deal in, dispense, or give away opium or coca leaves, their salts, derivatives, or preparations, and for other purposes."[6] With a title like that, it's no wonder that this historic law is usually referred to as the Harrison Act.

For the first time, dealers and dispensers of the opioids and cocaine had to register annually, pay a small fee, and use special order forms provided by the Bureau of Internal Revenue. Physicians, dentists, and veterinary surgeons were named as potential lawful distributors if they registered. In 1914 there would have been no support and no constitutional rationale for a federal law prohibiting an individual from possessing or using these drugs. Congress would not have considered such a law; if it had, the Supreme Court would probably have declared it unconstitutional. The Harrison Act was a tax law, constitutionally similar to the whiskey tax. It was not a punitive act, penalties for violation were not severe, and the measure contained no reference to users of "narcotics."

During congressional debate, some concern was expressed about the tax law's inconvenience to physicians and pharmacists, and it is doubtful that such a law would have been passed in the United States if its purpose had been merely to meet the rather weak treaty obligations of the 1912 Hague Conference. It was not meant to replace existing laws and, in fact, specifically supported the continuing legality of the 1906 Pure Food and Drugs Act and the 1909 Opium Exclusion Act. Dr. Wright had written and lectured extensively, waging an effective, emotional, and in some instances outright racist public campaign for additional controls over these drugs. For example, his claims about the practice of "snuffing" cocaine into the nose, which he said was popular among Southern blacks, caused a great deal of concern and fear.[7] Dr. Wright testified before Congress that this practice led to the raping of white women. Combining this depiction with the racially tinged fears about "those immoral Chinese opium

dens" added the necessary heat to make the difference, and the Harrison Act passed and was signed into law in 1914. This law was the seed, which has since sprouted into all of our federal controlled-substance regulations.

Two Bureaus, Two Types of Regulation

By 1914 the basic federal laws had been passed that would influence our nation's drug regulations up to the current time. The Pure Food and Drugs Act was administered within the Department of Agriculture, whereas the Harrison Act was administered by the Treasury Department—two different federal departments administering two different laws. Many of the drugs regulated by the two laws were the same, but the political issues to which each agency responded were different. The Agriculture Department was administering a law aimed at ensuring that drugs were pure and honestly labeled. On the other hand, the Treasury Department's experience was in taxing alcohol, and it would soon be responsible for enforcing Prohibition. The approach taken by each bureau was further shaped by court decisions, so that the actual effect of each law became something a bit different from what seems to have been intended.

Regulation of Pharmaceuticals

The pharmaceutical industry has grown into one of the most important sources of commerce in the world, with the U.S. market of more than $180 billion representing almost half the estimated total. Prescription and nonprescription drugs are subject to a complex set of regulations, but in the United States they all grew out of the Pure Food and Drugs Act. The 1906 law called for the government to regulate the purity of both foods and drugs, and evidence had been presented during the congressional debate that thousands of products in both categories were at fault. Where was the task of analyzing and prosecuting to begin? Dr. Harvey Wiley, chief chemist in the Department of Agriculture, had been a major proponent of the

Targeting Prevention

Prescribing Practices

Some prescription drugs have the potential for patients to abuse them or to become dependent on them. According to the logic of the Controlled Substances Act, a drug that has such potential should be listed as a Schedule II–V controlled substance. This triggers laws limiting the way in which these drugs can be prescribed, in an effort to prevent them from being abused or creating dependence in users. Prescribing rules vary, but one of the most common limitations is that the prescriptions may not be automatically refilled. In other words, the physician must write a new prescription if the patient wants to get more of the drug. Despite these rules, we sometimes hear about people who develop dependence on a prescription drug. Do you think the current limitations are effective? Could changes be made that would effectively reduce the chances of patients becoming dependent?

1906 law and had drafted most of it. He was in charge of administering the law, and he influenced the direction its enforcement would take. His first concern was adulterated food, so most of the initial cases dealt with food products rather than drugs.

Purity

Most large drug manufacturers made efforts to comply with the new law, although they were not given specific recommendations as to how this should be accomplished. The manufacturer of Cuforhedake Brane-Fude modified its label to show that it contained 30 percent alcohol and 16 grains of a widely used headache remedy. The government took the manufacturer to trial in 1908 on several grounds: the alcohol content was a bit lower than that claimed on the label, and the label seemed to claim that the product was a "cure" and food for the brain, both misleading claims. After much arguing about different methods of describing alcohol content and about the label claims, the manufacturer was convicted by the jury, proba-

bly because of the "brane-fude" claim, and paid a fine of $700.[8]

Dr. Wiley went on vigorously testing products and pursuing any that were adulterated or didn't properly list important ingredients, but he also went after many companies on the basis of their therapeutic claims. In 1911, government action against a claimed cancer cure was overturned by arguing that the ingredients were accurately labeled and that the original law had not covered therapeutic claims, only claims about the nature of the ingredients. Congress rapidly passed the 1912 Sherley amendment, which outlawed "false and fraudulent" therapeutic claims on the label. Even so, it was still up to the government to prove that a claim was not only false but also fraudulent in that the manufacturer knew it to be false. In a 1922 case, the claim that "B&M External Remedy" could cure tuberculosis was ruled not to be fraudulent because its manufacturer, who had no scientific or medical training, truly believed that its ingredients (raw eggs, turpentine, ammonia, formaldehyde, and mustard and wintergreen oils) were effective.[8] This seemed like an encouragement for the ignorant to become manufacturers of medicines!

From its beginning, the Food and Drug Administration (**FDA**) had adopted the approach of encouraging voluntary cooperation, which it could obtain from most of the manufacturers through educational and corrective actions rather than through punitive, forced compliance. As more and more cases were investigated, FDA officials determined that many of the violations of the 1906 law were unintentional and caused primarily by poor manufacturing techniques and an absence of quality-control measures. The FDA began developing assay techniques for various chemicals and products and collaborated extensively with the pharmaceutical industry to improve standards.

FDA: The United States Food and Drug Administration.

Despite these improvements, many smaller companies continued to bring forth quack medicines that were ineffective or even dangerous. The Great Depression of the 1930s increased competition for business, and the Roosevelt administration took a more critical view of the pharmaceutical industry. FDA surveys in the mid-1930s showed that more than 10 percent of the drug products studied did not meet the standards of the *United States Pharmacopoeia* or *The National Formulary*. Several attempts were made during the early 1930s to enact major reforms, but opposition by the manufacturers of proprietary medicines prevented these changes from happening.

Safety

The 1930s had seen an expansion in the use of "sulfa" drugs, which are effective antibiotics. In searching for a form that could be given as a liquid, a chemist found that *sulfanilamide* would dissolve in diethylene glycol. The new concoction looked, tasted, and smelled fine, so it was bottled and marketed in 1937. Diethylene glycol causes kidney poisoning, and within a short time 107 people died from taking "Elixir Sulfanilamide." The federal government could not intervene simply because the mixture was toxic—there was no legal requirement that medicine be safe. The FDA seized the elixir on the grounds that a true elixir contains alcohol, and this did not. The chemist committed suicide, the company paid the largest fine ever under the 1906 law, and a public crisis arose, which led to passage of the 1938 Food, Drug, and Cosmetic Act.[8]

A critical change in the 1938 law was the requirement that *before* a new drug could be marketed its manufacturer must test it for toxicity. The company was to submit a "new drug application" (**NDA**) to the FDA. This NDA was to include "full reports of investigations which have been made to show whether or not such a drug is safe for use." If the submitted paperwork was satisfactory, the application was allowed to become effective.

The new drug application provision was important in two ways: first, it changed the role of the FDA from testing and challenging some of the drugs already being sold to that of a gatekeeper, which must review every new drug before it is marketed. This increased power and responsibility led to a great expansion in the size of the FDA. Second, the requirement that companies conduct research before marketing a new drug greatly reduced the likelihood of new drugs being introduced by small companies run by untrained people.

The 1938 act also stipulated that drug labels either give adequate directions for use or state that the drug is to be used only on the prescription of a physician. Thus, the federal law now recognized a difference between drugs that could be sold over the counter and prescription-only drugs.

Effectiveness

In the late 1950s, Senator Estes Kefauver began a series of hearings investigating high drug costs and marketing collaboration between drug companies. One major concern was that some of the most widely sold over-the-counter medications were probably ineffective. For example, Carter's Little Liver Pills consisted of small bits of candy-coated dried liver. It was accurately labeled and made no unsubstantiated therapeutic claims on the label—if you concluded that it was supposed to help your liver, that wasn't the company's fault. And no law required the medicines to actually do anything. Amendments to the Food, Drug, and Cosmetic Act were written but were bottled up in committee. Again it took a disaster that raised public awareness and congressional concern before major reforms were implemented.

Thalidomide, a sedative and sleeping pill, was first marketed in West Germany in 1957. The drug was used by pregnant women because it reduced the nausea and vomiting associated with the morning sickness experienced early in pregnancy. An American company submitted an NDA in 1960 to market thalidomide, but luckily the FDA physician in charge of the application did not approve it quickly. In 1961 and early 1962, it became clear that thalidomide had been responsible for birth defects. In West Germany, hundreds of children had been born with deformed limbs. The American company had released some thalidomide for clinical testing, but, because its NDA was not approved, a major disaster was avoided in the United States.[8]

The 1962 Kefauver-Harris amendments added several important provisions, including the requirement that companies seek approval of any testing to be done with humans before the clinical trials are conducted. Another provision required advertisements for prescription drugs (mostly in medical journals) to contain a summary of information about adverse reactions to the drug.

The most important change was one requiring that every new drug be demonstrated to be *effective* for the illnesses mentioned on the label. As with the details of safety testing required by the 1938 law, this research on effectiveness was to be submitted to the FDA. The FDA was also to begin a review of the thousands of products marketed between 1938 and 1962 to determine their effectiveness. Any that were found to be ineffective were to be removed from the market. In 1966, the FDA began the process of evaluating the formulations of prescription drugs. In the next eight years, the FDA removed from the market 6,133 drugs manufactured by 2,732 companies.

Marketing a New Drug

The basic rules for introducing a new drug have been in place for more than 40 years, with procedural amendments reflecting other issues that have arisen since 1962. Companies are required to demonstrate, through extensive chemical, biological, animal, and human testing, that the new drug they want to sell is both safe and effective. According to the pharmaceutical industry, the entire research and approval process now takes on average more than 10 years and costs about $800 million.[9]

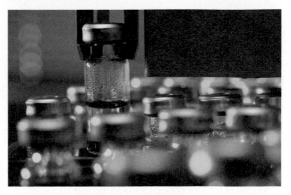

A new drug must move through three phases of clinical investigation before it reaches the market.

The FDA formally enters the picture only when a drug company is ready to study the effects of a compound on humans. At that time the company supplies to the FDA a "Notice of Claimed Investigational Exemption for a New Drug" (**IND**); it is also required to submit all information from preclinical (before human) investigations, including the effects of the drug on animals. The principal purpose of this preclinical work is to establish the safety of the compound.

As minimum evidence of safety, the animal studies must include acute, onetime administration of several dose levels of the drug to different groups of animals of at least two species. There must also be studies in which the drug is given regularly to animals for a period related to the proposed use of the drug in humans. For example, a drug to be used chronically requires two-year toxicology studies in animals. Again, two species are required. The method of drug administration and the form of the drug in these studies must be the same as that proposed for human use.

NDA: new drug application. Must be approved before a drug is sold.
IND: application to investigate a new drug in human clinical trials.

In addition to these research results, the company must submit a detailed description of the proposed clinical studies of the drug in humans. The company must also certify that the human research participants will be told they are receiving an investigational compound, and the participants will sign a form, stating they know they are to receive such a compound and this is acceptable to them. Finally, the company must agree to forward annually a comprehensive report and to inform the FDA immediately if any adverse reactions arise in either animals or humans receiving the investigational drug.

If the FDA authorizes the use of the drug in humans, the company can move into the first of *three phases of clinical investigation:*

1. *Phase One* encompasses studies with relatively low doses of the drug on a limited number of healthy people—typically, 20 to 80 company employees, medical school personnel, and others who volunteer for such trials. At this stage the researchers are primarily interested in learning how their drug is absorbed and excreted in healthy people, as well as the side effects it may trigger.
2. *Phase Two* of the human studies involves patients who have the condition the candidate drug is designed to treat. These studies involve about a few hundred patients who are chosen because the new agent might help them.
3. *Phase Three* administers the drug to larger numbers of individuals (typically, 1,000 to 5,000) with the disease or symptom for which the drug is intended. If the compound proves effective in phase three, the FDA balances its possible dangers against the benefits for patients before releasing it for sale to the public.

There have been a few changes to this basic procedure since 1962. In 1983, Congress passed the Orphan Drug Act, offering tax incentives and exclusive sales rights for a guaranteed seven years for any company developing a drug for rare disorders afflicting no more than 200,000 people. Up to that time, companies had stayed away from much research on rare disorders because they couldn't earn enough to recover the enormous research costs. By 2004, almost 240 drugs developed under this act had received FDA approval.[9] However, because of the limited market, many of these new drugs are extremely expensive, with some costing more than $100,000 per patient per year.

On the "drug war" front, the Prescription Drug Marketing Act of 1988 tightened the procedures whereby drug company salespeople could provide free samples to physicians, after Congress had heard testimony about widespread diversion of samples. Also, because counterfeit and adulterated drugs had found their way into the U.S. market from abroad as shipments of "American goods returned," new regulations were added covering the transfer and reimportation of drugs.

The 1997 FDA Modernization Act made several more procedural adjustments, including guidelines for annual postmarketing reporting by the companies of adverse reactions to some medications (so-called Phase IV reporting). Also, the act allowed companies to distribute information to physicians about other, less well-researched, uses for an approved medication. One example of such "off-label" prescribing is the drug carbamazepine, which was originally tested and approved for use as an anticonvulsant. Based on published research as well as clinical experience, the drug is also widely prescribed as a mood stabilizer (see Chapter 8) even though it has not received FDA approval for that use.

There is one big, continually debated issue surrounding the FDA drug approval system: Why does it take so long? The issue is not just of concern to the sick individual. Pharmaceutical manufacturers have a 20-year patent on a new drug. They usually patent the chemical as soon as there is some evidence that it is marketable. The manufacturers claim that, by the time a drug is cleared for marketing, they have only a few years left on the patent. From the mid-1980s to the late 1990s, the average approval time was reduced from 32 months to 12 months—but the increased speed of the FDA's approval process has been offset by an increased amount of time spent by companies in clinical trials—an average of almost seven years.[9]

From 1994 to 2003, the FDA approved an average of 32 new drugs per year.[9]

Dietary Supplements

Certain druglike products, such as vitamin pills, are not drugs but, rather, are considered dietary supplements and treated more as foods. They don't need to be proved to be effective for a specific intended purpose. Many questions arose about whether such new products needed to be reviewed for safety before marketing them and whether some of the beneficial claims made by people selling them constituted mislabeling. The 1994 Dietary Supplement Health and Education Act cleared up many of those issues. It broadened the definition of dietary supplements to include not only vitamins, minerals, and proteins but also herbs and herbal extracts. The labels are not allowed to make unsubstantiated direct claims, such as "cures cancer," but they are permitted to make general statements about the overall health and "well-being" that can be achieved by consuming the dietary ingredient. The label must then say, "This statement has not been evaluated by the Food and Drug Administration. This product is not intended to diagnose, treat, cure, or prevent any disease." Nevertheless, growth in sales of herbal products and other dietary supplements has been enormous, probably in large part because many consumers don't distinguish between the vague, general claims made by supplements and the specific, demonstrated effectiveness required of drugs.

One issue that should be of concern for users of dietary supplements is that, rather than the company demonstrating the safety of the supplement before it is marketed, the FDA must prove that the product is unsafe before its sale can be stopped. For example, the FDA became concerned in 1997 about *ephedra* (see Chapter 12), found in many herbal weight-loss products.

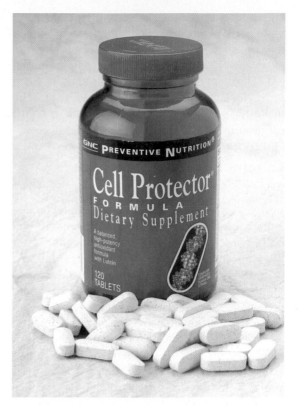

Dietary supplements are not regulated in the same way as drugs. They do not have to be proven safe and effective before they are marketed.

In high doses, this herbal product can cause dangerous increases in blood pressure and interfere with normal mechanisms for reducing body heat during exercise. It took seven years and the well-publicized deaths of some athletes before *ephedra* was banned in 2004.[10]

Controlled Substances

To most Americans the word *narcotics* means drugs that are manufactured and sold illegally. Pharmacologically, the term refers only to drugs having certain effects, with the prototype being the narcotic analgesics derived from opium, such as morphine and heroin. Although the Harrison Act controlled opioids, which are narcotics, and cocaine, which is not, the enforcement effort focused so much on the opioids that eventually the enforcement officers became known as narcotics officers, the office within the Treasury Department officially became the Narcotics Division, and people began to refer to the "Harrison Narcotics Act," though the word *narcotics* was not in the original title. The meaning of the term changed so much in political use that later federal laws incorrectly classified cocaine and then marijuana as narcotics.

After the Harrison Act

In 1914, it was estimated that about 200,000 Americans—1 in 400—were dependent on opium or its derivatives. One way to administer the Harrison Act would have been to allow a continued legal supply of opioids to those individuals through registered physicians and to focus enforcement efforts on the smugglers and remaining opium dens. After all, the Harrison Act stated that an unregistered person could purchase and possess any of the taxed drugs if they had been prescribed or administered by a physician "in the course of his professional practice and for legitimate medical purposes." Until the 1920s, most users continued to receive opioids quietly through their private physicians, and in most large cities public clinics dispensed morphine to users who could not afford private care.

Early enforcement efforts focused on smugglers and did not result in a large number of arrests. However, one very important arrest was to have later repercussions. It seems that a Dr. Webb was taking telephone orders for opioids, including some from people he had never seen in person. Evidence was presented that this physician would prescribe whatever amount the caller requested. He was arrested, convicted, and appealed the conviction all the way to the U.S. Supreme Court, which in 1919 upheld his conviction on the grounds that his activity did not constitute a proper prescription in the course of the professional practice of medicine. It's interesting to speculate whether fears about unexpected uses for the telephone, which most people did not yet have in their homes, might have contributed to Dr. Webb's prosecution. There is a parallel with today's Internet pharmacies, some of which provide medical consultation and prescription through home computers.

The single most important legislation that has shaped the federal government's approach to controlled substances wasn't a "drug law" at all but, rather, the 18th Amendment prohibiting alcohol. That law was also to be enforced by the Treasury Department, and a separate Prohibition unit was established in 1919. The Narcotics Division was placed within that unit, and Colonel Levi G. Nutt was appointed the first director, with 170 agents at his disposal.[5] Although the Harrison Act had not changed, the people enforcing it had. Just as with alcohol, these people believed that the cure for narcotic dependence was to prevent the user from having access to the drug (in other words, opioid "prohibition," at least for those who were dependent). The new enforcers interpreted the Webb case to mean that any prescription of a habit-forming drug to a dependent user was not a "legitimate medical purpose," and they began to charge many physicians under the Harrison Act.

Arresting Physicians and Pharmacists The Internal Revenue Service (IRS) moved to close municipal narcotics clinics in more than 30 cities from coast to coast. From 1919 to 1929, the Narcotics Division arrested about 75,000 people, including 25,000 physicians and druggists.[5] The American Medical Association supported the view that reputable physicians would not prescribe morphine or other opioids to dependent users. Because there was then no legal way to obtain the drug, the user was forced either to stop using drugs or to look for them in the illegal market. Thus, this new method of enforcing the Harrison Act resulted in the growth of an illicit drug trade, which charged users up to 50 times more than the legal retail drug price. Opioid dependence came increasingly to be viewed as a police, rather than a medical, problem.

Stiffer Penalties Partly in response to the growing illicit market, in 1922 Congress passed the Jones-Miller Act, which more than doubled the maximum penalties for dealing in illegally imported drugs to $5,000 and 10 years of imprisonment. Included also was the stipulation that the mere possession of illegally obtained opioids or cocaine was sufficient basis for conviction, thus officially making the user a criminal. Because illegal opioids were so expensive, many users came to prefer the most potent type available, heroin. In 1924, another act prohibited importing opium for the manufacture of heroin. Already by this time several important trends had been set: Users were criminals at odds with the regulatory agency, the growth of the illicit market was responded to with greater penalties and more aggressive enforcement, and the focus was on attempting to eliminate a substance (heroin) as though the drug itself were the problem. In the 1925 Linder case, the U.S. Supreme Court declared it could be legal for a physician to prescribe opioids for a dependent user if it were part of a curing program and did not transcend "the limits of that professional conduct with which Congress never intended to interfere."[6] However, the damage had been done, and most physicians would have nothing to do with drug-dependent patients.

Prison versus Treatment By 1928, individuals sentenced for drug violations made up one-third of the total population in federal prisons. Even though the 1920s were the period of alcohol prohibition, during those years twice as many people were imprisoned for drug violations as for liquor violations.[11] In 1929, Congress viewed this enormous expenditure for drug offenders as an indicator that something was wrong and decided that users should be cured rather than repeatedly jailed. It voted to establish two "narcotic farms" for the treatment of persons dependent on habit-forming drugs (including marijuana and peyote) who had been convicted of violating a federal law. The farm in Lexington, Kentucky, opened in 1935 and generally held about a thousand patients, two-thirds of whom were prisoners.

The Bureau of Narcotics Answering the call for new approaches to dependence, and in response to the end of Prohibition and to charges of corruption in the previous Narcotics Division, in 1930 Congress took several actions that culminated in the formation of a separate Bureau of Narcotics in the Treasury Department. Harry Anslinger became the first commissioner of that bureau in 1932 and took office with a pledge to stop arresting so many users and instead to go after the big dealers. Anslinger became the first "drug czar," although he wasn't called that at the time. To some extent, he followed the lead of J. Edgar Hoover, director of the Federal Bureau of Investigation (FBI). Each of these men was regularly reappointed by each new president, and each built up a position of considerable power and influence. Anslinger had almost total control of federal efforts in drug education, prevention, treatment, and enforcement for 30 years, from 1932 to 1962. No federal or state drug-control law was passed without his influencing it, and he also represented U.S. drug-control interests to international organizations, including the United Nations. He was tough-minded in the area of drug abuse and always opposed any form of ambulatory drug treatment (treatment outside a secure hospital environment).

The end of Prohibition, combined with Depression-era cutbacks, had reduced the number of agents available for enforcement, but not for long. After some newspaper reports linked marijuana smoking with crime, Anslinger adopted this new cause and began writing, speaking, testifying, and making films depicting the evils of marijuana. This effort succeeded in bringing public attention to the fight his bureau was waging against drugs and resulted in the 1937 passage of the Marijuana Tax Act. Marijuana came under the same type of legal control as cocaine and the opiates, in that one was supposed to register and pay a tax to legally import, buy, or sell marijuana. From 1937 until 1970, marijuana was referred to in federal laws as a narcotic.

World War II caused a decrease in the importation of both legal and illegal drugs. With the end of the war and the resumption of easy international travel, the illegal drug trade resumed and increased every year, despite the 1951 Boggs amendment to the Harrison Act, which established mandatory minimum sentences for drug offenses. Testimony before a subcommittee of the Senate Judiciary Committee in 1955 included the statement that inducing drug dependence in U.S. citizens was one of the ways Communist China planned to demoralize the United States. Remember that this was the height of the so-called McCarthy era, during which a mere hint by Senator Joseph McCarthy that someone associated with "known Communists" was enough to ruin that person's career. One interesting bit of history from that time was revealed years later. Anslinger and Hoover were aware that McCarthy, in addition to his widely known alcohol abuse, was dependent on morphine. Anslinger arranged for McCarthy to obtain a regular supply of his drug from a Washington, D.C., pharmacy without interference from narcotics officers.[5] With both crime and communism to combat, Congress passed the 1956 Narcotic Drug Control Act, with the toughest penalties yet. Under this law, any offense except first-offense possession had to result in a jail term, and no suspension, probation, or parole was allowed. Anyone caught selling heroin to a person younger than 18 could receive the death penalty. Anslinger commented on that particular provision by saying, "I'd like to throw the switch myself on drug peddlers who sell their poisons to minors."[12]

Drug Abuse Control Amendments of 1965

The early 1960s saw not only an increase in illegal drug use but also a shift in the type of drugs being used illegally. The trend was for the new drug users to be better educated and to emphasize drugs that alter mood and consciousness, such as amphetamines, barbiturates, and hallucinogens. Some hospitals in large cities reported that up to 15 percent of their emergency room calls involved individuals with adverse reactions to these drugs. Although amphetamines and barbiturates were legal prescription drugs, it was felt that they should be under the same types of controls as opioids, cocaine, and marijuana. The 1965 Drug Abuse Control amendments referred to these as dangerous drugs and included hallucinogens, such as LSD. The Bureau of Narcotics became the Bureau of Narcotics and Dangerous Drugs. Thus, the 1960s saw a number of major changes for this agency. Anslinger had retired, the bureau had new classes of drugs to control, and it was facing widespread disregard of the drug laws by large numbers of young people who were not all members of the underprivileged and criminal classes.

Comprehensive Drug Abuse Prevention and Control Act of 1970

The Comprehensive Drug Abuse Prevention and Control Act of 1970, usually referred to as the *Controlled Substances Act,* replaced or updated all previous laws concerned with both the narcotic and dangerous drugs. The law, still in effect, specifically states that the drugs controlled by the act are under federal jurisdiction regardless of involvement in interstate commerce. The law did not eliminate state regulations; it just made clear that federal enforcement and prosecution are possible in any illegal activity involving controlled drugs.

Prevention and Treatment The Controlled Substances Act dealt with the prevention and treatment of drug abuse by appropriating funds to expand the role of community mental health centers and Public Health Service hospitals in the treatment of those who misuse drugs. It authorized the development of educational material and drug education workshops for professional workers and in public schools.

Control Issues Resolved The control aspects of the Controlled Substances Act were the most debated portions, and several basic philosophical, ethical, and legal issues were resolved by the law. First, this was a law to control drugs directly rather than through taxes. Enforcement authority was moved from the Treasury Department to the new Drug Enforcement

Mind/Body Connection

Looking for More Humane Policies

If California is setting a trend, as it often does in fashion, entertainment, and politics, the United States may be having a change of heart in how it deals with drug dependence. In the November 7, 2000, election, more than 60 percent of California voters approved Proposition 36, requiring judges to sentence nonviolent first-time drug users to treatment instead of jail time.

It appears that Californians are prepared to give up "tough on crime" and "zero tolerance" policies for drug regulations they regard as more humane. Interestingly, the proposition was vigorously opposed by California law enforcement officials, many politicians in both parties, and the state's most influential newspapers, both conservative and liberal.

Opponents argue that giving a "free pass" to even first-time offenders will lead to more drug use, distribution, and crime. They say there's nothing in the proposition to encourage users to succeed in treatment.

Californians who favor the measure don't think the war on drugs is working. They prefer to see more money spent on treatment. Proposition 36 calls for the state Department of Alcohol and Drugs to spend $120 million a year on treatment.

In the 2001–2002 fiscal year, more than 30,000 offenders received treatment under this system, and over half said this was their first treatment opportunity. The increased funding produced a 50 percent increase in treatment capacity in California. In the next few years, further studies will determine the long-term success of these treatment clients in avoiding rearrest.

In May 2004, the California Supreme Court ruled that alcohol offenders (driving under the influence) could not use Proposition 36 to escape jail. The logic: It is simply too dangerous to allow people with a history of driving while intoxicated to be out of jail and on the highways.

Administration (**DEA**) in the Department of Justice. A second major issue was the separation of enforcement of the law from the scientific evaluation of the drugs considered for control. The attorney general is responsible for the administration of the control aspects of the law, but the secretary of the Department of Health and Human Services makes a binding recommendation about which drugs are to be controlled. This separation of enforcement from scientific and medical decisions about what should be controlled was, in theory, a major victory for those arguing for a rational drug law. In practice, the DEA usually develops the arguments for controlling a substance, and the Secretary of Health and Human Services is often under political pressure to make a positive recommendation for control.

Schedules The Controlled Substances Act begins by excluding "distilled spirits, wine, malt beverages, or tobacco." The logical reason for their exclusion is that they already had specific tax provisions separate from the substances being considered here. No doubt another reason was the political influence of the tobacco and liquor industries, which always strive to distinguish their "legal" products from other drugs such as heroin and marijuana. The law established five schedules of drugs that must be updated and published regularly. Table 3.1 summarizes the characteristics of drugs in each of the five schedules and gives a few examples. Perhaps the most important distinction is between Schedule I and the others: Schedules II through V consist primarily of prescription drugs that are further controlled by these regulations, whereas the substances in Schedule I by definition "have no medical use" and are therefore

DEA: Drug Enforcement Administration, a branch of the Department of Justice.

Table 3.1
Summary of Controlled Substance Schedules

Schedule	Criteria	Examples
Schedule I	a. High potential for abuse b. No currently acceptable medical use in treatment in the United States c. Lack of accepted safety for use under medical supervision.	Heroin Marijuana MDMA (Ecstasy)
Schedule II	a. High potential for abuse b. Currently accepted medical use c. Abuse may lead to severe psychological or physical dependence.	Morphine Cocaine Methamphetamine
Schedule III	a. Potential for abuse less than I and II b. Currently accepted medical use c. Abuse may lead to moderate physical dependence or high psychological dependence.	Anabolic steroids Most barbiturates Dronabinol
Schedule IV	a. Low potential for abuse relative to III b. Currently accepted medical use c. Abuse may lead to limited physical or psychological dependence relative to III.	Alprazolam (Xanax) Barbital Chloral hydrate Fenfluramine
Schedule V	a. Low potential for abuse relative to IV b. Currently accepted medical use c. Abuse may lead to limited physical or psychological dependence relative to IV.	Mixtures having small amounts of codeine or opium

not available by prescription. Notice that cocaine is on Schedule II and marijuana, which has no federally recognized medical uses, is on Schedule I.

Penalties for Possession The penalties for simply possessing a drug are more lenient than before and do not depend on the schedule. Therefore, an individual is guilty of the same crime whether he or she has a Valium tablet prescribed for another person or a bag of heroin. A first offense of illegal possession of a controlled drug or "distributing a small amount of marijuana for no remuneration" can be punished by up to one year's imprisonment and/or a fine of $1,000 to $5,000. In lieu of this, the court can place the individual on probation for up to a year. If there is no violation of the conditions of probation, the charge is dismissed and the conviction is "erased," except that a nonpublic record of the action is kept to prevent a person from being a "first offender" more than once.

Penalties for Selling The penalties for illegally making or selling controlled substances were not too complicated when the law passed in 1970, and the maximum first-offense penalty for distributing a Schedule I or II "narcotic" drug was 15 years and $25,000. In 1986, the penalties became much more complex, depending on the individual drug and the amount sold. Mandatory minimum penalties were again introduced, as they had been in the 1950s. First-offense sale of a large amount of heroin, cocaine, or several other drugs can, if the sale results in death or serious bodily injury, result in a life sentence and a fine of $4 million. First-offense sale of a small amount of marijuana can result in imprisonment for up to five years and a fine of up to $250,000. No parole is allowed.[13]

These 1986 amendments were passed at a time of maximum concerns about a "new" type of drug, crack cocaine (see Chapter 6). Because of this, the law established much lower quantities for crack cocaine to trigger the larger, dealer-level, penalties, and this has resulted in a large proportion of crack cocaine arrests meeting this lower minimum, and in turn triggering longer prison sentences.

One important feature of the 1986 law was the establishment of *mandatory minimum* sentences. This provision prevents a judge from considering such things as the defendant's character, work history, and so on, and requires that prison terms of 5 years or 10 years be imposed, depending on the offense. This provision has helped contribute to the huge growth in prison populations, and it has sometimes led to the paroling of other offenders to make space for the drug offenders who are subject to the mandatory sentencing provisions.

Omnibus Drug Act The 1988 Omnibus Drug Act made some interesting additions and adjustments to the Controlled Substances Act.[14] Components of this new law included the registration of airplanes, money laundering, firearms sales to felons, and chemicals used to manufacture drugs. One part allowed for the death penalty for anyone who murdered someone or orders the killing of someone in conjunction with a drug-related felony. A 1994 modification extends the death penalty to so-called drug kingpins, leaders of large-scale drug production and distribution organizations. Major sections of the 1988 law funded treatment and education programs. The most noteworthy change was a toughening of approaches toward drug users, aimed at reducing the *demand* for drugs (as opposed to putting all federal efforts into reducing the *supply* of drugs). Before this law, there were few penalties and little interest in convicting users for possessing small (personal-use) amounts of controlled substances. Under the new law, these are some of the unpleasant possibilities if convicted of possession:

- A civil fine of up to $10,000
- Forfeiture of the car, boat, or plane conveying the substance

- Loss of all federal benefits, including student loans and grants, for up to one year after the first offense and up to five years after a second offense.

The 1988 law also removes from public housing the entire family of anyone who engages in criminal activity, including drug-related activity, on or near public-housing premises.

Drug Precursors The Controlled Substances Act provides that the attorney general may include on the schedules any "immediate precursor" of a controlled substance. An immediate precursor would be the raw material that could be made in one step into the controlled substance. In addition, in 1988 Congress passed the Chemical Diversion and Trafficking Act, which allows the DEA to monitor chemicals that are not necessarily precursors, but are required for the illegal manufacturing of drugs (such as the acetic anhydride used in making heroin). One issue of current concern is that several over-the-counter drugs, such as ephedrine and pseudoephedrine (see Chapter 12) can be converted into methamphetamine. Some states have passed laws prohibiting unlicensed sales of large quantities of these otherwise legal products, but the manufacturers of legitimate medicines have opposed tighter federal controls.

Drug Paraphernalia In the mid-1970s, a small industry developed around the sale of legal items that were in some way related to the use of drugs. Sales of cigarette papers grew, whereas sales of loose cigarette tobacco declined, implying that something besides tobacco was being rolled up and smoked. Water pipes and "bongs" (pipes for concentrating marijuana smoke) were big items, as were "roach clips," sifters, and scales. These were mostly sold in places referred to as head shops, which sold legal items but catered to the drug-using subculture. Later, cocaine-related paraphernalia (mirrors, spoons, razor blades) appeared, and then small torches and glass pipes associated

Drugs in Depth

Americans in Prison

Fueled largely by the increases in drug-law arrests, the number of people held in state and local prisons in the United States has reached record levels. From the 1920s through the mid-1970s, about 1 person was in prison for every 1,000 people in the U.S. population. There were peaks and valleys, with the highest peak in 1939 (the end of the Depression) at 1.39 per 1,000 population. From 1974 to 1985, the rate doubled, from 1 to 2 per 1,000. By 2004, the imprisonment rate had more than doubled again to 4.9 per 1,000 population. Almost 5 million were on probation or parole, also record numbers and proportions.[19] The United States now has a greater proportion of its own citizens in prisons than does any other country.

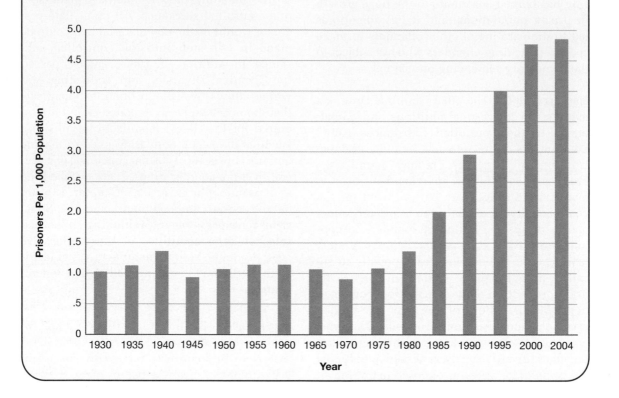

with heating and inhaling the vapors from crack cocaine, methamphetamine, or heroin. Several states began to pass laws regulating these items, and the 1988 revision of the Controlled Substances Act prohibited sales of drug **paraphernalia.**

How do you make an ordinary product, such as an alligator clip, mirror, or torch, illegal?

According to Congress, the legality is based on its intended use. Among the factors that may be considered are information provided with the item or in advertising about the item, how the item is displayed, and whether the person selling it is also a legitimate supplier of like or related items (e.g., an alligator clip sold at a store that also sells other electronic supplies).

The Internet has become a major marketing tool for drug paraphernalia, and in 2003 the DEA announced 50 arrests on paraphernalia charges resulting from "Operation Headhunter" and "Operation Pipe Dreams," displaying such items as a pipe concealed inside a felt-tip marker. These arrests resulted in the disappearance of 11 Web sites specializing in such products.[15]

Office of National Drug Control Policy To better co-ordinate all these federal efforts, the 1988 Omnibus Drug Act established the cabinet-level position of Director of National Drug Control Policy (commonly referred to as a "drug czar"). This individual is ordered by the legislation to prepare a national drug-control strategy and an annual consolidated drug-control budget for all federal agencies involved, to advise the National Security Council, and to report directly to the president. The Office of National Drug Control Policy was reauthorized and given additional authority in 1998.

State and Local Regulations

It is impossible to describe here all of the varied drug laws in the 50 states. Most states and many local communities had laws regulating sales of drugs before the federal government got into the act in 1906. Aspects of those old laws might still be in effect in some areas. Regarding the legal sales of prescription and over-the-counter drugs, there is considerable uniformity across the states, but some details do differ. For example, in some states licensed physician's assistants or psychologists are allowed to prescribe many types of medication, and in a few states pharmacists are now allowed to prescribe a few types of drugs that had previously required prescription by a physician or dentist.

After the passage of the federal 1970 Controlled Substance Act, states began to adopt the *Uniform Controlled Substances Act,* a model state law recommended by the DEA. The majority of states have adopted the same five schedules as in the federal law, but six states

have a different breakdown of schedules (four, six, or seven categories), and three states have a completely different method of categorizing illicit drugs that is not based on "schedules." Although the basic scheduling is similar in most states, there are large differences in the penalties. For example, possession of a small amount of cocaine can result in a maximum prison sentence ranging from less than one year up to 15 years, depending on the state.[16]

Violations of illicit drug laws may lead either to federal charges or to state charges, and this is important because federal mandatory minimum laws often mean much longer sentences than if the individual is convicted under most state laws. The greatest discrepancy between state and federal laws is in the 11 states that provide for some form of legal access to marijuana for medicinal purposes (see Chapter 15). There are several current instances of individuals being charged under federal law for conduct that is specifically protected by their state laws, and this conflict between jurisdictions seems to be increasing.

Federal Support for Drug Screening

Military and Federal Employees

It wasn't until the 1970s that relatively inexpensive screening tests were invented that could detect a variety of abused substances or their metabolites in urine. The Navy, followed by the other armed forces, was the first to use random urine screening on a large scale. Soon to follow were tests of people in various high-risk or high-profile positions, oil-field workers, air traffic controllers, and professional athletes. In 1986, President Reagan first declared that random urine tests should be performed on all federal employees in "sensitive" jobs. He also

paraphernalia (pare a fer *nail* ya): equipment used in conjunction with any activity.

Taking Sides

Prescription Marijuana?

The Controlled Substances Act lists substances under Schedules II through V based on their abuse potential. However, all substances with "no medical use" fall under Schedule I. The active ingredient in marijuana, delta-9-tetrahydrocannabinol (**THC**), has recently caused some classification headaches for the DEA. THC does now have a medical use—treating the nausea caused by cancer chemotherapy agents. Since 1986, under the generic name dronabinol, THC has been legally marketed as a prescription drug. The DEA's response to this has been to reschedule dronabinol *when dissolved in sesame oil and sealed in gelatin capsules,* as a Schedule III controlled substance. Any other preparation of THC is still Schedule I, as is marijuana itself. Marijuana is also being prescribed to some people for the treatment of glaucoma, and the government is even providing "official" marijuana cigarettes for this purpose. Marijuana has also been reported to provide some relief to multiple sclerosis patients. But marijuana cigarettes are not a generally available prescription drug. These prescriptions have been available only to about a dozen people under a "compassionate use" investigation of a new drug application. In 1992, the FDA stopped issuing new compassionate-use approvals for marijuana (see Chapter 15).

Since 1996, several states have passed citizen referenda allowing marijuana to be used for medical purposes. Because there are no legal sources of marijuana and because the federal government has actively opposed such measures, the referenda have not resulted in the widespread availability of legal medical marijuana in those states.

Visit the Online Learning Center for links to more information on medical marijuana.

urged companies doing business with the federal government to begin testing their employees if they had not already done so. Since then, most federal employees have become subject to at least the possibility of being asked to provide a random urine sample, although the actual frequency of such tests is rare in most federal occupations. In 2004, new guidelines were proposed that would allow federal agencies to use urine, sweat, saliva, or hair samples to test for drugs.[17]

Transportation Workers

In 1987, a collision between an Amtrak passenger train and a Conrail freight train near Baltimore, Maryland, resulted in the deaths of 16 people. The wreck was quickly blamed on drug use, because the Conrail engineer and brakeman had shared a marijuana joint shortly before the tragedy. The cause of the wreck can be argued: A warning indicator on the Conrail train was malfunctioning and the backup alarm had been silenced because it was too irritating. The marijuana use could be viewed as a symptom of a general "goofing off" attitude by the Conrail crew, who violated a number of safety procedures. Nevertheless, politicians and the news media saw this tragedy as a clear indication of the need for random drug testing. Transportation workers are now subject to surprise drug testing, and in 1992 this was expanded to interstate truck drivers. In addition, drug testing has become a common feature for prisoners, both while incarcerated and during probation or parole.

Private Employers

Private corporations, which may require drug testing before hiring a new employee and/or may periodically test employees, have two main reasons for adopting drug tests, but the bottom line in both cases is money. First, companies believe that drug-free workers will be absent less often, will make fewer mistakes, will have better safety records, and will produce more and better work. Second, by spending relatively few dollars on drug tests, they protect the company against negligence suits that might follow if a "stoned" employee hurt someone on the job or turned out a dangerously faulty product. Companies doing business with the federal government have an additional reason—they are required to have drug-free workplace rules in place.

Public Schools

Giving urine tests to high school students seems like a great idea to some parents and community officials. After all, society is most concerned about substance use and abuse among the young, and the belief is that if the students know testing is a possibility they will be less likely to use drugs in the first place. But many believe that such testing is an invasion of privacy, and to test students randomly without some evidence pointing to likely drug use by a particular individual destroys any sense of trust that might exist between the students and school officials. With all the concern about drug use by athletes, the first groups of students to be widely subjected to urine screening for drugs were those involved in team sports. In a legal challenge to this process, the U.S. Supreme Court in 1995 allowed drug testing of athletes, based partly on evidence from the school in question that its student athletes were at a higher than average risk for drug use. Many schools since have adopted policies that include other extracurricular activities, and a 2002 Supreme Court case upheld those programs as well. Students are required by law to attend school up to a certain age, but extracurricular activities are voluntary. Therefore, if a student wants to participate in football, band, or the debate team, he or she might have to agree to random urine screening as a condition of being part of that activity. In 2003, President George W. Bush endorsed random testing of all students, and has provided federal funds to assist school districts in implementing these programs. However, as of 2006, the legality of random, suspicionless urine testing for all public school students has not been established at the federal level.

Testing Methods

With so many pilots, truck drivers, federal workers, hospital employees, athletes, and students being tested, selling testing kits and lab analysis has become a big business. New methods for analyzing urine have combined with test kits for saliva, hair, and other kinds of samples to make a wide variety of choices available. What are the apparent advantages and disadvantages of the different kinds of samples? Urine testing, the standard method for many years, is said to be capable of detecting most kinds of drugs for up to three days, as the drug, or its metabolites, clears the system. But that depends on how much drug was used and on the detection levels set for triggering a positive result: The higher the amount required for a positive result, the shorter the detection time. Setting a lower threshold for a positive result makes the test sensitive for a longer period of time, but it increases the rate of false-positive results. The metabolites of marijuana can be detected in the urine for five days or more. For someone who has been smoking a lot of marijuana for a long time, urine tests may be positive for a couple of weeks or more after the last dose. One concern employers and officials have about urine testing is whether a drug user can beat the test, by substituting a clean urine sample from someone else, by diluting the urine, or by ingesting something that will mask the presence of a drug in the urine. With proper monitoring to avoid sample substitution or dilution, concerns about masking drug use do not seem to be too great. Although Internet companies offer a variety of products that are supposed to help users mask the drug in their urine, the value of these products is questionable.

Hair testing has increased in popularity in recent years. Hair samples are theoretically capable of detecting drug use (based on levels incorporated into the hair as it grows) for up to

THC: delta-9-tetrahydrocannabinol, the most important psychoactive chemical in marijuana.

90 days. That means that an occasional drug user will be more easily detected with this sampling method. Also, it seems less invasive to ask to take a small sample of someone's hair than to have someone watch while they "pee into the cup." Saliva samples also seem less invasive and are easy to collect. However, they detect only fairly recent drug use, up to one day, in most cases.

Although many employers treat the results of these tests as absolute proof of drug use, there should always be concern about their accuracy. In a large workplace testing program, proper procedure would call for splitting the sample and keeping half for a retest, and submitting known positive samples and known negative samples to the lab along with the actual samples. The biggest practical concern is the rate of false-positive results (the test results indicate drug use when the person did not actually take the drug being tested for. False positives can be caused by legal drugs, or even by some foods (e.g., poppy seeds contain trace amounts of opioids). If 4 percent of those tested actually use methamphetamine, and the test has a 5 percent false-positive rate, then a positive result is more likely due to an error than to actual drug use! The FDA has worked with reputable testing companies over the years to improve the accuracy of their tests, but none is perfect.

Most test kits look for marijuana, opioids, amphetamines, and cocaine. Often one or two other drugs (PCP, MDMA, benzodiazepines) may be included. These drug screens can detect the presence of a drug or its metabolite, but they can't tell anything about the state of impairment of the individual at the time of the test. One person might show up at work Monday morning with a terrible hangover from drinking the night before, be unable to perform well on the job, and pass the drug screen easily. Another person might have smoked marijuana on Friday night, have experienced no effect for the past day and a half, and yet fail the screen. The general idea of the screens seems to be to discourage illicit drug use more than to detect impairment of performance.

The Impact of Drug Enforcement

We can examine the current efforts at enforcing federal drug laws by asking ourselves three questions. What exactly are we doing to enforce drug laws? How much is it costing? How effective is it? Although there had been previous "wars" on illicit drugs, the largest efforts to date began in 1982, when President Reagan announced a renewed and reorganized effort to combat drug trafficking and organized crime. For the first time, all federal agencies were to become involved, including the DEA; FBI; IRS; Alcohol, Tobacco and Firearms Bureau; Immigration and Naturalization; U.S. Marshals; U.S. Customs Service; and Coast Guard. In some regions, Defense Department tracking and pursuit services were added. This last item had been legalized earlier in the Reagan administration and had signaled an important change in the role of the military. The idea of using our military forces to police our population had long been abhorrent to Americans, who had insisted that most police powers remain at the state and local levels. Because of the success of smugglers, we now use Air Force radar and aircraft and Navy patrol boats to detect and track aircraft and boats that might be bringing in drugs. These efforts have continued to expand, and in 2004 the Defense Department spent about $500 million on drug interdiction activities.

Budget

A good overview of the widespread federal efforts can be obtained from the National Drug Control Strategy review and budget prepared each year by the White House. The total requested for the 2003 budget was a record $19.2 billion. The White House restructured the drug-control budget request for 2004, removing the costs associated with agencies that did not have a *primary* drug control objective (e.g., drug control costs in the U.S. Postal Service, most items from the Defense Department, and most notably, about $3 billion of federal prison costs associated with imprisoning drug offenders). The restructured drug-control budget dropped from $19.2 billion to $11.4 billion (the actual budgets didn't change, just how they were counted). The proposed fiscal year 2007 budget was for $12.7 billion. No matter how you measure it, that's a big increase from less than $1 billion in 1980.[18]

International Programs

International efforts aimed at reducing the drug supply include State Department programs that provide aid to individual countries to help them with narcotics controls, usually working in conjunction with the DEA. The DEA has agents in more than 40 countries, and they assist the local authorities in eradicating drug crops, locating and destroying illicit laboratories, and interfering with the transportation of drugs out of those countries. The State Department's Bureau of International Narcotics and Law Enforcement Affairs budget for 2004 was over $1 billion. This included direct aid tied to drug enforcement and loans and support for South American countries to develop alternative crops and industries. The United States is providing increased military aid in the form of helicopters, "defensive" weapons, uniforms, and other supplies to be used in combating drug trafficking, plus military training to both army and police agencies. This program is supposedly restricted to countries that do not engage in a "consistent pattern of gross violations" of human rights.

Other Federal Agencies

Efforts within the United States have broadened to include activities related to drug trafficking. The Customs Service and IRS were joined in 1990 by a Financial Crimes Enforcement Network to combat the "laundering" of drug profits through banks and other investments. The Federal Aviation Administration is involved not only in the urine testing of pilots and other airline workers but also in keeping track of private aircraft and small airports that

might be used for transporting drug shipments. The Department of Agriculture, Bureau of Land Management, and National Park Service are on the lookout for marijuana crops planted on federal land.

Other Costs

Besides the direct budget for drug-control strategies, there are other costs, only some of which can be measured in dollars. We are paying to house a large number of prisoners: more than 230,000 drug-law violators in state prisons and local jails and more than 60,000 in federal prisons.[19] Add to this the cost of thousands on probation or parole, plus various forms of juvenile detention. We should also add the cost of crimes committed to purchase drugs at black-market prices and the incalculable price of placing so many of our state and local police, DEA, FBI, and other federal agents in danger of losing their lives to combat the drug trade, as some have done. A price that has been paid by many law enforcement agencies over the years is the corruption that is ever-present in drug enforcement. Because it is necessary for undercover officers to work closely with and to gain the trust of drug dealers, they must sometimes ignore an offense in hopes of gaining information about more and bigger deals in the future. They may even accept small favors from a drug dealer, and some officers have found it necessary to use drugs along with the suspects. Under those circumstances, and given the large amounts of money available to some drug dealers and the small salaries paid to most law officers, the possibility of accepting too large a gift and ignoring too many offenses is always there, and there might be no obvious "line" between doing one's job and becoming slightly corrupted.[20]

There are costs on the international level, too. The United States and most other countries work together to restrict international drug trafficking. However, there have been times when our interest in controlling illicit drug supplies is in conflict with national security issues and one or the other must be compromised. One recent example would be in Afghanistan, which has a long tradition of growing opium poppies and in recent years has been the primary source for the illicit heroin that reaches Europe. In May 2001, the U.S. Secretary of State announced a $43 million grant to the Taliban government as a reward for the crackdown on opium production in Afghanistan. Four months later, we were at war against the Taliban government following the attack on the World Trade Center. While we cannot say that U.S. drug-aid money was used to directly fund terrorist activities, the funds likely were spent in part to equip the Taliban army. Since the fall of the Taliban and the institution of a government friendly to the United States, opium production has increased. For now, it is probably more important for us to support that fragile government than to put too much pressure on the government to destroy one of the country's main sources of income.

Our drug-control efforts sometimes find us providing help to repressive governments, and it has been charged that some of our previous drug-control aid has been used for political repression, in both Latin America and Southeast Asia. To the extent that narcotics-control efforts place additional strains on our foreign policy needs in the East, the Caribbean, and Latin America, this also represents a significant cost to our country.

Finally, there is an unquantifiable cost in the loss of individual freedom that is inevitable when the government acquires increased powers. Because of increased drug-control efforts, American citizens are subjected to on-the-job urine tests; searches of homes, land, and vehicles; computer-coded passports that record each international visit; and increased government access to financial records. Americans are also threatened with seizure of their property and loss of federal benefits.

Given this effort and these costs, are our drug-enforcement efforts effective? Do they work? Critics have pointed out that, despite

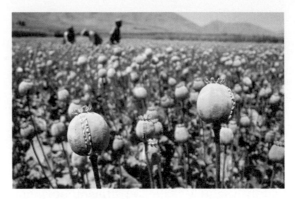

Afghanistan is the largest producer of opium poppies in the world.

escalating expenditures, more agents, and an increasing variety of supply-reduction efforts, the supplies of cocaine, heroin, and marijuana have not dried up; in fact, they may have increased. Although there have been record-breaking seizures of cocaine year after year, the price of cocaine has actually decreased since the 1980s. The U.S. government made a decision in 1924 to make heroin completely unavailable to users in this country, and after more than 75 years we can say only that it has been consistent in its failure to accomplish that goal. Our effort to eradicate illegal coca fields in South America was described as a failure by the General Accounting Office, which pointed out that many more new acres are being planted in coca each year than are being destroyed by our program.[21] An economic analysis indicated that, even if eradication and interdiction efforts could result in massive disruption of a particular source country's production, it would take only about two years for the market to push production back to the previous levels.[22]

Illicit drug trade remains a big business, even if most people avoid these substances. The United Nations estimates that only about 3 percent of the world's population uses illicit drugs, yet that amounts to 185 million people, and a total market value in the hundreds of billions of dollars.[23]

Effectiveness of Control

The laws do work at one level. It is estimated that 10 to 15 percent of the illegal drug supply is seized by federal agencies each year. In 2002, for example, U.S. government agencies seized 200 tons of cocaine, 2.5 tons of heroin, and more than 1,000 tons of cannabis.[18] These efforts have made it difficult and expensive to do business as a major importer. Evidence that supply is restricted can be found in the high prices charged on the streets. The price is many times more than the cost of the drug itself if sold legally. It is likely that the high cost influences the amount taken by some of these users. Local efforts make a difference, too. Small pushers forced to work out of sight are less able to contact purchasers, and both the buyer and the seller have a higher risk of being hurt or cheated in the transaction. This not only raises the cost of doing business, but it also probably deters some people from trying the drugs. For example, suppose you were curious about heroin and wanted to try some. You might take some money to a rough part of a larger city. If you are "lucky" enough to find a dealer, he might not be the sort of person you would trust. The transaction could take place in a nonpublic place, and if you were robbed, beaten, or just sold some worthless junk, you wouldn't be in a position to call the police!

Summary

- In the early 1900s, two federal laws were passed on which our current drug regulations are based.
- The 1906 Pure Food and Drugs Act, requiring accurate labeling, was amended in 1938 to require safety testing and in 1962 to require testing for effectiveness.
- A company wishing to market a new drug must first test it on animals, then file an IND. After a three-phase sequence of human testing, the company can file the NDA.
- The 1914 Harrison Act regulated the sale of opioids and cocaine.
- The Harrison Act was a tax law, but after 1919 it was enforced as a prohibition against providing drugs to dependent users.
- As drugs became more scarce and their price rose on the illicit market, the illicit market grew. Harsher penalties and increased enforcement efforts, which were the primary strategies of Commissioner of Narcotics Harry Anslinger, failed to reverse the trend.
- Marijuana was added to the list of controlled drugs in 1937, and in 1965 amphetamines, barbiturates, and hallucinogens were also brought under federal control.
- The Controlled Substances Act of 1970 first provided for direct federal regulation of drugs, not through the pretense of taxing their sale.
- Controlled substances are placed on one of five schedules, depending on medical use and dependence potential.
- Amendments in 1988 were aimed at increasing pressure on users, as well as on criminal organizations and money laundering.
- Federal support for drug screening began in the military and has since spread to other federal agencies, nonfederal transportation workers, and many private employers.
- Current federal enforcement efforts involve thousands of federal employees and include activities in other countries, along our borders, and within the United States.
- Most states have adopted some version of the DEA's recommended Uniform Controlled Substances Act.
- Federal, state, and local enforcement limits the supply of drugs and keeps their prices high, but the high prices attract more smugglers and dealers. It will never be possible to eliminate illicit drugs.

Review Questions

1. What four kinds of habit-forming drug use at the start of the 20th century caused social reactions leading to the passage of federal drug laws?

2. What were the two fundamental pieces of federal drug legislation passed in 1906 and 1914?

3. In about what year did it first become necessary for drug companies to demonstrate to the FDA that new drugs were effective for their intended use?

4. What three phases of clinical drug testing are required before a new drug application can be approved?

5. What historic piece of federal legislation did the most to shape our overall approach to the control of habit-forming drugs in the United States?

6. Who was Harry Anslinger, and what was his role in marijuana regulation?

7. What is the important difference between a Schedule I and a Schedule II controlled substance?

8. What are drug paraphernalia laws, and why have they been subject to court challenges?

9. What are the limitations of urine screening versus hair sample analysis?

10. Approximately how much is the United States spending per year on federal drug-control efforts?

References

1. Adams, S. H. "The Great American Fraud," *Collier's*, six segments, October 1905 to February 1906.
2. Kane, H. H. *Opium-smoking in America and China*. New York: G.P. Putnam's Sons, 1882.
3. Musto, D. F. *The American Disease: Origins of Narcotic Control*, 3rd ed. New York: University Press, 1999.
4. *Congressional Record* 40, no. 102 (Part 1), (December 4, 1905 to January 12, 1906).
5. Latimer, D., & J. Goldberg. *Flowers in the Blood: The Story of Opium*, New York: Franklin Watts, 1981.
6. Terry, C. E., & M. Pellens. *The Opium Problem*. New York: Bureau of Social Hygiene, 1928.
7. Courtwright, D. T. *Dark Paradise: Opiate Addiction in America Before 1940*. Cambridge, MA: Harvard University Press, 1982.
8. Young, J. H. *The Medical Messiahs: A Social History of Health Quackery in Twentieth-Century America*. Princeton, NJ: Princeton University Press, 1967.
9. *Industry profile 2004,* Washington, DC: Pharmaceutical Manufacturers Association, 2004.
10. Rados, C. "Ephedra Ban: No Shortage of Reasons." *FDA Consumer* 38 (2004).
11. Schmeckebier, L. F. *The Bureau of Prohibition*. Service Monograph No. 57, Institute for Government Research, 1929, Brookings Institute. Cited in R. King: "Narcotic Drug Laws and Enforcement Policies," *Law & Contemporary Problems* 22, no. 122 (1957).
12. *U.S. News & World Report* 41, no. 22 (1956).
13. *Controlled Substances Act as amended, with addenda.* Available from Drug Enforcement Administration, Washington, DC: U.S. Department of Justice.
14. Lawrence, C. "In Its Last Act, Congress Clears Anti-drug Bill," *Congressional Quarterly*, October 29, 1988, pp. 3145–51.
15. Drug Enforcement Administration. *Operations Pipe Dreams and Headhunter Put Illegal Drug Paraphernalia Sellers Out of Business*. Press release, February 24, 2003.
16. Impacteen Illicit Drug Team. *Illicit Drug Policies: Selected Laws from the 50 States*. Berrien Springs, MI: Andrews University, 2002.
17. Substance Abuse and Mental Health Services Administration. Proposed revisions to mandatory guidelines for federal workplace drug testing programs. *Federal Register* 69 (2004), pp. 19673–74.
18. Office of National Drug Control Policy. *National Drug Control Strategy FY2007 Budget Summary*. Washington, DC: The White House, 2006.
19. Beck, A. J. *Prisoners in 2004*. Bureau of Justice Statistics Bulletin, Washington, DC: U.S. Department of Justice, October 2005.
20. Gray, J. P. *Why Our Drug Laws Have Failed and What We Can Do About It*. Philadelphia: Temple University Press, 2001.
21. Culhane, C. "U.S. Fails in South American Drug War," *The U.S. Journal of Drug and Alcohol Dependence*, January 1989.
22. Riley, K. J. *Snow Job?* New Brunswick, NJ: Transaction, 1996.
23. United Nations Office on Drugs and Crime. *World Drug Report 2004*. Vienna: United Nations Publication E.04.XI.16, 2004.

Check Yourself

Consider the Consequences

One of the most damaging things that can occur to a person who is working toward a successful and happy life is to get into trouble with the law and establish a criminal record. Many people have done a few things for which they could have been apprehended and either fined or arrested. Perhaps it is only parking illegally for a few minutes or driving a few miles over the speed limit. We all know that we don't get caught every time, or perhaps even most of the time, so there's a certain amount of luck involved. Also, of course, the seriousness of the violation and the ensuing consequence vary quite a bit. Most people can afford to pay a parking fine and it is not considered much of a blemish on their record. However, some people seem to tempt fate more often than others and for higher stakes—in other words, they do things that risk more serious consequences, and they do those things more often. Many of the risks that people take involve the use of substances, and often it seems they have not considered the possible consequences. Create a confidential list of such behaviors in the following table. For each behavior, indicate whether you have done it; whether you have been caught; if so, what the consequences were; and how the consequence or lack of consequence influenced your likelihood of doing it again.

	Behavior			
	Underage smoking	**Underage drinking**	**Driving while intoxicated**	**Using an illegal drug**
Done it? (Y/N)				
Caught? (Y/N)				
Consequence				
Influence on future behavior: +, −, none				

How Drugs Work

A drug is nothing but a chemical substance until it comes into contact with a living organism. In fact, that's what defines the difference between drugs and other chemicals—drugs have specific effects on living tissue.

4   The Nervous System
How do drugs interact with the brain and the nervous system?

5   The Actions of Drugs
How do drugs move in the body, and what are the general principles of drug action?

Because this book is about psychoactive drugs, the tissue we're most interested in is the brain. We want to understand how psychoactive drugs interact with brain tissue to produce effects on behavior, thoughts, and emotions.

Obviously, we don't put drugs directly into our brains; usually we swallow them, inhale them, or inject them. In Section Two, we will find out how the drugs we take get to the brain, and what effects they might have on the other tissues of the body.

4

The Nervous System

Objectives

After you have studied this chapter, you should be able to:

- **Understand how psychoactive drugs alter communication among the billions of cells in the human brain.**

- **Explain the concept of homeostasis.**

- **Know the general properties of glia and neurons.**

- **Understand and describe the action potential.**

- **Describe the roles of the sympathetic and parasympathetic branches of the autonomic nervous system and associated neurotransmitters.**

- **Be able to associate important neurotransmitters with key brain structures and chemical pathways, and describe the major functions of the neurotransmitters.**

- **Describe the life cycle of a neurotransmitter molecule.**

- **Understand the importance of receptor subtypes in determining the action of a neurotransmitter at a particular site in the brain.**

- **Give examples of a drug that alters neurotransmitter availability and of a drug that interacts with neurotransmitter receptors.**

Drugs are psychoactive, for the most part, because they alter ongoing functions in the brain. To understand how drugs influence behavior and psychological processes, it is necessary to have some knowledge of the normal functioning of the brain and other parts of the nervous system and then to see how drugs can alter those normal functions. The goal of this chapter is not to turn you into a neuroscientist. Rather, the goal is to introduce basic concepts and terminology that will help you understand the effects of psychoactive drugs on the brain and on behavior. The knowledge acquired in this chapter should also make you aware of the limitations of applying an exclusively biological approach to the study of psychoactive drug effects.

Chemical Messengers

Since the first multicellular organisms oozed about in their primordial tidal pools, some form of cell-to-cell communication has been necessary to ensure the organism's survival.

Online Learning Center Resources

www.mhhe.com/ksir12e

Visit our Online Learning Center (OLC) for access to these study aids and additional resources.

- Learning objectives
- Glossary flashcards
- Web activities and links
- Self-scoring chapter quiz
- Audio chapter summaries

Those first organisms probably needed to coordinate only a few functions, such as getting nutrients into the system, distributing them to all of the cells, and then eliminating wastes. At that level of organization, perhaps one cell excreting a chemical that could act on neighboring cells was all that was necessary. As more complex organisms evolved with multicellular systems for sensation, movement, reproduction, and temperature regulation, the sophistication of these communication mechanisms increased markedly. It became necessary for many types of communication to go on simultaneously and over greater distances.

Although those early organisms were at the mercy of the sea environment in which they lived, we carry our own seawater-like cellular environment around with us and must maintain that internal environment within certain limits. This process is known as **homeostasis.** This word can be loosely translated as "staying the same," and it describes the fact that many biological factors are maintained at or near certain levels. For example, most of the biochemical reactions basic to the maintenance of life are temperature-dependent, in that these reactions occur optimally at temperatures near 37°C (98.6°F). Because we cannot live at temperatures too much above or below this level, our bodies have many mechanisms to either raise or lower temperature: perspiring, shivering, altering blood flow to the skin, and others. Similar homeostatic mechanisms regulate the

acidity, water content, and sodium content of the blood; glucose concentrations; and other physical and chemical factors that are important for biological functioning.

Components of the Nervous System

Although we often speak of the nervous system, several communication and control systems utilize nerve cells and chemical signals. Before discussing distinctions between these systems, we will describe the major components common to the entire nervous system.

Glia

The nervous system is comprised of two types of cells: (1) glial cells, often referred to as *glia,* and (2) nerve cells, often referred to as *neurons.* The nervous system has 10 to 50 times more glia than neurons. Unlike neurons, glia do not have information-processing capabilities (i.e., they do not communicate with other cells). However, these cells provide several important functions that help to ensure the survival of the organism, including providing firmness and structure to the brain, getting nutrients into the system, eliminating waste, and forming myelin. The myelin produced by glia is wrapped around the axons (described below) of some neurons to form a myelin sheath, which increases the information-processing speed of these neurons. The movement disorder multiple sclerosis occurs as a result of a lack of or damage to the myelin wrappings on some neurons.

Another important function of glia is to create the *blood-brain barrier,* a barrier between the blood and the fluid that surrounds

> **homeostasis:** maintenance of an environment of body functions within a certain range (e.g., temperature, blood pressure).

Drugs in the Media

Coverage of Chemical Causes of Mental Disorders

In the past, you may have been only vaguely aware of the number of reports that appear in newspapers and magazines indicating a possible breakthrough in some type of mental illness. Because new brain chemicals are being discovered rapidly, it is inevitable that our hopes are high for new understanding and possible new treatments for schizophrenia, depression, and other major disorders. Chapter 8 presents the current state of our understanding and treatment of these problems.

In this chapter you will learn some things about the brain and its neurotransmitters, and you will probably pay more attention to such media coverage in the future. If you want to test and sharpen your knowledge of this important approach to understanding human behavior, go to your college library and look back over the last year's issues of current magazines, such as *Time, Newsweek,* or *Scientific American,* or search their Web sites. The publications will probably include quite a few brief news reports relating chemicals to mental disorders.

In current fashion and daily news, you'll find reports about researchers testing new drugs to cure alcohol, nicotine, opioid, and cocaine dependence.

Just in the past few years, two medications have received FDA approval: one to treat alcohol dependence (acamprosate) and one to treat opioid dependence (buprenorphine). These and other substance abuse treatment medications are discussed in Chapter 18.

Covering health issues such as these follows careful consideration by magazine and newspaper editors. When surveyed, readers report that they want more coverage of health issues, and publishers have complied. Fortunately, the health editors and writers for major publications generally do an excellent job of preparing news reports. Most try to consult health researchers who are experts in their fields. But be inquisitive about whether there is more than one perspective on stories that interest you. You can find and read the original sources mentioned in the article. Many of these original sources are available at your library or on the Internet. If you have additional questions, ask professors, physicians, or someone else who is knowledgeable in the field. Magazines and newspapers can provide an ideal first step in your quest for new information concerning your health.

neurons. This *semipermeable* (allowing some, but not all, chemicals to pass) structure protects the brain from potentially toxic chemicals circulating in the blood. For a drug to be psychoactive, its molecules must be capable of passing through the blood-brain barrier. In general, only small *lipophilic* (the extent to which chemicals can be dissolved in oils and fats) molecules enter the brain. This feature has important implications for the effects of some psychoactive drugs on the brain, and ultimately on behavior. Take, for example, the opioid drugs morphine and heroin. Heroin (also known as diacetylmorphine) was synthesized by adding two acetyl groups to the morphine chemical. This slight modification of the morphine structure made the new chemical more lipophilic, thereby facilitating its movement across the blood-brain barrier and into the brain. As a result, heroin has a more rapid onset of effects and is about three times as potent as morphine.

Neurons

Neurons are the elements of the nervous system that are responsible for analyzing and transmitting information. In other words, everything that we see and understand as behavior is dependent upon the functioning of these cells. The nervous system contains more than 100 billion neurons, and each can influence or be influenced by hundreds of other neurons. Before we can understand how

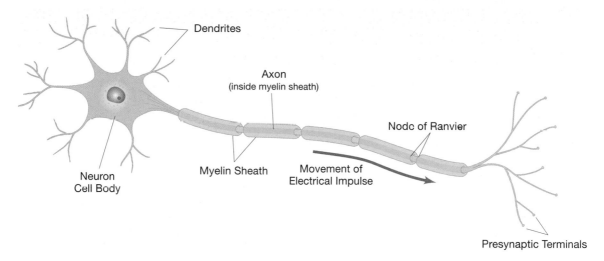

Figure 4.1 Every Neuron Has Four Regions: Cell Body, Dendrites, Axon, and Presynaptic Terminals

neurons produce behavior, we must first become familiar with a few basic facts about neurons. While neurons come in a variety of shapes and sizes, they all have four morphologically defined regions: cell body, dendrites, axon, and presynaptic terminals (see Figure 4.1). Each of these regions contributes to the neuron's ability to communicate with other neurons, and psychoactive drugs can exert effects within each of these regions. The *cell body* contains the nucleus and other substances that sustain the neuron. The drug MPP$^+$, a potential by-product of illicitly produced opioids, causes neuronal death via inhibition of certain components located in the cell body. The *dendrites* are treelike features extending from the cell body and contain within their membranes the specialized structures (**receptors**) that recognize and respond to specific chemicals' signals. (Some receptors are also found on cell regions other than dendrites.) Stimulation of specific receptors by psychoactive drugs can either activate or inhibit the neuron depending upon the type of receptor (see below). The long, slender *axon* extends from the cell body and is responsible for conducting the electrical signal

(action potential, described below) to the presynaptic terminals. Finally, the presynaptic terminals are the bulbous structures located at the end of the axon, where chemical messengers (neurotransmitters, discussed below) are stored in small, round packages, called *vesicles.*

Neurotransmission

Have you ever wondered how local anesthetics like those dentists use can block the perception of pain? After a brief discussion of the basic concepts of neurotransmission, you will be better able to understand how local anesthetics and other drugs work to alter perception, mood, and behavior.

Action Potential

The production of even simple behavioral acts requires complex interactions between the

receptors: recognition mechanisms that respond to specific chemical signals.

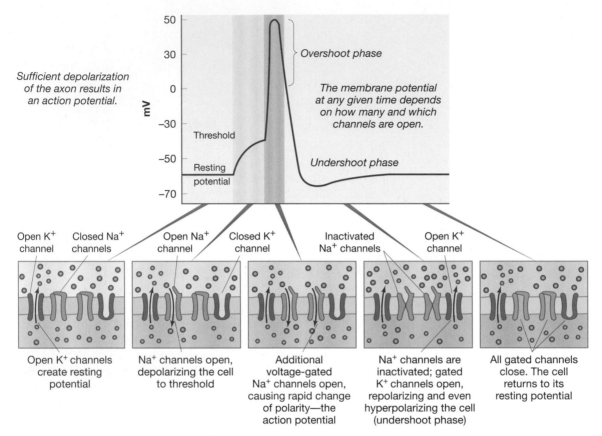

Figure 4.2 Action Potential

SOURCE: Reproduced from Rosenzweig, Leiman, & Breedlove, 1999, with permission from the publishers.

individual's environment and nerve cells. Here we focus on only one element of this complex interaction—the communication between neurons. Such communication is accomplished through a highly specialized, precise, and rapid method. An essential process for neuronal communication is the *action potential,* a brief electrical signal transmitted along a neuron's axon (see Figure 4.2). This electrical signal initiates a chain of events that allows one neuron to communicate with another through the release of **neurotransmitters.** The action potential occurs as a result of opening ion channels (pores in the membrane) that allow electrically charged particles (ions) access to the inside of the cell. This change moves the

cell's membrane away from its *resting potential* (about −65 mV) to a more positively charged voltage. When the cell membrane is at rest, there is an uneven distribution of ions between the inside and outside of the cell. Specifically, there are more potassium (K^+) ions and negatively charged organic anions on the inside of the cell, while there are more sodium (Na^+) and chloride (Cl^-) ions on the outside of the cell. This uneven distribution of ions is the source of the negative resting potential across the membrane.

The action potential occurs when Na^+ ion channels open, allowing Na^+ ions to move across the membrane, which rapidly shifts the membrane potential in a positive direction (depolarization). Adjacent areas on the neuron become sequentially depolarized, allowing propagation of the "all-or-none" action potential signal. The action potential is referred to as all or none because, once initiated, it will travel without decrement to the end of the axon in the presynaptic terminals where it will ultimately cause the release of a neurotransmitter.

Suppose we selectively blocked Na^+ channels? What would be the effect? Selective blockade of Na^+ channels prevents the action potential and thus disrupts communication between neurons. Selective blockade of Na^+ channels is the mechanism through which drugs such as cocaine and chlorprocaine reduce pain. Although many local anesthetics are used in clinical practice today, cocaine was the first. More recent local anesthetics are simple modifications of the cocaine molecule. In the case of chlorprocaine, the chemical alteration of the cocaine structure yielded a compound that does not readily cross the blood-brain barrier (i.e., it does not produce cocainelike psychoactive effects).

The Nervous System(s)

Somatic Nervous System

The nerve cells that are on the "front lines," interacting with the external environment, are referred to as the *somatic* system. These peripheral nerves carry sensory information into the central nervous system and carry motor (movement) information back out. The cranial nerves that relate to vision, hearing, taste, smell, chewing, and movements of the tongue and face are included, as are spinal nerves carrying information from the skin and joints and controlling movements of the arms and legs. We think of this system as serving voluntary actions. For example, a decision to move your leg results in activity in large cells in the motor cortex of your brain. These cells have long axons, which extend down to the spinal motor neurons. These neurons also have long axons, which are bundled together to form

nerves, which travel out directly to the muscles. The neurotransmitter at neuromuscular junctions in the somatic system is acetylcholine, which acts on receptors that excite the muscle.

Autonomic Nervous System

Your body's internal environment is monitored and controlled by the **autonomic** nervous system, (ANS), which regulates the visceral, or involuntary, functions of the body, such as heart rate and blood pressure. Many psychoactive drugs have simultaneous effects in the brain and on the ANS. The ANS is also where chemical neurotransmission was first studied. If the vagus nerve in a frog is electrically stimulated, its heart slows. If the fluid surrounding that heart is then withdrawn and placed around a second frog's heart, it, too, will slow. This is an indication that electrical activity in the vagus nerve causes a chemical to be released onto the frog's heart muscle. When Otto von Loewi first demonstrated this phenomenon in 1921, he named the unknown chemical "vagusstoffe." We now know that this is acetylcholine, the same chemical that stimulates muscle contraction in our arms and legs. Because a different type of receptor is found in the heart, acetylcholine inhibits heart muscle contraction.

The ANS is divided into **sympathetic** and **parasympathetic** branches. The inhibition of heart rate by the vagus nerve is an example of

---

neurotransmitters: chemical messengers released from neurons and having brief, local effects.

autonomic: the part of the nervous system that controls "involuntary" functions, such as heart rate.

sympathetic: the branch of the autonomic system involved in flight or fight reactions.

parasympathetic: the branch of the autonomic system that stimulates digestion, slows the heart, and has other effects associated with a relaxed physiological state.

Table 4.1
Sympathetic and Parasympathetic Effects on Selected Structures

Structure or function	Sympathetic reaction	Parasympathetic reaction
Pupil	Dilation	Constriction
Heart rate	Increase	Decrease
Breathing rate	Fast and shallow	Slow and deep
Stomach and intestinal glands	Inhibition	Activation
Stomach and intestinal wall	No motility	Motility
Sweat glands	Secretion	No effect
Skin blood vessels	Constriction	Dilation
Bronchi	Relaxation	Constriction

---

the parasympathetic branch; acetylcholine is the neurotransmitter at the end organ. In the sympathetic branch, norepinephrine is the neurotransmitter at the end organ. Table 4.1 gives examples of parasympathetic and sympathetic influences on various systems. Note that often, but not always, the two systems oppose each other.

Because the sympathetic system is interconnected, it tends to act more as a unit, to open the bronchi, reduce blood supply to the skin, increase the heart rate, and reduce stomach motility. This has been called the "fight or flight" response and is elicited in many emotion-arousing circumstances in humans and other animals. Amphetamines, because they have a chemical structure that resembles norepinephrine, stimulate these functions in addition to their effects on the brain. Those drugs that activate the sympathetic branch are referred to as sympathomimetic drugs.

Central Nervous System

The **central nervous system (CNS)** consists of the brain and spinal cord. These two structures form a central mass of nervous tissue, with sensory nerves coming in and motor nerves going out. This is where most of the integration of information, learning and memory, and coordination of activity occur.

The Brain

Major Structures

Knowing about a few of the major brain structures makes it easier to understand some of the effects of psychoactive drugs. When looking at the brain of most mammals, and especially of a human, much of what one can see consists of *cerebral cortex,* a layer of tissue that covers the top and sides of the upper parts of the brain (see Figure 4.3). Some areas of the cortex are known to be involved in processing visual information; other areas are involved in processing auditory or somatosensory information. Relatively smaller cortical areas are involved in the control of muscles (motor cortex), and large areas are referred to as association areas. Higher mental processes, such as reasoning and language, occur in the cerebral cortex. In an alert, awake individual, arousal mechanisms keep the cerebral cortex active. When a person is asleep or under the influence of sedating drugs, the cerebral cortex is much less active, whereas other parts of the brain might be equally active whether a person is awake or asleep.

Underneath the cerebral cortex on each side of the brain and hidden from external view are the basal ganglia, comprised of three primary components: the caudate nucleus, the putamen, and the globus pallidus. The **basal**

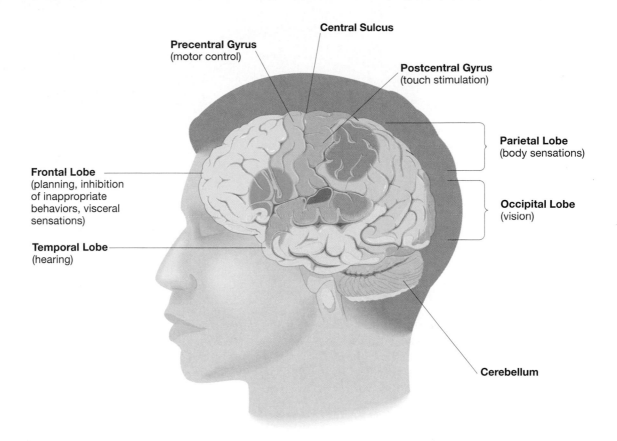

Figure 4.3   Major Subdivisions of the Human Cerebral Cortex

ganglia are important for the maintenance of proper muscle tone. For example, when you are standing still in a relaxed posture, your leg muscles are not totally relaxed. If they were, you would fall down in a slump. Instead, you remain standing, partly because of a certain level of muscular tension, or tone, that is maintained by the output of the basal ganglia. Too much output from these structures results in muscular rigidity in the arms, legs, and facial muscles. This can occur as a side effect of some psychoactive drugs that act on the basal ganglia, or it can occur if the basal ganglia are damaged by **Parkinson's disease.**

The *hypothalamus* is a small structure near the base of the brain just above the pituitary gland (see Figure 4.4). The hypothalamus

is an important link between the brain and the hormonal output of the pituitary and is thus involved in feeding, drinking, temperature regulation, and sexual behavior.

The *limbic system* consists of a number of connected structures that are involved in emotion, memory for location, and level of physical activity. Together with the hypothalamus, the limbic system involves important mechanisms

central nervous system (CNS): brain and spinal cord.
basal ganglia: subcortical brain structures controlling muscle tone.
Parkinson's disease: degenerative neurological disease involving damage to dopamine neurons.

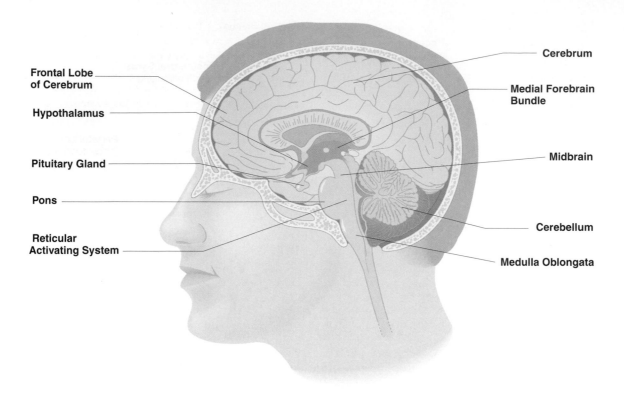

Frontal Lobe of Cerebrum

Hypothalamus

Pituitary Gland

Pons

Reticular Activating System

Cerebrum

Medial Forebrain Bundle

Midbrain

Cerebellum

Medulla Oblongata

Figure 4.4   Cross Section of the Brain: Major Structures

for behavioral control at a more primitive level than that of the cerebral cortex.

The midbrain, pons, and medulla are the parts of the brain stem that connect the larger structures of the brain to the spinal cord. Within these brain-stem structures are many groups of cell bodies (nuclei) that play important roles in sensory and motor reflexes as well as coordinated control of complex movements. Within these brain-stem structures also lie the nuclei that contain most of the cell bodies for the neurons that produce and release the neurotransmitters dopamine, norepinephrine, and serotonin. Virtually all of the brain's supply of these important neurotransmitters is produced by a relatively small number of neurons (a few thousand for each neurotransmitter) located in these brain-stem regions.

The lower *brain stem* contains a couple of small areas of major importance. One area is

the vomiting center. Often when the brain detects foreign substances in the blood, such as alcohol, this center is activated, and vomiting results. It is easy to see the survival value of such a system to animals, including humans, that have it. Another brain-stem center regulates the rate of breathing. This respiratory center can be suppressed by various drugs, resulting in respiratory depression, which can lead to death.

These structures and their functions have been understood in general terms for many years. Knowledge about such things comes partly from people who have suffered accidental brain damage and partly from experiments using animals. These basic structures exist in mammals other than humans, with functions and connections that are basically the same, so it is possible to learn a great deal about human brain function from animal experiments.

Chemical Pathways

Although many neurotransmitters have been identified, we are concerned mostly with those few we believe to be associated with the actions of the psychoactive drugs we are studying. Those neurotransmitters include dopamine, acetylcholine, norepinephrine, serotonin, GABA, glutamate, and the endorphins.

Dopamine In some cases, groups of cells in a particular brain region contain a particular neurotransmitter chemical, and axons from these cells are found grouped together and terminating in another brain region. We think of many psychoactive drug actions in terms of a drug's effect on one of these chemical pathways. For example, we know that cells in the basal ganglia receive input from **dopamine** fibers that arise in the substantia nigra in the midbrain, course together past the hypothalamus, and end in the corpus striatum (part of the basal ganglia). This **nigrostriatal dopamine pathway** is what is damaged in Parkinson's disease and what is affected by the tranquilizers that produce muscular rigidity as a side effect (see Chapter 8).

Another important dopamine pathway also begins in the midbrain but projects to the *nucleus accumbens,* which is part of the limbic system. This **mesolimbic dopamine pathway** has been proposed to play a role in some types of psychotic behavior. Also, the most widely studied neurochemical theory of drug dependence is based on the idea that all reinforcing drugs, from alcohol to nicotine, stimulate dopamine neurons in the mesolimbic system. The mesolimbic system is proposed to be the main component responsible for the "reward" properties of electrical stimulation of the midbrain or limbic system. Thus, according to this theory, drugs lead to dependence because they stimulate this reward system, which is responsible for telling the rest of the brain "that's good—do that again."[1] Recent data, however, suggest this view may be overly simplistic. For example, it has been reported that although initial depletion of dopamine in the nucleus accumbens produces profound reductions in cocaine self-administration by rodents, cocaine self-administration recovers long before restoration of nucleus accumbens dopamine levels.[2] This suggests that other brain mechanisms play a role in the maintenance of cocaine self-administration.

Acetylcholine Pathways containing **acetylcholine** arise from cell bodies in the *nucleus basalis* in the lower part of the basal ganglia and project to much of the cerebral cortex. In patients who have died from *Alzheimer's disease,* these cells are damaged and the cortex contains much less acetylcholine than normal. This degenerative disease affects millions of older Americans, causing personality changes, memory loss, and widespread mental deterioration. Because this link with an acetylcholine pathway was only recently discovered, much research activity is currently focused on finding chemical means to diagnose and treat Alzheimer's disease. Acetylcholine has also been one of the main neurotransmitters studied with regard to the initiation of REM (rapid eye movement) sleep, during which most dreaming occurs.

Norepinephrine Pathways arising from the *locus ceruleus* in the brain stem have numerous branches and project both up and down in the brain, releasing **norepinephrine** and influencing

---

dopamine (*dope* ah meen): neurotransmitter found in the basal ganglia and other regions.

nigrostriatal dopamine pathway: one of two major dopamine pathways; damaged in Parkinson's disease.

mesolimbic dopamine pathway (meh zo *lim* bick): one of two major dopamine pathways; may be involved in psychotic reactions and in drug dependence.

acetylcholine (eh see till *co* leen): neurotransmitter found in the parasympathetic branch in the cerebral cortex.

norepinephrine: neurotransmitter that may be important for regulating waking and appetite.

the level of arousal and attentiveness. It is perhaps through these pathways that stimulant drugs induce wakefulness. Norepinephrine pathways play an important role in the initiation of food intake, although other transmitter systems are also involved in the very important and therefore very complex processes of controlling energy balance and body weight.

Serotonin Serotonin-containing pathways arise from the brain-stem *raphe nuclei* and have projections both upward into the brain and downward into the spinal cord. Animal research has suggested one or more roles for serotonin in the complex control of food intake and the regulation of body weight. The diet drug Sibutramine causes its weight-reducing effects in humans by blocking the reuptake of serotonin and norepinephrine.[3] Research on aggressiveness and impulsivity has also focused on serotonin. In studies with monkeys, low levels of serotonin metabolites in the blood have been associated with impulsive aggression, as well as with excessive alcohol consumption. And recent studies indicate a role for serotonin system dysfunction in individuals who commit suicide.[4] The success of selective serotonin reuptake inhibitors, such as Prozac, in treating major depressive disorder has also led to theories linking serotonin to depression. In all these cases (food intake and weight control, aggression and impulsivity, alcohol use, and depression), environmental influences play important roles, and other drugs that work through different neurotransmitter systems can also influence these behaviors. Therefore, it is much too simple to attribute these behavioral problems to low serotonin levels alone. Hallucinogenic drugs, such as LSD, are believed to work by influencing serotonin pathways.

GABA (γ-amino butyric acid) GABA is one neurotransmitter that is *not* neatly organized into discrete pathways or bundles. GABA is found in most areas of the CNS and exerts generalized inhibitory functions. Many sedative drugs act by enhancing GABA inhibition (see Chapter 7). The club drug GHB (γ-hydroxy butyrate) is a close chemical relative of the neurotransmitter GABA. Interfering with normal GABA inhibition, such as with the GABA-receptor-blocking drug strychnine, can lead to seizures resembling those seen in epilepsy.

Glutamate Glutamate, like GABA, is found throughout the brain, and nearly all neurons have receptors that are activated by it. But, unlike GABA, stimulation of receptors that respond to glutamate makes cells more excitable. Thus, glutamate is often referred to as the brain's major excitatory neurotransmitter. In recent years, increasing amounts of evidence indicate that specific glutamate pathways may be important for the expression of some psychoactive drug effects. For instance, abnormal glutamate transmission, caused by prolonged chronic cocaine use, in the projection from the prefrontal cortex to the nucleus accumbens has been hypothesized to mediate relapse to cocaine use following a period of drug abstinence.[5] The overwhelming majority of the data supporting this hypothesis have been obtained using laboratory animals. Therefore, clinical implications of altered glutamate transmission in substance abuse remain unclear.

Endorphins Several chemicals in the brain produce effects similar to those of morphine and other drugs derived from opium. The term **endorphin** was coined in reference to endogenous (coming from within) morphinelike substances. These substances are known to play a role in pain relief, but they are found in several places in the brain as well as circulating in the blood, and not all their functions are known. Although it is tempting to theorize about the role of endorphins in drug abuse or dependence, the actual evidence linking dependence to endorphins has not been strong, and other neurotransmitter systems (particularly dopamine and serotonin systems) have also been shown to influence behaviors related to dependence.

Drugs and the Brain

A drug is carried to the brain by the blood supply. How does each drug know where to go once it gets into the brain? The answer is that the drug goes everywhere. But, because the drug molecules of LSD, for example, have their effect by acting on serotonin systems, LSD affects the brain systems that depend on serotonin. The LSD molecules that reach other types of receptors appear to have no particular effect. Because the brain is so well supplied with blood, an equilibrium develops quickly for most drugs, so that the drug's concentration in the brain is about equal to that in the blood and the number of molecules leaving the blood is equal to the number leaving the brain to enter the blood. As the drug is removed from the blood (by the liver or kidneys) and the concentration in the blood decreases, more molecules leave the brain than enter it, and the brain levels begin to decrease.

We are currently able to explain the mechanisms by which many psychoactive drugs act on the brain. In most of these cases, the drug has its effects because the molecular structure of the drug is similar to the molecular structure of one of the neurotransmitter chemicals. Because of this structural similarity, the drug molecules interact with one or more of the stages in the life cycle of that neurotransmitter chemical. We can therefore understand some of the ways drugs act on the brain by looking at the life cycle of a typical neurotransmitter molecule.

Life Cycle of a Neurotransmitter

Neurotransmitter molecules are made inside the cell from which they are to be released. If they were just floating around everywhere in the brain, then the release of a tiny amount from a nerve ending wouldn't have much information value. However, the raw materials, or **precursors,** from which the neurotransmitter will be made are found circulating in the blood supply and generally in the brain. A cell that is going to make a particular neurotransmitter needs to bring in the right precursor in a greater concentration than exists outside the cell, so machinery is built into that cell's membrane for active **uptake** of the precursor. In this process, the cell expends energy to bring the precursor into the cell, even though the concentration inside the cell is already higher than that outside the cell. Obviously, this uptake mechanism must be selective and must recognize the precursor molecules as they float by. Many of the precursors are amino acids that are derived from proteins in the diet, and these amino acids are used in the body for many things besides making neurotransmitters. In the example diagram of the life cycle of the neurotransmitter norepinephrine in Figure 4.5, the amino acid tyrosine is recognized by the norepinephrine neuron, which expends energy to take it in.

After the precursor molecule has been taken up into the neuron, it must be changed, through one or more chemical reactions, into the neurotransmitter molecule. This process is called **synthesis.** At each step in the synthetic chemical reactions, the reactions are helped along by **enzymes.** These enzymes are

---

serotonin (sehr o *tone* in): neurotransmitter found in the raphe nuclei; may be important for impulsivity, depression.

GABA: inhibitory neurotransmitter found in most regions of the brain.

glutamate: excitatory neurotransmitter found in most regions of the brain.

endorphin: opiate-like chemical that occurs naturally in the brain of humans and other animals.

precursors: chemicals that are acted on by enzymes to form neurotransmitters.

uptake: energy-requiring mechanism by which selected molecules are taken into cells.

synthesis: the forming of a neurotransmitter by the action of enzymes on precursors.

enzyme: large molecule that assists in either the synthesis or metabolism of another molecule.

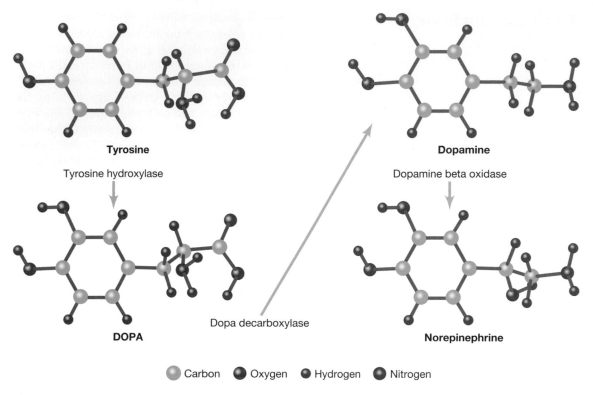

Tyrosine

Tyrosine hydroxylase

DOPA

Dopa decarboxylase

Dopamine

Dopamine beta oxidase

Norepinephrine

Carbon   Oxygen   Hydrogen   Nitrogen

Figure 4.5   Neurons Use Enzymes to Synthesize the Neurotransmitters Dopamine and Norepinephrine

themselves large molecules that recognize the precursor molecule, attach to it briefly, and hold it in such a way as to make the synthetic chemical reaction occur. Figure 4.6 provides a schematic representation of such a synthetic enzyme in action. In our example diagram of the life cycle of the catecholamine neurotransmitters dopamine and norepinephrine (Figure 4.5), the precursor tyrosine is acted on first by one enzyme to make DOPA and then by another enzyme to make dopamine. In dopamine cells the process stops there, but in our norepinephrine neuron, a third enzyme is present to change dopamine into norepinephrine.

After the neurotransmitter molecules have been synthesized, they are stored in small *vesicles* near the terminal from which they will be released. This storage process also calls for

recognizing the transmitter molecules and concentrating them inside the vesicles.

The arrival of the action potential in the presynaptic terminals causes calcium (Ca^{2+}) channels to open. Calcium enters the cells and assists the movement of the small vesicles filled with neurotransmitter toward the presynaptic terminal membrane so that the neurotransmitter is released into the *synapse,* the small space between two neurons. To give some idea of scale, the synaptic space is less than 1/10,000th of an inch across. Several thousand neurotransmitter molecules are released at once, and it takes only microseconds for these molecules to diffuse across the synapse. Once neurotransmitters are released into the synapse, they may bind with receptors on the membrane of the next neuron, sometimes referred to as the postsynaptic cell

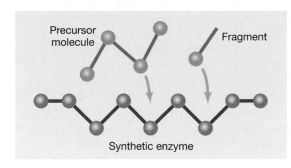

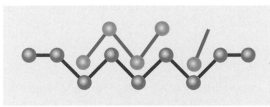

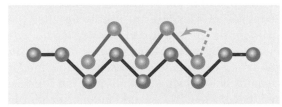

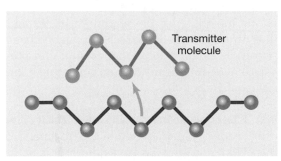

Figure 4.6 Schematic representation of the action of a synthetic enzyme. A precursor molecule and another chemical fragment both bind to the enzyme. The fragment has a tendency to connect with the precursor, but the connection is made much more likely because of the way the enzyme lines up the two parts. After the connection is made, the new transmitter molecule separates from the enzyme.

(see Figure 4.7). This receptor is the most important recognition site in the entire process, and it is one of the most important places for drugs to interact with the natural neurotrans-

mitter. With thousands of neurotransmitter molecules floating freely in the synapse, some will come near these receptors, bind to them briefly, then float away again. In the process of binding, the neurotransmitter distorts the receptor, so that a tiny passage is opened through the membrane, allowing ions to move through the membrane (Figure 4.7). As a result, the postsynaptic cell can either become more or less excitable, and thus more or less likely to initiate an action potential.

Whether the effect of a neurotransmitter is excitatory or inhibitory depends on the type of receptor. There are specific receptors for each neurotransmitter, and most neurotransmitters have more than one type of receptor in the brain. For example, the neurotransmitter GABA has at least three receptor subtypes—$GABA_A$, $GABA_B$, and $GABA_C$—and stimulation of all seem to make the cell less excitable. Therefore, GABA is often called an inhibitory neurotransmitter. Many of the sedativelike effects produced by drugs such as barbiturates and benzodiazepines are dependent upon their binding to the $GABA_A$ receptors. When $GABA_A$ receptors are stimulated, Cl^- channels open and Cl ions enter the cell; this process decreases the cell's ability to generate an action potential. Acetylcholine also acts at multiple receptors in the brain: muscarinic and nicotinic. At least five muscarinic receptor subtypes and at least 11 inicotinic receptor subtypes have been identified, and acetylcholine's action can be either excitatory or inhibitory, depending on the receptor stimulated.

Because signaling in the nervous system occurs at a high rate, once a signal has been sent in the form of neurotransmitter release, it is important to terminate that signal, so that the next signal can be transmitted. Thus, the thousands of neurotransmitter molecules released by a single action potential must be removed from the synapse. Two methods are used for this. The neurons that release the monoamine neurotransmitters serotonin, dopamine, and

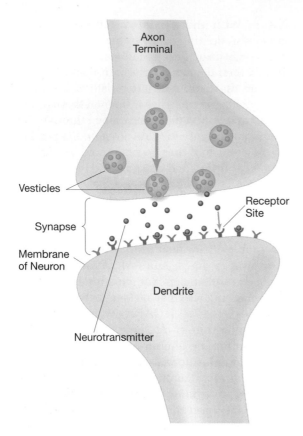

Figure 4.7 Schematic representation of the release of neurotransmitter molecules from synaptic vesicles in the axon terminal of one neuron and the passage of those molecules across across the synapse to receptors in the membrane of another neuron. A neurotransmitter molecule has bound to the center receptor and has distorted it so as to open a channel through the membrane of the second cell. This channel allows the flow of electrically charged ions through the membrane, thus altering the electrical charge on the membrane of the second cell.

cules are released into the synapse, some of them are being removed or metabolized and never get to bind to the receptors on the other neuron. All neurotransmitter molecules might be removed in less than one-hundredth of a second from the time they are released. In the case of our example neurotransmitter, norepinephrine, those molecules are rapidly taken back up into the neuron from which they were released. Once inside the neuron, the norepinephrine molecules are metabolized by an enzyme found in the cell.

Examples of Drug Actions

It is possible to divide the actions of drugs on neurotransmitter systems into two main types. Through actions on synthesis, storage, release, reuptake, or metabolism, drugs can alter the *availability of the neurotransmitter in the synapse.* Either the amount of transmitter in the synapse, when it is released, or how long it remains before being cleared from the synapse will be affected. The second main type of drug effect is *directly on the receptors.* A drug can mimic the action of the neurotransmitter and thus directly activate the receptor (an *agonistic* action), or it can occupy the receptor and prevent the neurotransmitter from activating it (an *antagonistic* action).

Drug Effects on Neurotransmitter Availability The drug L-dopa, which is used in the treatment of the CNS disorder Parkinson's disease, is actually the normal precursor for dopamine and is converted into dopamine by synthetic enzymes inside the neurons. This makes more dopamine available for release each time the neuron fires.

Perhaps one of the most interesting mechanisms is interference with the transporters that clear neurotransmitters, such as norepinephrine, serotonin, and dopamine, from the synapse by bringing them back into the neuron from which they were just released. Both the stimulant drug cocaine and most of the antidepressant drugs block one or more of these transporters

norepinephrine have specific **transporters** built into their terminals. The serotonin transporter recognizes serotonin molecules and brings them back into the releasing neuron, thus ending their interaction with serotonin receptors. The dopamine transporter and norepinephrine transporter are specific to their neurotransmitters, also. With other neurotransmitters, enzymes in the synapse **metabolize,** or break down, the molecules (see Figure 4.8). In either case, as soon as neurotransmitter mole-

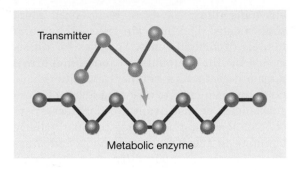

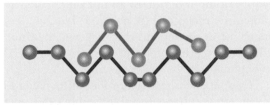

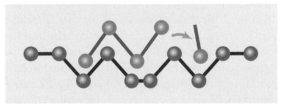

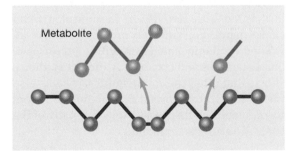

Figure 4.8 Schematic representation of the action of a metabolic enzyme. The transmitter molecule binds to the enzyme in such a way that the transmitter molecule is distorted and "pulled apart." The fragments then separate from the enzyme.

the neurotransmitter systems affected and the time course of the drug's action.

Drug Effects on Neurotransmitter Receptors One method by which a drug can influence a receptor is to mimic the action of the neurotransmitter molecules (act as a receptor agonist). For example, heroin mimics the action of endorphins at opioid receptors. Nicotine has effects very similar to the effects of the neurotransmitter acetylcholine at some types of cholinergic receptors (they are called *nicotinic* acetylcholine receptors for this reason).

When the neurotransmitter binds to its receptor, in the process of matching up the structure of the transmitter molecule with the structure of the receptor, the receptor has to bend or stretch slightly, thus opening a small pore in the membrane. Suppose a drug molecule matched up so well with the receptor that the receptor didn't have to bend or stretch during the binding process. That drug molecule would fit the receptor better than the natural neurotransmitter. However, because the receptor doesn't have to change, there would be no effect on the electrical activity of the cell. Such agents are called antagonists, or "blockers," because by occupying the site they prevent the normal neurotransmitters from having a postsynaptic effect. The antipsychotic (also called neuroleptic or major tranquilizer) drugs, such as haloperidol (Haldol), block receptors for dopamine. When we refer to *blocking receptors,* only enough drug is given to block some of the receptors some of the time, so the net effect is to modulate, or alter, the activity in an ongoing system. Generally, if enough drug were given to block most of the receptors most

and cause the normally released neurotransmitter to remain in the synapse longer than normal. One of the most exciting research areas in the neurosciences is the search for greater understanding of how altering these reuptake processes can produce either cocaine-like or antidepressant effects, depending perhaps on

transporter: mechanism in the nerve terminal membrane responsible for removing neurotransmitter molecules from the synapse by taking them back into the neuron.
metabolize: to break down or inactivate a neurotransmitter (or a drug) through enzymatic action.

of the time, the result would be highly toxic or even lethal.

What would happen if we tried to treat a psychotic patient who has Parkinson's disease with both L-dopa and haloperidol? The L-dopa is used to counteract damage to the dopamine systems in Parkinson's disease by making more dopamine available at the synapses. Haloperidol is used to control psychotic behavior, and it acts by blocking dopamine receptors. Thus, the drugs seem to have opposing actions. In fact, haloperidol often produces side effects that resemble Parkinson's disease, and L-dopa often produces hallucinations in its users. The two drugs are not used in the same patient because each tends to reduce the effectiveness of the other.

Chemical Theories of Behavior

Drugs that affect existing biochemical processes in the brain often affect behavior, and this has led to many attempts to explain normal (not drug-induced) variations in behavior in terms of changes in brain chemistry. For example, differences in personality between two people might be explained by a difference in the chemical makeup of their brains, or changes in an individual's reactions from one day to the next might be explained in terms of shifting tides of chemicals. The ancient Greek physician Hippocrates believed that behavior patterns reflected the relative balances of four *humors:* blood (hot and wet, resulting in a sanguine or passionate nature); phlegm (cold and wet, resulting in a phlegmatic or calm nature); yellow bile (hot and dry, resulting in a choleric, bilious, or bad-tempered nature); and black bile (cold and dry, resulting in a melancholic or gloomy nature). The Chinese made do with only two basic dispositions: *yin,* the moon, representing the cool, passive, "feminine" nature; and *yang,* the sun, representing the warm, active, "masculine" nature. Thus, any personality could be seen as a relative mixture of these two opposing forces. Unfortunately, most of the chemical-balance theories that have been proposed based on relative influences of differ-

ent transmitters have not really been more sophisticated than these yin-yang and humoral notions of ancient times. Searches for differences in the amounts of norepinephrine, dopamine, serotonin, or other transmitters have not found evidence to relate the levels of these substances to personality differences, psychopathology, or mood swings. It is particularly tempting to speculate that alcohol- and drug-dependent individuals differ from "normal" people in the function of an enzyme or neurotransmitter receptor, but, no single biochemical theory of drug dependence has yet obtained sufficient experimental support to be considered an explanation.

One biochemical theory that still seems to have merit continues to guide people's thinking about major alterations in moods, such as those seen in clinical depression. Drugs that interfere with the monoamines (norepinephrine, serotonin, and dopamine) are able to bring on a depressed mood, and drugs such as cocaine and amphetamines that stimulate activity in these monoamine systems produce a temporary mood elevation. Thus, the *monoamine theory of mood* is that too little activity in these systems can cause depression and too much can cause an excited or manic state (seen with high doses of amphetamines and cocaine). Although evidence shows that other neurotransmitter systems also play a role in the normal modulation of mood, the monoamine theory accounts for many of the basic drug effects on mood.

Brain Imaging Techniques

Two techniques were developed during the 1980s for obtaining chemical maps of the brains of living humans. These techniques offer exciting possibilities for furthering our understanding of brain chemistry, abnormal behavior, and drug effects.

One of the techniques is positron emission tomography (PET) (see Figure 4.9). In this technique, a radioactively labeled chemical is injected into the bloodstream, and a computerized scanning device then maps out the relative

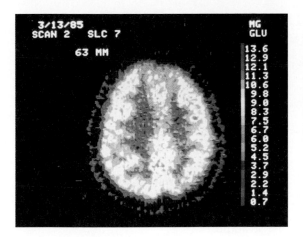

Figure 4.9   PET Scan

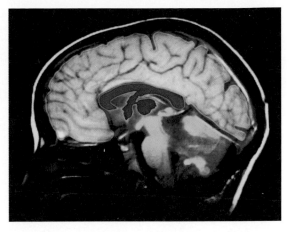

Figure 4.10   MRI Scan

amounts of the chemical in various brain regions. Because all neurons in the brain rely on blood glucose for their energy, a labeled form of glucose can be used to see which parts of the brain are most active, and these vary depending on what the person is doing. Similarly, blood flow to a particular brain region reflects the activity there, and labeled oxygen or other gases can map regional cerebral blood flow, which also changes depending on what the person is doing. More recently, labeled drugs that bind to dopamine, serotonin, or opiate receptors have been used, and it is therefore possible to see where the binding of those chemicals takes place in a living human brain. Our understanding of normal and abnormal brain function and of psychoactive drug effects will be advanced by these techniques over the next several years. Because these systems are very expensive to operate, they are found predominately in well-financed research hospitals.

Magnetic resonance imaging (MRI) is another brain imaging technique (see Figure 4.10). Rather than using radioactive labels, the technique relies on applying a strong magnetic field and then measuring the energy released by various molecules as the field is collapsed. The signals are complex, but with the aid of computers it is possible to detect certain chemical "fingerprints" in the signals.

This technique gives a high-resolution image and does not require the administration of expensive radiochemicals; because it can provide much information not attainable with simple X-ray studies, it has been rapidly adopted by the medical community. MRI systems have been installed in most major hospitals. A refinement of this technique (functional MRI), using higher-energy magnetic fields and more complex computational techniques, is beginning to be used to study apparent changes in metabolic activity in specific brain regions.

Summary

- Chemical signals in the body are important for maintaining homeostasis. The two types of chemical signals are hormones and neurotransmitters.

- Neurotransmitters act over brief time periods and very small distances because they are released into the synapse between neurons and are then rapidly cleared from the synapse.

- Receptors are specialized structures that recognize neurotransmitter molecules and, when activated, cause a change in the electrical activity of the neuron.

- The nervous system can be roughly divided into the central nervous system, the somatic system, and the autonomic system.

- The autonomic system, with its sympathetic and parasympathetic branches, is important because so many psychoactive drugs also have autonomic influences on heart rate, blood pressure, and so on.

- Specialized chemical pathways contain the important neurotransmitter dopamine, acetylcholine, norepinephrine, and serotonin.

- The nigrostriatal dopamine system is damaged in Parkinson's disease, leading to muscular rigidity and tremors.

- The mesolimbic dopamine system is thought by many to be a critical pathway for the dependence produced by many drugs.

- The neurotransmitter GABA is inhibitory and is found in most parts of the brain.

- The life cycle of a typical neurotransmitter chemical involves uptake of precursors, synthesis of the transmitter, storage in vesicles, release into the synapse, interaction with the receptor, reuptake into the releasing neuron, and metabolism by enzymes.

- Psychoactive drugs act either by altering the availability of a neurotransmitter at the synapse or by directly interacting with a neurotransmitter receptor.

Review Questions

1. What are some examples of homeostasis in the human body?
2. What are the similarities and differences between glia and neurons?
3. Describe the process of neurotransmitter release and receptor interaction.
4. Give some examples of the opposing actions of the sympathetic and parasympathetic branches of the autonomic nervous system. What is the neurotransmitter for each branch?
5. What is the function of the basal ganglia, and which neurotransmitter is involved?
6. What is the proposed role of the mesolimbic dopamine system in drug dependence?
7. Alzheimer's disease produces a loss of which neurotransmitter from which brain structure?
8. What neurotransmitter seems to have only inhibitory receptors?
9. After a neurotransmitter is synthesized, where is it stored while awaiting release?
10. What are the two main ways in which drugs can interact with neurotransmitter systems?
11. PET and MRI are two examples of what technology?

References

1. Koob, G.F., & M. LeMoal. "Drug Abuse: Hedonic Hemostatic Dysregulation." *Science* 278 (1997), pp. 52–58.
2. Sizemore, G.M., and others. "Time-Dependent Recovery from the Effects of 6-Hydroxydopamine Lesions of the Rat Nucleus Accumbens on Cocaine Self-administration and the Levels of Dopamine in Microdialysates." *Psychopharmacology* 171 (2004), pp. 413–20.
3. Ryan, D.H. "Clinical Use of Sibutramine." *Drugs Today* 40 (2004), pp. 41–54.
4. Lin, P.Y., & G. Tsai. "Association Between Serotonin Transporter Gene Promoter Polymorphism and Suicide: Results of a Meta-analysis." *Biological Psychiatry* 55 (2004), pp. 1023–30.
5. Kalivas, P.W. "Glutamate Systems in Cocaine Addiction." *Current Opinions in Pharmacology* 4 (2004), pp. 23–29.

Check Yourself

What's Your Body's Natural Cycle?

Can your behavior affect your brain chemistry? You bet! One of the more interesting aspects of brain biochemistry being studied is the daily changes in serotonin and other brain chemicals that follow a regular pattern, known as a circadian rhythm. The term *circadian* means "approximately daily" and reflects the fact that humans deprived of any information about time of day tend to follow a pattern of waking, sleeping, and eating that varies somewhat from day to day but usually averages out to a cycle just a bit more than 24 hours. Most people under normal circumstances report that they have certain peak times of the day when they feel most energetic and mentally sharper, and people are more likely to be hungry around their normal mealtimes and sleepy at their normal bedtimes. We also know that people whose jobs keep them on irregular schedules of sleeping and waking (repeated shift changes) and people who have recently flown across several time zones (jet lag) do not perform at their best. Also, most people who suffer from major depressive disorder show some disruption of normal patterns of sleeping, waking, and eating.

Thus, one thing you can do to help your brain chemistry maintain its natural cycles is to keep a fairly consistent schedule. Following is a checklist to help you:

1. On most days of the week, do you wake up at approximately the same time each day (within 30 minutes or so)? Yes No
2. Do you spend at least a few minutes outdoors in the morning every day? Even on a cloudy day, sunlight is usually brighter than most indoor lighting, and light is an important stimulus to your brain's circadian rhythms. Yes No
3. Do you eat breakfast every morning, at about the same time each day? Yes No
4. Do you get some physical exercise on most days, and is it usually at about the same time of day? Yes No
5. On most days of the week, do you usually go to sleep at about the same time each night? The timing of when you go to sleep is apparently somewhat less important than consistency in when you wake up. Yes No

If your own pattern is quite variable from day to day, try being more consistent and see if it helps you feel more energetic and able to focus your attention. If your pattern is fairly consistent from day to day, try to determine when you feel the most mentally alert, and see if you can schedule your most challenging mental activities close to that time of day.

5

The Actions of Drugs

Objectives

When you have finished this chapter, you should be able to:

- **Explain why plants produce so many of the chemicals we use as drugs.**

- **Distinguish between generic, brand, and chemical names for a drug.**

- **Understand and describe the typical effects of drugs in each of six categories.**

- **Understand the importance of placebo effects and the necessity of double-blind studies.**

- **Define and explain dose-response relationship, ED_{50}, LD_{50}, and therapeutic index.**

- **Explain why pharmacological potency is not synonymous with effectiveness.**

- **Explain how lipid solubility influences passage through the blood-brain barrier.**

- **Compare and contrast the most important routes of drug administration.**

- **Explain the potential influence of protein binding on interactions between different drugs.**

- **Describe ways psychoactive drugs interact with neurons to produce effects in the brain.**

- **Explain the role of homeostatic mechanisms in pharmacodynamic tolerance and withdrawal symptoms.**

Sources and Names of Drugs

Sources of Drugs

Most of the drugs in use 50 years ago originally came from plants. Even now, most of our drugs either come from plants or are chemically derived from plant substances. Why do the plants of this world produce so many drugs? Suppose a genetic mutation occurred in a plant so that one of its normal biochemical processes was changed and a new chemical was produced. If that new chemical had an effect on an animal's biochemistry, when the animal ate the plant the animal might become ill or die. In either case, that plant would be less likely to be eaten and more likely to reproduce others of its own kind. Such a selection process must have occurred many thousands of times in various places all over the earth. Many of those plant-produced chemicals have effects on the intestines or muscles; others alter brain biochemistry. In large doses the effect is virtually always unpleasant or dangerous, but in controlled doses those chemicals might alter the biochemistry just enough to

Online Learning Center Resources

www.mhhe.com/ksir12e

Visit our Online Learning Center (OLC) for access to these study aids and additional resources.

- Learning objectives
- Glossary flashcards
- Web activities and links
- Self-scoring chapter quiz
- Audio chapter summaries

produce interesting or even useful effects. In primitive cultures, the people who learned about these plants and how to use them safely were important figures in their communities. Those medicine men and women were the forerunners of today's pharmacists and physicians, as well as being important religious figures in their tribes.

Today the legal pharmaceutical industry is one of the largest and most profitable industries in the United States, with sales exceeding $160 billion a year.[1] With such extensive sales, many people expect that there are zillions of drugs. Not so. More than half of all prescriptions are filled with only 200 drugs.

Names of Drugs

Commercially available compounds have several kinds of names: *brand, generic,* and *chemical.* The *chemical* name of a compound gives a complete chemical description of the molecule and is derived from the rules of organic chemistry for naming any compound. Chemical names of drugs are rarely used except in a laboratory situation where biochemists or pharmacologists are developing and testing new drugs.

Generic names are the official (i.e., legal) names of drugs and are listed in the *United States Pharmacopoeia (USP).* Although a **generic** name refers to a specific chemical, it is usually shorter and simpler than the complete chemical name. Generic names are in the public domain, meaning they cannot be trademarked.

The *brand* name of a drug specifies a particular formulation and manufacturer, and the trademark belongs to that manufacturer. A brand name is usually quite simple and as meaningful (in terms of the indicated therapeutic use) as the company can make it. For example, the name *Elavil* was chosen for an antidepressant drug to indicate that it would elevate mood. However, brand names are controlled by the FDA, and overly suggestive ones are not approved.

When a new chemical structure, a new way of manufacturing a chemical, or a new use for a chemical is discovered, it can be patented. Patent laws in the United States now protect drugs for 20 years, and after that time the finding is available for use by anyone. Therefore, for 20 years a company that has discovered and patented a drug can manufacture and sell it without direct competition. After that, other companies can apply to the FDA to sell the "same" drug. Brand names, however, are copyrighted and protected by trademark laws. Therefore, the other companies have to use the drug's generic name or their own brand name. The FDA requires these companies to submit samples to demonstrate that their version is chemically equivalent and to do studies to demonstrate that the tablets or capsules they are making will dissolve appropriately and result in blood levels similar to those of the original drug. When a drug "goes generic," the original manufacturer might reduce the price of the brand name product to remain competitive.

Categories of Drugs

Physicians, pharmacologists, chemists, lawyers, psychologists, and users all have drug classification schemes that best serve their own purposes. A drug such as amphetamine might be categorized as a weight-control aid by a physician, because it reduces food intake for a period of time. It might be classed as a phenylethylamine by a

Drugs in the Media

The Grapefruit-Juice Effect

Reports about the "grapefruit-juice effect"—the observation that grapefruit juice may boost the absorption of some commonly prescribed drugs—recently resurfaced in the news, leaving some citrus fans wondering if it's OK to pop pills with their morning glass of juice. Drinking grapefruit juice to wash down some prescription medications may be dangerous because the juice can raise blood concentrations of the drug beyond what the dosage calls for.

Unlike other citrus juices, grapefruit juice inhibits one of the body's intestinal enzyme systems and can result in marked increases in serum levels of some prescription drugs, such as calcium-channel blockers used to control blood pressure and protease inhibitors given to treat HIV. An unknown chemical in grapefruit juice lowers the levels of a specific intestinal enzyme, allowing more of the drug to be absorbed. This enzyme normally breaks down drug molecules before they reach the bloodstream.

Researchers say grapefruit juice enhances the absorption of the cancer drug Vinblastine; the allergy medication Fexofenadine; the drug Digoxin, which is used to treat congestive heart failure; the blood pressure drug Losartan; and the drug Cyclosporine, an immunosuppressant medication used by organ transplant recipients. Interactions between grapefruit juice and certain drugs—which have been known but not extensively studied—are particularly worrisome for elderly people, who are more likely to take medications and may drink calcium-fortified grapefruit juice.

Although some drugs are prescribed with others to enhance their effects, grapefruit juice should not be used for this purpose because its effects can be unpredictable and potentially dangerous. Only about one in 10 people are affected, but in those who are, the juice has boosted a drug's potency as much as 40 percent.

Researchers are working to identify exactly what gives grapefruit juice this unusual property. Better understanding of this phenomenon might lead to improvement in the effectiveness of some kinds of drugs, potentially lowering the amount of drug needed. It may also lead to more consistency in doses from patient to patient, because individual variations in the activity of this intestinal enzyme account for big differences in the effective dose from one person to another.

---

pharmacologist, because its basic structure is a phenyl ring with an ethyl group and an amine attached. The chemist says amphetamine is 2-amino-1-phenylpropane. To the lawyer, amphetamine might be only a controlled substance falling in Schedule II of the federal drug law, whereas the psychologist might say simply that it is a stimulant. The user might call it a diet pill or an upper. Any scheme for categorizing drugs has meaning only if it serves the purpose for which the classification is being made.

The scheme presented here organizes the drugs according to their effects on the user, with first consideration given to the psychological effects. The basic organization and examples of each type are given in Figure 5.1, but it is worthwhile to point out some of the defining characteristics of each major grouping.

At moderate doses, *stimulant drugs* produce wakefulness and a sense of energy and well-being. The more powerful stimulants, such as cocaine and amphetamines, can at high doses produce a manic state of excitement combined with paranoia and hallucinations.

If you know about the behavioral effects of alcohol, then you know about the *depressant drugs*. At low doses they appear to depress

generic (juh *ner* ic): a name that specifies a particular chemical but not a particular brand.

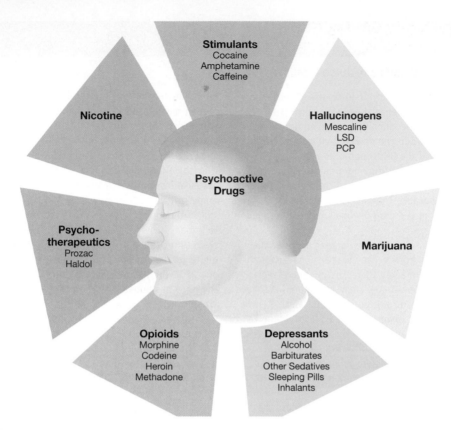

Figure 5.1 Classification of Psychoactive Drugs

inhibitory parts of the brain, leading to disinhibition or relaxation and talkativeness that can give way to recklessness. As the dose is increased, other neural functions become depressed, leading to slowed reaction times, uncoordinated movements, and unconsciousness. Stimulants and depressants do not counteract one another. Although it may be possible to keep a drunk awake with cocaine, he or she would still be reckless, uncoordinated, and so on. Regular use of depressant drugs can lead to a withdrawal syndrome characterized by restlessness, shakiness, hallucinations, and sometimes convulsions.

Opioids are a group of analgesic (painkilling) drugs that produce a relaxed, dreamlike state; moderately high doses often induce sleep. Pharmacologically, this group is also known as the narcotics, and it is important to distinguish

them from the "downers," or depressants. With opioids there is a clouding of consciousness without the reckless abandon, staggering, and slurred speech produced by alcohol and other depressants. Regular use of any of the opioids can lead to a withdrawal syndrome different from that of depressants and characterized by diarrhea, cramps, chills, and profuse sweating.

The *hallucinogens* produce altered perceptions, including unusual visual sensations and quite often changes in the perception of one's own body.

The *psychotherapeutic drugs* include a variety of drugs prescribed by psychiatrists and other physicians for the control of mental problems. The *antipsychotics,* such as haloperidol, are also called neuroleptics. They can calm psychotic patients and over time help them control hallucinations and illogical thoughts.

The *antidepressants,* such as fluoxetine (Prozac), help some people recover more rapidly from seriously depressed mood states. Lithium is used to control manic episodes and to prevent mood swings in bipolar disorder.

As with any classification system, some things don't seem to fit into the classes. Nicotine and marijuana are two such drugs. Nicotine is often thought of as being a mild stimulant, but it also seems to have some of the relaxant properties of a low dose of a depressant. Marijuana is often thought of as a relaxant, depressive type of drug, but it doesn't share most of the features of that class. It is sometimes listed among the hallucinogens because at high doses it can produce altered perceptions, but that classification doesn't seem appropriate for the way most people use it.

Drug Identification

There are many reasons to identify exactly what drug is represented by a tablet, capsule, or plant substance. The *Physician's Desk Reference (PDR)* has for many years published color photographs of many of the legally manufactured pharmaceuticals.[2] In this way a physician can determine from the pills themselves what drugs a new patient has been taking and in what doses. More critically, in emergency rooms it is possible to determine what drugs a person has just taken, if some of the pills are available for viewing. Police chemistry labs also use the *PDR* to get a preliminary indication of the nature of seized tablets and capsules.

Even illicit drugs can sometimes be identified by visual appearance. Often the makers of illicit tablets containing amphetamines or MDMA mark them, however crudely, in a consistent way, so that they can be recognized by their buyers. Such visual identification is far from perfect, of course. Cocaine or heroin powder can also be wrapped and labeled in a consistent way by street dealers. Some plant materials, such as psilocybin mushrooms, peyote cactus, or coca or marijuana leaves, can be fairly easy to identify visually, although again not with perfect accuracy.

If a case involving illicit drugs is to be prosecuted in court, the prosecution will usually be expected to present the testimony of a chemist indicating that the drug had been tested and identified using specific chemical analyses.

Drug Effects

No matter what the drug or how much of it there is, it can't have an effect until it is taken. For there to be a drug effect, the drug must be brought together with a living organism. After a discussion of the basic concepts of drug movement in the body, you will be better able to understand such important issues as blood alcohol level, the dependence potential of crack cocaine, and urine testing for marijuana use.

Nonspecific (Placebo) Effects

The effects of a drug do not depend solely on chemical interactions with the body's tissues. With psychoactive drugs in particular, the influences of expectancy, experience, and setting are also important determinants of the drug's effect. For example, a good "trip" or a bad trip on LSD seems to be more dependent on the experiences and mood of the user before taking the drug than on the amount or quality of drug taken. Even the effect of alcohol depends on what the user expects to experience. *Nonspecific* effects of a drug are those that derive from the user's unique background and particular perception of the world. In brief, the nonspecific effects include anything except the chemical activity of the drug and the direct effects of this activity. Nonspecific effects are also sometimes called **placebo** effects, because they can often be produced by an inactive chemical (placebo) that the user believes to be a drug.

placebo (pluh *see* bo): an inactive drug.

The effects of a drug that depend on the presence of the chemical at certain concentrations in the target tissue are called *specific* effects. One important task for psychopharmacologists is to separate the specific effects of a drug from the nonspecific effects.

Suppose you design an experiment with two conditions: One group of people receives the drug you're interested in testing, in a dose that you have reason to believe should work. Each person in the second condition, or control group, receives a capsule that looks identical to the drug but contains no active drug molecules (a placebo). The people must be randomly assigned to the groups and be treated and evaluated identically except for the active drug molecules in the capsules for the experimental group. For this reason, tests for the effectiveness of a new drug must be done using a **double-blind procedure.** Neither the experimental participant nor the person evaluating the drug's effect knows whether a particular individual is receiving a placebo or an experimental drug. Only after the experiment is over and the data have all been collected is the code broken, so that the results can be analyzed.

Placebo effects have been shown to be especially important in two major kinds of therapeutic effects: treating pain, and treating psychological depression. The size of the placebo response in studies of depression has led to some recent controversy about just how effective the "real" antidepressants are. It has been known for the past 50 years that at least one-third of psychologically depressed patients treated with placebos show improvement—in some published studies the rates of placebo response have been even higher. One group of scientists reviewed all the data submitted to the Food and Drug Administration between 1987 and 1999 in support of new drug applications for six of the most popular antidepressant medications on the U.S. market.[3] They concluded about 80 percent of the effectiveness attributed to the antidepressant drugs could be obtained from a placebo!

Nonspecific effects are not caused by the chemicals in drugs, but they are still "real" effects that in some cases might have a biological basis. A recent study used a technique known as quantitative electroencephalography, in which electrical activity was recorded from multiple electrodes placed on patients' heads. In a group of patients who were initially depressed, 38 percent of those treated with a placebo showed improved mood scores during the nine-week study. Those who showed improvement after placebo treatment were also likely to show changes in the electrical responses from the prefrontal cortex. Among the patients treated with either of two active antidepressant drugs, 52 percent were improved, and they showed a different pattern of electrical changes from the patients treated with a placebo.[4]

Dose-Response Relationships

Perhaps the strongest demonstration of the specific effects of a drug is obtained when the dose of the drug is varied and the size of the effect changes directly with the drug dose. A graph showing the relationship between the dose and the effect is called a **dose-response curve.** Typically, at very low doses no effect is seen. At some low dose, an effect on the response system being monitored is observed. This dose is the *threshold,* and as the dose of the drug is increased, there are more molecular interactions and a greater effect on the response system. At the point where the system shows maximal response, further additions of the drug have no effect.

In some drug-response interactions, the effect of the drug is all or none, so that when the system does respond, it responds maximally. There might, however, be variability in the dosage at which individual organisms respond, and as the dose increases, there is a rise in the percentage of individuals who show the response.

As the drug dose increases, sometimes new response systems are affected by the drug. This fact suggests that some response systems have

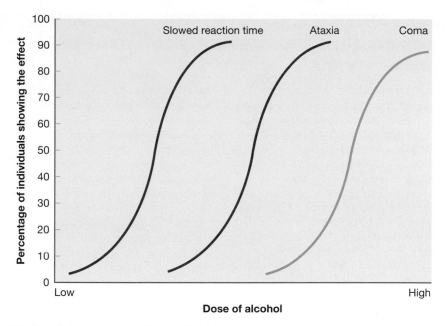

Figure 5.2   Relationship between Alcohol Dose and Multiple Responses

higher drug thresholds than others. Figure 5.2 shows a series of dose-response curves for three different effects of alcohol. As the dose increases from the low end, first a few and then more and more of the individuals show a slowing of their reaction times. If we also have a test for **ataxia** (staggering or inability to walk straight), we see that, as the alcohol dose reaches the level at which most individuals are showing slowed reaction times, a few are also beginning to show ataxia. As the dose increases further, more people show ataxia, and some become **comatose** (they pass out and cannot be aroused). At the highest dose indicated, all of the individuals would be comatose. We could draw curves for other effects of alcohol on such a figure; for example, at the high end we would begin to see some deaths from overdose, and a curve for lethality could be placed to the right of the coma curve.

In the rational use of drugs, four questions about drug dosage must be answered. First, what is the effective dose of the drug for a desired goal? For example, what dose of morphine is necessary to reduce pain? What amount of marijuana is necessary for an individual to feel euphoric? How much aspirin will make the headache go away? The second question is what dose of the drug will be toxic to the individual? Combining those two, the third question is what is the safety margin—how different are the effective dose and the toxic dose? Finally, at the effective dose level, what other effects, particularly adverse reactions, might develop? Leaving aside for now this last question, a discussion of the first three deals with basic concepts in understanding drug actions.

double-blind procedure: experiment in which neither the doctor nor the patient knows which drug is being used.

dose-response curve: a graph comparing the size of response to the amount of drug.

ataxia (ay _tax_ ee ah): uncoordinated walking.

comatose (_co_ mah tose): unconscious and unable to be aroused.

Taking Sides

Animal Toxicity Tests

Increasing interest in the welfare of laboratory animals has resulted in improved standards for housing, veterinary care, and anesthesia. Some animal rights groups have suggested that most types of animal research should be stopped because the experiments are either unnecessary or even misleading. The use of the LD_{50} test by drug companies, in which the researchers estimate the dose of a drug required to kill half the animals (usually mice), has been a particular target. The groups have claimed that these tests are outmoded and that toxicity could be predicted from computer models or work on isolated cell cultures.

A pamphlet published by People for the Ethical Treatment of Animals (PETA), one of the most well-known animal rights groups, claims on the one hand that the laboratory animals are sensitive beings with "distinct personalities. Just like you and me," but on the other hand that toxicity tests on animals are not relevant to humans because of basic biological differences. In reality, most basic biological functions are quite similar among all mammals, whereas the greatest differences between laboratory mice and humans would probably be found in the areas of thoughts, emotions, and "personality."

A specific case cited by PETA was thalidomide testing (see Chapter 3), which it claims "passed animal safety tests with flying colors" and later caused thousands of human deformities. Some critical points in that argument were omitted, however. Thalidomide caused birth defects when taken during pregnancy. Otherwise, its human toxicity was quite low. Thalidomide was not tested on pregnant animals. If it had been, the birth defects would have been detected. And because of thalidomide, the laws were changed 30 years ago to *require* that drugs to be used by humans during pregnancy first undergo testing in pregnant animals.

Admittedly, giving drugs to pregnant animals to see if they produce birth defects or spontaneous abortions may seem cruel. Would you volunteer to be the first living animal to take a new drug whose toxicity had been estimated by a computer model?

Estimating the safety margin is an important part of the preclinical (animal) testing that is done on any new drug before it is tried in humans. To determine an *effective dose (ED)*, it is necessary to define an effect in animals that is meaningful in terms of the desired human use, although in some cases this is difficult. Say we will test a new sleeping pill (hypnotic), on several groups of 20 mice each. Each group will receive a different dose, and an hour later we will check to see how many mice in each group are sleeping. Let us assume that at the lowest dose we tested, only one of the 20 mice was asleep, and at the highest doses all were asleep, with other values in between. By drawing a line through these points, we can estimate the dose required to put half of the mice to sleep (the ED_{50}, or the effective dose for 50 percent of the animals).

Toxicity is usually measured in at least one early animal study by determining how many mice die as a result of the drug. Let's say we check each cage the next day to see how many mice in each group died. From such a study we can estimate the LD_{50} (lethal dose for 50 percent of the mice). The **therapeutic index (TI)** is defined as LD_{50}/ED_{50}. Since the *lethal dose* should be larger than the *effective dose*, the TI should always be greater than 1. How large should the TI be if the company is going to go forward with expensive clinical trials? It depends partly on the TIs of the drugs already available for the same purpose. If the new drug has a greater TI than existing drugs, it is likely to be safer when given to humans.

This approach of estimating the dose to affect 50 percent of the mice is used in early animal tests because it is statistically more reliable to estimate the 50 percent point using a small number of mice per group than it is to estimate the 1 percent or 99 percent points. However, with humans we don't do LD_{50}

Targeting Prevention

Avoiding Withdrawal Symptoms

Withdrawal symptoms may appear after ceasing the use of many psychoactive drugs if the user has been taking high doses for a prolonged period. When a hospital patient needs to be treated with an opioid for pain control (analgesia), how can the drug be given in such a way as to reduce the chances of developing physical dependence, as evidenced by withdrawal symptoms? Obviously, keeping doses as low as possible and giving the drug for as short a time as possible are two important keys. One way to keep the dose as low as necessary while still obtaining adequate pain control is the use of a PCA (patient-controlled anesthesia or analgesia) pump. Within limits, each patient is allowed to administer just the amount of narcotic needed to control his or her pain. This prevents two problems: (1) giving more of the drug than is necessary just to make sure the pain is controlled, and (2) not giving quite enough of the drug, so that the patient experiences pain and has to request and wait for more of the drug before the pain is relieved. Dependence may be less of a problem when the patient is allowed to take the drug as needed.

experiments. Also, with some disorders, perhaps the best drugs we have can help only half of the people. What we ultimately want is to estimate the dose that will produce a desired effect in most patients and the lowest dose producing some unacceptable toxic reaction. The difference between these doses would be called the **safety margin.**

Most of the psychoactive compounds have an LD_1 well above the ED_{95} level, so the practical limitation on whether or not, or at what dose, a drug is used is the occurrence of **side effects.** With increasing doses there is usually an increase in the number and severity of side effects—the effects of the drug that are not relevant to the treatment. If the number of side effects becomes too great and the individual begins to suffer from them, the use of the drug will be discontinued or the dose lowered, even though the drug may be very effective in controlling the original symptoms. The selection of a drug for therapeutic use should be made on the basis of effectiveness in treating the symptoms with minimal side effects.

Potency

The **potency** of a drug is one of the most misunderstood concepts in the area of drug use. Potency refers only to the *amount of drug* that must be given to obtain a particular response. The smaller the amount needed to get a particular effect, the more potent the drug. Potency does not necessarily relate to how effective a drug is or to how large an effect the drug can produce. *Potency* refers only to relative effective dose; the ED_{50} of a potent drug is lower than the ED_{50} of a less potent drug. For example, it has been said that LSD is one of the most potent psychoactive drugs known. This is true in that hallucinogenic effects can be obtained with 50 micrograms (µg), compared with several milligrams (mg) required of other hallucinogens (a µg is 1/1,000 of a mg, which is 1/1,000 of a gram [g]). However, the effects of LSD are relatively limited—it doesn't

ED_{50}: effective dose for half of the animals tested.
LD_{50}: lethal dose for half of the animals tested.
therapeutic index (TI): ratio of LD_{50} to ED_{50}.
safety margin: dosage difference between an acceptable level of effectiveness and the lowest toxic dose.
side effects: unintended effects that accompany therapeutic effects.
potency: measured by the amount of drug required to produce an effect.

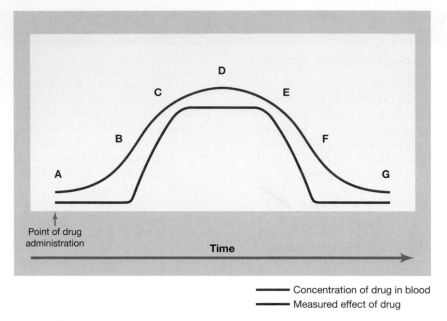

Point of drug administration

Time

——— Concentration of drug in blood
——— Measured effect of drug

Figure 5.3   Possible Relationship between Drug Concentration in the Body and Measured Effect of the Drug

lead to overdose deaths the way heroin and alcohol do. Alcohol has a greater variety of more powerful effects than LSD, even though in terms of the *dose* required to produce a psychological effect LSD is thousands of times more *potent*.

Time-Dependent Factors in Drug Actions

In the mouse experiment, we picked one hour after administering the drug to check for the sleeping effect. Obviously, we would have had to learn a bit about the **time course** of the drug's effect before picking one hour. Some very rapidly acting drug might have put the mice to sleep within 10 minutes and be wearing off by one hour, and we would pick a 20- or 30-minute time to check the effect of that drug. The time course of a drug's action depends on many things, including how the drug is administered, how rapidly it is absorbed, and how it is eliminated from the body.

Figure 5.3 describes one type of relationship between administration of a drug and its effect over time. Between points *A* and *B* there is no observed effect, although the concentration

of drug in the blood is increasing. At point *B* the threshold concentration is reached, and from *B* to *C* the observed drug effect increases as drug concentration increases. At point *C* the maximal effect of the drug is reached, but its concentration continues increasing to point *D*. Although deactivation of the drug probably begins as soon as the drug enters the body, from *A* to *D* the rate of absorption is greater than the rate of deactivation. Beginning at point *D* the deactivation proceeds more rapidly than absorption, and the concentration of the drug decreases. When the amount of drug in the body reaches *E*, the maximal effect is over. The action diminishes from *E* to *F*, at which point the level of the drug is below the threshold for effect, although the drug is still in the body up to point *G*.

If the relationship described in Figure 5.3 is true for a particular drug, then increasing the dose of the drug will not increase the magnitude of its effect. Aspirin and other headache remedies are probably the most misused drugs in this respect—if two are good, four should be better, and six will really stop this headache. No way! When the maximum possible therapeutic effect has been reached, increasing the dose primarily adds to the number of side effects.

The usual way to obtain a prolonged effect is to take an additional dose at some time after the first dose has reached its maximum concentration and started to decline. The appropriate interval varies from one drug to another. If doses are taken too close together, the maximum blood level will increase with each dose and can result in **cumulative effects.**

One of the important changes in the manufacture of drugs is the development of time-release preparations. These compounds are prepared so that after oral ingestion the active ingredient is released into the body over a 6- to 10-hour period. With a preparation of this type, a large amount of the drug is initially made available for absorption, and then smaller amounts are released continuously for a long period. The initial amount of the drug is expected to be adequate to obtain the response desired, and the gradual release thereafter is designed to maintain the same effective dose of the drug even though the drug is being continually deactivated. In terms of Figure 5.3, a time-release preparation would aim at eliminating the unnecessarily high drug level at *C–D–E* while lengthening the *C–E* time interval.

Getting the Drug to the Brain

A Little "Chemistry"

The chemistry of the drug molecules determines if some drugs act quickly and others more slowly. One of the most important considerations is the **lipid solubility** of the molecules. Shake up some salad oil with some water, let it stand, and the oil floats on top. When other chemicals are added, sometimes they "prefer" to be concentrated more in the water or in the oil. For example, if you put sodium chloride (table salt) in with the oil and water and shake it all up, most of the salt will stay with the water. If you crush a garlic clove and add it to the mix, most of the chemicals that give garlic its flavor will remain in the oil. The extent to which a chemical can be dissolved in oils and fats is called its lipid

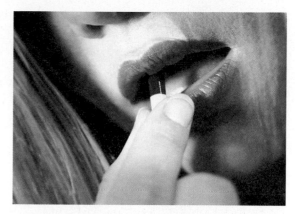

Absorption of a drug into the bloodstream through the gastrointestinal tract is a complicated process.

solubility. Most psychoactive drugs dissolve to some extent in either water or lipids, and in our oil-and-water experiment some fraction of the drug would be found in each. The importance of lipid solubility will become clear as we see how molecules get into the brain.

Routes of Administration

We rarely put chemicals directly into our brains. All psychoactive drugs reach the brain tissue by way of the bloodstream. Most psychoactive drugs are taken by one of three basic routes: by mouth, injection, or inhalation.

Oral Administration Most drugs begin their grand adventure in the body by entering through the mouth. Even though oral intake might be the simplest way to take a drug, absorption from the gastrointestinal tract is the most complicated way to enter the bloodstream. A chemical in the digestive tract must withstand the actions of stomach acid and digestive enzymes and not be deactivated by food before it is absorbed.

> **time course:** timing of the onset, duration, and termination of a drug's effect.
> **cumulative effects:** effects of giving multiple doses of the same drug.
> **lipid solubility:** tendency of a chemical to dissolve in fat, as opposed to in water.

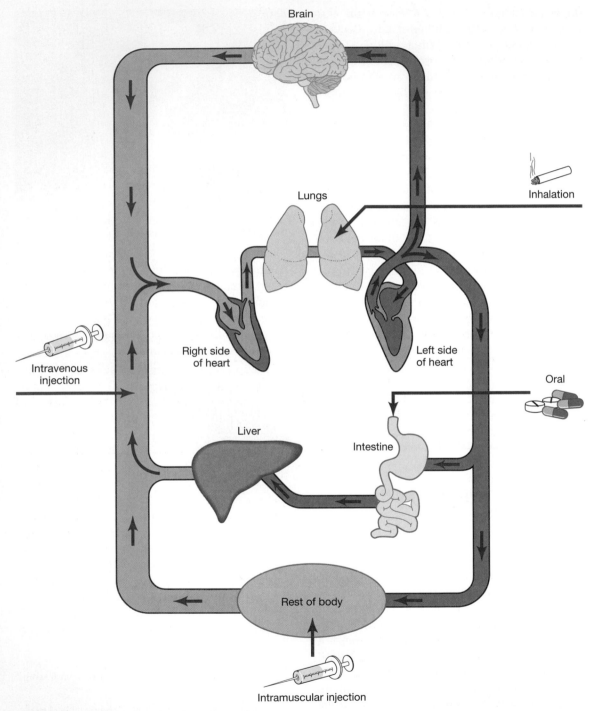

Figure 5.4 Distribution of Drugs through the Body

The antibiotic tetracycline provides a good example of the dangers in the gut for a drug. This antibiotic readily combines with calcium ions to form a compound that is poorly absorbed. If tetracycline is taken with milk (calcium ions), blood levels will never be as high as if it were taken with a different beverage.

The drug molecules must next get through the cells lining the wall of the gastrointestinal tract and into the blood capillaries. If taken in capsule or tablet form, the drug must first dissolve and then, as a liquid, mix into the contents of the stomach and intestines. However, the more other material there is in the stomach, the greater the dilution of the drug and the slower it will be absorbed. The drug must be water soluble for the molecules to spread throughout the stomach. However, only lipid-soluble and very small water-soluble molecules are readily absorbed into the capillaries surrounding the small intestine, where most absorption into the bloodstream occurs.

Once in the bloodstream, the dangers of entering through the oral route are not over. The veins from the gut go first to the liver (see Figure 5.4). If the drug is the type that is metabolized rapidly by the liver (nicotine is one example), very little may get into the general circulation. Thus, nicotine is much more effective when inhaled than when swallowed.

Injection Chemicals can be delivered with a hypodermic syringe directly into the bloodstream or deposited in a muscle mass or under the upper layers of skin. With the **intravenous (IV)** injection, the drug is put directly into the bloodstream, so the onset of action is much more rapid than with oral administration or with other means of injection. Another advantage is that irritating material can be injected this way, because blood vessel walls are relatively insensitive. Also, it is possible to deliver very high concentrations of drugs intravenously, which can be both an advantage and a danger. A major disadvantage of IV injections is that the vein wall loses some of its strength and elasticity in the area around the injection site.

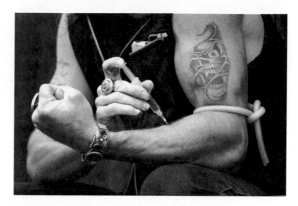

For many heroin users, the preferred route of administration is by intravenous injection.

If there are many injections into a small segment of a vein, the wall of that vein eventually collapses, and blood no longer moves through it, necessitating the use of another injection site. The greatest concern about IV drug use is the danger of introducing infections directly into the bloodstream, either from bacteria picked up on the skin as the needle is being inserted or from contaminated needles and syringes containing traces of blood. This risk is especially great if syringes and needles are shared among users. This has been a significant means by which AIDS and other blood-borne diseases have been spread (see Chapter 2).

Subcutaneous and **intramuscular** injections have similar characteristics, except that absorption is more rapid from intramuscular injection. Muscles have a better blood supply than the underlying layers of the skin and thus more area over which absorption can occur. Absorption is most rapid when the injection is into the deltoid muscle of the arm and least rapid when the injection is in the buttock. Intermediate between these two areas in speed of

intravenous (IV) (in trah *vee* nuss): injection directly into a vein.
subcutaneous (sub cue *tay* nee us): injection under the skin.
intramuscular: injection into a muscle.

drug absorption is injection into the thigh. There is less chance of irritation if the injection is intramuscular because of the better blood supply and faster absorption. Another advantage is that larger volumes of material can be deposited in a muscle than can be injected subcutaneously. Sometimes it is desirable to have a drug absorbed very slowly (over several days or even weeks). A form of the drug that dissolves very slowly in water might be injected into a muscle, or the drug might be microencapsulated (tiny bits of drug coated with something to slow its absorption).

One disadvantage of subcutaneous injection is that, if the material injected is extremely irritating to the tissue, the skin around the site of injection might die and be shed. This method of injection is not very common in medical practice but has long been the kind of injection used by beginning opioid users. This is commonly called "skin popping."

Inhalation Inhalation is the drug delivery system used for smoking nicotine, marijuana, and crack cocaine, and for "huffing" gasoline, paints, and other inhalants; it is used medically with various anesthetics. It is a very efficient way to deliver a drug. Onset of drug effects is quite rapid because the capillary walls are very accessible in the lungs, and the drug thus enters the blood quickly. For psychoactive drugs, inhalation can produce more rapid effects than even intravenous administration. This is because of the patterns of blood circulation in the body (review Figure 5.4). The blood leaving the lungs moves fairly directly to the brain, taking only five to eight seconds to do so. By contrast, blood from the veins in the arm must return to the heart, then be pumped through the lungs before moving on to the brain, and this takes 10 to 15 seconds. Aerosol dispensers have been used to deliver some drugs via the lungs, but three considerations make inhalation of limited value for medical purposes. First, the material must not be irritating to the mucous membranes and lungs. Second, control of the dose is more difficult than

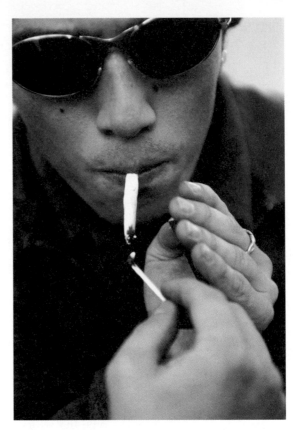

Inhalation is a very effective means of delivering a drug to the brain.

with the other drug delivery systems. Last, and perhaps the prime advantage for some drugs and disadvantage for others, there is no depot of drug in the body. This means the drug must be given as long as the effect is desired and that, when drug administration is stopped, the effect rapidly decreases.

Other Routes Topical application of a drug to the skin is not widely used because most drugs are not absorbed well through the skin. However, for some drugs this method can provide a slow, steady absorption over many hours. For example, a skin patch results in the slow absorption of nicotine over an entire day. This patch has been found to help prevent relapse in people who have quit smoking. Application to mucous membranes results in more rapid absorption than through the skin because these membranes are moist and have a rich blood supply. Both rectal and vaginal suppositories take advantage of these characteristics, although suppositories are used only rarely. The mucous membranes of the nose are used by most cocaine users, who "snort" or "sniff" cocaine powder into the nose, where it dissolves and is absorbed through the membranes. Also, the mucosa of the oral cavity provide for the absorption of nicotine from chewing tobacco directly into the bloodstream without going through the stomach, intestines, and liver.

Transport in the Blood

When a drug enters the bloodstream, often its molecules will attach to one of the protein molecules in the blood, albumin being the most common protein involved. The degree to which drug molecules bind to plasma proteins is important in determining drug effects. As long as there is a protein-drug complex, the drug is inactive and cannot leave the blood. In this condition, the drug is protected from inactivation by enzymes.

An equilibrium is established between the free (unbound) drug and the protein-bound forms of the drug in the bloodstream. As the unbound drug moves across capillary walls to sites of action, there is a release of protein-bound drug to maintain the proportion of bound to free molecules. Considerable variation exists among drugs in the affinity that the drug molecules have for binding with plasma proteins. Alcohol has a low affinity and thus exists in the bloodstream primarily as the unbound form. In contrast, most of the molecules of THC, the active ingredient in marijuana, are bound to blood proteins, with only a small fraction free to enter the brain or other tissues. If two drugs were identical in every respect except protein binding, the one with greater affinity for blood proteins would require a higher dose to reach an effective tissue concentration. On the other hand, the duration of that drug's effect would be longer because of the "storage" of molecules on blood proteins.

Because different drugs have different affinities for the plasma proteins, one might expect that drugs with high affinity would displace drugs with weak protein bonds, and they do. This fact is important because it forms the basis for one kind of drug interaction. When a high-affinity drug is added to blood in which there is a weak-affinity drug already largely bound to the plasma proteins, the weak-affinity drug is displaced and exists primarily as the unbound form. The increase in the unbound drug concentration helps move the drug out of the bloodstream to the sites of action faster and can be an important influence on the effect the drug has. At the very least, the duration of action is shortened.

Blood-Brain Barrier

The brain is very different from the other parts of the body in terms of drugs' ability to leave the blood and move to sites of action. As described in Chapter 4, a barrier keeps certain classes of compounds in the blood and away from brain cells. Thus, some drugs act only on neurons outside the central nervous system—that is, only on those in the peripheral nervous system, whereas others may affect all neurons.

The **blood-brain barrier** is not well developed in infants; it reaches complete development only after one or two years of age in humans. Although the nature of this barrier is not well understood, several factors are known to contribute to the blood-brain barrier. One is the makeup of the capillaries in the brain. They are different from other capillaries in the body, because they contain no pores. Even small water-soluble molecules cannot leave the capillaries in the brain; only lipid-soluble substances can pass the lipid capillary wall.

If a substance can move through the capillary wall, another barrier unique to the brain is

blood-brain barrier: structure that prevents many drugs from entering the brain.

met. About 85 percent of the capillaries are covered with glial cells; there is little extracellular space next to the blood vessel walls. With no pores and close contact between capillary walls and glial cells, almost certainly an active transport system is needed to move chemicals in and out of the brain. In fact, known transport systems exist for some naturally occurring agents.

A final note on the mystery of the blood-brain barrier is that cerebral trauma can disrupt the barrier and permit agents to enter that normally would be excluded. Concussions and cerebral infections frequently cause enough trauma to impair the effectiveness of this screen, which normally permits only selected chemicals to enter the brain.

Mechanisms of Drug Actions

Many types of actions are suggested in Chapters 6 to 16 as ways in which specific drugs can affect physiochemical processes, neuron functioning, and ultimately thoughts, feelings, and other behaviors. It is possible for drugs to affect all neurons, but many exert actions only on very specific presynaptic or postsynaptic processes.

Effects on All Neurons

Chemicals that have an effect on all neurons must do it by influencing some characteristic common to all neurons. One general characteristic of all neurons is the cell membrane. It is semipermeable, meaning that some agents can readily move in and out of the cell, but other chemicals are held inside or kept out under normal conditions. The semipermeable characteristic of the cell membrane is essential for the maintenance of an electric potential across the membrane. It is on this membrane that some drugs seem to act and, by influencing the permeability, alter the electrical characteristics of the neuron.

Most of the general anesthetics have been thought to affect the central nervous system by a general influence on the cell membrane. The classical view of alcohol's action on the nervous system was that it has effects similar to the general anesthetics through an influence on the neural membrane. However, evidence has pointed to more specific possible mechanisms for alcohol's effects (see Chapter 9), and even the gaseous anesthetics might be more selective in their action than was previously thought. Thus, the entire notion that some drugs act nonspecifically through altering the nerve membrane's electrical properties is in dispute.[5]

Effects on Specific Neurotransmitter Systems

The various types of psychoactive drugs (e.g., opioids, stimulants, depressants) produce different types of effects primarily because each type interacts in a different way with the various neurotransmitter systems in the brain. Chapter 4 pointed out that the brain's natural neurotransmitters are released from one neuron into a small space called a *synapse,* where they interact with receptors on the surface of another neuron. Psychoactive drugs can alter the *availability* of a neurotransmitter by increasing or decreasing the transmitter chemical's rate of synthesis, metabolism, release from storage vesicles, or reuptake into the releasing neuron. Or the drug might act directly on the *receptor,* either to activate it or to prevent the neurotransmitter chemical from activating it. With the existence of more than 50 known neurotransmitters, and considering that different drugs can interact with several of these in different combinations, and given the variety of mechanisms by which each drug can interact with the life cycle of a natural neurotransmitter, the potential exists for an endless variety of drugs with an endless variety of actions. However, all of these actions are nothing more mysterious than a modification of the ongoing (and quite complex) functions of the brain.

Drugs in Depth

Drug Interactions

Various drugs can interact with one another in many ways: They may have similar actions and thus have additive effects, one may displace another from protein binding and thus one drug may enhance the effect of another even though they have different actions, one drug may stimulate liver enzymes and thus reduce the effect of another, and so on.

Even restricting ourselves to psychoactive drugs, there is such a variety of possible interactions that it would not make sense to try to catalog them all here. Instead, a few of the most important interactions are described.

Respiratory Depression (Alcohol, Other Depressants, Opioids)

The single most important type of drug interaction for psychoactive drugs is the effect on respiration rate. All depressant drugs (sedatives such as Valium and Xanax, barbiturates, sleeping pills), alcohol, and all narcotics tend to slow down the rate at which people breathe in and out, because of effects in the brain stem. Combining any of these drugs can produce effects that are additive and in some cases may be more than additive. Respiratory depression is the most common type of drug overdose death: People simply stop breathing.

Stimulants and Antidepressants

Although antidepressant drugs such as amitriptyline (Elavil) and Prozac are not in themselves stimulants, they can potentiate the effects of stimulant drugs, such as cocaine and amphetamine, possibly leading to manic overexcitement, irregular heartbeat, high blood pressure, or other effects.

Stimulants and Depressants

It might seem that the "uppers" and "downers" would counteract one another, but that's generally not the case when it comes to behavior. Drugs such as Valium, Xanax, and alcohol may lead to disinhibition and recklessness. When combined with the effects of stimulants, explosive and dangerous behaviors are possible.

Cocaine + Alcohol = Cocaethylene

Although this may sound like a special case of combining a depressant and a stimulant (it is), there is another possible interaction in that cocaine can combine chemically with ethyl alcohol to produce a substance called cocaethylene—a potent stimulant that animal studies indicate may be 20 times as toxic as cocaine. The ramifications of this recent discovery are not yet clear (see Chapter 6).

Drug Deactivation

Before a drug can cease to have an effect, one of two things must happen to it. It may be excreted unchanged from the body (usually in the urine), or it may be chemically changed so that it no longer has the same effect on the body. Although different drugs vary in how they are deactivated, the most common way is for enzymes in the liver to act on the drug molecules to change their chemical structure. This usually has two effects: one, the **metabolite** no longer has the same action as the drug molecule; two, the metabolite is more likely to be excreted by the kidneys.

The kidneys operate in a two-stage process. In the first step, water and most of the small and water-soluble molecules are filtered out. Second, most of the water is reabsorbed, along with some of the dissolved chemicals. The more lipid-soluble molecules are more likely to be reabsorbed, so one way in which the liver enzymes can increase the elimination of a drug is by changing its molecules to a more water-soluble and less lipid-soluble form.

The most important drug-metabolizing enzymes found in the liver belong to a group known as the CYP450 family of enzymes. The

---

metabolite (muh *tab* oh lite): product of enzyme action on a drug.

CYP450 enzymes seem to be specialized for inactivating various general kinds of foreign chemicals that the organism might ingest. This is not like the immune system, in which foreign proteins stimulate the production of antibodies for that protein—the CYP450 enzymes already exist in the liver and are waiting for the introduction of certain types of chemicals. Various plants have evolved the ability to produce chemicals that do nothing directly for the plant but kill or make ill any animals that eat the plant. In defense, apparently many animals have evolved CYP450 enzymes for eliminating these toxic chemicals once they are eaten.

Although the CYP450 enzymes are always available in the liver, the introduction of drugs can alter their function. Many drugs, including alcohol and the barbiturates, have been shown to induce (increase) the activity of one or more of these drug-metabolizing enzymes. Once the body's cells detect the presence of these foreign molecules, they produce more of the enzyme that breaks down that molecule, in an effort to normalize the cell's chemistry (homeostasis—see Chapter 4). Enzyme induction has important potential not only for tolerance to that particular drug, but also for interactions with other drugs that might be broken down by the same enzyme. The increased rate of metabolism could mean that a previously effective dose of an antibiotic or heart medicine can no longer reach therapeutic levels. The enzyme activity typically returns to normal some time after the inducing drug is no longer being taken. For example, the FDA has warned that the herbal product Saint-John's-wort can decrease blood concentrations of several drugs, presumably by inducing CYP450 enzymes. Other drugs, including fluoxetine (Prozac) and other modern antidepressant drugs, have a high affinity for one of the CYP450 enzymes and "occupy" the enzyme molecules, so that they effectively inhibit the enzyme's action on any other drug. Now a previously safe dose of blood-pressure medication or cough suppressant results in much higher blood levels that could be dangerous. Prescribing physicians

have to be aware of the potential for these types of drug interactions, either to avoid using certain drugs together or to adjust doses upward or downward to compensate for enzyme induction or inhibition.

Not all of the metabolites of drugs are inactive. Both diazepam (Valium) and marijuana have **active metabolites** that produce effects similar to those of the original (parent) drug and prolong the effect considerably. In fact, so-called **prodrugs** are being developed that are inactive in the original form and become active only after they are altered by the liver enzymes.

Mechanisms of Tolerance and Withdrawal Symptoms

The phenomena of tolerance and withdrawal symptoms have historically been associated with drug dependence. *Tolerance* refers to a situation in which repeated administration of the same dose of a drug results in gradually diminishing effects. There are at least three mechanisms by which a reduced drug response can come about: drug disposition tolerance, behavioral tolerance, and pharmacodynamic tolerance.

Drug Disposition Tolerance

Sometimes the use of a drug increases the drug's rate of metabolism or excretion. This is referred to as **drug disposition tolerance,** or pharmacokinetic tolerance. For example, phenobarbital induces increased activity of the CYP450 enzymes that metabolize the drug. Increased metabolism reduces the effect of subsequent doses, perhaps leading to increased dosage. But additional amounts of the drug increase the activity of the enzymes even more, and the cycle continues. Another possible mechanism for increased elimination has to do with the pH (acidity) of the urine. Amphetamine is excreted unchanged in the urine, and the rate of excretion can be increased by making the urine more acidic. Both amphetamine itself and the decreased food intake that often accompanies heavy ampheta-mine use tend to make the urine more acidic. Amphetamine is excreted 20 times as rapidly in urine with a pH of 5 as in urine with a pH of 8.

Behavioral Tolerance

Particularly when the use of a drug interferes with normal behavioral functions, individuals may learn to adapt to the altered state of their nervous system and therefore compensate somewhat for the impairment. In some ways, this is analogous to a person who breaks a wrist and learns to write with the nonpreferred hand—the handwriting probably won't be as good that way, but with practice the disruptive effect on writing will be reduced. A person who regularly drives a car after drinking alco-hol will never be as good a driver as he or she would be sober, but with experience the im-pairment may be reduced. In this type of toler-ance, called **behavioral tolerance,** the drug may continue to have the same biochemical ef-fect but with a reduced effect on behavior.

Pharmacodynamic Tolerance

In many cases the amount of drug reaching the brain doesn't change, but the sensitivity of the neurons to the drug's effect does change. This is best viewed as an attempt by the brain to maintain its level of functioning within normal limits (an example of homeostasis). There are many possible mechanisms for this. For exam-ple, if the central nervous system is constantly held in a depressed state through the regular use of alcohol or another depressant drug, the brain might compensate by reducing the amount of the inhibitory neurotransmitter GABA that is released, or by reducing the number of in-hibitory GABA receptors (many studies show that the brain does regulate the numbers of specific types of receptors). This adjustment might take several days, and after it occurs the depressant drug doesn't produce as much CNS depression as it did before. If more drug is taken, the homeostatic mechanisms might further de-crease the release of GABA or the number of

GABA receptors. If the drug is abruptly stopped, the brain now does not have the proper level of GABA inhibition, and the CNS becomes overex-cited, leading to wakefulness, nervousness, possibly hallucinations, and the sensation that something is crawling on the skin. In severe cases, brain activity becomes uncontrolled and seizures can occur. These withdrawal symptoms are the defining characteristic of physical de-pendence. Thus, **pharmacodynamic tolerance** leads not only to a reduced effectiveness of the drug but also to these withdrawal reactions. After several days the compensating homeosta-tic mechanisms return to a normal state, the withdrawal symptoms cease, and the individ-ual is no longer as tolerant to the drug's effect.

Summary

- Most drugs are derived directly or indi-rectly from plants.

- The legal pharmaceutical industry is one of the largest and most profitable indus-tries in the United States.

- Brand names belong to one company; the generic name for a chemical may be used by many companies.

- Most psychoactive drugs can be categorized as stimulants, depressants, opioids, hallu-cinogens, or a psychotherapeutic agent.

- Drugs can be identified by the appearance of commercial tablets or capsules, in some

---

active metabolites: metabolites that have drug actions of their own.

prodrugs: drugs that are inactive until acted on by enzymes in the body.

drug disposition tolerance: tolerance caused by more rapid elimination of the drug.

behavioral tolerance: tolerance caused by learned adaptation to the drug.

pharmacodynamic tolerance: tolerance caused by altered nervous system sensitivity.

cases by the packaging or appearance of illicit drugs, or by a variety of chemical assays.

- Specific drug effects are related to the concentration of the chemical; nonspecific effects can also be called placebo effects.

- Because each drug is capable of producing many effects, many dose-effect relationships can be studied for any given drug.

- The ratio of LD_{50} to ED_{50} is called the therapeutic index and is one indication of the relative safety of a drug for a particular use or effect.

- The potency of a drug is the amount needed to produce an effect, not the importance of the effect.

- The time course of a drug's effect is influenced by many factors, including route of administration, protein binding in the blood, and rate of elimination.

- The blood-brain barrier prevents many drugs from reaching effective concentrations in the brain.

- Virtually all psychoactive drugs have relatively specific effects on one neurotransmitter system or more, either through altering availability of the transmitter or by interacting with its receptor.

- The liver microsomal enzyme system is important for drug deactivation and for some types of drug interactions.

- Drug tolerance can result from changes in distribution and elimination, from behavioral adaptations, or from changes in the responsiveness of the nervous system caused by compensatory (homeostatic) mechanisms. Physical dependence (withdrawal) can be a consequence of this last type of tolerance.

Review Questions

1. Morton's makes table salt, also known as sodium chloride. What is the chemical name, what is the generic name, and what is the brand name?
2. Into which major category does each of these drugs fall: heroin, cocaine, alcohol, LSD, Prozac?
3. Why might nonspecific factors influence psychoactive drug effects more than the effect of an antibiotic?
4. Why should LD_{50} always be greater than ED_{50}?
5. Why do people say that LSD is one of the most potent psychoactive drugs?
6. Which route of administration gets a drug to the brain most quickly?
7. If an elderly person has less protein in the blood than a younger person, how would you adjust the dose of a drug that has high protein binding?
8. How might two drugs interact with each other through actions on the CYP450 enzyme system?
9. Which type of tolerance is related to physical dependence, and why?

References

1. *Industry Profile 2005*. Washington, DC: Pharmaceutical Research and Manufacturing Association.
2. *Physician's Desk Reference*. Oradell, NJ: Medical Economics Company.
3. Kirsch, I., T.J. Moore, A. Scoboria, and S.S. Nicholls. "The Emperor's New Drugs: An Analysis of Antidepressant Medication Data Submitted to the U.S. Food and Drug Administration." *Prevention & Treatment* 5 (2002), p. 23.
4. Gottlieb, S. "Placebo Response Not All in the Mind." *The Scientist*, January 11, 2002.
5. Hu, H., & M. Wu. "Mechanism of Anesthetic Action: Oxygen Pathway Perturbation Hypothesis." *Medical Hypotheses* 57 (2001), p. 619.

Check Yourself

How Do Drugs Work?

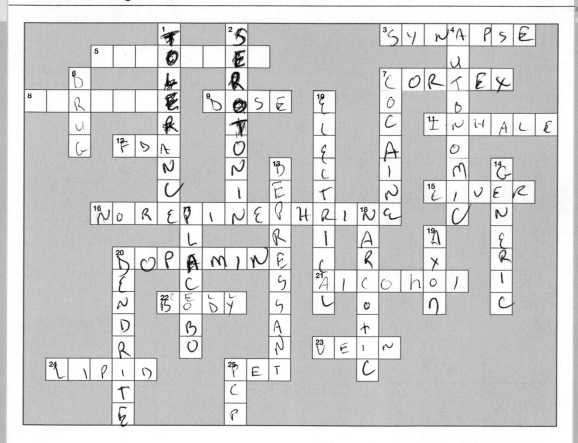

ACROSS

3. Space between two neurons
5. Cause for tobacco dependence
7. Brain part for integration of information, planning
8. Chemical signal carried through the blood
9. Amount of drug given
11. Fastest way to get a drug to the brain
12. Agency responsible for regulating pharmaceuticals
15. Where most drugs are broken down
16. Transmitter in the sympathetic branch
20. Transmitter in the mesolimbic system
21. Most widely used depressant
22. Axons, dendrites are part of the nerve _____.
23. Most rapid method of injection is into a _____.
24. Potent CNS drugs must be _____ soluble.
25. Type of modern brain scan using radioactive chemicals

DOWN

1. Reduced effect of a drug after repeated use
2. Opiate-like substance found in the brain
4. Nervous system controlling heart, pupils of the eye, etc.
6. Chemical that affects a living organism
7. Powerful stimulant derived from a South American plant
10. An _____ signal travels along the axon.
13. Drug that makes you drowsy, drunk, uncoordinated
14. Drug name used by several companies
17. Inactive or "fake" drug
18. Opium, morphine, heroin, etc.
19. Neuron part that carries electrical signals to the terminals
20. Neuron part that picks up signals from other neurons
25. Hallucinogen sometimes smoked on marijuana

Uppers and Downers

We start our review of drugs by studying two types that have straightforward actions on behavior. Stimulants generally excite the central nervous system, whereas depressants generally inhibit it. In Section Three, we find that most drugs used in treating mental disorders are not simply uppers or downers—their action is more complicated. However, this can best be appreciated by comparing them with the stimulants and depressants. Antidepressant drugs, used in treating psychological depression, are not stimulants. When taken for several weeks they can help raise a depressed mood into the normal range, but they don't produce excited, sleepless effects as stimulants do. Likewise, the tranquilizers used in treating psychotic behavior are not depressants and do not always produce the drowsiness that sedatives and sleeping pills do.

6 Stimulants
How do the stimulant drugs, cocaine and amphetamines, act on the body?

7 Depressants and Inhalants
How do the depressants work as sedatives and hypnotics?

8 Medication for Mental Disorders
Which drugs are used in treatment of depression, schizophrenia, and other mental disorders?

6

Stimulants

Objectives

When you have finished this chapter, you should be able to:

- Discuss the history of cocaine and amphetamine use and how their rates of use are related.

- Describe how cocaine hydrochloride and crack cocaine are processed from coca.

- Describe early psychiatric uses of cocaine and its current use for local anesthesia.

- Explain the concerns about the selective racial impact of federal sentencing requirements for crack vs. powder cocaine.

- Compare and contrast the mechanism of action and route of administration of cocaine and amphetamine.

- Discuss the dependence potential of cocaine and amphetamines.

- Compare and contrast the supply sources for illicit cocaine and illicit methamphetamine.

- Compare the chemical structure of amphetamine to the catecholamine neurotransmitters and to ephedrine.

- Discuss the medical uses and names of new stimulant drugs.

- Compare and contrast acute and chronic toxicity concerns associated with cocaine and amphetamines.

Stimulants are the drugs that can keep you going, both mentally and physically, when you should be tired. There have been lots of claims about the other things these drugs can do for (and to) people. Do they really make you smarter, faster, or stronger? Can they sober you up? Improve your sex life? Do they produce dependence?

We can divide the stimulants somewhat arbitrarily: The readily available stimulants nicotine and caffeine are discussed in Chapters 10 and 11, and the restricted stimulants cocaine and the amphetamines are covered in this chapter. Since the widespread introduction of cocaine into Western Europe and the United States in the 19th century, a fair-sized minority of individuals has always been committed to the regular recreational use of the stimulants, but neither cocaine nor the amphetamines have ever achieved widespread social acceptance as recreational drugs.

Cocaine

History

The origin of the earliest civilization in the Americas, the beginning around 5000 B.C. of what was to become the Inca Empire in Peru, has been traced to the use of **coca.** Natives of

Online Learning Center Resources

www.mhhe.com/ksir12e

Visit our Online Learning Center (OLC) for access to these study aids and additional resources

- Learning objectives
- Glossary flashcards
- Web activities and links
- Self-scoring chapter quiz
- Audio chapter summaries

the Andes mountains in Bolivia and Peru today still use coca as their ancestors did: chewing the leaves and holding a ball of coca leaf almost continually in the mouth. The freedom from fatigue provided by the drug is legendary in allowing these natives to run or to carry large bundles great distances over high mountain trails. The psychoactive effects can be made stronger by adding some calcified lime to raise the alkalinity inside the mouth—this increases the extraction of **cocaine** and allows greater absorption into the blood supplying the inside of the mouth. It appears that humans in the Andes first settled down and formed communities around places where this calcified lime could be mined.[1] Eventually they took up the planting and harvesting of crops in the nearby fields—and one of those important crops was, of course, coca.

The terrain of the Andes in Bolivia and Peru is poorly suited for growing almost everything. *Erythroxylon coca,* however, seems to thrive at elevations of 2,000 to 8,000 feet (600 to 2,400 meters) on the Amazon slope of the mountains, where more than 100 inches (254 centimeters) of rain fall annually. The shrub is pruned to prevent it from reaching the normal height of six to eight feet (1.8 to 2.4 meters), so that the picking, which is done three or four times a year, is easier to accomplish. The shrubs are grown in small, two- to three-acre patches called cocals, some of which are known to have been under cultivation for over 800 years.

Before the 16th-century invasion by Pizarro, the Incas had built a well-developed civilization in Peru. The coca leaf was an important part of the culture, and although earlier use was primarily in religious ceremonies, coca was treated as money by the time the conquistadors arrived. The Spanish adopted this custom and paid coca leaves to the native laborers for mining and transporting gold and silver. Even then the leaf was recognized as increasing strength and endurance while decreasing the need for food.

Early European chroniclers of the Incan civilization reported on the unique qualities of this plant, but it never interested Europeans until the last half of the 19th century. At that time the coca leaf contributed to the economic well-being and fame of three individuals. They, in turn, brought the Peruvian shrub to the notice of the world.

Coca Wine

The first of the individuals was Angelo Mariani, a French chemist. His contribution was to introduce the coca leaf indirectly to the general public. Mariani imported tons of coca leaves and used an extract from them in many products. You could suck on a coca lozenge, drink coca tea, or obtain the coca leaf extract in any of a large number of other products. It was Mariani's coca wine, though, that made him rich and famous. Assuredly, it had to be the coca leaf extract in the wine that prompted the pope to present a medal of appreciation to Mariani. Not only the pope but also royalty and the general public benefited from the Andean plant. For them, as it had for the Incas for a thousand years and was to do for Americans who drank early versions of Coca-Cola (see Chapter 11), the extract of the coca leaf lifted their spirits, freed them from fatigue, and gave them a generally good feeling.

coca: a bush that grows in the Andes and produces cocaine.
cocaine: the active chemical in the coca plant.

Drugs in the Media

The Drug War in Tulia: Aberration or Representative?

On the morning of July 23, 1999, 46 alleged cocaine dealers were arrested in Tulia, Texas, a desolate town of about 5,000 residents located in the Texas panhandle. Each suspect was charged with selling varying amounts of cocaine to Officer Tom Coleman, the agent who single-handedly conducted the 18-month undercover investigation. This was the biggest drug bust in Swisher County's history. On the morning of the arrests, Agent Coleman and other town law enforcement officials notified the local media to publicize the event. This public display is a common practice for many law enforcement agencies throughout the United States. Publicizing such major drug busts serves at least two functions: (1) it highlights the extent of the apparent drug problem, thereby justifying the allocation of funds to decrease the problem; and (2) it demonstrates the effectiveness of the enforcement strategies employed.

As half-clothed and disheveled arrestees were awakened and paraded in front of television cameras, a few things quickly became apparent. The overwhelming majority was poor and black. In fact, 40 of those arrested were black, comprising almost 15 percent of the town's black population. The remaining six defendants were either Hispanic or had an intimate relationship with a black person. No drugs, money, or weapons were confiscated during the early-morning raids. Despite this, the headline in the local newspaper, the *Tulia Sentinel,* read: "Tulia's Streets

Cleared of Garbage." This seemed to be the sentiment of many Tulia residents. Another article in the defunct paper quoted a local resident as saying, "We don't like these scumbags doing business in our town."

The stage was now set for the trials. Nearly all-white juries (only one juror was black) quickly convicted the first eight defendants in separate trials. The penalties were severe, ranging from 20 to 341 years in prison, even though the convictions were based solely on the uncorroborated and unsubstantiated testimony of Agent Coleman, who is white. He wore no wire, recorded no video or still images of illicit activity, and had no partner to support his story. The only record of the alleged drug deals were notes of names, times, dates, and places that Agent Coleman had scrawled on his leg. Joe Moore, a 60-year-old hog farmer who lived in a one-room shack, described by authorities as Tulia's drug kingpin, was one of the first individuals convicted, receiving a sentence of 90 years. On July 29, 2002, writing in *The New York Times,* Bob Herbert noted, "If these were major cocaine dealers, as alleged, they were among the oddest in the U.S. None of them had any money to speak of." Awaiting trial and watching the number of convictions accumulate, many of the defendants, all of them poor, decided to accept plea bargains in

continued

Local Anesthesia

Coca leaves contain, besides the oils that give them flavor, the active chemical cocaine (up to almost 2 percent). Cocaine was isolated before 1860, but there is still debate over who did it first and exactly when. Simple and inexpensive processing of 500 kilograms of coca leaves yields 1 kilogram of cocaine. An available supply of pure cocaine and the newly developed hypodermic syringe improved the drug delivery system, and in the 1880s physicians began to experiment with it. In the United States, the second famous cocaine proponent, Dr. W. S. Halsted, who was later referred to as "the father of modern surgery," experimented with the ability of cocaine to produce local anesthesia.

Early Psychiatric Uses

The third famous individual to encourage cocaine use was a young Viennese physician named Sigmund Freud, who studied the drug for its potential as a treatment medication in a variety of ailments including depression and morphine dependence. In 1884, Freud wrote to his fiancée that he had been experimenting with "a magical drug." He wrote, "If it goes

Drugs in the Media

The Drug War in Tulia: Aberration or Representative?—*continued*

hopes of receiving lesser sentences. They were given sentences ranging from one year of probation to 18 years in prison, and in August 1999, Agent Coleman was given the Texas Lawman of the Year award.

All of the cases, however, did not result in convictions. And a few cases began to raise suspicions about Agent Coleman's integrity. The case against Billy Wafer was dismissed when he presented time cards showing he was at work at the same time that Agent Coleman testified Mr. Wafer was selling him cocaine. Tonya White's case was also dismissed when she provided a time-stamped bank record demonstrating that she was more than 300 miles away in Oklahoma City when Agent Coleman swore she was selling him cocaine. Reports began surfacing about Agent Coleman's less than honorable past. In 1996, Sheriff Ken Burke, his former employer, wrote a letter of complaint to the Texas Commission on Law Enforcement in which he stated, "Mr. Coleman should not be in law enforcement," because he had left his previous law enforcement job abruptly without paying thousands of dollars owed to local merchants. Moreover, Agent Coleman was arrested in the middle of his Tulia investigation for abuse of official capacity and theft in his previous job. The arresting officer, Agent Coleman's current employer, Sheriff Larry Stewart, permitted him to continue his undercover cocaine operations in Tulia.

As knowledge of the above events became more widely known, the national and international media began focusing on the Tulia arrests, thereby drawing further attention to this issue. The CBS news show, "60 Minutes;" the PBS show "Now with Bill Moyers;" and the BBC News all produced television stories about the events, while Bob Herbert wrote at least five editorials in *The New York Times*. In one such piece, Herbert wrote, "The idea that people could be rounded up and sent away for what are effectively lifetime terms solely on the word of a police officer like Tom Coleman is insane." Texas Governor Rick Perry agreed. On August 22, 2003, he pardoned 35 individuals who were arrested during the drug sting, noting, "Questions surrounding testimony from the key witness in these cases weighed heavily on my final decision." Of the remaining 11 individuals who were not pardoned, seven had their cases dismissed before trial, two were on probation at the time of their arrests and so were ineligible for pardons, one's conviction was not final, and one had died. Agent Coleman was found guilty of perjury charges and was sentenced to 7 years of probation.

While some contend that the Tulia undercover drug operation was an extreme aberration of the war on drugs, others argue that these events are representative of U.S. drug policies that target people of color disproportionately. Do you think the events of Tulia raise serious concerns about the current drug war? Is the drug war unfairly targeting people of color?

---

well I will write an essay on it and I expect it will win its place in therapeutics by the side of morphium, and superior to it. . . . I take very small doses of it regularly against depression and against indigestion, and with the most brilliant success." He urged his fiancée, his sisters, his colleagues, and his friends to try it, extolling the drug as a safe exhilarant, which he himself used and recommended as a treatment for morphine dependence. For emphasis he wrote in italics, "*inebriate asylums can be entirely dispensed with.*"[2]

In an 1885 lecture before a group of psychiatrists, Freud commented on the use of cocaine as a stimulant, saying, "On the whole it must be said that the value of cocaine in psychiatric practice remains to be demonstrated, and it will probably be worthwhile to make a thorough trial as soon as the currently exorbitant price of the drug becomes more reasonable"—the first of the consumer advocates!

Freud was more convinced about another use of the drug, however, and in the same lecture said,

> We can speak more definitely about another use of cocaine by the psychiatrist. It was first discovered in America that cocaine is capable of alleviating the serious withdrawal symptoms

observed in subjects who are abstaining from morphine and of suppressing their craving for morphine. . . . On the basis of my experiences with the effects of cocaine, I have no hesitation in recommending the administration of cocaine for such withdrawal cures in subcutaneous injections of 0.03–0.05 g per dose, without any fear of increasing the dose. On several occasions, I have even seen cocaine quickly eliminate the manifestations of intolerance that appeared after a rather large dose of morphine, as if it had a specific ability to counteract morphine.[3]

Even great people make mistakes. The realities of life were harshly brought home to Freud when he used cocaine to treat a close friend, Fleischl, to remove his dependence on morphine. Increasingly larger doses were needed, and eventually Freud spent a frightful night nursing Fleischl through an episode of cocaine psychosis. After that experience he generally opposed the use of drugs in the treatment of psychological problems.

Besides Mariani, Halsted, and Freud, one well-known fictional character revealed that the psychological effects of cocaine, both the initial stimulation and the later depression, had been well appreciated by 1890:

> Sherlock Holmes took his bottle from the corner of the mantelpiece, and his hypodermic syringe from its neat morocco case. With his long, white nervous fingers, he adjusted the delicate needle and rolled back his left shirtcuff. For some little time his eyes rested thoughtfully upon the sinewy forearm and wrist, all dotted and scarred with innumerable puncture-marks. Finally, he thrust the sharp point home, pressed down the tiny piston, and sank back into the velvet-lined armchair with a long sigh of satisfaction.
>
> Three times a day for many months I had witnessed this performance, but custom had not reconciled my mind to it. . . .
>
> "Which is it today," I asked, "Morphine or cocaine?"
>
> He raised his eyes languidly from the old black-letter volume which he had opened.
>
> "It is cocaine," he said, "a seven-per-cent solution. Would you care to try it?"

> "No, indeed," I answered brusquely. "My constitution has not got over the Afghan campaign yet. I cannot afford to throw any extra strain upon it."
>
> He smiled at my vehemence. "Perhaps you are right, Watson," he said. "I suppose that its influence is physically a bad one. I find it, however, so transcendently stimulating and clarifying to the mind that its secondary action is a matter of small moment."[4]

Although physicians were well aware of the dangers of using cocaine regularly, nonmedical and quasimedical use of cocaine was widespread in the United States around the start of the 20th century. It was one of the secret ingredients in many patent medicines and elixirs but was also openly advertised as having beneficial effects. The Parke-Davis Pharmaceutical Company noted in 1885 that cocaine "can supply the place of food, make the coward brave, and silent eloquent" and called it a "wonder drug."[5]

Early Legal Controls on Cocaine

With so much going for cocaine, and its availability in a large number of products for drinking, snorting, or injection, it may seem strange that, between 1887 and 1914, 46 states passed laws to regulate the use and distribution of cocaine. One historian provided extensive documentation and concluded

> All the elements needed to insure cocaine's outlaw status were present by the first years of the 20th century: it had become widely used as a pleasure drug, and doctors warned of the dangers attendant on indiscriminate sale and use; it had become identified with despised or poorly regarded groups—blacks, lower-class whites, and criminals; it had not been long enough established in the culture to insure its survival; and it had not, though used by them, become identified with the elite, thus losing what little chance it had of weathering the storm of criticism.[6]

Although many articles were written, both in the popular press and medical journals, solidifying the association of cocaine use with one "despised" group, blacks, a 1914 *New York Times* article entitled "Negro Cocaine 'Fiends' are a New Southern Menace" summarized the fears expressed by many whites.[7] The article's author made several unsubstantiated assertions, including: (1) rates of cocaine use by blacks in the South had reached epidemic proportions, and as a result, the South was experiencing psychiatric hospital admissions at record rates; (2) cocaine increased "homicidal tendencies" and improved marksmanship among blacks (he wrote: "a cocaine nigger* near Ashville dropped five men dead in their tracks, using only one cartridge for each . . . the deadly accuracy of the cocaine user has become axiomatic in Southern police circles"); and (3) cocaine made blacks almost unaffected by mere .32-caliber bullets. He wrote, "Knowing that he must kill the man or be killed himself, the Chief drew his revolver, placed the muzzle over the negro's heart, and fired—'intending to kill him right quick.' As the officer tells it. But the shot did not even stagger the man. And a second shot that pierced the arm and entered the chest had just as little effect in stopping the negro or checking his attack." The author concluded by stating that such incidences provided the impetus for Southern police departments to switch to the more powerful .38-caliber revolvers. Despite the questionable veracity of such accounts, they were recounted often, even at the highest levels of government. During congressional hearings regarding the control of cocaine and opium, for instance, a report from President Taft was read: "It has been authoritatively stated that cocaine is often the direct incentive to the crime of rape by the negroes of the South . . . the cocaine vice, the most serious that has to be dealt with, has proved to be a creator of criminals and unusual forms of violence, and it has been a potent incentive in driving the humbler negroes all over the country to abnormal crimes."[8]

*This word was used in the original *New York Times* article, and is included here only to convey accurately the emotional tone of that article.

Such negative publicity was a major influence on the passage of the 1914 Harrison Act, which taxed the importation and sale of coca and cocaine along with opium.

Not that cocaine went away: It was sometimes mixed with heroin and injected intravenously (the combination was called a "speedball"), and some of the carefree and wealthy young people of the era dabbled in its use. "Cocaine Lil," a song written in the 1920s, included the line "Lil went to a 'snow' party one cold night, and the way she sniffed was sure a fright." Cole Porter's "I Get a Kick Out of You" in 1934 originally contained the verse:

> I get no kick from cocaine
> I'm sure that if
> I took even one sniff
> It would bore me terrifically too
> But I get a kick out of you.

Forms of Cocaine

As was pointed out in Chapter 1, it is important to understand *how* a drug is taken when determining the potential effects of that drug. This issue has spurred intense debates on the fairness of the U.S. cocaine sentencing policy.

As a part of the process of making illicit cocaine, the coca leaves are mixed with an organic solvent, such as kerosene or gasoline. After thorough soaking, mixing, and mashing, the excess liquid is filtered out to form a substance known as **coca paste.** In South America, this paste is often mixed with tobacco and smoked. The paste can be made into **cocaine hydrochloride,** a salt that mixes easily in water and is so stable that it cannot be heated to form vapors for inhalation. Recreational users of this form of cocaine either "snort" (sniff) or inject the drug intravenously. Some users who

coca paste: a crude extract containing cocaine in a smokable form.
cocaine hydrochloride: the most common form of pure cocaine, it is stable and water soluble.

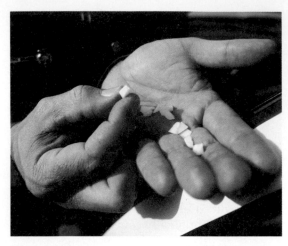

Crack cocaine.

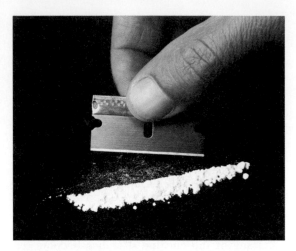

Cocaine in powdered form.

wanted to smoke cocaine used to convert it into **freebase** by extracting it into a volatile organic solvent, such as ether. The freebase can be heated and the vapors inhaled. This method of smoking cocaine can be very dangerous because the combination of fire and ether fumes is extremely explosive. The popularity of this form of freebasing began to decline in the early 1980s when it was discovered that mixing cocaine with simple household chemicals, including baking soda and water, and then drying it resulted in a lump of smokable cocaine (**crack** or **rock**).

Contemporary Legal Controls on Cocaine

Little concern was given to cocaine until the end of the 1960s when amphetamines became harder to obtain, and cocaine use again began to increase. As had occurred nearly a century before, the virtues of cocaine were now being touted by a number of individuals, ranging from physicians to celebrities. America's second era of flirtation with cocaine was under way. In 1974, psychiatrist Peter Bourne, who would soon become President Jimmy Carter's chief drug advisor, wrote, "Cocaine . . . is probably the most benign of illicit drugs currently in widespread use. At least as strong a case could be made for legalizing it as for legalizing mari-

juana. Short acting—about 15 minutes—not physically addicting, and acutely pleasurable, cocaine has found increasing favor at all socioeconomic levels in the last year."[9] A respected psychiatrist, writing in a premier psychiatric text echoed the above remarks: "Used no more than two or three times a week, cocaine creates no serious problems. . . . Daily in fairly large amounts it can . . . produce minor psychological disturbance. . . . Chronic cocaine abuse does not usually appear as a medical problem."[10] These endorsements of cocaine use bore a striking resemblance to those of Sigmund Freud in 1884, who wrote in his famous essay titled, "Über Coca," "Opinion is unanimous that the euphoria induced by coca is not followed by any feeling of lassitude or other state of depression. . . . It seems probable . . . that coca, if used protractedly but in moderation, is not detrimental to the body."[11] Had we forgotten our experience with cocaine a century earlier? If so, it wouldn't take long for Americans to become alarmed.

Cocaine use before 1985 had come to symbolize wealth and fame, in part, because street sales of the drug were mainly in the hydrochloride form in quantities that made the price relatively expensive. As a result, those with substantial amounts of discretionary income comprised the primary consumer base.

Because a convenient method for smoking cocaine was not yet widely available, the overwhelmingly majority of these individuals snorted cocaine. The abuse potential of snorted cocaine is lower than that of smoked cocaine or intravenous cocaine. The infrequent use of smoked cocaine changed in the mid- to late-1980s when enterprising dealers began selling smokable cocaine in the form of crack. The cocaine experience was now available to anyone with $5 to $10, a lighter, a glass pipe, and access to a dealer. With the availability of a seemingly cheaper form of cocaine, use increased among some groups. Because the majority of crack cocaine sold by street-level dealers is considerably adulterated, it is actually more expensive than powder cocaine.

The media focus on cocaine, especially the use of crack cocaine by black urbanites, dramatically intensified. In the months leading up to the 1986 congressional elections, more than 1,000 stories appeared about cocaine in the national media, including five cover stories in *Time* and *Newsweek*.[12] Although the language had been tempered, the message was clear and similar to that of a century earlier: (1) cocaine use was widespread; (2) cocaine caused people to engage in violent behavior; and (3) cocaine produced an unparalleled dependency, one that was nearly impossible to overcome.

By the summer of 1986, Americans believed that substance abuse in general, and smoked cocaine in particular, had become a problem of overwhelming dimensions and something had to be done. Congress responded by passing the Anti-Drug Abuse Act of 1986. Ostensibly, this law targeted high-level crack cocaine dealers and manufacturers (kingpins). It created a 100:1 quantity ratio between the amounts of powder cocaine and crack needed to trigger certain mandatory minimum sentences for trafficking cocaine. That is, an individual convicted of selling five grams of crack cocaine would be required to serve a *minimum* sentence of five years in prison. To receive the same sentence for trafficking in powder cocaine, that individual would need to possess 500 grams of cocaine—100 times the 5 gram crack cocaine amount. Two years later the Anti-Drug Abuse Act of 1988 was passed, which extended the five-year minimum penalty to individuals convicted of possession of five grams of crack cocaine, including first-time offenders. Simple possession of any other illicit drug, including powder cocaine, by a first-time offender carries a *maximum* penalty of one year in prison.

In recent years, these laws have been criticized extensively because of the belief that they have had selective effects on black communities. In response to increasing concerns about the resulting number of black Americans incarcerated, the U.S. Sentencing Commission studied this issue and released its findings to Congress in 1995, 1997, and 2002.[13] The findings can be summarized as the following: (1) the current penalties exaggerate the relative harmfulness of crack cocaine; (2) current penalties sweep too broadly and apply most often to lower-level offenders; (3) current quantity-based penalties overstate the seriousness of most crack cocaine offenses and fail to provide adequate proportionality; and (4) current penalties' severity mostly impacts blacks (see Table 6.1).

Congress has failed to act on any of the commission's recommendations. At the time of this writing, no changes have been made to the federal cocaine sentencing policy.

Mechanism of Action

The chemical structure of cocaine is shown in Figure 6.1. This is a fairly complicated molecule, which doesn't resemble any of the known transmitters in an obvious way. In fact, the

---

freebase: a method of preparing cocaine as a chemical base so that it can be smoked.
crack: a street name for simple and stable preparation of cocaine base for smoking.
rock: another name for crack.

Table 6.1
Racial Characteristics of Federal Cocaine Offenders

	1992		2000	
	Number	**Percent**	**Number**	**Percent**
Powder cocaine				
Black	1,778	27.2%	1,596	30.5%
Hispanic	2,601	39.8	2,662	50.8
White	2,113	32.3	932	17.8
Other	44	0.7	49	0.9
Crack cocaine				
Black	2,096	91.4%	4,069	84.7%
Hispanic	121	5.3	434	9.0
White	74	3.2	269	5.6
Other	3	0.1	33	0.7

Source: U.S. Sentencing Commission, *Report to Congress: Cocaine and Federal Sentencing Policy,* May 2002.

structure of cocaine doesn't give us much help at all in understanding how the drug works on the brain.

The more we learn about cocaine's effects on the brain, the more complex the drug's actions seem. Cocaine blocks the reuptake of dopamine, norepinephrine, and serotonin, causing a prolonged effect of these neurotransmitters. The observation that the blockage of dopamine receptors or the destruction of dopamine-containing neurons lessened the amount of cocaine that laboratory animals self-administered led many cocaine researchers to focus on dopamine neurons. After several years of intense scientific research, enthusiasm regarding dopamine's exclusive role in cocaine-related behaviors has been tempered, in part, because drugs that block only dopamine reuptake do not produce the same behavioral effects as cocaine. Additionally, these drugs have been unsuccessful in treating cocaine dependence. Because cocaine is a complex drug, affecting many neurotransmitters, the latest bet is that cocaine's behavioral effects depend on an interaction of multiple neurotransmitters, including dopamine, serotonin, GABA, and glutamate.[14]

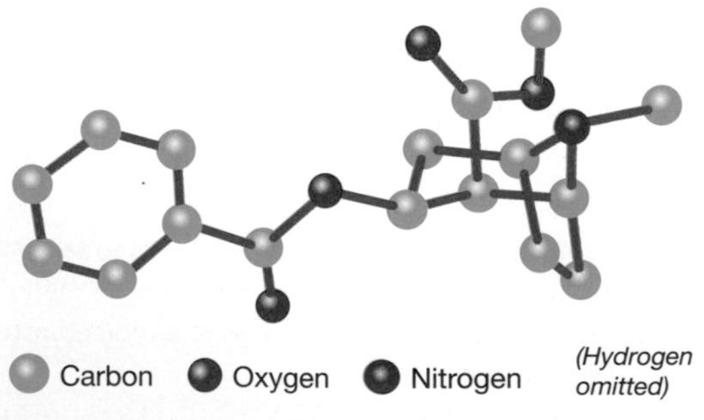

Absorption and Elimination

People can, and do, use cocaine in many ways. Chewing and sucking the leaves allows the cocaine to be absorbed slowly through the mucous membranes. This results in a slower onset of effects and much lower blood levels than are usually obtained via snorting, the most common route by which the drug is used recreationally.

Carbon   Oxygen   Nitrogen   *(Hydrogen omitted)*

Figure 6.1   Cocaine

In snorting, the intent is to get the very fine cocaine hydrochloride powder high into the nasal passages—right on the nasal mucosa. From there it is absorbed quite rapidly and, through circulatory mechanisms that are not completely understood, reaches the brain rather quickly.

The intravenous use of cocaine delivers a very high concentration to the brain, producing a rapid and brief effect. For that reason, intravenous cocaine used to be a favorite among compulsive users, many of whom switched from intranasal to intravenous use. However, the smoking of crack is now preferred by most compulsive users because this route is less invasive (no needles) and the onset of its effects is just as fast.

The cocaine molecules are metabolized by enzymes in the blood and liver, and the activity of these enzymes is variable from one person to another. In any case, cocaine itself is rapidly removed, with a half-life of about one hour. The major metabolites, which are the basis of urine screening tests, have a longer half-life of about eight hours.

Beneficial Uses

Local Anesthesia The local anesthetic properties of cocaine—its ability to numb the area to which it is applied—were discovered in 1860 soon after its isolation from coca leaves. It was not until 1884 that this characteristic was used medically; the early applications were in eye surgery and dentistry. The use of cocaine spread rapidly because it apparently was a safe and effective drug. The potential for misuse soon became clear, though, and a search began for synthetic agents with similar anesthetic characteristics but little or no potential for misuse. This work was rewarded in 1905 with the discovery of procaine (Novocain), which is still in wide use.

Many drugs have been synthesized since 1905 that have local anesthetic properties similar to those of cocaine but have little or no ability to produce CNS stimulation. Those

drugs have largely replaced cocaine for medical use. However, because cocaine is absorbed so well into mucous membranes, it remains in use for surgery in the nasal, laryngeal, and esophageal regions.

Other Claimed Benefits Because cocaine produces a feeling of increased energy and well-being, it enjoyed an important status among achievers of the 1980s who self-prescribed it to overcome fatigue. Many athletes and entertainers felt that they could not consistently perform at their peak without the assistance of cocaine, and this resulted in increased cocaine use among these groups. Cocaine has not been used medically for its CNS effects for many years, in part because its effects are brief, but mostly because of concern about the development of dependence.

Causes for Concern

Acute Toxicity There is no evidence that occasional use of small amounts of cocaine is a threat to the individual's health. However, many people have increased the amount they use to the point of toxicity. Acute cocaine poisoning leads to profound CNS stimulation, progressing to convulsions, which can lead to respiratory or cardiac arrest. This is in some ways similar to amphetamine overdose, with the exception that there is much greater individual variation in the uptake and metabolism of cocaine, so that a lethal dose is much more difficult to estimate. In addition, there are very rare, severe, and unpredictable toxic reactions to cocaine and other local anesthetics, in which individuals die rapidly, apparently from cardiac failure. Cocaine can trigger the chaotic heart rhythm called ventricular fibrillation by preventing the vagus nerve from controlling the heartbeat.[15] Intravenous cocaine users might also experience an allergic reaction either to the drug or to some additive in street cocaine. The lungs fill rapidly with fluid, and death can occur.

It was reported in 1992 that the combination of cocaine and alcohol (ethanol) in the body could result in the formation of a chemical called **cocaethylene,** which was subsequently shown to be more toxic than cocaine in mice. However, this finding is inconsistent with results from studies that have compared the effects of cocaine and cocaethylene in humans. These studies have shown that cocaethylene is less potent than cocaine with respect to its cardiovascular and subjective effects.[16]

Chronic Toxicity

Regularly snorting cocaine, and particularly cocaine that has been "cut" with other things, can irritate the nasal septum, leading to a chronically inflamed, runny nose. Use of cocaine in a binge, during which the drug is taken repeatedly and at increasingly high doses, can lead to a state of increasing irritability, restlessness, and paranoia. In severe cases, this can result in a full-blown paranoid psychosis, in which the individual loses touch with reality and experiences auditory hallucinations.[17] This experience is disruptive and quite frightening. However, most individuals seem to recover from the psychosis as the drug leaves the system.

There has been concern for several years about the effects of chronic cocaine use on the heart muscle. It appears that, in some users, frequent, brief disruption of the heart's function can damage the heart muscle itself.[18] It is not clear how often such damage occurs.

Dependence Potential Cocaine can produce dependence in some users, particularly among those who inject it or inhale the vapors of smokable cocaine. This phenomenon is substantiated by the fact that cocaine accounts for the largest proportion of admissions for drug treatment in most major U.S. cities.[19] Additionally, in laboratory experiments, human research volunteers will perform rigorous tasks in order to receive a dose of cocaine.[20] Virtually every species of laboratory animal, when given the opportunity, will readily self-administer

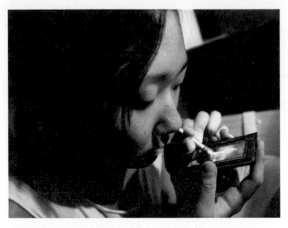

Regularly snorting cocaine can irritate the nasal septum, cause psychological effects including paranoia, and damage the heart muscle.

cocaine and if given unlimited access to cocaine they will self-administer the drug until their eventual death.[21] Thus, it appears that cocaine can be a powerfully reinforcing drug: Take it and it will make you want to take it again.

Throughout the 1970s, the importance of this dependence potential went unrecognized, partly because cocaine was expensive and in short supply and largely because the only common method of using cocaine during this time was snorting it. The 1980s saw an increase in freebasing and then of the more convenient form of smokable cocaine, crack or rock. As relatively large numbers of people began to smoke cocaine in the mid-1980s, the dependence potential of this form of use became clear to the American public and to the users themselves.

Because at one time drug dependence was linked to the presence of physical withdrawal symptoms (when the abused substance was removed), a number of experiments have studied whether physical withdrawal symptoms appear upon abrupt cessation after repeated cocaine use. After prolonged daily cocaine administration in animals, there were no obvious withdrawal signs (for example, no diarrhea or convulsions), and many scientists concluded that cocaine produces no physical dependence and is therefore not a dependence-producing drug. More recent experience has led to a different way of looking at this issue. Abuse potential of a drug is no longer defined solely by the presence of physical withdrawal symptoms during drug abstinence. As was discussed in Chapter 2, a person may be diagnosed with a cocaine use disorder if he or she exhibits a set of maladaptive behaviors listed in the *DSM-IV-TR,* which may or may not include physical withdrawal symptoms. Following several days of cocaine use (a binge), a constellation of withdrawal symptoms may be present, including cocaine craving, irritability, anxiety, depressed mood, increased appetite, and exhaustion. However, these symptoms vary greatly among individuals, with some individuals exhibiting little or no symptoms.

Reproductive Effects Early reports of babies being born under the influence of cocaine resulted in lurid media accounts of the "crack baby" phenomenon, which unfortunately overstated both the number of such children (see the Drugs in the Media, Chapter 2) and the expected long-term effects. However, more recent data from well-controlled human studies indicate that, among children six years old and younger, there are no consistent negative associations between prenatal cocaine exposure and several developmental measures, including physical growth, test scores, and language.[22] The long-term effects of prenatal cocaine exposure on older children are less well known because limited data are available. Nevertheless, the use of cocaine during pregnancy is not recommended because of more immediate problems associated with cocaine use during pregnancy—the risk increases for both spontaneous abortions (miscarriages) and a torn placenta.

Supplies of Illicit Cocaine

Cocaine is readily available on the illicit market in all major U.S. metropolitan areas. The U.S. Drug Enforcement Administration develops annual estimates of the prices of these illicit drugs and their purity, both indicators of supply. Theoretically, if supplies become scarce, street prices will increase and the purity of seized samples will decrease as the available drug is diluted by street traffickers. Both measures vary widely from one place to another, so what is important is the annual trend in estimated average price and purity. Both price and purity have remained relatively stable for the past decade. A kilogram of cocaine sells for $13,000 to $25,000 in most U.S. cities, and the average purity of samples purchased or seized by DEA agents was 75 percent. As has been the case for many years, increased efforts to disrupt the supply of cocaine have been countered by changes in production and smuggling practices.[23]

Illicit cocaine comes to the United States primarily from three South American countries: Peru, Bolivia, and Colombia. Each year, more than 250,000 tons of coca leaf are produced in South America, enough to produce about 650 tons of cocaine hydrochloride. Bolivia typically produces about half as much coca as Peru, and Colombia somewhat less than Bolivia. In all of these countries, attempts to control production are complex: U.S. DEA agents assist local police, who may be in conflict with army units fighting against local guerrillas. Often the price and availability of coca in these countries are determined more by local politics than by the DEA's eradication and interdiction efforts. Although we might pay some farmers to grow alternative crops, the high profits from growing illicit cocaine draw others to plant new fields. An economic analysis of the impact of eradication efforts indicates that even the most successful projects result in at best only temporary shortages.[24]

> **cocaethylene (co cah *eth* eh leen):** a chemical formed when ethanol and cocaine are co-administered.

Large shipments of cocaine were traditionally routed by boat or plane to any of hundreds of islands in the Caribbean, and from there to Miami or other ports in the Eastern United States, again by small boat or airplane. Although sea routes continue to be important, the pressure brought by Navy, Air Force, and Coast Guard interdiction efforts has shifted trafficking somewhat more to land routes through Central America and Mexico. Now, more than half of the cocaine smuggled into the United States crosses the U.S.–Mexico border.

Current Patterns of Cocaine Use

Throughout the early 1980s, the national household survey conducted by the National Institute on Drug Abuse (NIDA) (see Chapter 1) found that 7 to 9 percent of young adults reported use of cocaine within the past month. In 2002, the comparable figure was less than 1 percent, and the use of cocaine had dropped significantly in the general population. Data from the Monitoring the Future study (Chapter 1) show that cocaine use decreased substantially among high school seniors between 1985 and 1994. Although the number reporting use increased somewhat during the mid-1990s, only about 3 percent now report use in the past year, compared to 12 percent at the peak of cocaine use in the early 1980s.

Cocaine's Future

In attempting to predict the future, we can learn from two writers who have made successful predictions about cocaine use in the past. The first, writing in the early 1970s, pointed out that historically, as cocaine use declined, amphetamine use increased. Looking at the decline in amphetamine use in the late 1960s, he predicted the increased use of cocaine that we saw in the 1970s and early 1980s.[25] The other writer[5] pointed out that at the height of cocaine use in 1986 we were reliving an earlier cycle of cocaine use that occurred around the start of the 20th century.

Targeting Prevention

Cocaine and Friendship

Imagine you have a good friend, Terry, who has been using cocaine off and on for a year. However, in the past couple of months it seems that Terry's use has become more and more frequent. You have had to stop lending her money because she never pays it back. When you hinted that her cocaine use might be getting out of hand, she did not respond. When you tried direct confrontation, she angrily denied that she had a problem. You are still good friends. You certainly don't want to turn Terry in to the police, but you are getting pretty worried. What do you think you should do?

There is no correct answer to this problem, but it might be interesting to discuss this hypothetical situation with a group of friends. Find out how they would want to be treated under the circumstances.

When cocaine was introduced in the 1880s, the experts had mostly positive opinions about its effects, and it was regarded as a fairly benign substance. In the second stage (1890s), more and more people used cocaine, and its dangers and side effects became well known. In the third stage, in the early 1900s, society turned against cocaine and passed laws to control it. After many years with little cocaine use, in the early 1970s the drug again had the reputation of being fairly benign and not capable of producing "real" dependence. In the 1980s, we were in the second stage, in which increasing use eventually made us all aware of the potential dangers. This comparison led to the prediction that Americans would again turn away from cocaine and would pass increased legal restrictions on it. This prediction came true during the late 1980s. Cocaine use increased slightly since then, but the more interesting story has been the reemergence of another illicit stimulant drug, amphetamine (and in particular, methamphetamine). Once again, it seems that as use of cocaine decreased, the market shifted somewhat toward amphetamines.

Amphetamines

History

Development and Early Uses For centuries the Chinese have made a medicinal tea from herbs they call *ma huang,* which American scientists classify in the genus *Ephedra.* The active ingredient in these herbs is called **ephedrine,** and it is used to dilate the bronchial passages in asthma patients. Bronchial dilation can be achieved by stimulating the sympathetic branch of the autonomic nervous system, and that is exactly what ephedrine does (it is referred to as a **sympathomimetic** drug). This drug also has other effects related to its sympathetic nervous system stimulation, such as elevating blood pressure. In the late 1920s, researchers synthesized and studied the effects of a new chemical that was similar in structure to ephedrine: **Amphetamine** was patented in 1932.

All major effects of amphetamine were discovered in the 1930s, although some of the uses were developed later. Amphetamine's first use was as a replacement for ephedrine in the treatment of asthma. Quite early it was shown that amphetamine was a potent dilator of the nasal and bronchial passages and could be efficiently delivered through inhalation. The Benzedrine (brand name) inhaler was introduced as an over-the-counter (OTC) product in 1932 for treating the stuffy noses caused by colds.

Some of the early work with amphetamine showed that the drug would awaken anesthetized dogs. As one writer put it, amphetamine is the drug that won't let sleeping dogs lie! This led to the testing of amphetamine for the treatment of **narcolepsy** in 1935. Narcolepsy is a condition in which the individual spontaneously falls asleep as many as 50 times a day. Amphetamine enables these patients to remain awake and function almost normally. In 1938, however, two narcolepsy patients treated with amphetamine developed acute *paranoid psychotic* reactions. The paranoid reaction to amphetamine has reappeared regularly and has been studied (discussed later in this chapter).

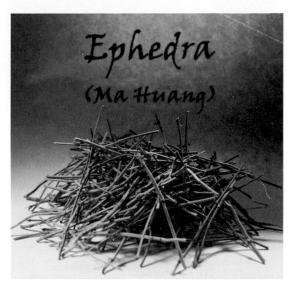

The active ingredient in the herb *ma huang* is ephedrine, which is chemically similar to amphetamine.

In 1937, amphetamine became available as a prescription tablet, and a report appeared in the literature suggesting that amphetamine, a stimulant, was effective in reducing activity in hyperactive children. Two years later, in 1939, notice was taken of a report by amphetamine-treated narcolepsy patients that they were not hungry when taking the drug. This *appetite-depressant* effect became the major clinical use of amphetamine. A group of psychology students at the University of Minnesota began experimenting with various drugs in 1937 and found that amphetamine was ideal for

ephedrine (eh *fed* rin): a sympathomimetic drug used in treating asthma.
sympathomimetic (sim path o mih *met* ick): a drug that stimulates the sympathetic branch of the autonomic nervous system.
amphetamine: a synthetic CNS stimulant and sympathomimetic.
narcolepsy: a disease that causes people to fall asleep suddenly.

"cramming," because it allowed them to stay awake for long periods of time. Truck drivers also noted this effect, and they used "bennies" to stay awake during long hauls.

Wartime Uses In 1939, amphetamine went to war. There were many reports that Germany was using amphetamines to increase the efficiency of its soldiers. Such statements provided the basis for other countries to evaluate the utility of amphetamines. A 1944 report in the *Air Surgeon's Bulletin,* titled "Benzedrine Alert," stated, "This drug is the most satisfactory of any available in temporarily postponing sleep when desire to sleep endangers the security of a mission."[26] Some early studies were reported, including one in which

> 100 Marines were kept active continuously for 60 hours in range firing, a 25-mile forced march, a field problem, calisthenics, close-order drill, games, fatigue detail and bivouac alerts. Fifty men received seven 10-milligram tablets of benzedrine at six hour intervals following the first day's activity. Meanwhile, the other 50 were given placebo (milk sugar) tablets. None knew what he was receiving. Participating officers concluded that the benzedrine definitely "pepped up" the subjects, improved their morale, reduced sleepiness and increased confidence in shooting ability. . . . It was observed that men receiving benzedrine tended to lead the march, tolerate their sore feet and blisters more cheerfully, and remain wide awake during "breaks," whereas members of the control group had to be shaken to keep them from sleeping.

Amphetamines were widely used in Japan during World War II to maintain production on the home front and to keep the fighting men going. To reduce large stockpiles of methamphetamine after the war, the drug was sold without prescription, and the drug companies advertised them for "elimination of drowsiness and repletion of the spirit." Such widespread use was accompanied by considerable overuse and abuse. In 1948 and again in 1955, strict amphetamine controls were enacted, along with treatment and education programs. Although the Japanese government claimed to have "eliminated" the amphetamine-abuse problem before 1960, there were smaller Japanese "epidemics" of methamphetamine use in the 1970s and 1980s.

The "Speed Scene" of the 1960s Most of the misuse of amphetamines until the 1960s was through the legally manufactured and legally purchased oral preparation. In 1963, the AMA Council on Drugs stated, "At this time, compulsive abuse of the amphetamines is a small problem."[27] But at exactly this time, trouble was brewing in California. It is difficult to pinpoint exactly when intravenous abuse of amphetamines began in the United States, but it was probably among IV users of heroin and cocaine. In the 1920s and 1930s, when IV use of those drugs was spreading among the drug subculture, the combination of heroin and cocaine injected together was known as the speedball, presumably because the cocaine rush or flash occurs rapidly after injection, thus speeding up the high. So, on the streets, one name for cocaine was "speed." When the amphetamines became so widely available after World War II, some of these enterprising individuals discovered that they could get an effect similar to that of cocaine if they injected amphetamine along with the heroin. Thus, amphetamines came to be known as **speed** by that small drug underground that used heroin intravenously. By the 1960s, amphetamines had become so widely available at such a low price that more IV drug users were using them, either in combination with heroin or alone. Although they were prescription drugs, it was not difficult to obtain a prescription to treat depression or obesity.

The most desired drug on the streets was methamphetamine, which was available in liquid form in ampules for injection. Hospital emergency rooms sometimes used this drug to stimulate respiration in patients suffering from overdoses of sleeping pills (no longer considered an appropriate treatment), and physicians also used injectable amphetamines intramuscularly to treat obesity. In the San Francisco Bay area, reports appeared in the early 1960s of "fat doctors" who had large numbers of patients coming in regularly for no treatment other than an injection of methamphetamine.

Because some heroin users would inject amphetamines alone when they could not obtain heroin, some physicians also felt that methamphetamine could serve as a legal substitute for heroin and thus be a form of treatment. In those days, amphetamines were not considered to produce dependancy, so these physicians were quite free with their prescriptions.[25] Reports of those abuses led to federal regulation of amphetamines within the new concept of dangerous drugs in the 1965 law. Unfortunately, the publicity associated with these revelations and the ensuing legislation caught the attention of young people whose identity as a generation was defined largely by experimentation with drugs their parents and government told them were dangerous. To the Haight-Ashbury district of San Francisco came the flower children, to sit in Golden Gate Park, smoke marijuana, take LSD, and discuss peace, love, and the brotherhood of humanity. They moved in next door to the old, established drug subculture, in which IV drug use was endemic. That mixture resulted in the speed scene and young people who became dependent on IV amphetamines. Although in historical perspective the speed scene of the late 1960s was relatively short-lived and only a small number of people were directly involved, it was the focus of a great deal of national concern, and it helped change the way the medical profession and society at large viewed these drugs, which had been so widely accepted.

As the abuse of amphetamines began to be recognized, physicians prescribed less and less of the drugs. Their new legal status as dangerous drugs put restrictions on prescriptions and refills, and in the 1970s the total amount of these drugs that could be manufactured was limited. Thus, within less than a decade, amphetamines went from being widely used and accepted pharmaceuticals to being less widely used, tightly restricted drugs associated in the public mind with drug-abusing hippies.

As controls tightened on legally manufactured amphetamines, at least three reactions continued to affect the drug scene. The first reaction was that a market began to develop for "look-alike" pills: legal, milder stimulants (usually caffeine or ephedrine) packaged in tablets and capsules that were virtually identical in color, shape, and markings to prescription amphetamines. Later the makers of look-alikes began to expand the variety of shapes and sizes to attract a wider market. Because these pills contained legally available, OTC ingredients, their sellers could not be prosecuted. By the early 1980s, the odds were good that if someone bought "speed" pills from a street dealer they were actually getting look-alikes. The national high school survey had to apply a correction factor to its data to account for these look-alikes and get a more accurate measure of actual amphetamine use. The FDA began to crack down on manufacturers and distributors of pills containing large amounts of caffeine or mixtures of caffeine and other legal stimulants, and states passed regulations making it illegal to distribute any substance that is misrepresented to be a controlled substance.

The reduced availability of legally manufactured amphetamines had a second important effect. As the price went up and the quality of the available speed became more questionable, the drug subculture began, slowly and without fanfare, to rekindle its interest in a more "natural," reportedly less dangerous stimulant—cocaine. In 1970, federal agents in Miami reported that "the traffic in cocaine is growing by leaps and bounds."[25] And as we now know, they were seeing only the small beginnings of a cocaine trade that would swell to much greater size by the mid-1980s.

speed: street name for amphetamine.

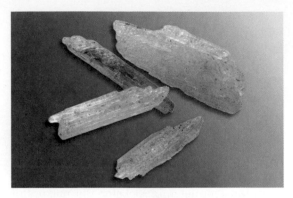
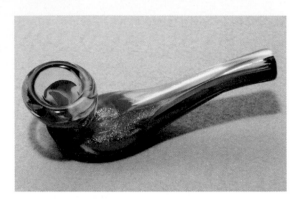

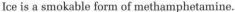

Ice is a smokable form of methamphetamine.

The Return of Methamphetamine The third reaction to limited amphetamine availability was an increase in the number of illicit laboratories making methamphetamine, which acquired the name **crank.** Most illicit methamphetamine consumed in the United States is produced in small "stovetop laboratories," which might exist for only a few days in a remote area before moving on. The process for making methamphetamine has been on the streets since the 1960s, and illicit laboratories have been raided every year. By the late 1990s, however, the number of illicit methamphetamine laboratories confiscated by the authorities had increased more than eight-fold, a clear indication that methamphetamine was the next drug fad. A major concern with clandestine methamphetamine laboratories is that fumes and residue associated with these laboratories are dangerous.[28]

In 1989, the media began warning of the next American drug epidemic: the "smoking" of methamphetamine hydrochloride crystals, also know by the street names **ice** and **crystal meth.** Although many media accounts regarding methamphetamine-related effects and its dependence-producing potential were exaggerated, methamphetamine abuse rose dramatically during the 1990s. By 1999, more than 9 million Americans had used methamphetamine at least once. Five years earlier this number was less than 4 million. In recent history, methamphetamine abuse has been viewed as a Western U.S. phenomenon; methamphetamine is the most common primary drug of abuse cited for treatment admissions in Honolulu and San Diego. In addition, methamphetamine users represent a sizable minority of treatment admissions in other Western states, including Colorado and Washington. There is evidence that methamphetamine use is spreading eastward. For instance, treatment admissions for methamphetamine abuse have increased in Atlanta, Minneapolis/St. Paul, New York, and St. Louis.[29] The drug of the 1960s urban hippie has now become associated with other subgroups, including biker gangs, rural Americans, and urban gay communities. Other indicators of increased methamphetamine use include data from DAWN, which show methamphetamine-associated emergency department admissions and deaths have remained considerably higher than any other "club drug," a term derived from the association of certain drugs with dance clubs, for more than a decade.[30]

Basic Pharmacology

Chemical Structures Figure 6.2 illustrates some similarities in the structures of amphetamines and related drugs. First, note the likeness between the molecular structures of the catecholamine neurotransmitters (dopamine and norepinephrine) and the basic amphetamine molecule. It appears that amphetamine produces its effects because it is recognized as one

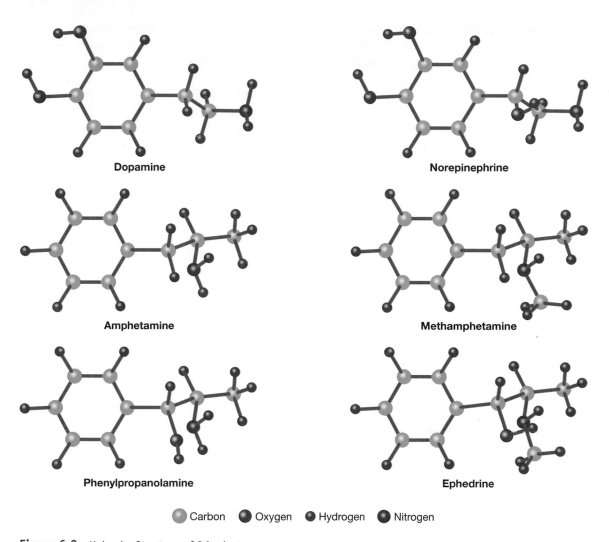

Dopamine

Norepinephrine

Amphetamine

Methamphetamine

Phenylpropanolamine

Ephedrine

⬤ Carbon ⬤ Oxygen ⬤ Hydrogen ⬤ Nitrogen

Figure 6.2 Molecular Structures of Stimulants

of these catecholamines at many sites in both the central and the peripheral nervous systems. The amphetamine molecule has both "left-handed" and "right-handed" forms (*l* and *d* forms). The original Benzedrine was an equal mixture of both forms. The *d* form is several times more potent in its CNS effects, however, and in 1945 d-amphetamine was first marketed as Dexedrine for use as an appetite suppressant.

Next, look at the methamphetamine molecule, which simply has a methyl group added to the basic amphetamine structure. This

methyl group seems to make the molecule cross the blood-brain barrier more readily and thus further increase the CNS potency. (If more of the molecules get into the brain, then fewer total molecules have to be given.) However, the

crank: street name for illicitly manufactured methamphetamine.
crystal meth; ice: street names for crystals of methamphetamine hydrochloride.

behavioral significance of this in humans has yet to be determined, as studies directly comparing the two compounds report no difference on many measures, including subjective drug-effect ratings and heart rate. Notice the structures for ephedrine, the old Chinese remedy that is still used to treat asthma, and for phenylpropanolamine (PPA). Before 2000, PPA was an ingredient in OTC weight-control preparations (see Chapter 12) and in many of the look-alikes. Both of these molecules have a structural addition that makes them not cross the blood-brain barrier as well; therefore, they produce peripheral effects without as much CNS effectiveness.

Mechanism of Action Like cocaine, amphetamines increase the activity of monoamine neurotransmitters (dopamine, norepinephrine, and serotonin), although amphetamines accomplish this effect via a different mechanism. Amphetamines augment the activity of these neurotransmitters by stimulating release rather than by inhibiting reuptake. Findings from studies of laboratory animals strongly implicate dopamine in mediating amphetamine-related reinforcement. For example, researchers have reported that amphetamines produce substantial increases in dopamine levels in nucleus accumbens, a brain region thought to be important for drug-related reinforcement. In humans, while amphetamine-induced euphoria and brain dopamine elevations have been positively correlated, dopamine antagonists do not block the euphoria produced by amphetamine.[31] These observations suggest that exclusive focus on dopamine might be overly simplistic. Recent evidence shows that amphetamines are more potent releasers of norepinephrine than of dopamine and serotonin. As a result, some researchers speculate that norepinephrine activity mediates the euphoric effects of amphetamines.[32] Nevertheless, it is unlikely that complex drug effects, such as subjective effects and drug taking, are mediated via one neurotransmitter system. As we are learning from our experience with

cocaine, amphetamine-related effects are probably the result of interactions with multiple neurotransmitters.

Absorption and Elimination Like cocaine, amphetamines are consumed through a variety of routes: oral, intranasal, intravenous, and smoked. When taken orally, peak effects occur about 1.5 hours after ingestion. In contrast, intranasal peak effects occur between 15 and 30 minutes after administration; peak effects following the intravenous and smoked routes occur within 5 to 10 minutes. The half-life of amphetamine is 10 to 12 hours, and the half-life for methamphetamine is four to five hours. Virtually complete elimination of the drug occurs within two days of the last dose.

With high doses a tachyphylaxis (rapid tolerance) may be seen. Because amphetamine produces its effects largely by displacing the monoamine transmitters from their storage sites, with large doses the monoamines might be sufficiently depleted, so that another dose within a few hours may not be able to displace as much neurotransmitter, and a reduced effect will be obtained.

Beneficial Uses

Previous Use for Depression During the 1950s and early 1960s, amphetamines were prescribed for depression and feelings of fatigue. If we look at an individual's mood as potentially ranging from very depressed, up through sadness into a normal range, and then into euphoria and finally the excited, manic range (Figure 6.3), we can better understand amphetamine's effects on mood. The person who is seriously depressed is not just sad; he or she feels helpless and hopeless with no energy and might think of suicide. Amphetamines are capable of temporarily moving the mood up the scale, so that a depressed person might, for a few hours, move into a normal range. But when the drug wears off, that person doesn't stay "up." The mood drops, often below the predrug level. To keep the mood up, one needs to keep taking

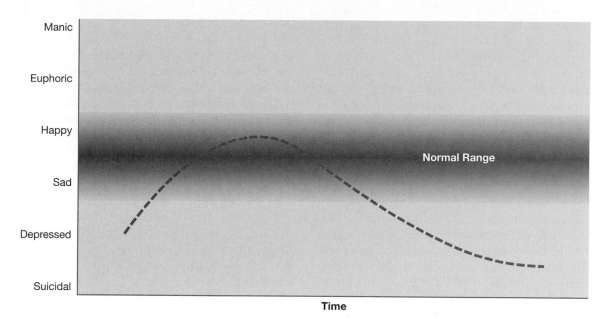

Figure 6.3 Mood Changes Over Time

amphetamine. Amphetamine does interfere with sleep, so some physicians prescribed sleeping pills for nighttime. These patients often went for a daily "ride" on an emotional roller coaster, waking up depressed and taking a pill to get going in the morning, and either coming off the drug or taking a "downer" at night. As we will see in Chapter 8, other treatments are now used for depression, and amphetamines are not recommended.

Weight Control Probably the most common medical use for amphetamines through the mid-1960s was for weight control. Studies show that amphetamine use reduces food intake and body weight in human research participants. With one-third of Americans overweight, the market is vast for a pill that would help us lose weight. For years the common medical response was some form of amphetamine or related sympathomimetic stimulant. Physicians dispensed prescriptions for pills and some gave injections, and a number of people did lose weight. But in the 1960s, when people began to view the amphetamines with greater

concern, it was also clear that some people who took these stimulants regularly were still overweight.

To understand the role of stimulant drugs in weight control, let's imagine a typical experiment to test the value of amphetamine in treating obesity. Patients who meet some criterion for being overweight are recruited for the study. All are brought to a hospital or clinic, where they are weighed, interviewed, examined, and given a diet to follow. Half are given amphetamine and half a placebo in a double-blind design. Each week the patients return to the hospital, where they are interviewed, weighed, and given their supply of drug for the next week. After two months the drug code is broken and the amount of weight loss in each group is calculated. This type of study virtually always finds that both groups lose weight, mostly in the first two or three weeks. After that, the weight loss is much slower. This initial weight loss by both groups probably is a result of beginning a new diet and being involved in a medical study in which they know they will be weighed each week. Over the first two or three weeks the amphetamine group will lose a little more weight than the placebo group. The difference between the two groups after two or three weeks might be about two or three pounds, which is statistically significant but probably not medically or cosmetically important. As the study continues, the gap stays about the same. In other words, in such studies the amphetamine effect is real but small and limited in duration. Even with moderate dose increases, four to six weeks seems to be the limit before tolerance occurs. Increasing to high doses might produce some further effect, but these experiments don't allow that, and it would be foolhardy as a treatment approach. The use of amphetamines for weight reduction came under attack from various sources, and the FDA in 1970 restricted the legal use of amphetamines to three types of conditions: narcolepsy, hyperkinetic (hyperactive) behavior, and "short-term" weight-reduction programs.

Amphetamine and several related stimulant drugs are still used for weight control. Preparations of *d*-amphetamine and methamphetamine are available by prescription for short-term weight loss, as are the other sympathomimetics diethylpropion, phentermine, phenmetrazine, phendimetrazine, and some related but slightly different drugs, fenfluramine and mazindol. The FDA allows the sale of all these drugs even though experts point out that the drugs make a clinically trivial contribution to the overall weight reduction seen in the experiments. The package insert for each of these drugs includes the following FDA mandated statements:

> The natural history of obesity is measured in years, whereas most studies cited are restricted to a few weeks duration; thus, the total impact of drug induced weight loss over that of diet alone must be considered clinically limited. . . . [Drug name] is indicated in the management of exogenous obesity as a short-term (a few weeks) adjunct in a regimen of weight reduction based on caloric restriction. The limited usefulness of agents of this class must be weighed against possible risk factors inherent in their use.[33]

The introduction in 1992 of a new combination of two old drugs, fenfluramine and phentermine, as a more effective aid to weight loss started the well-known "fen-phen" craze and renewed public interest in the use of prescription stimulants as appetite suppressants. This was followed in 1996 by the introduction of a new relative of fenfluramine, dexfenfluramine (Redux). However, in August 1997 the FDA began warning physicians and the public that the fen-phen combination had been associated with damage to heart valves and that several patients had also developed a serious lung disease. By September 1997, it was clear that the culprit was fenfluramine (Pondimin) and that its new relative, dexfenfluramine (Redux), might have the same effects. As warnings went out from the FDA to stop taking these medications, the manufacturer removed them from the market.

Then in November 1997, another new weight-control drug, sibutramine (Meridia), was introduced. Intended for use only in those who are extremely overweight, this drug is believed to act by blocking reuptake of both norepinephrine and serotonin.

Narcolepsy Narcolepsy is a sleep disorder in which individuals do not sleep normally at night and in the daytime experience uncontrollable episodes of muscular weakness and falling asleep. Although interest has increased in sleep disorders in general, and sleep-disorder clinics are now associated with almost every major medical center in the United States, the best available treatment for a long time was to keep the patient awake during the day with amphetamine or methylphenidate, a related stimulant. Recently, the FDA approved modafinil (Provigil) to promote wakefulness in patients with narcolepsy. This medication is chemically and pharmacologically distinct from other psychostimulants such as amphetamines. Modafinil's mechanism of action is complex and not completely understood, but increasing evidence indicates that its therapeutic effects depend upon increasing the activity of glutamate and the catecholamine neurotransmitters nor-epinephrine and dopamine. Unlike amphet-amines and other stimulants, modafinil appears to have low abuse potential,[34] and has been demonstrated to be effective in the treatment of narcolepsy and excessive daytime sleepiness for up to 40 weeks, suggesting a lack of tolerance development.[35]

Hyperactive Children Even though it has been more than 50 years since the first report that amphetamine could reduce activity levels in hyperactive children, and even though hun-dreds of thousands of children are currently being treated with stimulant drugs for this problem, we still have controversy over the nature of the disorder being treated, we still don't understand what the drugs are doing to reduce hyperactivity, and we still don't have a widely accepted solution to the apparent para-dox: Why does a "stimulant" drug appear to produce a "calming" effect?

The disorder itself was referred to as child-hood hyperactivity for many years, and the children who received that label were the ones who seemed absolutely incapable of sitting still and paying attention in class. Many of these children had normal or even above-average IQ scores yet were failing to learn. Dur-ing the 1960s, lead toxicity or early oxygen deprivation were proposed as the possible cause of a small amount of brain damage. Pointing out that many of these children ex-hibit "soft" neurological signs (impairments in coordination or other tests that are not local-izable to a particular brain area), the term *minimal brain dysfunction* (MBD) became pop-ular. By 1980, there was a belief that there had been too much focus on activity levels and that the basic disorder was a deficit in attention, which usually, but not always, was accompa-nied by hyperactivity. Thus, the *Diagnostic and Statistical Manual* of the American Psychiatric Association used the term *attention deficit dis-order*. However, the current revision of that manual, the *DSM-IV-TR,* recognized the strong relationship between attention deficit and hy-peractive behavior by using the term *attention-deficit hyperactivity disorder* (**ADHD**).[36] The criteria used to diagnose this disorder are listed in the DSM-IV-TR box.

The cause or causes of ADHD are not well understood. The fact that it is at least three times more common in boys than in girls hasn't helped us understand its cause. Also, in many cases the problems seem to lessen once the child reaches puberty. It was once thought that this was an absolute developmental change, but now we recognize that as many as one-third of the children continue to have hyperac-tivity problems into adulthood.

Some progress has been made toward a better understanding of the etiology of the disorder. Data from twin studies, for example, indicate that genetic factors contribute sub-stantially to the expression of ADHD. Findings from other studies suggest the disorder is asso-ciated with prefrontal cortex deficits, espe-cially in catecholamine-rich regions.[37] The clear evidence demonstrating the beneficial effects of amphetamines and **methylphenidate (Ritalin)** in the treatment of ADHD bolsters this latter finding. These medications increase brain catecholamine activity, which would, in theory, reverse catecholamine-associated deficits. Although this theory is plausible, there are other theories and none has yet been widely accepted.

One concern is that treatment with stimu-lant medications will lead to substance abuse, even though findings from controlled studies show that stimulant therapy is protective against substance abuse (i.e., the occurrence of substance-use disorders is actually decreased). Despite this, an increasing number of nonstim-ulant medications are being assessed for utility. Atomoxetine (Strattera) has been shown to be efficacious in the treatment of ADHD.[38]

ADHD: attention-deficit hyperactivity disorder.
methylphenidate (Ritalin) (meth il *fen* ih date): a stimulant used in treating ADHD.

DSM-IV-TR

Diagnostic Criteria for Attention-Deficit Hyperactivity Disorder

A. Either (1) or (2):

(1) Six (or more) of the following symptoms of inattention have persisted for at least six months to a degree that is maladaptive and inconsistent with developmental level:

Inattention

   a. Often fails to give close attention to details or makes careless mistakes
   b. Often has difficulty sustaining attention in tasks or play
   c. Often does not seem to listen when spoken to directly
   d. Often does not follow through on instructions and fails to finish schoolwork, chores, or duties
   e. Often has difficulty organizing tasks and activities
   f. Is often easily distracted by extraneous stimuli
   g. Is often forgetful in daily activities

(2) Six (or more) of the following symptoms of hyperactivity-impulsivity have persisted for at least six months to a degree that is maladaptive and inconsistent with developmental level:

Hyperactivity

   a. Often fidgets with hands or feet or squirms in seat
   b. Often leaves seat in classroom or in other situations in which remaining seated is expected
   c. Often runs about or climbs excessively in situations in which it is inappropriate
   d. Often has difficulty playing or engaging in leisure activities quietly
   e. Is often "on the go" or often acts as if "driven by a motor"
   f. Often talks excessively

Impulsivity

   g. Often blurts out answers before questions have been completed
   h. Often has difficulty awaiting turn
   i. Often interrupts or intrudes on others

B. Some hyperactive-impulsive or inattentive symptoms that caused impairment were present before age seven years.

C. Some impairment from the symptoms is present in two or more settings.

D. There must be clear evidence of clinically significant impairment in social, academic, or occupational functioning.

E. The symptoms do not occur exclusively during the course of a Pervasive Developmental Disorder or other disorder and are not better accounted for by another mental disorder.

Atomoxetine's ability to increase catecholamines in the prefrontal cortex has been hypothesized to be the basis for these effects. Unlike stimulant therapies used to treat ADHD, atomoxetine does not increase dopamine transmission in the nucleus accumbens and does not appear to have abuse potential. Modafinil (Provigil) has also been under review for the treatment of ADHD.

One of the more disturbing side effects of stimulant therapy is a suppression of height and weight increases during drug treatment. Amphetamine produces a slightly greater effect in most studies than methylphenidate. If drug treatment is stopped over the summer vacation, a growth spurt makes up for most of the suppressed height and weight gain.

The seemingly indiscriminate but medically prescribed use of stimulant drugs to influence the behavior of school-age children has evoked much social protest and commentary. (See the Mind/Body Connection.)

"Smart Pills" A number of studies in the 1960s seemed to show that rats learned faster and performed better if they were given amphet-

Mind / Body Connection

How Far Should We Go to Enhance Human Abilities?

New drugs, as well as increasing or innovative use of old drugs, are causing medical professionals to confront a spiritual and ethical question that has dogged the age of pharmacology: How far does our society want to go in its efforts to enhance human abilities?

One example is the popularity of the stimulant Ritalin, a common treatment for children with attention-deficit hyperactivity disorder (ADHD), who are impulsive, easily distracted, and unable to sit still and concentrate in school. After more than three decades of use, Ritalin's sales boomed throughout the 1990s, increasing by more than 500 percent, according to Drug Enforcement Administration reports. Physicians and others, such as Senator Hillary Rodham Clinton, have expressed concern that Ritalin is being prescribed for children whose symptoms do not clearly meet the specific diagnostic criteria for ADHD but who have difficulty paying attention and for adults who find themselves easily distracted.

Pediatricians and psychiatrists say that Ritalin can help anyone concentrate, whether or not he or she has a neurological problem. Some people, though no one knows how many, are using the drug simply to improve their mental performance. Although it is clear that a learning disorder can disrupt one's life, some experts say it is too easy to see ADHD everywhere we look. Anxiety, stress, and depression can also cause kids to be inattentive or somewhat hyperactive. And some experts fear that the diagnosis of adult ADHD is becoming an excuse for any sort of

psychological problem. Adults may want to believe that problems with their families or their jobs are caused by problems with impulsivity and attention. Is it more socially acceptable now to have ADHD than depression or anxiety?

There is no single definitive test for ADHD. A medical expert makes a diagnosis after evaluating the patient. Symptoms, including restlessness, a short attention span, distractability, and impulsiveness, must cause a significant impairment in school performance or home behavior and must have appeared by the age of seven. Not every person with ADHD has every symptom, and no one symptom leads to a diagnosis.

There are concerns that parents and others are misusing Ritalin as a Band-Aid approach to therapy and that, in doing so, they may be treating the symptoms, not the problem. But as consumer demand for choice allows market forces to take more and more control of the health care industry, patients are redefining the purpose of "medicine." Rather than just being prevention or treatment oriented, we now want to enhance the average.

Is it appropriate to medicate children without a clear diagnosis in the hope that they will do better in school? Should the drug be prescribed for adults who are failing in their careers, who are procrastinators, or who are otherwise not living up to their potential? Does the use of drugs to enhance mental performance, sexual performance, and athletic performance really make us better human beings?

amine or some other stimulant. Abbott Laboratories obtained a patent for the stimulant it named Cylert, which it was testing as a "smart pill." Much animal and human research has since been done on the role of stimulants in improving mental performance. One way to represent the effects of stimulants can be seen in Figure 6.4, which schematically relates degree of mental performance to the arousal level of the CNS. At low levels of arousal, such as when the individual is sleepy, performance

suffers. Increasing the arousal level into the normal range with a stimulant can then improve performance. At the very high end of the arousal scale the person is so maniacal or so involved in repetitive, stereotyped behavior that performance suffers, even on the simplest of tasks. The region of the graph labeled "Excited" shows that some simple tasks can be improved above normal levels, but complex or difficult tasks are disrupted because of difficulty in concentrating, controlling attention, and

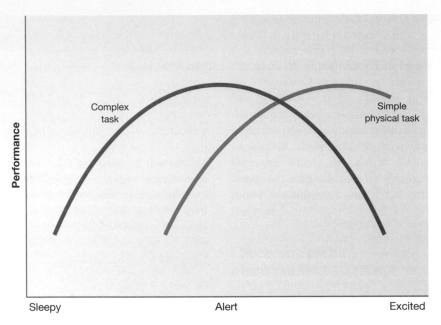

Figure 6.4   Effects of Stimulants on Performance

making careful decisions. Cylert never made it to the market as a smart pill, but the company later introduced it as an alternative to Ritalin in the treatment of ADHD.

Figure 6.4 reveals that anyone trying to improve his or her mental performance level with amphetamines or other stimulants is taking a chance. Depending on the type of task, predrug performance level, and dose, one might obtain improvement or disruption. A small dose could be beneficial to a tired person driving alone at night on a deserted interstate highway but would probably only add to the confusion of a school bus driver trying to negotiate a Los Angeles freeway interchange at 7:30 A.M. with a load of noisy students. As for the students, a small dose of a stimulant might help keep them awake to study when they should be sleeping, but a larger dose? An old piece of college folklore recounts something that probably never happened but has the ring of possible truth to it. It involves a student who stayed awake for days studying with the help of amphetamines, went into a final exam "wired up," wrote feverishly and eloquently for two hours, and only

later when she received her exam back with an *F* saw that she had written the entire answer on one line, using the line over and over, so that it was solid black and the rest of the paper was blank.

Athletics   Under some conditions the use of amphetamines or other stimulants at an appropriate dose can produce slight improvements in athletic performance. The effects are so small as to be meaningless for most athletes, but at the highest levels of competition even a 1 percent improvement can mean the difference between winning a medal or coming in sixth. The temptation has been strong for athletes to use amphetamines and other stimulants to enhance their performances, and this topic is discussed in more detail in Chapter 16.

Causes for Concern

Acute Toxicity   During the period of amphetamine intoxication with above-normal doses, the altered behavior patterns (acute behavioral toxicity) can cause some dangers. As we have seen, even at moderate doses complex decision making can be temporarily impaired. At higher doses, especially administered for extended periods, the user tends to be easily panicked and to become suspicious to the point of paranoia. Combine this with increased feelings of power and capability, and there is concern that incidents of violence may increase.

There were multiple reports of the association of amphetamine use and violence and aggression in the late 1960s and early 1970s. Those reports returned along with increased amphetamine use in the 1990s. But violence is a lifestyle characteristic of many methamphetamine users, and a causal relationship between violent behavior and methamphetamine use is not well established. In addition, the amount of demonstrated violence due to methamphetamine use is considerably lower than that resulting from alcohol use.

At one time there was concern that large doses of amphetamines would push the blood pressure so high that small strokes would occur and cause slight brain damage, which would be cumulative for repeated high-dose users. However, no direct human evidence has been obtained indicating this to be a problem.

It has been shown in rats that high doses of methamphetamine result in the production in the brain of a chemical that selectively destroys catecholamine neurons.[39] The possible long-term behavioral consequences for humans are unclear because the dosing regimens used in animal studies have been excessive and do not mimic the use of amphetamines by humans. What is clear, however, is that contaminants formed during the manufacturing of illicit methamphetamine have been shown to produce toxic effects on brain cells.[40] Some have expressed concern that, as abusers of amphetamine-like drugs age, they may be at a greater risk of developing movement disorders, such as Parkinson's disease (see Chapter 4). Only time and better-controlled studies will tell.

Chronic Toxicity The development of a paranoid psychosis has long been known to be one of the effects of sustained cocaine use. The first amphetamine psychosis was described in 1938, but little attention was given this syndrome until the late 1950s. Possible reasons for the psychosis included that heavy methamphetamine users have schizoid personalities or that the psychosis is really caused by sleep deprivation, particularly dream-sleep deprivation. The question of the basis for the amphetamine psychosis was resolved by the demonstration that it could be elicited in the laboratory in individuals who clearly were not prepsychotic and who did not experience great sleep deprivation. The paranoid psychosis after high-dose IV use of amphetamine is primarily the result of the drug and not the personality predisposition of the user. Evidence shows that the paranoid psychosis results from dopaminergic stimulation, probably in the mesolimbic system. In some cases in which paranoid psychoses have been produced by amphetamines, the paranoid thinking and loss of touch with reality have been slow to return to normal, persisting for days or even weeks after the drug has left the system. There is no good evidence for permanent behavioral or personality disruption.

Another behavior induced by high doses of amphetamine is compulsive and repetitive actions. The behavior might be acceptable (the individual might compulsively clean a room over and over) or it might be bizarre (one student spent a night counting corn flakes). There is a precedent for this stereotyped behavior in animal studies using high doses of amphetamine; it probably results from an effect of amphetamine on dopaminergic systems in the basal ganglia.

Dependence Potential Theories about the abuse potential of amphetamines parallel the history of such theories regarding cocaine. For years experts argued about whether the amphetamines were truly "addicting." Because abrupt cessation of amphetamine use didn't produce the kind of obvious physical withdrawal symptoms seen with barbiturate or heroin withdrawal, most people decided amphetamines did not produce "real" dependence. By today's standards, as defined by the DSM-IV-TR, amphetamine-like compounds are capable of producing dependence, although the empirical evidence demonstrating a withdrawal syndrome (the "crash") in humans upon cessation of amphetamines use is limited. Anecdotally, amphetamine-related withdrawal has been described to be analogous to cocaine-related withdrawal. Symptoms may include craving, lethargy, depressed mood, and so on.

It has been known for years that amphetamines could be habit forming—that is, they could produce psychological dependence. Until a few years ago, that was not considered important. Amphetamines were even considered by some to be a so-called soft drug. They were available by prescription, and most users did not develop psychological dependence. The idea seemed to be that, although it could be habit forming in some individuals, its potential for abuse was limited. Now we realize that important factors such as dose and route of administration were not being considered. Small doses (5 or 10 mg) taken orally by people acting under their physician's orders for some purpose other than achieving a high rarely result in dependence. A larger dose injected intravenously for the purpose of getting high can result in a rapid development of dependence. Taken in this way, amphetamine is as potent a reinforcer as any known drug. Data from studies of laboratory animals reveal that rats and monkeys will quickly learn to press a lever that produces IV injections of amphetamine. If required to do so, an animal will press hundreds of times for a single injection.[41]

Summary

- The stimulants can reverse the effects of fatigue, maintain wakefulness, decrease appetite, and temporarily elevate the mood of the user.
- Cocaine is derived from the coca plant. Coca leaves have been chewed for centuries.
- Cocaine's earliest uses in the United States were as a local anesthetic and in psychiatry.
- Coca paste and crack are smokable forms of illicit cocaine.
- Cocaine and amphetamines appear to act by interacting with several neurotransmitters, including dopamine, norepinephrine and serotonin.
- Excessive cocaine or amphetamine use can result in a paranoid psychotic reaction.
- Cocaine and amphetamines can produce dependence.
- Use of cocaine has declined in the general population since 1985.
- Amphetamines are a synthetic sympathomimetic similar to ephedrine.
- The amphetamine-like drugs are similar in structure to dopamine and norepinephrine.
- Amphetamines are used in short-term weight reduction, narcolepsy, and ADHD (methylphenidate is preferred for ADHD, however).
- Illicit methamphetamine is primarily made in small laboratories.
- Illicit methamphetamine use has increased over the past several years.

Review Questions

1. At about what periods in history did cocaine reach its first and second peaks of popularity, and when was amphetamine's popularity at its highest?
2. How did Mariani, Freud, and Halsted popularize the use of cocaine?
3. How are coca paste, freebase, crack, and ice similar?
4. What similarities and what differences are there in the toxic effects of cocaine and amphetamine?
5. How would medical practice be affected if both cocaine and amphetamine were placed on Schedule I?

6. Contrast the typical "speed freak" of the 1960s with the typical cocaine user of the early 1980s and with our stereotype of a modern crack smoker.

7. How does the chemical difference between methamphetamine and amphetamine relate to the behavioral effects of the two drugs?

8. Compare the dependence potential of cocaine with that of amphetamine.

References

1. Dillehay, T.D., and others. "The Nanchoc Tradition: The Beginnings of Andean Civilization" *American Scientist* 85 (1997), pp. 46–55.

2. Taylor, N. *Flight from Reality*. New York: Duell, Sloan & Pearce, 1949.

3. Freud, S. *On the General Effect of Cocaine.* Lecture before the Psychiatric Union on March 5, 1885. Reprinted in *Drug Dependence* 5 (1970), p. 17.

4. Doyle, A.C. "The Sign of the Four." In *The Complete Sherlock Holmes*. New York: Garden City, 1938.

5. Musto, D.F. "Opium, Cocaine and Marijuana in American History" *Scientific American,* July 1991, p. 40.

6. Ashley, R. *Cocaine: Its History, Uses and Effects*. New York: Warner Books, 1976.

7. Williams, E.H. "Negro Cocaine 'Fiends' Are a New Southern Menace." *The New York Times,* February 8, 1914.

8. Wright, H. "Report on the International Opium Commission and the Opium Problem as Seen Within the United States and Its Possessions." *61st Congress, 2nd Session, Senate Document No. 377,* February 21, 1910, pp. SO-SI.

9. Bourne, P.G. "The Great Cocaine Myth." *Drugs and Drug Abuse Education Newsletter* 5 (1974).

10. Grinspoon, L., and others. *The Comprehensive Textbook of Psychiatry,* February 21, 1980, pp. 50–51.

11. Freud, S. "Über Coca" *St. Louis Med. Surg. Journal* 47 (1884), pp. 502–50. This complete paper and Freud's other two cocaine studies are translated and published in S. A. Edminster, et al, *The Cocaine Papers* (Vienna: Dunquin, 1963).

12. Johnson, B.D., and others. "Careers in Crack, Drug Use, Drug Distribution, and Nondrug Criminality" *Crime and Delinquency* 41 (1995), p. 275.

13. United States Sentencing Commission. *Report to Congress: Cocaine and Federal Sentencing Policy,* May 2002.

14. Feldman, R.S., J.S. Meyer, and L.F. Quenzer. *Principles of Neuropsychopharmacology.* Sunderland, MA: Sinauer, 1997.

15. Williams, S. "Cocaine's Harmful Effects." *Science* 248: (1990), p. 166.

16. Hart, C.L., and others. "Comparison of Intravenous Cocaethylene and Cocaine in Humans." *Psychopharmacology* 149: (2000), p. 153.

17. Brady, K.T., and others. "Cocaine-Induced Psychosis." *Journal of Clinical Psychiatry* 52: (1991), p. 509.

18. Bunn, W.H., & A.J. Giannini. "Cardiovascular Complications of Cocaine Abuse." *American Family Physician* 46 (1992), p. 769.

19. Substance Abuse and Mental Health Services Administration. "Overview of Findings from the 2002 National Survey on Drug Use and Health." *NHSDA Series H-21, DHHS Publication No. SMA 03–3774.* Rockville, MD: Office of Applied Studies, 2003.

20. Haney, M., and others. "Effects of Pergolide on Intravenous Cocaine Self-administration in Men and Women." *Psychopharmacology* 137 (1998), p. 15.

21. Johanson, C.E., and others. "Self-Administration of Psychomotor Stimulant Drugs: The Effects of Unlimited Access." *Pharmacology Biochemistry & Behavior* 4 (1976), p. 45.

22. Frank, D.A., and others. "Growth, Development, and Behavior in Early Childhood Following Prenatal Cocaine Exposure: A Systematic Review." *Journal of the American Medical Association* 285 (2001), p. 1613.

23. *Drug Trafficking in the United States*. Washington, DC: U.S. Drug Enforcement Administration, 2002. www.usdoj.gov/dea.

24. Riley, K. J. *Snow Job?* New Brunswick, NJ: Transaction, 1996.

25. Brecher, E.M. *Licit and Illicit Drugs*. Boston: Little, Brown, 1972.

26. "Benzedrine Alert." *Air Surgeon's Bulletin* 1, no.2 (1944), pp. 19–21.

27. *Journal of the American Medical Association* 183 (1963), p. 363.

28. Burgess, J.L. "Phosphine Exposure from a Methamphetamine Laboratory Investigation." *Journal of Toxicology and Clinical Toxicology* 39 (2001), p. 165.

29. Community Epidemiology Work Group (CEWG). "Epidemiologic Trends in Drug Abuse, Volume I." *Proceedings of the Community Epidemiology Work Group, NIH Pub. No. 04-5364*. Washington, DC: U.S. Government Printing Office, 2004.

30. Drug Abuse Warning Network. *The DAWN Report: Club Drugs*. October 2002.

31. Brauer, L.H., & H. deWit. "High Dose Pimozide Does Not Block Amphetamine-induced Euphoria in Normal Volunteers." *Pharmacology Biochemistry and Behavior* 56 (1997), p. 265.

32. Rothman, R.B., and others. "Amphetamine-type Central Nervous System Stimulants Release Norepinephrine More Potently Than They Release Dopamine and Serotonin." *Synapse* 39 (2001), p. 32.

33. *Physician's Desk Reference Medical Economics*. Ordell, NJ. Annual.

34. Rush, C.R., and others. "Acute Behavioral and Physiological Effects of Modafinil in Drug Abusers." *Behavioural Pharmacology* 13: (2002), p. 1055.

35. U.S. Modafinil in Narcolepsy Multicenter Study Group. "Randomized Trial of Modafinil as a Treatment for the Excessive Daytime Somnolence of Narcolepsy." *Neurology* 54 (2002), p. 1166.

36. American Psychiatric Association. *Diagnostic and Statistical Manual of Mental Disorders,* 4th ed. Washington, DC: American Psychological Association, 2000.

37. Spencer, T.L., and others. "Overview and Neurobiology of Attention-Deficit/Hyperactivity Disorder." *Journal of Clinical Psychiatry* 63 Supplement 12, (2003).

38. Caballero, J., & M.C. Nahata. "Atomoxetine Hydrochloride for the Treatment of Attention-Deficit/Hyperactivity Disorder." *Clinical Therapeutics* 25 (2003), p. 3065.

39. Marek, G.J., and others. "Dopamine Uptake Inhibitors Block Long-term Neurotoxic Effects of Methamphetamine upon Dopaminergic Neurons" *Brain Res* 513 (1990), p. 274.

40. Moore, K.A., and others. "Alpha-Benzyl-N-methylphenethylamine (BNMPA), an Impurity of Illicit Methamphetamine Synthesis: Pharmacological Evaluation and Interaction with Methamphetamine." *Drug and Alcohol Dependence* 39 (1995), p 83.

41. Griffiths, R.R., and others. "Predicting the Abuse Liability of Drugs with Animal Self-Administration Procedures: Psychomotor Stimulants and Hallucinogens." In T. Thompson, P. Dews, editors. *Advances in Behavioral Pharmacology* (Vol. 2). New York: Academic Press, 1979.

Check Yourself

For each of the 13 items, select the choice that best describes your likes or dislikes, or the way that you feel. Select only one statement for each item.

Question 1:
A. I would like a job that requires a lot of traveling.
B. I would prefer a job in one location.

Question 2:
A. I am invigorated by a brisk, cold day.
B. I can't wait to get indoors on a cold day.

Question 3:
A. I get bored seeing the same old faces.
B. I like the comfortable familiarity of everyday friends.

Question 4:
A. I would prefer living in an ideal society in which everyone is safe, secure, and happy.
B. I would have preferred living in the unsettled days of our history.

Question 5:
A. I sometimes like to do things that are a little frightening.
B. A sensible person avoids activities that are dangerous.

Question 6:
A. I would not like to be hypnotized.
B. I would like to have the experience of being hypnotized.

Question 7:
A. The most important goal of life is to live it to the fullest and experience as much as possible.
B. The most important goal of life is to find peace and happiness.

Question 8:
A. I would like to try parachute jumping.
B. I would never want to try jumping out of a plane, with or without a parachute.

Question 9:
A. I enter cold water gradually, giving myself time to get used to it.
B. I like to dive or jump right into the ocean or a cold pool.

Question 10:
A. When I go on vacation, I prefer the comfort of a good room and bed.
B. When I go on vacation, I prefer the change of camping out.

Question 11:
A. I prefer people who are emotionally expressive even if they are a bit unstable.
B. I prefer people who are calm and even-tempered.

Question 12:
A. A good painting should shock or jolt the senses.
B. A good painting should give one a feeling of peace and security.

Question 13:
A. People who ride motorcycles must have some kind of unconscious need to hurt themselves.
B. I would like to drive or ride a motorcycle.

To Score:
Give yourself one point for each of the following items you circled: 1A, 2A, 3A, 4B, 5A, 6B, 7A, 8A, 9B, 10B, 11A, 12A, 13B. Add up your points, and compare the total to the following scale: 1–3 (very low in sensation seeking), 4–5 (low), 6–9 (average), 10–11 (high), 12–13 (very high).

Adapted from M. Zuckerman, Behavioral Expressions and Biosocial Bases of Sensation Seeking. (New York: Cambridge University Press, 1994).

7

Depressants and Inhalants

Objectives

When you have finished this chapter, you should be able to:

- **Give several examples of depressant drugs and describe the general set of behavioral effects common to them.**

- **Understand how concerns about barbiturate use led to acceptance of newer classes of sedative-hypnotics.**

- **Describe the differences in dose and duration of action that are appropriate for daytime anxiolytic effects as opposed to hypnotic effects of prescription depressants.**

- **Describe how the time of onset of a depressant drug relates to abuse potential and how duration of action relates to the risk of withdrawal symptoms.**

- **Describe the mechanism of action for barbiturates and benzodiazepines.**

- **Explain why it is not recommended that people use sleeping pills for more than a few days in a row.**

- **Describe several types of substances that are abused as inhalants.**

- **Describe GHB's typical dose range and behavioral effects, as well as its effects when combined with alcohol.**

Downers, depressants, sedatives, hypnotics, gin-in-a-pill: Known by many names, these prescription drugs all have a widespread effect in the brain that can be summed up as decreased neural activity. What are the behavioral effects? As suggested by one of the names, if you know what alcohol does, you know what these drugs do. They come from several different chemical classes but are grouped because of their common psychological effects. At low doses these drugs might be prescribed for daytime use to reduce anxiety (as **sedatives**). At higher doses many of the same drugs are prescribed as sleeping pills (**hypnotics**). This group of prescription drugs is often referred to as *sedative-hypnotics,* part of a larger group of substances considered to be CNS **depressants.** The most widely *used* depressant is alcohol, which is discussed in detail in Chapter 9. The most widely *prescribed* types of sedative-hypnotics fall into the chemical grouping called the **benzodiazepines,** which in the past 40 years have largely replaced the **barbiturates.** A similar depressant effect is produced by most of the **inhalants**—the glues, paints, solvents, and gasoline fumes that some young people (and a few older people) breathe to get "high."

Online Learning Center Resources

www.mhhe.com/ksir12e

Visit to our Online Learning Center (OLC) for access to these study aids and additional resources.

- Learning objectives
- Glossary flashcards
- Web activities and links
- Self-scoring chapter quiz
- Audio chapter summaries

History and Pharmacology

Before Barbiturates

Chloral Hydrate The "knockout drops" (or "Mickey Finn") they slipped in the sailor's drink in those old movies were a solution of chloral hydrate. First synthesized in 1832, chloral hydrate was not used clinically until about 1870. It is rapidly metabolized to trichloroethanol, which is the active hypnotic agent. When taken orally, chloral hydrate has a short onset period (30 minutes), and 1 to 2 grams will induce sleep in less than an hour.

In 1869, Dr. Benjamine Richardson introduced chloral hydrate to Great Britain. Ten years later he called it "in one sense a beneficent, and in another sense a maleficent substance, I almost feel a regret that I took any part whatever in the introduction of the agent into the practice of healing."[1] He had learned that what humankind can use, some will abuse. As early as 1871, he referred to its nontherapeutic use as "toxical luxury" and lamented that chloral hydrate abusers had to be added to "alcohol intemperants and opium-eaters." Chloral hydrate abuse is a tough way to go; it is a gastric irritant, and repeated use causes considerable stomach upset.

Paraldehyde Paraldehyde was synthesized in 1829 and introduced clinically in 1882. Paraldehyde would probably be in great use today because of its effectiveness as a CNS depressant

with little respiratory depression and a wide safety margin, except for one characteristic: It has an extremely noxious taste and an odor that permeates the breath of the user. Its safety margin and its ability to sedate patients led to widespread use of paraldehyde in mental hospitals before the 1950s. Anyone who ever worked in, was a patient in, or even visited one of the large state mental hospitals during that era probably still remembers the odor of paraldehyde.

Bromides Bromide salts were used so widely in patent medicines to induce sleep in the 19th century that the word *bromide* entered our language as a reference to any person or story that was tiresome and boring. Bromides accumulate in the body, and the depression they cause builds up over several days of regular use. Serious toxic effects follow repeated hypnotic doses of these agents. Dermatitis and constipation are minor accompaniments; with increased intake, motor disturbances, delirium, and psychosis can develop. Very low (ineffective) doses of bromides remained in some OTC medicines until the 1960s.

Barbiturates

More than 2,500 barbiturates have been synthesized. Barbital (Veronal) was the first to be used clinically, in 1903. Its name gave rise to the practice of giving barbiturates names ending in *-al*. The second barbiturate in clinical use, phenobarbital (Luminal), was introduced in 1912. Amobarbital (Amytal), as well as pentobarbital (Nembutal) and secobarbital (Seconal), are other examples of the barbiturates.

As Table 7.1 indicates, barbiturates are typically grouped on the basis of the duration of their activity. In general, the most lipid-soluble drugs have both the shortest time of onset (i.e., they are absorbed and enter the brain rapidly) and the shortest duration of action (i.e., they leave the brain quickly and tend to be more rapidly metabolized). These varying time courses are important for our understanding of

Drugs in the Media

The Legacy of Samantha Reid

We have previously discussed the importance of emotional "prairie fires" in the passage of many of the U.S. drug laws. From the time of the 1906 Pure Food and Drugs Act to the present, the media have played a critical role in spreading the word about the tragic consequences related to the use of one or another type of drug. That publicity often leads to legislation generated in the heat of emotion. A recent example is the passage of a law requiring that gamma hydroxybutyrate (**GHB**) be listed as a Schedule I controlled substance. President Clinton quickly signed the law, and it went into effect in March 2000. This is an unusual process; decisions about the scheduling of drugs are supposed to be made in a nonpolitical way on the basis of scientific evidence. Previous reviews of GHB by the federal agency responsible for making these decisions had determined that the substance, although posing risks of abuse and the possibility of overdose deaths, should not be listed on Schedule I. Why did Congress take this decision out of the hands of the Department of Health and Human Services and the Drug Enforcement Administration?

The answer to that question is Samantha Reid, a 15-year-old Michigan student who died after some male friends apparently put GHB into her soft drink without her knowledge. When she and another young woman passed out, the young men waited to see whether they would recover, rather than getting them quickly to the hospital. One eventually recovered from her coma; Samantha did not. This tragic death and the subsequent formation of the Samantha Reid Foundation, dedicated to exposing the dangers of GHB, were widely reported by the *Detroit News* and other U.S. news media. Testimony by Samantha's mother left no doubt about her message that young people needed more protection from this potentially dangerous substance. The result was the toughest thing Congress knew how to do—not only list the drug as a federal controlled substance but also list it on Schedule I, even though it was currently undergoing clinical testing as a treatment for narcolepsy.

Regardless of the merits of this decision, it is important to realize how much of our current legacy of drug laws evolved through a similar series of emotional responses to tragic events.

the different uses of these drugs and their different tendencies to produce dependence.

Suppose you want a drug to keep a person calm and relaxed during the daytime (a sedative). You don't want the person to become drowsy, and you want to produce as stable and smooth a drug effect as possible. Therefore, you would choose a *low* dose of a *long-acting* barbiturate, say 30 to 50 mg of phenobarbital. For a sleeping-pill (hypnotic) effect, you want the person to become drowsy, you want the drug to act fairly quickly after it is taken, and you don't want the person to still be groggy the next morning. Therefore, you would choose a *higher* dose of a *shorter-acting* drug, say 100 to 200 mg of amobarbital or secobarbital. Both of these types of prescription were fairly common 40 years ago, before the introduction of the benzodiazepines.

The barbiturates are one of the classes of drugs that stimulate the activity of the CYP450 enzymes of the liver. Some of the tolerance that develops to the barbiturates is the result of an increased rate of deactivation caused by this

sedatives: drugs used to relax, calm, or tranquilize.
hypnotics: drugs used to induce sleep.
depressants: drugs that slow activity in the CNS.
benzodiazepines (ben zo die *ay* zah peens): a chemical grouping of sedative-hypnotics.
barbiturates (bar *bitch* er ates): a chemical group of sedative-hypnotics.
inhalants: volatile solvents inhaled for intoxicating purposes.
(GHB): gamma hydroxybutyrate; chemically related to GABA; used recreationally as a depressant.

Table 7.1
Groupings of Barbiturates

Type	Time of Onset	Duration of Action
Short-acting	15 minutes	2 to 3 hours
Pentobarbital (Nembutal)		
Secobarbital (Seconal)		
Intermediate-acting	30 minutes	5 to 6 hours
Aprobarbital (Alurate)		
Amobarbital (Amytal)		
Butabarbital (Butisol)		
Long-acting	1 hour	6 to 10 hours
Mephobarbital (Merbaral)		
Phenobarbital (Luminal)		

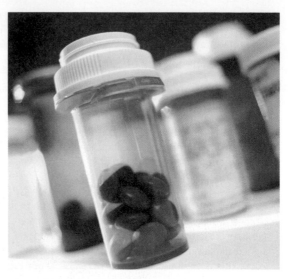

The risk of dependence on prescription sedatives depends on the timing of their effects and on the dose.

stimulation. The induction of these enzymes by the barbiturates might also cause the more rapid metabolism of other drugs, perhaps requiring an adjustment of the dose.

Tolerance can develop to the barbiturates, as well as both psychological and physical dependence. In addition, they depress respiration and, in large doses or in combination with alcohol, can completely stop one's breathing. For many years barbiturate sleeping pills were chosen above all others by people wishing to commit suicide. Also, accidental overdoses occurred when sleeping pills were taken after an evening of heavy drinking.

Although the majority of individuals who took barbiturates were not harmed by them, there was a great deal of concern about both the abuse potential and the danger of overdose. These concerns led to the ready acceptance of new sedative or hypnotic agents that appeared to be safer.

Meprobamate

The first modern antianxiety agents (*anxiolytics*) developed from a muscle relaxant called mephenesin, which was patented in 1946 and was a commercial success but had a short duration of action. One compound patented in 1952 not only was longer lasting but also was believed to be a unique type of CNS depressant. Clinical trials in 1953 supported this belief, and the compound was approved by the FDA and released for prescription use in 1955. Meprobamate became widely prescribed, and it represented the drug revolution of the 1950s to many people.

The boom in meprobamate use was tremendous. In the year it was introduced, sales went from $7,500 in May to more than $500,000 in December. The happy pills had arrived! A publicity agency and excessive prescribing by physicians combined to make meprobamate a public nuisance.

It gradually became clear that meprobamate, like the barbiturates, can also produce both psychological and physical dependence.

Physical dependence can result from taking a bit more than twice a normal daily dose. In 1970, meprobamate became a Schedule IV controlled substance, and although it is still available for prescriptions under several brand names, the benzodiazepines have largely replaced it.

In retrospect, it seems ironic that the medical community so readily accepted meprobamate as being safer than barbiturates. By deciding that the "barbiturates" were dangerous, the focus was on the chemical class, rather than on the dose and the manner in which the drug was used. Thus, a new, "safer" chemical was accepted without considering that its safety was not being judged under the same conditions. This mistake has occurred frequently with psychoactive drugs. It occurred again with methaqualone.

Methaqualone

With continued reports of overdoses and physical dependence associated with secobarbital and amobarbital sleeping pills, in the 1960s the market was wide open for a hypnotic that would be less dangerous. Maybe it was too wide open.

The methaqualone story is one where everyone was wrong—the pharmaceutical industry, the FDA, the DEA, the press, and the physicians. Methaqualone was originally synthesized in India, tested, and found to be ineffective as an antimalarial drug. But it was a good sedative, so in 1959 it was introduced as a prescription drug in Great Britain. It never sold well, but after the thalidomide disaster, interest increased in a "safe" nonbarbiturate sleeping pill. Mandrax (250 mg of methaqualone and 25 mg of an antihistamine) was introduced in 1965 in a massive advertising campaign to physicians. The campaign worked, and 2 million prescriptions were issued for Mandrax in 1971 in Great Britain. The drug had already found its way into the street, where it was widely abused: by heroin users, by high school students, by anyone who wanted a cheap but potent "down." Misuse was so great

that Great Britain tightened controls on it in 1970 and then again in 1973.

Germany introduced methaqualone in 1960 as a nonprescription drug, had its first methaqualone suicide in 1962, and discovered that 10 to 22 percent of the drug overdoses treated in this period were a result of this drug. In 1963, Germany reduced the problem by making methaqualone a prescription drug. From 1960 to 1964, Japan experienced a major epidemic of methaqualone abuse, causing more than 40 percent of all overdoses admitted to hospitals. Japan tightened controls almost to the maximum possible on methaqualone and stemmed the tide.

Apparently no one in the United States was paying much attention to these problems in other countries, because in 1965, after three years of testing, Quaalude and Sopor, brand names for methaqualone, were introduced in the United States as prescription drugs with a package insert that read "Addiction potential not established." In June 1966, the FDA Committee on the Abuse Potential of Drugs decided there was no need to monitor methaqualone, since there was no evidence of abuse potential! Thus, from 1967 to 1973 the package insert read "Physical dependence has not clearly been demonstrated."

In the early 1970s in this country, *ludes* and *sopors* were familiar terms in the drug culture and in drug-treatment centers. Physicians were overprescribing a hypnotic drug that they believed to be safer than the barbiturates. Most of the methaqualone sold on the street was legally manufactured and then either stolen or obtained through prescriptions. Sales zoomed, and front-page reporting of its effects when misused helped to build its reputation as a drug of abuse. In 1973, 8 years after it was introduced into this country, 4 years after American scientists began saying it produced dependence, 11 years after the first suicide, methaqualone was put on Schedule II. By 1985, methaqualone was no longer available as a prescription drug, and it is now listed on Schedule I.

Was methaqualone really very different from the barbiturates? For a while physicians thought it was safer. Street users referred to it as the "love drug" (one of many drugs to have been called this) or "heroin for lovers," implying an *aphrodisiac* effect. In reality the effect is probably not different from the disinhibition produced by alcohol or other depressants. Methaqualone causes the same kind of motor incoordination as alcohol and the barbiturates. Both psychological and physical dependence can develop to methaqualone as easily and rapidly as with the barbiturates, and for a few years methaqualone was also near the top of the charts for drug-related deaths (DAWN coroners' reports, Chapter 2). If it was different, it wasn't much different.

Benzodiazepines

The first of the benzodiazepines was chlordiazepoxide, which was marketed under the trade name Librium (possibly because it "liberates" one from anxieties). Chlordiazepoxide was synthesized in 1947, but it was 10 years before its value in reducing anxiety was suggested, and it was not sold commercially until 1960. The discovery of this class of drugs was a triumph for behavioral research; a drug-company pharmacologist found that mice given the right dose of chlordiazepoxide would loosen their grip on an inclined wire screen and fall to the floor of the test cage. When this experiment had been done with barbiturates, the mice promptly fell asleep. With Librium, the relaxed mouse continued to walk around, sniffing the cage in a normal manner.[2]

This drug was marketed as a more selective "antianxiety" agent that produced less drowsiness than the barbiturates and had a much larger safety margin before overdose death occurred in animals. Clinical practice bore this out: Physical dependence was almost unheard of, and overdose seemed not to occur except in combination with alcohol or other depressant drugs. Even strong psychological dependence seemed rare with this drug. The conclusion

was reached that the benzodiazepines were as effective as the barbiturates and much safer. Librium became not only the leading psychoactive drug in sales but also the leading prescription drug of all. It was supplanted in the early 1970s by diazepam (Valium), a more potent (lower-dose) agent made by the same company. From 1972 until 1978, Valium was the leading seller among all prescription drugs. Since then no single benzodiazepine has so dominated the market, but alprazolam is currently the most widely prescribed among this class of drugs.

As these drugs became widely used, reports again appeared of psychological dependence, occasional physical dependence, and overdose deaths. Diazepam was one of the most frequently mentioned drugs in the DAWN system coroners' reports, although almost always in combination with alcohol or other depressants. What happened to the big difference between the barbiturates and the benzodiazepines? One possibility is that it might not be the chemical class of drugs that makes the big difference but the dose and time course of the individual drugs. *Overdose* deaths are more likely when a drug is sold in higher doses, such as those prescribed for hypnotic effects. *Psychological dependence* develops most rapidly when the drug hits the brain quickly, which is why intravenous use of heroin produces more dependence than oral use, and why smoking crack produces more dependence than chewing coca leaves. So a drug that has a rapid onset of action will be more likely to produce psychological dependence than a slow-acting drug. *Physical dependence* occurs when the drug leaves the system more rapidly than the body can adapt—one way to reduce the severity of withdrawal symptoms is to reduce the dose of a drug slowly over time. Drugs with a shorter duration of action leave the system quickly and are much more likely to produce withdrawal symptoms than are longer-acting drugs.

Figure 7.1 provides a schematic look at the time course of the depressant actions of some

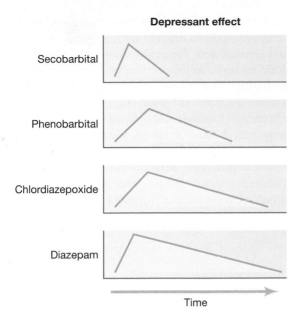

Figure 7.1 Schematic diagram of the relative time courses of two barbiturates and two benzodiazepines after oral administration.

of these drugs. Secobarbital, a short-acting barbiturate, has a relatively rapid onset, which should make it more likely than other barbiturates to produce psychological dependence. Also, because its depressant action is terminated fairly quickly, withdrawal symptoms would be quite dramatic if the person had been taking large doses. Because this drug was used primarily as a sleeping pill, relatively large doses were prescribed. Thus, in the days when barbiturates were widely prescribed, secobarbital was associated with overdoses and both physical and psychological dependence. Phenobarbital, a long-acting barbiturate, has a slower onset of action, which should be less likely to produce psychological dependence. Because the depressant action is terminated more slowly, drug clearance occurs slowly and withdrawal symptoms are minimized. Because phenobarbital was prescribed mostly in low sedative doses, it was rarely associated with overdose.

The first benzodiazepine was chlordiazepoxide, which was sold in low doses for daytime use and has a slow onset of action and an even longer duration of action than phenobarbital. Chlordiazepoxide produced few problems with either compulsive use or withdrawal symptoms, and overdoses were almost unheard of. Diazepam has a more rapid onset than chlordiazepoxide, but because of slow metabolism and the presence of active metabolites, it also has a long duration of action. We might expect a drug with these characteristics to produce more psychological dependence than chlordiazepoxide but only rarely to produce withdrawal symptoms. This is exactly what happened. To summarize this pharmacology object lesson, there might be greater differences among the barbiturates and among the benzodiazepines than there are between these two classes.

As if to underscore the basic similarity that exists among all the depressant drugs, in the 1990s a new version of the "Mickey Finn" was popularized. **Rohypnol** (flunitrazepam), a benzodiazepine sold as a hypnotic in many countries around the world but not in the United States, hit the news when reports surfaced of its being put into the drinks of unsuspecting women by their dates. The combination of Rohypnol and alcohol was reputed to produce a profound intoxication, during which the woman would be highly suggestible and unable to remember what had happened to her. Thus, Rohypnol became widely known as a "date-rape" drug (see Targeting Prevention). In 1997, the drug's manufacturer changed the formulation of the pill so that when it dissolves in a drink it produces a characteristic color.[3]

Mechanism of Action

An important key to understanding the effects of these sedative-hypnotic agents was found in 1977 when it was reported that diazepam molecules had a high affinity for specific receptor sites in brain tissue. Other benzodiazepine types of sedatives also bound to these receptors, and the binding affinities of these various drugs

Rohypnol: a benzodiazepine; the "date-rape drug."

Targeting Prevention

The Drug-Induced Rape Prevention and Punishment Act

In 1996, the U.S. Congress debated what to do in response to widespread concerns about the use of rohypnol as a "date-rape" drug. One proposal was to make the drug a Schedule I controlled substance—it was not a prescription drug in the United States and therefore could be considered to have "no medical use," one of the defining criteria for inclusion in Schedule I. However, the drug was legally available in more than 60 other countries, and Schedule I status would compel the United States to pressure those countries to outlaw it also. Instead, Congress passed the Drug-Induced Rape Prevention and Punishment Act. This act makes it a federal crime to give someone a controlled substance without the recipient's knowledge, with the intent of committing a violent crime. During the debate it was affirmed that rape is considered to be a crime of violence. Under this law, the maximum penalty is 20 years in prison and a $250,000 fine. A urine test is available for rohypnol, so any woman who suspects that she may have been given the drug can request that the test be conducted. It would then be possible, under this act, to charge the person suspected of giving her the drug. Even if no rape occurred, it might be difficult for the drug-giver to argue that such was not his intention, given the reputation this drug has.

Start a discussion among a group of your friends about date rape. What is their perception of this problem? What drugs have they heard about in conjunction with date rape? Are they aware of this federal law and its implications?

correlated with their behavioral potencies in humans and other animals. It was soon noticed that the benzodiazepine receptors were always near receptors for the amino acid neurotransmitter **GABA.** It now appears that when benzodiazepines bind to their receptor site, they enhance the normally inhibitory effects of GABA on its receptors. The barbiturates act at a separate binding site nearby and increase the actions of GABA on its receptors. The picture emerges of a GABA receptor *complex*, which includes the barbiturate binding site and the benzodiazepine receptor.[4] Drug companies quickly began developing new drugs based on their ability to bind to these sites, and several new sedative-hypnotics have reached the market in recent years. A study using genetically altered mice appears to have separated the antianxiety effect from the hypnotic effect, based on isolating different subtypes of the GABA receptor. This could lead to more selective antianxiety drugs.[5]

Nonbenzodiazepine Hypnotics

The most recent additions to the class of depressant drugs do not have the chemical structure of the benzodiazepines, but they have similar effects. Because they are more selective for the GABA-A type of receptor, they seem to be better as sleeping pills than as antianxiety drugs. Zolpidem (Ambien) was introduced in 1993, followed later by zaleplon (Sonata) and eszopiclone (Lunesta).

Beneficial Uses

Anxiolytics

> Raze out the written troubles of the brain,
> and with some sweet oblivious antidote
> Cleanse the stuff'd bosom of that perilous stuff
> Which weighs upon the heart . . .

As these lines from Shakespeare's *Macbeth* reveal, humans have often sought a "sweet oblivious antidote" to the cares and woes of living. Alcohol has most frequently been used for that purpose, but the sedative drugs also play a major role in modern society. In the United States in recent decades, the barbiturates, then meprobamate, and then the benzodiazepines have been among the most widely prescribed medications. Four benzodiazepines are listed among the top 100 most commonly prescribed medications in the United States: alprazolam (Xanax), lorazepam (Ativan), clonazepam (Klonopin), and diazepam (Valium) (Table 7.2). These are all relatively long-lasting drugs used primarily as **anxiolytics** (to reduce anxiety).

The combined sales of these anxiolytics make them one of the most widely prescribed

Table 7.2	
Some Popular Sedative-Hypnotics	
Type	**Half-Life (Hours)**
Anxiolytics	
Alprazolam (Xanax)	6 to 20
Chlordiazepoxide (Librium)	5 to 30
Clonazepam (Klonopin)	30 to 40
Diazepam (Valium)	20 to 100
Lorazepam (Ativan)	10 to 20
Hypnotics	
Temazepam (Restoril)	5 to 25
Zolpidem (Ambien)	1
Eszopiclone (Lunesta)	6

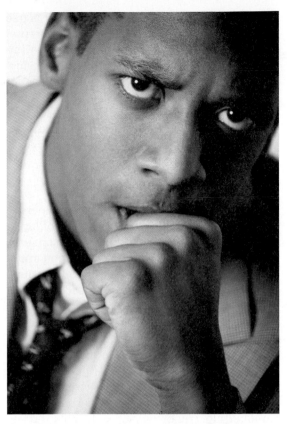

Benzodiazepines are commonly prescribed for anxiety disorders.

drug classes. Most physicians used to accept the widely held view that various types of dysfunctional behavior (e.g., phobias, panic attacks, obsessive-compulsive disorders, psychosomatic problems) result from various forms of psychological stress that can be lumped under the general classification of "anxieties." So if anxieties produce dysfunctional behavior and these drugs can reduce anxieties, then the drugs will be useful in reducing the dysfunctional behavior. Although this approach seems logical, in reality not all of these conditions respond well to antianxiety drugs. For specific phobias (e.g., fear of spiders), behavior therapy is a more effective treatment. And for obsessive-compulsive disorder and most of the official "anxiety disorders" (Chapter 8), certain antidepressant drugs seem to be most effective. Most of the prescriptions for antianxiety medications are not written by psychiatrists, nor are they written for patients with clearly defined anxiety disorders. In addition, many patients take the drugs daily for long periods. Galen, a second-century Greek physician, estimated that about 60 percent of the patients he saw had emotional and psychological, as opposed to physical, illness. It is currently estimated that for a typical general practitioner, about half of the patients have no treatable physical ailment. Many of these patients who complain of nervousness, distress, or vague aches and

pains will be given a prescription for an anxiolytic, such as Xanax. One way to look at this is that the patients may be suffering from a low-level generalized anxiety disorder, and the sedative is reducing the anxiety. A more cynical way of looking at it is that some patients are asking to be protected from the cares and woes of daily living. The physician prescribes something that can make the patient feel better in a general way. The patient doesn't complain as much and comes back for more pills, so everyone is happy.

GABA: an inhibitory neurotransmitter.

anxiolytics Drugs, such as Valium, used in the treatment of anxiety disorders. Literally, "anxiety-dissolving."

Although most physicians would agree that the benzodiazepines are probably overprescribed, in any individual case it may be impossible to know whether the patient just enjoys getting a "feel-good pill" or feels better because of a specific antianxiety effect. Whatever the reason for each individual, based on history the market for prescription anxiolytics will continue to be very large and profitable.

As Sleeping Pills

Although one or two beers might relax a person and reduce inhibitions a bit, the effect of larger amounts is more dramatic. If you consume several beers at an active, noisy party, you might become wild and reckless. But if you consume the same number of beers, go to bed, and turn off the lights, you will probably fall asleep fairly quickly. This is essentially the principle on which hypnotic drug therapy is based: a large enough dose is taken to help you get to sleep more quickly.

Insomnia is a fairly common symptom, and in one multisite survey about one out of three adults reported some trouble falling asleep, staying asleep, or both.[6] About half of these people felt that their insomnia was serious, but fewer than 10 percent had used a prescription hypnotic drug within the past year. People who complain of insomnia often overestimate how long it takes them to get to sleep and underestimate how much time they actually sleep. Partly because physicians know this and partly because of concern about tolerance, rebound insomnia, dependence, and "hangover" effects, fewer hypnotics are prescribed now than 30 years ago, and they are usually taken for only a few nights at a time rather than continually.

After 1976, the benzodiazepines displaced the barbiturates in the sleeping-pill market. By the early 1990s, triazolam (Halcion) sales had reached $100 million per year in the United States and $250 million worldwide. However, concerns were raised about the safety of the drug, and Upjohn, the drug's manufacturer,

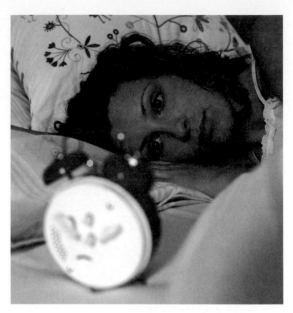

About one-third of adults report trouble sleeping.

was sued by a woman who claimed the drug made her so agitated and paranoid that she had killed her own mother. That case was settled out of court, but it brought attention to the drug and to other claims that it produced an unusual number of adverse psychiatric reactions in patients. Halcion has been banned in five countries because of these side effects. It has survived two FDA reviews in the United States and remains on the market, but its sales have declined markedly.

The nonbenzodiazepine drug zolpidem (Ambien) binds selectively to the GABA-A receptor and has therefore been suggested to be a more specific hypnotic agent. Clinically it appears to be similar to Halcion, with rapid onset and short duration of action. Ambien was the sales leader among sleeping pills in 2004, but in 2006 concerns were raised about people driving impaired while still under the influence of the drug, some because they failed to heed the warning to devote eight hours to sleep after taking it. Lunesta (eszopiclone) seems likely to take over the top position based on a big direct-to-consumer advertising campaign and the fact that it is approved for long-term use.

Targeting Prevention

Falling Asleep Without Pills

The following procedures are recommended ways of dealing with insomnia. If you occasionally have trouble sleeping, ask yourself which of these rules you typically follow, and which ones you often don't. Could you adopt some of these procedures?

- Establish and maintain a regular bedtime and a regular arising time. Try to wake up and get out of bed at the appointed time, even if you had trouble sleeping the night before. Avoid excessive sleep during holidays and weekends.
- When you get into bed, turn off the lights and relax. Avoid reviewing in your mind the day's stresses and tomorrow's challenges.
- Exercise regularly. Follow an exercise routine, but avoid heavy exercise late in the evening.
- Prepare a comfortable sleep environment. Too warm a room disturbs sleep; too cold a room does not solidify sleep. Occasional loud noises can disturb sleep without fully awakening you. Steady background noise, such as a fan may be useful for masking a noisy environment.

- Watch what you eat and drink before bedtime. Hunger may disturb sleep, as may caffeine and alcohol. A light snack may promote sleep, but avoid heavy or spicy foods at bedtime.
- Avoid the use of tobacco.
- Do not lie awake in bed for long periods. If you cannot fall asleep within 30 minutes, get out of bed and do something relaxing before trying to fall asleep again. Repeat this as many times as necessary. The goal is to avoid developing a paired association between being in bed and restlessness.
- Do not nap during the day. A prolonged nap after a night of insomnia may disturb the next night's sleep.
- Avoid the chronic use of sleeping pills. Although sedative-hypnotics can be effective when used as part of a coordinated treatment plan for certain types of insomnia, chronic use is ineffective at best and can be detrimental to sound sleep.

If you or someone you know has trouble sleeping, before resorting to the use of medication it would be wise to follow the suggestions given in the Targeting Prevention box. These tactics will probably help most people deal with their concerns about sleeplessness.

As Anticonvulsants

A thorough description of seizure disorders (the **epilepsies**) is beyond the scope of this book. Both the barbiturates and the benzodiazepines are widely used for the control of epileptic seizures. They are effective in reasonably low doses and are often combined with other anticonvulsant drugs for even better effectiveness. Some practical problems are associated with this use.

Anticonvulsant medications are given chronically, so tolerance tends to develop. The dose should be kept high enough to control

the seizures without producing undesirable drowsiness. Abrupt withdrawal of these drugs is likely to lead to seizures, so medication changes should be done carefully. Despite these problems, the sedative drugs are currently a necessary and useful treatment for epilepsy.

Causes for Concern

Dependence Liability

Psychological Dependence Most people who have used either barbiturates or benzodiazepines have not developed habitual use patterns. However, it was clear with the barbiturates

epilepsies: disorders characterized by uncontrolled movements (seizures).

that some individuals do become daily users of intoxicating amounts. Again, the short-acting barbiturates seemed to be the culprits. When Librium, the first benzodiazepine, was in its heyday, relatively little habitual use was reported. As Librium was displaced by the newer, more potent Valium, we saw increasing reports of habitual Valium use, perhaps because its onset, although slower than that of the short-acting barbiturates, is more rapid than that of Librium. Then Xanax, another rapid-acting benzodiazepine, became the most widely prescribed sedative, and reports of Xanax dependence appeared.[7]

Animals given the opportunity to press a lever that delivers intravenous barbiturates will do so, and the short-acting barbiturates work best for this. Animals will also self-inject several of the benzodiazepines, but at lower rates than with the short-acting barbiturates.[8] When human drug abusers were allowed an opportunity to work for oral doses of barbiturates or benzodiazepines on a hospital ward, they developed regular patterns of working for the drugs. When given a choice between pentobarbital and diazepam, the subjects generally chose pentobarbital.[9] These experiments indicate that these sedative drugs can serve as reinforcers of behavior but that the short-acting barbiturates are probably more likely to lead to dependence than are any of the benzodiazepines currently on the market.

Physical Dependence A characteristic withdrawal syndrome can occur after chronic use of large enough doses of any of the sedative-hypnotic drugs. This syndrome is different from the narcotic withdrawal syndrome and quite similar to the alcohol withdrawal syndrome. An early description of the withdrawal from barbiturates is an excellent example:

> Upon abrupt withdrawal of barbiturates from individuals who have been ingesting 0.8 gm or more daily of one of the shorter-acting barbiturates (secobarbital, pentobarbital, amobarbital), signs of barbiturate intoxication disappear in the first 8 to 12 hours of abstinence, and, clini-

cally, the patient seems to improve. Thereafter, increasing anxiety, insomnia, tremulousness, weakness, difficulty in making cardiovascular adjustments on standing, anorexia, nausea and vomiting appear. One or more convulsions of *grand mal* type usually occur during the second or third day of abstinence. Following the seizures a psychosis characterized by confusion, disorientation in time and place, agitation, tremulousness, insomnia, delusions and visual and auditory hallucinations may supervene. The psychosis clinically resembles alcoholic delirium tremens, usually begins and is worse at night, and terminates abruptly with a critical sleep.[10]

This syndrome is different in character from the narcotic withdrawal syndrome, longer lasting, and probably more unpleasant. In addition, withdrawal from the sedative-hypnotics or alcohol is potentially life-threatening, with death occurring in as many as 5 percent of those who withdraw abruptly after taking large doses.

Animal experiments using large intravenous doses of benzodiazepines show clearly that a barbiturate-like withdrawal syndrome can be produced with an onset that varies with the half-life of the drug. In humans, benzodiazepine withdrawal symptoms are rarely as severe as those seen with barbiturates and often consist of increased anxiety, irritability, or insomnia, which can be confused with a return to the predrug conditions of anxiety or insomnia for which the drug was initially prescribed.

Although it is said that withdrawal symptoms are less common after abrupt cessation of the newer nonbenzodiazepine hypnotics, there is at least one case report of a woman experiencing seizures during withdrawal after extended use of zolpidem.[11]

Because there is a cross-dependence among the barbiturates, the benzodiazepines, and alcohol, it is theoretically possible to use any of these drugs to halt the withdrawal symptoms from any other depressant. Drug treatment is often used, and a general rule is to

Mind/Body Connection

Learning to Relax

Most people shouldn't need pills to relax or to sleep. Here's a procedure suggested by the University of Texas Learning Center you can use to relax before you study or as a refreshing study break. You can also use it to help you go to sleep at night.

Sit in a comfortable chair in a quiet room. Tense or contract each muscle group for a slow count of 10, then relax slowly for a count of 10. For each group, notice the difference between the feeling of tension and the warm, soft feeling of relaxation. Go from tension to relaxation slowly. Think of a balloon slowly leaking air and collapsing, or of a flower bud opening and folding back.

1. Tense and slowly relax your fists and forearms.
2. Bend your elbows and tense and relax your biceps.
3. Straighten your arms and tense and relax your triceps.
4. Wrinkle up and relax your forehead.
5. Clench and relax your jaw.
6. Shrug and relax your shoulders.
7. Fill your lungs and let air out slowly.
8. Pull in and relax your stomach.
9. Push down your feet to tense and relax your thighs.
10. Tip up your toes to tense and relax your shins.
11. Raise your heels to tense and relax your calves.

The whole procedure should take about 20 minutes the first time; it will take much less time later. Eventually, you will be able to put your body in a state of complete relaxation almost at will.

use a long-acting drug, given in divided doses until the withdrawal symptoms are controlled. Typically, one of the benzodiazepines is used during detoxification from any of the CNS depressants.[12]

Toxicity

The major areas of concern with these depressant drugs are the behavioral and physiological problems encountered when high doses of the drug are present in the body (acute toxicity). Behaviorally, all these drugs are capable of producing alcohol-like intoxication with impaired judgment and incoordination. Obviously, such an impaired state vastly multiplies the dangers involved in driving and other activities, and the effects of these drugs combined with alcohol are additive, so that the danger is further increased. On the physiological side, the major concern is the tendency of these drugs to depress the respiration rate. With large enough doses, as in accidental or intentional overdose, breathing ceases. Again, the combination of these depressants and alcohol is quite dangerous. Although benzodiazepines are usually quite high on the list of

drugs associated with deaths in the DAWN coroners' reports, in almost every case the culprit is the drug in combination with alcohol or another drug, rather than the benzodiazepine alone.[13]

Patterns of Abuse

Almost all of the abuse of the sedative-hypnotic agents has historically involved the oral use of legally manufactured products. Two characteristic types of abusers have been associated with barbiturate use, and these two major types probably still characterize a large fraction of sedative abusers. The first type of abuser is an older adult who obtains the drug on a prescription, either for daytime sedative use or as a sleeping pill. Through repeated use, tolerance develops and the dose is increased. Even though some of these individuals visit several physicians to obtain prescriptions for enough pills to maintain this level of use, many would vehemently deny that they are "drug abusers." This type of chronic use can lead to physical dependence.

The other major group tends to be younger and consists of people who obtain the drugs

Table 7.3
Some Chemicals Abused by Inhalation

Substances	Chemical Ingredients
Volatile solvents	
Paint and paint thinners	Petroleum distillates, esters, acetone
Paint removers	Toluene, methylene chloride, methanol, acetone
Nail polish remover	Acetone, ethyl acetate
Correction fluid and thinner	Trichloroethylene, trichloroethane
Glues and cements	Toluene, ethyl acetate, hexane, methyl chloride, acetone, methyl ethyl ketone, methyl butyl ketone, trichloroethylene, tetrachloroethylene
Dry-cleaning agents	Tetrachloroethylene, trichloroethane
Spot removers	Xylene, petroleum distillates, chlorohydrocarbons
Aerosols, propellants, gases	
Spray paint	Butane, propane, toluene, hydrocarbons
Hair spray	Butane, propane
Lighters	Butane, isopropane
Fuel gas	Butane, propane
Whipped cream, "whippets"	Nitrous oxide
Anesthetics	
Current medical use	Nitrous oxide, halothane, enflurane
Former medical use	Ether, chloroform
Nitrites	
Locker room, Rush, poppers	Isoamyl, isobutyl, isopropyl nitrite, butyl nitrite

simply to get high. Sleeping pills might be taken from the home medicine cabinet, or the drugs might be purchased on the street. These younger abusers tend to take relatively large doses, to mix several drugs, or to drink alcohol with the drug, all for the purpose of becoming intoxicated. With this type of use, the possibility of acute toxicity is particularly high.

Inhalants

Some people will do almost anything to escape reality. Gasoline, glue, paint, lighter fluid, spray cans of almost anything, nail polish, and Liquid Paper all contain volatile solvents that, when inhaled, can have effects that are similar in an overall way to the depressants. High-dose exposure to these fumes makes users intoxicated, often slurring their speech and causing

them to have trouble walking a straight line, as if they were drunk on alcohol.

Although most people think first of the abuse of volatile solvents such as glues, paints, and gasoline, other types of substances can be abused through sniffing or inhaling in a similar manner (Table 7.3). Two major groups are the gaseous anesthetics and the nitrites, as well as volatile solvents.

Gaseous Anesthetics

Gaseous anesthetics have been used in medicine and surgery for many years, and abuse of these anesthetics occurs among physicians and others with access to these gases. One of the oldest, nitrous oxide, was first used in the early 1800s and quite early acquired the popular name "laughing gas" because of the hilarity exhibited by some of its users. During the 1800s,

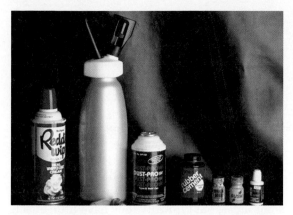

Chemicals abused by inhalation can be found in a variety of household products.

traveling demonstrations of laughing gas enticed audience members to volunteer to become intoxicated for the amusement of others. Nitrous oxide is also one of the safest anesthetics when used properly, but it is not possible to obtain good surgical anesthesia unless the individual breathes almost pure nitrous oxide, which leads to suffocation through a lack of oxygen. Nitrous oxide is still used for light anesthesia, especially by dentists. It is also often used in combination with one of the more effective inhaled anesthetics, allowing the use of a lower concentration of the primary anesthetic. Nitrous oxide is also found as a propellant in whipping-cream containers and is sold in small bottles ("whippets") for use in home whipping-cream dispensers. Recreational users have obtained nitrous oxide from both sources.

Nitrites

The chemicals amyl nitrite and butyl nitrite cause a rapid dilation of the arteries and reduce blood pressure to the brain, resulting in a brief period of faintness or even unconsciousness. These chemicals have an unpleasant odor and were sold under such suggestive brand names as "Locker Room" and "Aroma of Men." The male-sounding names might also reflect the popularity of these products among some homosexual males who used these "poppers"

during sex to enhance the sense of lightheadedness at orgasm. Although many surveys have not separated nitrites from other inhalants, the high school survey began to do so in 1979. It appears that the popularity of the nitrites declined throughout the 1980s and 1990s. Since 1988, the Consumer Product Safety Commission has taken steps to remove these various nitrites from the market.

Volatile Solvents

The modern era of solvent abuse, or at least of widely publicized solvent abuse, can be traced to a 1959 investigative article in the Sunday supplement of a Denver, Colorado, newspaper. This article reported that young people in a nearby city had been caught spreading plastic model glue on their palms, cupping their hands over their mouths, and inhaling the vapors to get high. The article warned about the dangers of accidental exposure to solvent fumes, and an accompanying photograph showed a young man demonstrating another way to inhale glue vapors—by putting the glue on a handkerchief and holding it over the mouth and nose. The article described the effects as similar to being drunk.

That article both notified the police, who presumably began looking for such behavior, and advertised and described the practice to young people: Within the next six months, the city of Denver went from no previously reported cases of "glue-sniffing" to 50 cases. More publicity and warnings followed, and by the end of 1961 the juvenile authorities in Denver were seeing about "30 boys a month." The problem expanded further in Denver over the next several years, while similar patterns of publicity, increased use, and more publicity followed in other cities. In 1962, the magazines *Time* and *Newsweek* both carried articles describing how to sniff model glue and warning about its dangers, and the Hobby Industry Association of America produced a film for civic groups that warned about glue sniffing and recommended that communities make it

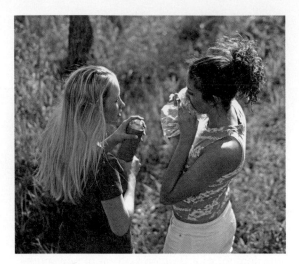

Most "huffers" are young. Risks include suffocation and damage to nerves, kidneys, and the brain.

illegal to sniff any substance with an intoxicating effect. Sales of model glue continued to rise as the publicity went nationwide.[14]

Since then, recreational use of various solvents by young people has occurred mostly as more localized fads. One group of kids in one area might start using cooking sprays, the practice will grow and then decline over a couple of years, and meanwhile in another area the kids might be inhaling a specific brand and even color of spray paint.

Although some "huffers" are adults (e.g., alcoholics without the funds to buy alcohol), most are young. The ready availability and low price of these solvents make them attractive to children. In the high school senior class of 2003, 4 percent of the students reported having used some type of inhalant in the past year, whereas 9 percent of the eighth-graders reported using an inhalant within the past year.[15] Inhalant use has traditionally been more common among poor Hispanic youth and on Indian reservations.[16]

Because so many different solvents are involved, it is impossible to characterize the potential harm produced by abuse of glues, paints, correction fluids, and so on. Several of the solvents have been linked to kidney damage,

brain damage, and peripheral nerve damage, and many of them produce irritation of the respiratory tract and result in severe headaches. However, several users of various inhalants have simply suffocated. Although most of the children who inhale solvents do so only occasionally and give it up as they grow older and have more access to alcohol, some become dependent and a few will die.

Laws to limit sales of these household solvents to minors or to make it illegal to use them to become intoxicated have been passed in some areas, but typically they have little effect. Too many products are simply too readily available. Look around your own home or on the shelves of a supermarket or discount store—how many products have a warning about using them in an enclosed place? That warning is used by some people to indicate an inhalant to try! This is one type of substance abuse that families and communities should attack with awareness, information, and direct social intervention.

GHB (Gamma Hydroxybutyric Acid)

Gamma hydroxybutyrate (GHB) occurs naturally in the brain as well as in other parts of the body. Its structure is fairly close to the inhibitory neurotransmitter GABA. GHB has been known for some time to be a CNS depressant, and has been used in other countries as an anesthetic. Because it appears to play a role in general cellular metabolism, for a time it was sold as a dietary supplement and taken (mostly in fairly low doses) by athletes and bodybuilders hoping to stimulate muscle growth. There is no good evidence that GHB is effective for this use, but its widespread availability in the 1980s led some to "rediscover" its powerful CNS depressant effects. Taking larger quantities of GHB alone, or combining GHB with alcohol, produces a combined depressant effect similar to what would be produced by combining alcohol with any of the other depressants discussed in this chapter, from chloral hydrate to the benzodiazepines.

The usual recreational dose of GHB taken alone ranges from 1 to 5 grams. It has a fairly short half-life of about one hour. The behavioral effects are similar to alcohol, and higher doses produce muscular incoordination and slurring of speech. Increasing recreational use led the FDA to ban the inclusion of GHB in dietary supplements in 1990. As mentioned in the Drugs in the Media, publicity about deaths associated with the use of GHB and alcohol as a date-rape combination led in 2000 to congressional action directing that it be listed as a Schedule I controlled substance. Evidence from the Monitoring the Future survey indicated that in 2003 only about 1.5 percent of high school seniors reported using GHB in the past year, down from about 2 percent in 2000, the first year GHB use was studied.[15]

In 2000, Congress directed that GHB be placed on Schedule I. However, in 2002, the FDA approved Xyrem, an oral solution of GHB for use in narcolepsy. For reasons that are not well understood, GHB tends to reduce the frequency of *cataplexy,* one common symptom of narcolepsy. Cataplexy refers to muscular weakness or paralysis, and in narcolepsy it is usually experienced as a brief, unpredictable episode. Thus, Xyrem, under the generic name sodium oxybate, is now available for prescription as a Schedule III controlled substance. Any other form of GHB remains listed on Schedule I.

Summary

- The barbiturates, benzodiazepines, inhalants, and other depressant drugs all have many effects in common with each other and with alcohol.

- Depressants may be prescribed in low doses for their sedative effect or in higher doses as sleeping pills (hypnotics).

- Over the past 40 years, the barbiturates have been mostly displaced by the benzodiazepines.

- The barbiturates and benzodiazepines both increase the inhibitory neural effects of the neurotransmitter GABA.

- Drugs that have a rapid onset are more likely to produce psychological dependence.

- Drugs that have a short duration of action are more likely to produce withdrawal symptoms.

- Overdoses of these depressant drugs can cause death by inhibiting respiration, particularly if the drug is taken in combination with alcohol.

- The abused inhalants include gaseous anesthetics, certain nitrites, and volatile solvents.

- Abuse of inhalants, especially of the volatile solvents, can lead to organ damage, including neurological damage, more readily than with alcohol or other psychoactive substances.

Review Questions

1. What was the foul-smelling drug that was so widely used in mental hospitals before the 1950s?
2. A prescription of 30 mg of phenobarbital would probably have been for which type of use?
3. What is the relationship between psychological dependence and the time course of a drug's action?
4. The barbiturates and benzodiazepines act at which neurotransmitter receptor?
5. Why should hypnotic drugs usually be prescribed only for a few nights at a time?
6. What is zolpidem (Ambien)?
7. What are the characteristics of the sedative-hypnotic withdrawal syndrome?
8. What happens to a person who takes an overdose of a sedative-hypnotic?
9. How are the effects of the nitrites different from the effects of inhaled solvent fumes?
10. What are the effects of combining GHB with alcohol?

References

1. Richardson, B.W. "Chloral and Other Narcotics, I." *Popular Science* 15: (1879), p. 492.

2. Rosenblatt, S., & R. Dobson. *Beyond Valium*. New York: G.P. Putnam's Sons, 1981.

3. "Drug Linked to Assaults Is Reformulated." *The New York Times,* October 19, 1997.

4. Julien, R.M. *A Primer of Drug Action,* 10th ed. New York: Worth, 2005.

5. Low, K., and others. "Molecular and Neuronal Substrate for the Selective Attenuation of Anxiety." *Science* 290 (2000), pp. 131–34.

6. Hatoum, H.T., S.X. Kong, C.M. Kania, J.M. Wong, and W.B. Mendelson. "Insomnia, Health-Related Quality of Life and Healthcare Resource Consumption. A Study of Managed-Care Organization Enrollees." *Pharmacoeconomics* 14 no. 6 (1998), pp. 629–37.

7. Longo, L.P., & B. Johnson. "Addiction: Part I. Benzodiazepines—Side Effects, Abuse Risk and Alternatives." *American Family Physician* 61 (2000), pp. 2121–28.

8. Griffiths, R.R. and others. "Self-injection of Barbiturates and Benzodiazepines in Baboons." *Psychopharmacology* 75: (1981), pp. 101–09.

9. Griffiths, R.R., G. Bigelow, and I. Liebson. "Human Drug Self-administration: Double-blind Comparison of Pentobarbital, Diazepam, Chlorpromazine and Placebo." *The Journal of Pharmacology and Experimental Therapeutics* 210 (1979), pp. 301–10.

10. Fraser, H.F., and others. "Death Due to Withdrawal of Barbiturates." *American Journal of Internal Medicine* 38 (1953), pp. 1319–25.

11. Tripodianakis, J., and others. "Zolpidem-related Epileptic Seizures: A Case Report." *European Psychiatry* 18 (2003), pp. 140–41.

12. Shader, R.I., and others. "Treatment of Physical Dependence on Barbiturates, Benzodiazepines, and Other Sedative-Hypnotics." In *Manual of Psychiatric Therapeutics,* 3rd ed. R.I. Shader, ed. Philadelphia: Lipincott Williams & Wilkins, 2003.

13. Substance Abuse and Mental Health Services Administration. "Drug Abuse Warning Network, 2003: Area Profiles of Drug-Related Mortality" DAWN Series D–27, DHHS Publication No. (SMA) 05-4023, Rockville, MD, 2005.

14. Brecher, E. M., *Licit and illicit drugs.* Boston: Little, Brown, 1972.

15. Johnston, L.D., P.M. O'Malley, J.G. Bachman, and J.E. Schulenberg. "Monitoring the Future, National Survey Results on Drug Use, 1975–2003: Volume I, Secondary School Students." *NIH Publication No. 04-5507.* Bethesda, MD: National Institute on Drug Abuse, 2004.

16. Beauvais, E., and others. "Inhalant Abuse among American Indian, Mexican American, and Non-Latino White Adolescents." *American Journal of Drug & Alcohol Abuse* 28 (2002), pp. 477–95.

8

Medication for Mental Disorders

Objectives

When you have finished this chapter, you should be able to:

- Discuss the medical model of mental disorders and why many professionals oppose it.

- Describe the typical characteristics of anxiety disorders, schizophrenia, and mood disorders.

- Explain the historical context and the importance of the discovery of the phenothiazine antipsychotics.

- Recognize the names of a number of currently available antipsychotic drugs.

- Distinguish between conventional and atypical antipsychotics.

- Discuss theories of antipsychotic drug action and why it is difficult to understand the mechanism of action for these and other classes of psychoactive drugs.

- Explain the sales trend of antidepressants since 1987 and what is expected in the future.

- Explain why it is simplistic to say that antidepressant drugs work by restoring serotonin activity to normal.

- Describe how lithium and anticonvulsant drugs are used in treating bipolar disorder.

- Describe arguments for and against giving prescription privileges to psychologists.

For most of today's mentally ill, the primary mode of therapy is drug therapy. Powerful psychoactive medications help control psychotic behavior, depression, and mania in thousands of patients, reducing human suffering and health care costs, yet these drugs are far from cures, and many have undesirable side effects. Should mental disorders be approached with chemical treatments? Do these treatments work? How do they work? What can these drugs tell us about the causes of mental illness? Although we don't yet have complete answers for any of these questions, we do have partial answers for all of them.

Mental Disorders

The Medical Model

The use of the term *mental illness* seems to imply a particular model for behavioral disorders or dysfunctions. The medical model has been attacked by both psychiatrists (who are medical doctors) and psychologists (who generally hold nonmedical doctorates such as a PhD or PsyD).

According to this model, the *patient* appears with a set of *symptoms,* and on the basis of these symptoms a *diagnosis* is made as to

Online Learning Center Resources

www.mhhe.com/ksir12e

Visit our Online Learning Center (OLC) for access to these study aids and additional resources.

- Learning objectives
- Glossary flashcards
- Web activities and links
- Self-scoring chapter quiz
- Audio chapter summaries

which *disease* the patient is suffering from. Once the disease is known, its *cause* can be determined and the patient provided with a *cure.* In general terms the arguments for and against a medical model of mental illness are similar to those for and against a medical model of dependence, presented in Chapter 2. For an infectious disease such as tuberculosis or syphilis, a set of symptoms suggests a particular disorder, but a specific diagnostic test for the presence of certain bacteria or antibodies is used to confirm the diagnosis, identify the cause, and clarify the treatment approach. Once the infection is cleared up, the disorder is cured.

For mental disorders a set of behavioral symptoms is about all we have to define and diagnose the disorder. A person might be inactive, not sleep or eat well, and not say much, and what little is said might be quite negative. This behavior might lead us to call the person depressed. Does that mean the person has a "disease" called depression, with a physical cause and a potential cure? Or does it really only give a description of how he or she is acting, in the same way as we might call someone "crabby," "friendly," or "nerdy"? The behaviors that we refer to as indicating depression are varied and probably have many different causes, most of them not known. And we are far from being able to prescribe a cure for depression that will be generally successful in eliminating these symptoms.

Despite these attacks on the medical model, it still seems to guide much of the current thinking about behavioral disorders. The fact that psychoactive drugs can be effective in controlling symptoms, if not in curing diseases, has lent strength to supporters of the medical model. If chemicals can help normalize an individual's behavior, a natural assumption might be that the original problem resulted from a chemical imbalance in the brain—and that measurements of chemicals in urine, blood, or cerebrospinal fluid could provide more specific and accurate diagnoses and give direction to efforts at drug therapy. This kind of thinking gives scientists great hope, and many experiments have attempted to find the searched-for chemical imbalances, so far with very little success.

Classification of Mental Disorders

Because human behavior is so variable and because we do not know the causes of most mental disorders, classification of the mentally ill into diagnostic categories is difficult. Nevertheless, some basic divisions are widely used and important for understanding the uses of psychotherapeutic drugs. In 2000, the American Psychiatric Association published the revised fourth edition of its *Diagnostic and Statistical Manual of Mental Disorders* (referred to as the DSM-IV-TR).[1] This manual provides criteria for classifying mental disorders into hundreds of specific diagnostic categories. Partly because this classification system has been adopted by major health insurance companies, its terms and definitions have become standard for all mental health professionals.

Anxiety is a normal and common human experience: Anticipation of potential threats and dangers often helps us avoid them. However, when these worries become unrealistic, resulting in chronic uneasiness, fear of impending doom, or bouts of terror or panic, they can interfere with the individual's daily life. Physical symptoms may also be present, often

Drugs in the Media

Mental Illness at the Movies

Most of us know at least one person who is being treated with medication for depression or for ADHD (Chapter 6). Because these and most other mental disorders can be controlled to some degree with medication means we do not experience firsthand many of the most troubling behavior problems that lead to a diagnosis of a serious mental disorder. Films and television programs have attempted to portray characters struggling with mental disorders, and some of these portrayals can be informative. The book *Movies and Mental Illness*[2] uses the viewing of popular films as an instructional aid to learning about abnormal psychology.

These films can also teach us about how medications are used in treating those disorders. Two of the best film depictions of mental institutions, for example, are *The Snake Pit* (1948), starring Olivia de Havilland, and *One Flew over the Cuckoo's Nest* (1975), starring Jack Nicholson. Both films are available in video stores and provide an interesting contrast. Although neither portrays the mental institution in a positive light, one is set in the period before antipsychotic and antidepressant medications were available, and the later film is set at a time when some of the early drugs of those types were widely used.

A more recent portrayal of mental illness by actor Jack Nicholson can be found in the 1998 film *As Good as It Gets*. Nicholson's character suffers from obsessive-compulsive disorder, and for most of the film he refuses to treat the problem with medication. Although the medication itself plays a minor role, it is shown to be an important part of his later improvement. In the 2001 film *A Beautiful Mind,* a Princeton math professor and Nobel laureate's lifelong struggle with schizophrenia is portrayed in convincing fashion, along with the usefulness, limitations, and side effects of the antipsychotic medications he used to control the symptoms.

Next time you are discussing movies with your friends, see if you can come up with other examples of films or television programs that depict the use of psychoactive drugs in the treatment of mental disorders. Are the medications generally treated inappropriately as either cures or as a way to force conformity and compliance? Or are they treated more realistically as beneficial in some ways, yet with both limited effectiveness and unwanted side effects?

---

associated with activation of the autonomic nervous system (e.g., flushed skin, dilated pupils, gastrointestinal problems, increased heart rate, or shortness of breath). The DSM-IV-TR refers to these and other problems as **anxiety disorders** (see the DSM-IV-TR box).

Perhaps because these disorders all seem to have some form of anxiety associated with them, and perhaps because for many years psychiatrists classified benzodiazepines and other depressants as *antianxiety drugs* (see Chapter 7), we tend to think of anxiety not as a behavioral symptom but rather as an internal state that *causes* the disorders. That view fits well with the medical model, but we should guard against easy acceptance of the view that these disorders are caused by anxiety and that therefore we can treat them using antianxiety drugs. In recent years, psychiatrists have increasingly used selective reuptake inhibitors, classified as "antidepressants" to treat obsessive-compulsive disorder and other anxiety disorders.

Psychosis refers to a major disturbance of normal intellectual and social functioning in which there is loss of contact with reality. Not knowing the current date, hearing voices that aren't there, and believing that you are Napoleon or Christ are some examples of this

> **anxiety disorders:** mental disorders characterized by excessive worry, fears, or avoidance.
> **psychosis (sy *co* sis):** a serious mental disorder involving loss of contact with reality.

DSM-IV-TR

Anxiety Disorders

Panic Disorder (With or Without Agoraphobia)

Panic disorder is defined by recurrent, unexpected panic attacks and by subsequent concern about future attacks or about the meaning of the attacks. Panic attacks may include shortness of breath, dizziness or faintness, palpitations or accelerated heart rate, trembling, sweating, choking, numbness, fear of dying, or fear of going crazy or doing something uncontrolled.

The agoraphobia (*fear of the marketplace*) that often accompanies panic disorders is a fear of being in places or situations from which escape might be difficult or where help might not be available in the event of either a panic attack or some other incapacitating or embarrassing situation (e.g., fainting or losing bladder control). The person with agoraphobia might avoid going outside the home alone or be afraid of being in a public place or standing in a line.

Specific Phobia

Specific phobia is excessive or unreasonable fear of a specific object or situation (e.g., elevators, flying, heights, or some type of animal).

Social Phobia

Social phobia is a marked and persistent fear of social or performance situations (e.g., speaking in public, entering a room full of strangers, or using a public restroom).

Obsessive-Compulsive Disorder

Obsessions are recurrent and persistent thoughts, impulses, or images that are intrusive and inappropriate and that cause marked anxiety or distress. Compulsions are urgent, repetitive behaviors, such as hand washing, counting, or repeatedly "checking" to make sure that some dreaded event will not occur (e.g., checking that all doors and windows are locked, then checking again and again).

Posttraumatic Stress Disorder

The person has been exposed to an event that involved actual or threatened death or serious injury, and the person reacted with intense fear, helplessness, or horror. The traumatic event is persistently reexperienced through recollections, dreams, or a sudden feeling as if the event were occurring.

Generalized Anxiety Disorder

Generalized anxiety disorder is excessive anxiety and worry about a number of events or activities, such as school or work performance or finances, lasting for a period of six months or longer.

---

withdrawal from reality. Many people refer to psychosis as reflecting a primary disorder of *thinking,* as opposed to mood or emotion.

Psychotic behavior may be viewed as a group of symptoms that can have many possible causes. One important distinction is between the *organic* psychoses and the *functional* psychoses. An organic disorder is one that has a known physical cause. Psychosis can result from many things, including brain tumors or infections, metabolic or endocrine disorders, degenerative neurological diseases, chronic alcohol use, and high doses of stimulant drugs, such as amphetamine or cocaine.

Functional disorders are simply those for which there is no known or obvious physical cause. A person suffering from a chronic (long-lasting) psychotic condition for which there is no known cause will probably receive the diagnosis of **schizophrenia.** There is a popular misconception that schizophrenia means "split personality" or refers to individuals exhibiting multiple personalities. Instead, schizophrenia should probably be translated as *shattered mind.* See the DSM-IV-TR box for the diagnostic criteria for schizophrenia.

Mood disorder refers to the appearance of depressed or manic symptoms. Look at

DSM-IV-TR

Diagnosis of Schizophrenia

A. Characteristic symptoms: Two or more of the following:
  1. Delusions (irrational beliefs)
  2. Hallucinations (e.g., hearing voices)
  3. Disorganized speech (incoherent, frequent changes of topic)
  4. Grossly disorganized behavior (inappropriate, unpredictable) or catatonic (withdrawn, immobile)
  5. Negative symptoms (lack of emotional response, little or no speech, doesn't initiate activities)
B. Interference with social or occupational function
C. Duration of at least six months

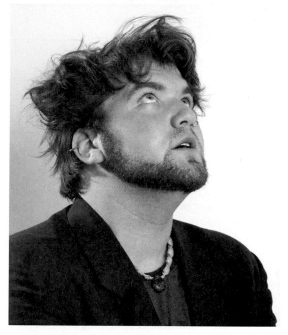

Mental disorders are typically categorized by behavioral symptoms; for example, schizophrenia is characterized by delusions, hallucinations, and disorganized speech and behavior.

Figure 6.3 on page 143 for one schematic representation of mood in which depression is shown as an abnormally low mood and mania as an abnormally high mood. The important distinction in *DSM-IV-TR*, and in the drug treatment of mood disorders, is between **bipolar disorder,** in which both manic and depressive episodes have been observed at some time, and major **depression,** in which only depressive episodes are reported. See the DSM-IV-TR box "Diagnosis of Mood Disorders" for diagnostic criteria for manic episode and major depressive episode.

Individual human beings often don't fit neatly into one of these diagnostic categories, and in many cases assigning a diagnosis and selecting a treatment are as much a matter of experience and art as they are of applying scientific descriptions. For example, suppose a person displays both abnormal mood states and bizarre thinking. If it is assumed that the disturbance of thinking is the primary problem and that the person is elated or depressed because of a bizarre belief, then the individual may be diagnosed as schizophrenic. Another

professional might see the mood disorder as primary, with the "crazy" talk supporting a negative view of the world, and give the individual a primary diagnosis of depression.

Treatment of Mental Disorders

Before 1950

Over the centuries, mental patients have been subjected to various kinds of treatment, depending on the views held at the time regarding the causes of mental illness. Because we are

schizophrenia (skitz o *fren* ee yah): a type of chronic psychosis.
bipolar disorder: a type of mood disorder also known as manic-depressive disorder.
depression: a major type of mood disorder.

DSM-IV-TR

Diagnosis of Mood Disorders

I. Manic Episode
   A. Abnormally and persistently elevated, expansive, or irritable mood
   B. At least three of the following:
      1. Inflated self-esteem or grandiosity
      2. Decreased need for sleep
      3. More talkative than usual or pressure to keep talking
      4. Flight of ideas or feeling that thoughts are racing
      5. Distractibility
      6. Increase in activity
      7. Excessive involvement in pleasurable activities that have a high potential for painful consequences (shopping, sex, foolish investments)
   C. Mood disturbance is sufficiently severe to cause marked impairment in functioning

II. Major Depressive Episode
   A. Five or more of the following, including either No. 1 or No. 2:
      1. Depressed mood most of the day, nearly every day
      2. Markedly diminished interest or pleasure in most activities
      3. Significant changes in body weight or appetite (increased or decreased)
      4. Insomnia or hypersomnia nearly every day
      5. Psychomotor agitation (increased activity) or retardation (decreased activity)
      6. Fatigue or loss of energy
      7. Feelings of worthlessness or excessive guilt
      8. Diminished ability to think or concentrate
      9. Recurrent thoughts of death or suicide, or a suicide attempt or plan for committing suicide
   B. The symptoms cause clinically significant distress or impairment
   C. Not due to a drug or medical condition and not a normal reaction to the loss of a loved one

concerned with drug therapy, a good place to begin our history is in 1917, when a physical treatment was first demonstrated to be effective in serious mental disease. In those days a great proportion of the psychotic patients were suffering from *general paresis,* a syphilitic infection of the nervous system. It was noticed that the fever associated with malaria often produced marked improvement, and so in 1917 "malaria therapy" was introduced in the treatment of general paresis. The later discovery of antibiotics that could cure syphilis virtually eliminated this particular type of treatment.

In the 1920s, wealthier patients could afford a course of "narcosis therapy," in which barbiturates and other depressants were used to induce sleep for as long as a week or more. Another use for sedative drugs was in conjunction with psychotherapy: an intravenous dose of thiopental sodium, a rapid-acting barbiturate, would relax a person and produce more talking during psychotherapy. The theory was that such a reduction in inhibitions would enable the patient to express repressed thoughts; thus, the term *truth serum* came to be used for thiopental sodium and for scopolamine, an anticholinergic drug used similarly. Anyone who has ever listened to a person who has drunk a good bit of alcohol will tell you that although the talk might be less inhibited, it isn't always more truthful. So-called truth serum apparently worked about as well.

In 1933, Manfred Sakel of Vienna induced comas in some schizophrenics by administering insulin. The resulting drop in blood glucose level caused the brain's neurons to first increase their activity and produce convulsions and then decrease their activity and leave the patient in a coma. A course of 30 to 50 of these treatments over two to three months was believed to be highly effective, and discharge rates of 90 percent were reported in the early years of insulin-shock therapy. Later studies demonstrated that the relapse rate was quite high, and this treatment was abandoned.

Ladislas von Meduna believed, incorrectly, that no epileptic was schizophrenic and no schizophrenic ever had epilepsy. Reasoning that epileptic convulsions prevented the development of schizophrenia, he felt that inducing convulsions might have therapeutic value for schizophrenic patients. His first convulsant drug was camphor, but it had the disadvantage of a lag time of several hours between injection and the convulsions. In 1934, he started using pentylenetetrazol (Metrazol), which induced convulsions in less than 30 seconds and reported improvement in 50 to 60 percent of patients.

The use of a drug was not ideal for inducing convulsions, because even a 30-second interval between injection and loss of consciousness (with the convulsion) produced much anguish in the patient. Ugo Cerletti, after experimenting on pigs in a slaughterhouse, developed the technique of using electric shock to induce convulsions. This method has the advantage of inducing loss of consciousness and convulsion at the moment the electric shock is applied. *Electroconvulsive therapy (ECT)* is hardly ever used now with schizophrenia. Although early work in the 1930s and 1940s suggested high improvement rates, later studies found a reduction of schizophrenic symptoms in only about half of the patients, and the relapse rates were quite high. However, ECT is still used with severely depressed patients who do not respond to medication.[3]

By the 1950s, probably the major drug in use for severely disturbed patients in the large mental hospitals was paraldehyde, a sedative, (see Chapter 6). Although it produces little respiratory depression and therefore is safer than the barbiturates, the drug has a characteristic odor, which is still well remembered by those who worked in or visited the hospitals of that era. Sedation of severely disturbed pa-tients by drugs that make them drowsy and slow them down has been referred to as the use of a "chemical straitjacket."

Antipsychotics

A number of people were involved in the discovery that a group of drugs called the **phenothiazines** had special properties when used with mental patients. Credit is usually given to a French surgeon, Henri Laborit, who first tested these compounds in conjunction with surgical anesthesia. He noted that the most effective of the phenothiazines, chlorpromazine, did not by itself induce drowsiness or a loss of consciousness, but it seemed to make the patients unconcerned about their upcoming surgery. He reasoned that this effect might reduce emotionality in psychiatric patients and encouraged his psychiatric colleagues to test the drug. The first report of these French trials of chlorpromazine in mental patients mentioned that not only were the patients calmed, but the drug also seemed to act on the psychotic process itself. This new type of drug action attracted a variety of names: in the United States the drugs were generally called tranquilizers, which some now think is an unfortunate term that focuses on the calming action and seems to imply sedation. Another term used was **neuroleptic,** meaning "taking hold of the nervous system," a term implying an increased amount of control. Although both of these terms are still in use, most medical texts now refer to this group of drugs as **antipsychotics,** reflecting their ability to reduce psychotic symptoms without necessarily producing drowsiness and sedation.

---

phenothiazines (feen o *thigh* uh zeens): a group of drugs used to treat psychosis.
neuroleptic (noor o *lep* tick): a general term for antipsychotic drugs.
antipsychotics: a group of drugs used to treat psychosis; same as neuroleptic.

One of the early reports (1955) dealing with the side effects of chlorpromazine on a large number of hospitalized psychotic patients stated:

It produces marked quieting of the motor manifestations. Patients cease to be loud and profane, the tendency to hyperbolic associations diminished, and the patients can sit still long enough to eat and take care of normal physiological needs. . . .

In the more chronic psychotic states, the effect of the drug is much less immediately dramatic, but for those experienced with the relief of psychotic symptoms from other measures, the use of the drug produces results that are equally gratifying when compared with results in the more acute situations.[4]

The tremendous impact of phenothiazine treatment on the management of hospitalized patients is clear from a 1955 statement by the director of the Delaware State Hospital:

We have now achieved . . . the reorganization of the management of disturbed patients. With rare exceptions, all restraints have been discontinued. The hydrotherapy department, formerly active on all admission services and routinely used on wards with disturbed patients, has ceased to be in operation. Maintenance EST (electroshock treatment) for disturbed patients has been discontinued. . . . There has been a record increase in participation by these patients in social and occupational activities.

These developments have vast sociological implications. I believe it is fair to state that pharmacology promises to accomplish what other measures have failed to bring about—the social emancipation of the mental hospital.[5]

Treatment Effects and Considerations Along with an increase in the use of phenothiazines in the treatment of the mentally ill came an increase in the sophistication of experimental programs that evaluate the effectiveness of various drugs. Results of these studies show clearly that phenothiazine-treated patients improve more than patients receiving placebo or no treatments. In an NIMH study, after six weeks 75 percent of acute schizophrenics

receiving phenothiazines showed either moderate or marked improvement, whereas of those receiving placebos, only 23 percent improved. Over the years many more studies have demonstrated consistently that, although phenothiazines are far from a complete cure for every patient, they are significantly better than placebo treatments in reducing psychotic behaviors. The issue of what to call this new type of drug arose early:

The inappropriateness of the term "tranquilizer" is evident when the pattern of response produced by antipsychotic drugs is examined. They certainly do more than simply calm patients or put them in a "chemical straitjacket." The core symptoms of schizophrenia are consistently improved: emotional withdrawal, hallucinations, delusions and other disturbed thinking, paranoid projection, belligerence, hostility and blunted affect. On the other hand, somatic complaints, anxiety and tension, symptoms which might ordinarily be favorably affected by a "tranquilizer," are not much changed.[6]

Another aspect of evaluating the effectiveness of drug treatment is determining the incidence of relapse, or symptom recurrence, when treatment is discontinued. It is most likely that discontinuation of drug therapy will lead to relapse in 75 to 95 percent of patients within a year and in more than 50 percent of patients in six months. Almost all studies report that when medication is resumed, there is again a reduction in symptoms.

In the years since 1950, many new phenothiazines have been introduced and several completely new types of antipsychotic drugs have been discovered. Table 8.1 lists those on the U.S. market. We now refer to antipsychotic drugs as either being *conventional* antipsychotics (the phenothiazines and most of the other drug types introduced before the mid-1990s) or *atypical* (all antipsychotics introduced in the past 10 years are atypical antipsychotics).

Mechanism of Antipsychotic Action The first clue to the mechanism of action for antipsychotics was that virtually all of the phenotriazines and

Table 8.1
Antipsychotic Drugs

Generic Name	Brand Name	Usual Dose Range (mg/day)
Conventional antipsychotics		
fluphenazine	generic	5–60
haloperidol	generic	2–100
loxapine	Loxitane	30–250
mesoridazine	Serentil	100–400
molindone	Moban	10–225
perphenazine	generic	8–64
prochlorperazine	Compazine	10–150
thioridazine	generic	100–600
thiothixene	Navane	5–60
trifluoperazine	generic	5–60
Atypical antipsychotics		
aripiprazole	Abilify	10–30
clozapine	Clozaril	100–900
olanzepine	Zyprexa	5–20
risperidone	Risperdal	4–16
ziprasidone	Geodon	40–160

Source: *Physician's Desk Reference* (Oradell, NJ: Medical Economics, 2004).

other conventional antipsychotics produce *pseudoparkinsonism.* Patients treated with these medications exhibit symptoms similar to Parkinson's disease (tremors and muscular rigidity). Because Parkinson's disease is known to be caused by a loss of dopamine neurons in the nigrostriatal dopamine pathway (see Chapter 4), scientists focused on the ability of antipsychotic drugs to block dopamine receptors. Although the conventional antipsychotics are generally fairly "dirty" drugs pharmacologically (they block other types of receptors as well), the doses required for the different drugs to produce antipsychotic effects do not correlate well with the ability of the different drugs to bind to any receptor except dopamine receptors (specifically, the D2 type of dopamine receptor). It is now well accepted that the initial effect of antipsychotic drugs is to block D2 dopamine receptors. However, this effect

occurs with the first dose, but the antipsychotic effect of these drugs is not seen for at least 10 to 14 days (the "lag period"). Thus, the ultimate mechanism of antipsychotic action is some (as yet unknown) response of the nervous system to repeated administration of dopamine antagonists.

When clozapine was introduced, it differed from the other antipsychotics in two interesting ways. First, it produced much less pseudoparkinsonism than the other drugs. Second, some patients who had failed to improve with the other antipsychotics showed improvement when treated with clozapine. Clozapine was very promising, but it unfortunately has a risk of producing a deadly suppression of white blood cell production. The drug was withdrawn from the market, but then made available again as long as patients have periodic blood samples taken to monitor their white cells. Clozapine produces effects on a wide range of receptor types, but eventually it was determined that its unique properties were probably related to its ability to block both D2 dopamine and 5HT2A serotonin receptors. Risperidone, olanzepine, and the other atypical antipsychotics were developed with these two actions in mind, and none of the newer drugs carries the risk of suppressing white blood cell production. The atypical antipsychotics are sometimes referred to as serotonin-dopamine antagonists. Pseudoparkinsonism is reduced because of serotonin-dopamine interactions in the nigrostriatal pathway. These drugs are also said to be capable not only of reducing the *positive* symptoms of schizophrenia (hallucinations, delusions, disorganized speech and behavior), but also of improving the *negative* symptoms (lack of emotion, social isolation, lack of initiative). In contrast, the conventional antipsychotics were known primarily for reducing positive symptoms.[3]

Side Effects of Antipsychotics Two positive aspects of the antipsychotics are that they are not addictive and it is extremely difficult to use them to commit suicide. Some allergic reactions might be noted, such as jaundice or skin rashes. Some patients exhibit photosensitivity, a tendency for the skin to darken and burn easily in sunlight. These reactions have a low incidence and usually decrease or disappear with a reduction in dosage. *Agranulocytosis,* low white blood cell count of unknown origin, can develop in the early stages of treatment. Because white blood cells are needed to fight infection, this disorder has a high mortality rate if it is not detected before a serious infection sets in. It is extremely rare with most of the antipsychotics other than clozapine.

The most common side effect of antipsychotic medication involves the nigrostriatal dopamine pathway (see Chapter 4). The major effects include a wide range of movement disorders from facial tics to symptoms that resemble those of Parkinson's disease (tremors of the hands when they are at rest; muscular rigidity, including a masklike face; and a shuffling walk). As noted above, this pseudoparkinsonism is less of a problem with the newer atypical antipsychotics.

Tardive dyskinesia is the most serious complication of antipsychotic drug treatment. Although first observed in the late 1950s, it was not viewed as a major problem until the mid-1970s, 20 years after these drugs were introduced. The term *tardive dyskinesia* means "late-appearing abnormal movements" and refers primarily to rhythmic, repetitive sucking and smacking movements of the lips; thrusting of the tongue in and out ("fly-catching"); and movements of the arms, toes, or fingers. The fact that this syndrome usually occurs only after years of antipsychotic drug treatment, and that the symptoms persist and sometimes increase when medication is stopped, raised the possibility of irreversible changes. The current belief is that tardive dyskinesia is the result of supersensitivity of the dopaminergic receptors. Although reversal of the symptoms is possible in most cases, the best treatment is prevention, which can be accomplished through early detection and an immediate lowering of the medication level.

A meta-analysis of several large trials of long-term conventional antipsychotic drug treatment using more than 1,600 patients found that pseudoparkinsonism was reported as an adverse reaction in about 20 percent of the patients, whereas tardive dyskinesia was reported for only about 2 percent.[7] Tardive dyskinesia is also less likely to appear during treatment with atypical antipsychotics.

Antidepressants

Monoamine Oxidase Inhibitors The story of the antidepressant drugs starts with the fact that tuberculosis was a major chronic illness until about 1955. In 1952, preliminary reports suggested that a new drug, isoniazid, was effective in treating tuberculosis; isoniazid and similar drugs that followed were responsible for the emptying of hospital beds. One of the antituberculosis drugs was iproniazid, which was introduced simultaneously with isoniazid but was withdrawn as too toxic. Clinical reports on its use in tuberculosis hospitals emphasized that there was considerable elevation of mood in the patients receiving iproniazid. These reports were followed up, and the drug was reintroduced as an antidepressant agent in 1955 on the basis of early promising studies with depressed patients.

Iproniazid is a **monoamine oxidase (MAO) inhibitor,** and its discovery opened up a new class of compounds for investigation. Although several MAO inhibitors have been introduced over the years, toxicity and side effects have limited their use and have reduced their number. Iproniazid was removed from sale in 1961 after being implicated in at least 54 fatalities. Currently two MAO inhibitors are on the U.S. market (see Table 8.2). A major limitation of the use of the MAO inhibitors is that they alter the normal metabolism of a dietary amino acid, tyramine, such that if an individual consumes foods with a high tyramine content while taking MAO inhibitors, a hypertensive (high blood pressure) crisis can result. Because aged cheeses are one source of tyramine, this is often

Table 8.2
Antidepressant Drugs

Generic Name	Brand Name	Usual Dose Range (mg/day)
MAO inhibitors		
phenelzine	Nardil	45–75
tranylcypromine	Parnate	20–30
Tricyclics		
amitriptyline	generic	100–200
amoxapine	generic	200–300
desipramine	Norpramin	75–200
doxepin	Sinequan	100–200
imipramine	Tofranil	100–200
nortriptyline	Pamelor	75–150
protriptyline	Vivactil	15–40
Selective Reuptake Inhibitors		
citalopram	Celexa	20–40
escitalopram	Lexapro	10–20
fluoxetine	Prozac	20–40
paroxetine	Paxil	20–50
sertraline	Zoloft	50–200
venlafaxine	Effexor	75–375
Others		
bupropion	Wellbutrin	200–300
mirtazapine	Remeron	15–45
trazodone	generic	150–200

referred to as the "cheese reaction." A severe headache, palpitations, flushing of the skin, nausea, and vomiting are some symptoms of this reaction, which has in some cases ended in death from a stroke (cerebrovascular accident). Besides avoiding foods and beverages that contain tyramine (aged cheeses, chianti wine, smoked or pickled fish, and many others), patients taking MAO inhibitors must also avoid sympathomimetic drugs, such as amphetamines, methylphenidate, and ephedrine.

MAO is an enzyme involved in the breakdown of serotonin, norepinephrine, and dopamine, and its inhibition results in increased availability of these neurotransmitters at the synapse. This was the first clue to the possible mechanism of antidepressant action.

Tricyclic Antidepressants Sometimes when you are looking for one thing, you find something entirely different. The MAO inhibitors were found among antituberculosis agents, and the phenothiazine antipsychotics were found while looking for a better antihistamine. The **tricyclic** antidepressants were found in a search for better phenothiazine antipsychotics. The basic phenothiazine structure consists of three rings, with various side chains for the different antipsychotic drugs. Imipramine resulted from a slight change in the middle of the three rings and was tested in 1958 on a group of patients. The drug had little effect on psychotic symptoms but improved the mood of depressed patients. This was the first tricyclic antidepressant, and many more have followed (see Table 8.2). Although these drugs are not effective in all patients, most controlled clinical trials do find that depressive episodes are less severe and resolve more quickly if the patients are treated with one of the tricyclic antidepressants than if they are given a placebo.

The first tricyclics were discovered to interfere with the reuptake into the terminal of the neurotransmitters norepinephrine, dopamine, and serotonin. This results in an increased availability of these neurotransmitters at the synapse. Because MAO inhibition also results in increased availability of the same neurotransmitters, there has been considerable speculation that the antidepressant actions of both classes of drugs result from increased synaptic availability of one or more of these neurotransmitters. One of the effective antidepressants, desipramine, was found to have a much greater effect on the reuptake of norepinephrine than on the reuptake of either dopamine or serotonin, so for a time most theories of antidepressant action focused on norepinephrine.

monoamine oxidase (MAO) inhibitor: a type of antidepressant drug.
tricyclic (try *sike* lick): a type of antidepressant drug.

Selective Reuptake Inhibitors The introduction in 1987 of fluoxetine (Prozac) ushered in the era of the *selective serotonin reuptake inhibitors* (**SSRIs**). Trazodone had already been available and was known to have a greater effect on serotonin than on norepinephrine reuptake, calling the norepinephrine theory into question. Prozac soon became the most widely prescribed antidepressant drug ever marketed. Prozac is safer than the tricyclic antidepressants in that it is less likely to lead to overdose deaths, so physicians felt more confident about prescribing it. Despite some reports in the early 1990s of unusual violent or suicidal reactions, sales of Prozac continued at a high rate, and several other SSRIs were introduced by other companies. Sales of antidepressants continued to increase, and the growing practice of prescribing antidepressants to children and adolescents helped to fuel sales. In 2003, eight different antidepressants were among the 100 most prescribed drugs in the United States, led by Zoloft, generic fluoxetine, and Effexor (venlafaxine), which is a selective reuptake inhibitor for both serotonin and norepinephrine.

Although the worldwide value of antidepressant sales exceeded $15 billion in 2003, this is expected to decline over the next few years for two reasons.[8] First, several of the most profitable drugs will become available in generic form, so their prices will drop. Second, concerns are growing about both the effectiveness and safety of these medications. A study that questioned the effectiveness of SSRIs has not received as much notice as it probably deserves. After studying unpublished reports of the clinical trials submitted to the FDA by manufacturers seeking approval for six antidepressants approved between 1987 and 1999, the researchers concluded that about 80 percent of the effectiveness demonstrated for the antidepressants was duplicated in placebo groups.[9] While overall the active drug groups showed statistically greater improvement than the placebo groups, the magnitude of the difference was small. In other words, they concluded

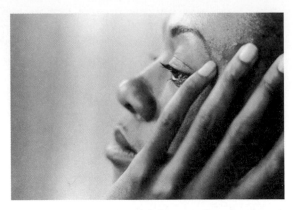

Depression is a serious, debilitating disorder that often responds to antidepressant medication.

that even the newest antidepressant drugs are only a little better than placebo.

The biggest impact on antidepressant prescriptions will come from action by the FDA in response to concerns that children and adolescents treated with antidepressants are at greater risk for suicide. Analysis of data submitted to the FDA for approval of nine drugs found higher rates of suicidal thoughts among the drug groups than among the placebo control groups, although there were no actual suicides in the studies. The FDA is not prohibiting the prescribing of these drugs, but it is now requiring a printed warning about the increased risk of suicidal tendencies in children and adolescents.[10]

Mechanism of Antidepressant Action It seems that most antidepressants work by increasing the availability of either norepinephrine or serotonin at their respective synapses. However, the antidepressant effect of MAO inhibitors, tricyclics, and SSRIs exhibits a "lag period": The patients must be treated for about two weeks before improvement is seen, even though the biochemical effects on MAO or on reuptake occur in a matter of minutes. Although it has been suggested that some patients might benefit more from one type than from another, experiments have so far failed to reveal any rational basis for choosing among

Taking Sides

Should Psychologists Be Allowed to Prescribe?

Currently, the professionals who are best prepared to understand the complexities of prescribing psychoactive medications for mental disorders are psychiatrists. Following their medical training, these specialists have intensive training in the diagnosis and treatment of mental disorders, and especially in the use of medications such as antipsychotics and antidepressants. However, most patients who receive prescriptions for psychoactive medications do not see psychiatrists; the prescriptions are written by family practitioners, internal medicine specialists, or other nonpsychiatrist medical doctors. This may be partly because patients are unwilling to visit a psychiatrist, but often it is due to a shortage of psychiatrists, particularly in rural settings or in low-income urban neighborhoods.

Basic medical training includes very little formal coursework or experience in understanding, diagnosing, and treating mental disorders. Sometimes patients are seeing the medical doctor for prescriptions, and also seeing a psychologist. Professional clinical psychologists have extensive training in understanding, diagnosing, and treating mental disorders with behavioral or psychotherapy, but they typically have little background in medicine. If the psychologist and the medical doctor have developed an effective collaboration, this arrangement can often work well for the patient. But in many cases it seems that the two professions have so little common ground that effective collaboration is difficult.

New Mexico and Louisiana have addressed this problem by setting up conditions under which licensed clinical psychologists can obtain prescription privileges. These psychologists must complete about two years of additional coursework in physiology, pharmacology, and related medical topics. They then spend about a year prescribing medications and following the patients under the supervision of a licensed physician. After passing examinations and obtaining the necessary coursework and experience, they can obtain a license to write their own prescriptions.

Many believe that this can improve the delivery of mental health services, while many others are opposed to the idea. Medical doctors are concerned that psychologists might miss some important medical consideration, such as interactions with other types of drugs, and put the patient's health at risk. And many psychologists are concerned about the resulting impact on the field of psychology, possibly turning practitioners into "pill pushers" who ignore other approaches to treatment or who do not take the time to get a more complete psychological understanding of the problem. Not every clinical psychologist will be interested in or willing to undertake the extensive additional training required to obtain prescription privileges, so it remains to be seen how much impact these prescribing psychologists will have on mental health services in these two states. Meanwhile, efforts are under way in other states to pass similar legislation. Do you know if such a bill is being considered where you live? Do you think it should be supported or opposed? What are the critical questions that should be answered by proponents of prescription privileges for psychologists?

the drugs in any individual case, and overall the effectiveness of the drug does not seem to depend on which of the neurotransmitters is more affected.

Current theories of the antidepressant action of these agents focus less on the initial biochemical effects of the drugs than on the reaction of the neurons to repeated drug exposure. As is the case with antipsychotics, we do not yet know the complete story of how long-term exposure to antidepressant drugs eventu-

ally results in improving the symptoms of depression. In addition to the MAO inhibitors, tricyclics, and selective reuptake inhibitors, drugs such as Wellbutrin and Remeron act through somewhat different mechanisms. The fact that drugs with a wide variety of initial

SSRI: selective serotonin reuptake inhibitors, a type of antidepressant drug.

biochemical effects are all about equally effective (they reduce depressive symptoms for some people, but not for all) means it is possible that there is not a single biochemical mechanism to explain the effects of all these drugs.

Electroconvulsive Therapy

Probably the single most effective treatment for the depressed patient is electroconvulsive shock therapy (ECT). One report summarized the available good studies and showed that in seven of eight studies ECT was more effective in relieving the symptoms of depression than was placebo. Further, in four studies ECT was more effective than the most effective class of antidepressant drugs, and in three other studies the two treatments were equal. One factor that makes ECT sometimes the clear treatment of choice is its more rapid effect than that found with current antidepressant drugs. Reversal of depression might not occur for two or three weeks with drug treatment, but with ECT results sometimes are noticed almost immediately. When there is a possibility of suicide, ECT is thus the obvious choice, and it is possible to use both drug and ECT treatment simultaneously.[3]

Mood Stabilizers

In the late 1940s, two medical uses were proposed for salts of the element **lithium.** In the United States, lithium chloride, which tastes much like sodium chloride (table salt), was introduced as a salt substitute for heart patients. However, above a certain level lithium is quite toxic, and because there was no control over the dose, many users became ill and several died. This scandal was so great in the minds of American physicians that a proposed beneficial use published in 1949 by an Australian, John Cade, produced little interest in this country.

Cade had been experimenting with guinea pigs, examining the effects of lithium on urinary excretion of salts. Lithium appeared to have sedative properties in some of the animals, so he administered the compound to several disturbed patients. The manic patients all improved, whereas there seemed to be no effect on depressed or schizophrenic patients. This was followed up by several Danish studies in the 1950s and early 1960s, and it became increasingly apparent that the large majority of manic individuals showed dramatic remission of their symptoms after a lag period of a few days when treated with lithium carbonate or other salts.

Three factors slowed the acceptance of lithium in the United States. First was the salt-substitute poisonings, which gave lithium a bad reputation as a potentially lethal drug. Second, mania was not seen as a major problem in the United States. Manic patients feel energetic and have an unrealistically positive view of their own abilities, and such people are unlikely to seek treatment on their own. Also, patients who became quite manic and lost touch with reality would probably have been called schizophrenic in those days, perhaps at least partly because a treatment existed for schizophrenia. The antipsychotic drugs can control mania in most cases. The third and possibly most important factor is economic and relates to the way new drugs are introduced in the United States: by companies that hope to make a profit on them. Lithium is one of the basic chemical elements (number 3 on the periodic chart) and its simple salts had been available for various purposes for many years, so it would be impossible for a drug company to receive an exclusive patent to sell lithium. A company generally must go to considerable expense to conduct the research necessary to demonstrate safety and effectiveness to the FDA. If one company had done this, as soon as the drug was approved any other company could also have sold lithium, and it would have been impossible for the first company to recoup its research investment. After several years of frustration, the weight of the academically conducted research and the clinical experience in Europe was such that several companies received approval to sell lithium in 1970.

Table 8.3
Drug Treatment Two-Year Outcome in Unipolar and Bipolar Patients

	PERCENTAGE OF PATIENTS WITH RELAPSES DURING TREATMENT	
	First 4 Months	Next 20 Months
Unipolar Subjects		
Lithium	30	41
Imipramine	32	29
Placebo	73	85
Bipolar Subjects		
Lithium	22	18
Imipramine	46	67
Placebo	54	67

Treatment with lithium requires 10 to 15 days before symptoms begin to change, and once again the ultimate mechanism for its action is not yet known. Lithium is both safe and toxic. It is safe because the blood level can be monitored routinely and the dose adjusted to ensure therapeutic, but not excessive, blood levels. Patients develop tolerances to the minor side effects of gastrointestinal disturbances and tremors. Excessively high levels in the blood cause confusion and loss of coordination, which can progress to coma, convulsions, and death if lithium is not stopped and appropriate treatment instituted.

Of primary importance in the therapeutic use of lithium is the realization that lithium acts as a mood-normalizing agent in individuals with bipolar (manic-depressive) illness. Lithium will prevent both manic and depressed mood swings. It has only moderate effects on unipolar depressions. (See Table 8.3.)

In addition to lithium, three drugs that were initially developed as anticonvulsants (to treat epileptic seizures) are being used as mood stabilizers (to treat bipolar disorder). Valproic acid (Depakote), carbamazepine (Tegretol), and lamotrigine (Lamictal) have received FDA approval for use in bipolar disorder, based on published evidence of their effectiveness. These drugs are particularly useful in people who might be susceptible to epileptic seizures. They are probably not quite as effective as lithium, but they have the advantage that monitoring of blood levels is not required.[3]

Consequences of Drug Treatments for Mental Illness

The use of modern psychopharmaceuticals, which began in the mid-1950s in the United States, has affected the lives of millions of Americans who have been treated with them. But the availability of these effective medications has also brought about revolutionary changes in our society's treatment of and relationship with our mentally ill citizens. Figure 8.1 depicts what happened to the population of our large mental hospitals from 1946 to 2004. These hospitals had grown larger and larger and held a total of over half a million people in the peak years of the early 1950s. The year in which chlorpromazine was introduced in the United States, 1955, was the last year in which the population of these hospitals increased. Since then the average population has continued to decline. The antipsychotics do not cure schizophrenia or other forms of psychosis, but they can control the symptoms to a great degree, allowing the patients to leave the hospital, live at home, and often earn a living. These drugs began the liberation of mental patients from hospitals, where many of them had previously stayed year after year, committed for an indefinite time.

The movement out of mental hospitals was accelerated in the 1960s with the establishment of federally supported community mental health centers. The idea was to treat mental

lithium (*lith* ee um): a drug used in treating mania and bipolar disorder.

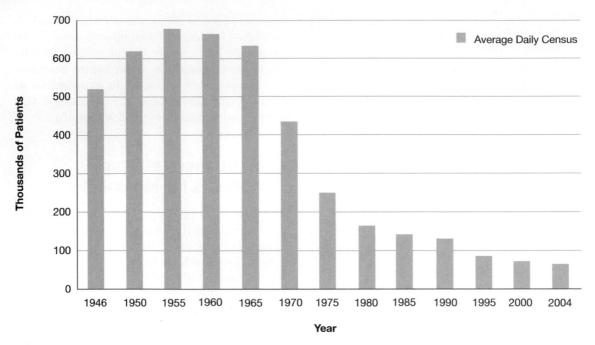

Figure 8.1   Number of Patients in Nonfederal Psychiatric Hospitals, 1946–2004

SOURCE: American Hospital Association, *Hospital Statistics, 2006* (Chicago: Health Forum, 2006).

patients closer to home in a more natural environment, at lesser expense, and on an outpatient basis. The opportunity for such a program to work was greatly enhanced by the availability of potent, effective psychopharmaceuticals, especially the antipsychotics.

The mental health professions have been greatly affected by these drugs. The majority of psychiatrists in practice today spend less time doing psychotherapy than did their colleagues in the 1950s. In fact, for many psychiatrists the first issue is to establish an appropriate drug regimen, and only after the initial symptoms are controlled will they engage in much talk therapy. For some psychiatrists the prescription pad has replaced the couch as their primary tool. This may be sensible in terms of overall cost effectiveness, but it has altered the doctor/patient relationship.

Concomitant with the liberation of patients from hospitals and their return to the

communities came a concern for their civil rights. Indefinite commitment to a hospital had been declared unconstitutional, and all states have since developed procedures to protect the rights of individual patients. Hearings are required before a person can be committed for treatment against his or her will, and it is usually necessary to demonstrate a clear and present danger to the patient's own person or to others. Periodic reviews of the patient's status are called for, and if at any time the immediate danger is not present, the patient must be released. No one would want to argue that mental patients should not have these rights, but the availability of psychoactive medications helps create difficult situations. A patient who is dangerously psychotic might be admitted for treatment, and after a few weeks on an antipsychotic drug might be sufficiently in control to be allowed to leave the hospital. However, if the patient remains suspicious or

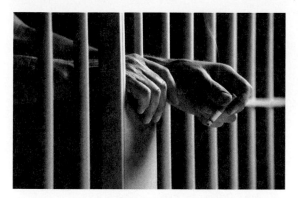

Prisons may hold more mentally ill persons than do state mental hospitals.

simply doesn't like to take the medication, he or she will eventually stop taking it and again become psychotic. Or patients might be released into the community, perhaps functioning with medication or perhaps not, too sick to really take care of themselves but not sick enough to present an immediate danger. Often, the eventual result is violation of a law, leading to imprisonment. According to an August 31, 2000, ABC news report, more mentally ill persons are jailed each year than are admitted to state mental hospitals. About one-third of all homeless people in the United States have some form of serious mental illness. The plight of our homeless, rootless, mentally ill citizens has been the subject of magazine and television reports, and efforts are being made to change the way these people are treated.

Summary

- The medical model of mental illness has been widely criticized, yet psychotherapeutic drugs are often discussed in the context of this model.

- Diagnosis of mental disorders is difficult and controversial, but the *DSM-IV-TR* provides a standard diagnostic approach for most purposes.

- The introduction of antipsychotics in the mid-1950s started a revolution in mental health care and increased interest in psychopharmacology.

- The antipsychotics are helpful for the majority of schizophrenics, but they often produce movement disorders, some of which resemble Parkinson's disease.

- The major groups of antidepressant drugs are the MAO inhibitors, the tricyclics, and the SSRIs.

- Fluoxetine (Prozac) quickly became the largest-selling antidepressant drug in history.

- Lithium is useful in treating mania and in preventing mood swings in bipolar disorder.

- The number of people occupying beds in mental hospitals has declined since 1955, largely because psychotherapeutic drugs allow people to be released after shorter stays.

Review Questions

1. Give two examples of anxiety disorder.
2. Is schizophrenia a functional or an organic psychosis?
3. Besides sadness, what are some other indicators of a major depressive episode?
4. What type of drug is chlorpromazine, and where was it first tested on patients?
5. What is tardive dyskinesia, and how does it respond to a reduction in the dose of an antipsychotic drug?
6. Which type of drug was discovered while testing an antituberculosis agent?
7. How do the SSRIs differ from the older tricyclics in terms of their actions in the brain?
8. What were two of the three reasons it took so long for lithium to be available for use in the United States?
9. If clozapine is so dangerous, why is it prescribed at all?
10. Why was Prozac the most widely prescribed antidepressant drug ever marketed?

References

1. American Psychiatric Association. *Diagnostic and Statistical Manual of Mental Disorders* (4th ed.). Washington, DC: 2000.

2. Wedding, D., & M. Boyd. *Movies and Mental Illness.* New York: McGraw-Hill, 1999.

3. Stahl, S.M. *Essential Psychopharmacology.* Cambridge, UK: Cambridge University Press, 2000.

4. Goldman, D. "Treatment of Psychotic States with Chlorpromazine." *Journal of the American Medical Association* 157 (1955), pp. 1274–78.

5. Freyhan, F.A. "The Immediate and Long-range Effects of *Chlorpromazine on the Mental Hospital.*" In Smith, Kline and French Laboratories, Chlorpromazine and Mental Health. Philadelphia: Lea & Febiger, 1955.

6. Veterans Administration. *Drug Treatment in Psychiatry,* Washington, DC: U.S. Government Printing Office, 1970.

7. Bollini, P., and others. "Antipsychotic Drugs: Is More Worse? A Meta-analysis of the Published Randomized Control Trials." *Psychological Medicine* 24 (1994), p. 307.

8. Pharmaceutical Business Review Online, "Commercial Insight: Antidepressants-Sliding SSRI Sales Inevitable." www.pharmaceutical-business-review.com/research.asp?guid=DMHC1942. Accessed February 2004.

9. Kirsch, L., and others. "The Emperor's New Drugs: An Analysis of Antidepressant Medication Data Submitted to the U.S. Food and Drug Administration." *Prevention & Treatment* 5 (2002), p. 23.

10. U.S. Food and Drug Administration. "FDA Launches a Multi-pronged Strategy to Strengthen Safeguards for Children Treated with Antidepressant Medications." *FDA News,* October 15, 2004.

Check Yourself

Track Your Daily Mood Changes

Some days are better than others—we all experience that. Try using this psychological "instrument" to measure how your outlook on life changes on a day-to-day basis. Decide on a particular time to mark the scales and try to do them at the same time each day, because your mood also varies with time of day. Mark a spot on each vertical scale that corresponds to how you're feeling at the moment.

After you've finished the week, look back and see if you can relate the highs and lows to particular events or activities that happened at that time. Do all your scores tend to vary together, or are some areas unrelated to others?

1. How optimistic do you feel about accomplishing something useful or meaningful in the next 24 hours?

	Day 1	Day 2	Day 3	Day 4	Day 5	Day 6	Day 7
Quite certain I will							
Probably will							
Not sure							
Probably won't							
Quite certain I won't							

2. How energetic do you feel at the moment?

	Day 1	Day 2	Day 3	Day 4	Day 5	Day 6	Day 7
Have lots of energy							
Fairly energetic							
About average							
Not much energy							
Almost no energy							

continued

3. How happy or sad are you today?

	Day 1	Day 2	Day 3	Day 4	Day 5	Day 6	Day 7
Very happy							
Happy							
Neither happy nor sad							
Sad							
Very sad							

4. How mentally sharp do you feel today (ability to remember things, ability to think)?

	Day 1	Day 2	Day 3	Day 4	Day 5	Day 6	Day 7
Quite sharp							
Pretty sharp							
Average							
A bit dull							
Very dull and slow							

5. How satisfied are you with yourself today?

	Day 1	Day 2	Day 3	Day 4	Day 5	Day 6	Day 7
Quite satisfied							
Fairly satisfied							
Not sure							
Fairly dissatisfied							
Quite dissatisfied							

Alcohol

Alcohol: social lubricant, adjunct to a fine meal, or demon rum? People today are no different from people throughout the centuries; many use alcohol, and

9   Alcohol
What is alcohol and how does it affect the body and brain? How does alcohol influence an individual's relationship with others and what is its impact on society?

many others condemn its use. This love-hate relationship with alcohol has been ongoing for a long time. The last two decades have brought a slight swing of the pendulum: Health-conscious Americans are opting for low-alcohol or no-alcohol drinks, consumption of hard liquor is down, and we receive frequent reminders to use alcohol responsibly, not to drink and drive, and not to let our friends drive if they've been drinking. Let's take a closer look at the world's number one psychoactive substance.

9

Alcohol

Objectives

When you have finished this chapter, you should be able to:

- **Understand the production and approximate alcohol content of the major beverage types.**

- **Relate the history and effectiveness of temperance and prohibition movements in the U.S.**

- **Know recent alcohol consumption trends.**

- **Describe how alcohol is processed by the body.**

- **Understand how consumption rate and body size influence BAC and know the legal BAC.**

- **Discuss the likely role of GABA in alcohol's mechanism of action.**

- **Explain the role of the balanced placebo study design in understanding alcohol's effects.**

- **Describe "alcohol myopia," acute alcohol poisoning, and alcohol withdrawal symptoms.**

- **Describe the impact of alcohol on traffic fatalities.**

- **Discuss the role of alcohol in sexual behavior and violence.**

- **Discuss alcohol exposure vs. malnutrition in the effects of chronic alcohol use on the brain and liver.**

- **Understand the role of AA in promoting the disease model of alcohol dependence.**

- **Discuss genetic influences on the risk of developing alcohol dependence.**

Alcoholic Beverages

Fermentation and Fermentation Products

Many thousands of years ago Neolithic humans discovered "booze." Beer and berry wine were known and used about 6400 BC and grape wine dates from 300 to 400 BC. Mead, which is made from honey, might be the oldest alcoholic beverage; some authorities suggest it appeared in the Paleolithic Age, about 8000 BC. Early use of alcohol seems to have been worldwide: Beer was drunk by the Native Americans whom Columbus met.

Fermentation forms the basis for all alcoholic beverages. Certain yeasts act on sugar in the presence of water, and this chemical action is fermentation. Yeast recombines the carbon, hydrogen, and oxygen of sugar into ethyl alcohol and carbon dioxide. Chemically, $C_6H_{12}O_6$ (glucose) is transformed into C_2H_5OH (ethyl alcohol) + CO_2 (carbon dioxide).

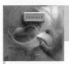

Online Learning Center Resources

www.mhhe.com/ksir12e

Visit our Online Learning Center (OLC) for access to these study aids and additional resources.

- Learning objectives
- Glossary flashcards
- Web activities and links
- Self-scoring chapter quiz
- Audio chapter summaries

Most fruits, including grapes, contain sugar, and the addition of the appropriate yeast (which is pervasive in the air wherever plants grow) to a mixture of crushed grapes and water will begin the fermentation process. The yeast has only a limited tolerance for alcohol; when the concentration reaches 15 percent, the yeast dies and fermentation ceases.

Cereal grains can also be used to produce alcoholic beverages. However, cereal grains contain starch rather than sugar, and before fermentation can begin the starch must be converted to sugar. This is accomplished by making *malt,* which contains enzymes that convert starch into sugar. In American beer the primary grain is barley, which is malted by steeping it in water and allowing it to sprout. The sprouted grain is then slowly dried to kill the sprout but preserve the enzymes formed during the growth. This dried, sprouted barley is called malt, and when crushed and mixed with water, the enzymes convert the starch to sugar. Only yeast is needed then to start fermentation.

Distilled Products

To obtain alcohol concentrations above 15 percent, distillation is necessary. **Distillation** is a process in which the solution containing alcohol is heated, and the vapors are collected and condensed into liquid form again. Alcohol has a lower boiling point than water, so there is a higher percentage of alcohol in the distillate

(the condensed liquid) than there was in the original solution.

There is still debate over who discovered the distillation process and when the discovery was made, but many authorities place it in Arabia around AD 800. The term *alcohol* comes from an Arabic word meaning "finely divided spirit" and originally referred to that part of the wine collected through distillation—the essence, or "spirit," of the wine. In Europe, only fermented beverages were used until the 10th century, when the Italians first distilled wine, thereby introducing "spirits" to the Western world. These new products were studied and used in the treatment of many illnesses, including senility. The initial feeling about their medicinal value is best seen in the name given these condensed vapors by a 13th-century professor of medicine at the French University of Montpelier: *aqua vitae,* "the water of life." Around the end of the 17th century, the more prosaic Dutch called the liquid *brandy,* meaning "burnt wine."

The name *whiskey* comes from the Irish-Gaelic equivalent of *aqua vitae* and was already commonplace around 1500. The distillation of whiskey in America started on a large scale toward the end of the 18th century. The chief product of the area just west of the Appalachian Mountains—western Pennsylvania, western Virginia, and eastern Kentucky—was grain. It was not profitable for the farmers to ship the grain or flour across the mountains to the markets along the eastern seaboard. But 10 bushels of corn could be converted to one barrel of whiskey, which could be profitably shipped east, so distillation started on a grand scale.

In the United States the alcoholic content of distilled beverages is indicated by the term

fermentation (fer men *tay* shun): the production of alcohol from sugars through the action of yeasts.
distillation (dis ti *lay* shun): the evaporation and condensing of alcohol vapors to produce beverages with higher alcohol content.

Drugs in the Media

Advertising Alcohol on Television

When it comes to the world portrayed on television, both in programs and in advertising, it seems that beer is OK (there are lots of beer ads and a few more or less positive references to beer drinking on some programs), wine is a little less OK, but distilled spirits are apparently not OK. Advertising of beer on television has not been particularly restricted. But, depending on where you live, you might never see television ads for distilled spirits.

After Prohibition, purveyors of distilled spirits did not advertise on radio, and later they did not advertise on television. This was a voluntary ban by the radio, television, and liquor industries, not something mandated by any federal agency. In 1996, Seagram became the first liquor manufacturer to break the voluntary ban, and a few other companies followed suit. The ads are shown on local TV stations in several large cities, usually later at night. According to a December 7, 2000, article in *The New York Times*, in 1999 $18 million was spent to advertise liquor on television and radio combined—not much in comparison to beer advertising or to the amount spent to advertise distilled spirits in magazines and newspapers.

In December 2001, NBC announced it would begin "limited" advertising for liquor, only after 9 PM, and only on shows with primarily adult viewers. The plan was to start the ads in April 2002. This announcement generated quite a response from a wide variety of watchdog groups. Several of NBC's local affiliates promised to block those ads when they appeared, public opinion polls showed most Americans opposed the idea of televised liquor ads, 13 members of Congress wrote NBC a letter promising to hold hearings on the matter. In March, only a couple of weeks before the first ads were to appear, NBC reversed its earlier decision and agreed not to advertise hard liquor. Apart from the embarrassment of explaining how these ads target mature adults rather than those under 21, the networks and their current advertisers worry that federal legislation might restrict the advertising of wine and beer along with hard liquor.

proof. The percentage of alcohol by volume is one-half of the proof number: for instance, 90-proof whiskey is 45 percent alcohol. The word *proof* developed from a British Army procedure to gauge the alcohol content of distilled spirits before there were modern techniques. The liquid was poured over gunpowder and ignited. If the alcohol content was high enough, the alcohol would burn and ignite the gunpowder, which would go "poof" and explode. That was proof that the beverage had an acceptable alcohol content, about 57 percent.

Beer

Beer is made by adding barley malt to other cereal grains, such as ground corn or rice. The enzymes in the malt change the starches in these grains into sugar; then the solids are filtered

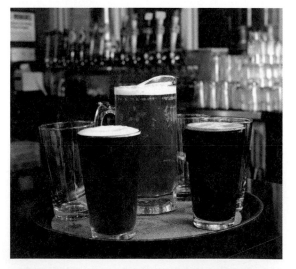

Brewpubs have become increasingly popular, but most beer consumed in the United States is produced by the two largest brewers.

out before the yeast is added to the mash to start fermentation. Hops (dried blossoms from only the female hop plant) are added with the yeast to give beer its distinctive, pungent flavor. One-fourth pound of hops is enough to flavor a 31-gallon barrel of beer. Most of the beer sold today in America is *lager,* from the German word *lagern,* meaning "to store." To brew lager, a type of yeast is used that settles to the bottom of the mash to ferment. After fermentation and before packaging, the beer is stored for a period to age. In most commercial beers today, alcohol content is a little over 4 percent. Because most American beer is sold in bottles or cans, the yeast must be removed to prevent it from spoiling after packaging. This is usually accomplished by heating it (pasteurization), but some brewers use microfilters to remove the yeasts while keeping the beer cold. The carbonation is added at the time of packaging.

Ale requires a top-fermentation yeast, warmer temperatures during fermentation, and more malt and hops, which produce a more flavorful beverage. *Malt liquor* is brewed much like lager but is aged longer, and it has less carbonation, more calories, and 1 percent to 3 percent more alcohol. If you were asked to produce a "light" beer, with fewer calories, a lighter taste, and less alcohol, what would you do—add water? That's only part of the answer, because light beers have about 10 percent less alcohol and 25 to 30 percent fewer calories. The mash is fermented at a cooler temperature for a longer time, so that more of the sugars are converted to alcohol. *Then* the alcohol content is adjusted by adding water, resulting in a beverage with considerably less remaining sugar and only a bit less alcohol.

The beer-drinking, free-lunch saloon with nickel beer and bucket-of-suds-to-go disappeared forever with Prohibition. And so did a couple of thousand breweries. Two years after Prohibition ended there were 750 brewers, but by 1941 that number had dwindled to 507. From 1960 to the mid-1970s, about 10 beer makers vanished each year, until in 1976 there were fewer than 50. This declined to about 40

Table 9.1
Largest-Selling Beer Brands (2003)

Brand	Market Share	Brewer
Bud Light	18.3%	Anheuser-Busch
Budweiser	14.9	Anheuser-Busch
Coors Light	8.0	Adolph Coors
Miller Light	7.6	Miller
Natural Light	4.0	Anheuser-Busch
Busch	3.4	Anheuser-Busch
Corona Extra	3.4	Modelo
Busch Light	2.8	Anheuser-Busch
Miller High Life	2.6	Miller
Miller Genuine Draft	2.2	Miller

Source: Data from AdAge.com, 2004.

in the early 1980s and then began to increase again as small, local "boutique" breweries began to sprout up. These were followed by the increasing popularity of *microbreweries,* or *brewpubs,* which make beer for sale only on the premises. As of 2005, there were over 1,300 specialty brewers, but their total sales represented less than 5 percent of the U.S. beer market.[1]

Table 9.1 points out a couple of interesting things about beer sales in the United States. The two largest brewers produce 8 of the top 10 beer brands. In fact, Anheuser-Busch's top two brands, Bud Light and Budweiser, vie for the leading spot and together represent more than 30 percent of all U.S. beer sales. Light beers have been popular for a number of years, but the recent interest in "low-carb" foods and beverages has pushed their sales even higher, to 45 percent of all U.S. sales in 2003.

Imported beers have become increasingly popular in the past 20 years. The largest-selling

proof: a measure of a beverage's alcohol content; twice the alcohol percentage.

imported beer is Corona, from Mexico. Mexican and Canadian beers are the biggest imports. Despite this increased appetite for foreign beers, imports still represent only about 7 percent of total U.S. sales. The craft beers produced by new, small breweries combined with an increased variety of imports and the no-alcohol beers add many new choices for the beer connoisseur, but Bud Light alone outsells all of these specialty beers combined.

Wine

Wine is one of humankind's oldest beverages, a drink that for generations has been praised as a gift from heaven and condemned as a work of the devil. Although a large volume of wine is now produced in mechanized, sterilized wine "factories," many small wineries operate alongside the industry giants, and the tradition continues that careful selection and cultivation of grapevines, good weather, precise timing of the harvest, and careful monitoring of fermentation and aging can result in wines of noticeably higher quality. An interesting ecological story resulted from the fact that most American wine grapes were originally transplanted from France and Spain. After a late-19th-century disease destroyed almost all of the European vineyards, it became necessary to transplant American vines, which had been protected by isolation, back into Europe. Today most of the French, Italian, and Spanish wine grapes are grown from descendants of those American vines.

There are two basic types of American wines. *Generics* usually have names taken from European land areas where the original wines were produced: Chablis, Burgundy, and Rhine are examples. These are all blended wines, made from whatever grapes are available, and during processing they are made to taste something like the traditional European wines from those regions. However, there is little guarantee of quality in these generic names among American wines. *Varietals* are named after one variety of grape, which by law must make up at least 51 percent of the grapes used

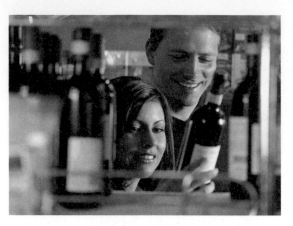

Wine consumption has increased considerably during the past 35 years.

in producing the wine. Chardonnay, merlot, and zinfandel are some examples. There are many varietal wines, and traditionally they have been sold in individual bottles and are more expensive than the generics. Some other countries have more restrictive rules for naming wines. For example, in France the name *Chablis* is carefully protected by law. A French Chablis must come from the Chablis region and be made only from the chardonnay grape. In America many inexpensive dry white wines are labeled Chablis, and they are likely to include a considerable amount of juice from table grapes such as the Thompson seedless. Thus, it is illegal to sell American "Chablis" wines in France without relabeling them. Most white wines are made from white grapes, although it is possible to use red grapes if the skins are removed before fermentation. Red wines are made from red grapes by leaving the skins in the crushed grapes while they ferment. "Blush" wines such as white zinfandel have become quite popular. With the zinfandel grape, which is red, the skins are left in the crushed grapes for a short while, resulting in a wine that is just slightly pink.

Besides red versus white and generic versus varietal, another general distinction is dry versus sweet. The sweeter wines are likely to have a "heavier" taste overall, with the sweetness balancing out flavors that might be considered harsh in a dry wine.

Because carbon dioxide is produced during fermentation, it is possible to produce naturally carbonated sparkling wines by adding a small amount of sugar as the wine is bottled and then keeping the bottle tightly corked. French champagnes are made in this way, as are the more expensive American champagnes, which might be labeled "naturally fermented in the bottle," or "methode Champagnoise." A cheaper method is used on inexpensive sparkling wines: Carbon dioxide is injected into a generic wine during bottling. Champagnes vary in their sweetness, also, with brut being the driest. Sweet champagnes are labeled "extra dry." The *extra* means "not," as in *extraordinary.*

It was discovered many years ago in Spain that, if enough brandy is added to a newly fermented wine, the fermentation will stop and the wine will not spoil (turn to vinegar). Sealing the wine in charred oak casks for aging further refined its taste, and soon *sherry* was in great demand throughout Europe. Other fortified wines, all of which have an alcohol content near 20 percent, include port, Madeira, and Muscatel. Dry sherry is typically consumed before dinner, whereas the sweeter fortified wines may be drunk as a dessert wine.

Distilled Spirits

Although brandy, distilled from wine, was probably the first type of spirits known to Europeans, the Celts of Ireland and the Scottish highlands were distilling a crude beverage known as *uisgebaugh*—"water of life"—before 1500. Today's Scotch whisky (without the *e;* it's *whiskey* in the United States and in Ireland, *whisky* in Scotland and Canada) is the distillate of fermented malted barley. The distinctive smoky flavor comes from two sources: The malted barley is dried in kilns in which burning peat provides the heat, so some of the distinctive characteristics of peat are picked up by the malt. With so many casks of sherry wine being sent to the British Isles after the 17th

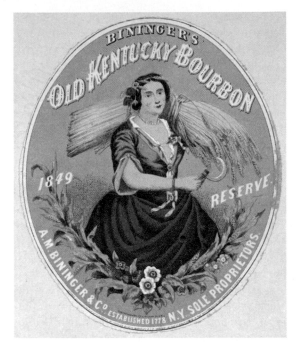

Bourbon whiskey is a distilled spirit first produced in the eighteenth century in Kentucky.

century, the Scots began to use the empty casks to age their whisky, and current practice calls for this storage in old sherry casks for at least three years. Pure malt whisky of this type is more popular in the Highlands than elsewhere because of its strong flavors. Most commercial Scotch whisky is blended with lighter-tasting grain spirits to provide a more pleasing drink.

In America the economics of trade resulted in an expanding production of spirits distilled from grain just as our new federal government was forming. In 1789, one of the early distillers who established a good reputation was Elijah Craig, a Baptist minister living in what was then Bourbon County, Kentucky. He began storing his whiskey in charred new oak barrels, originating a manufacturing step still used with American bourbon whiskeys.

By the 17th century, improved distillation techniques had made possible the production of relatively pure alcohol. Today's standard product from many large commercial distilleries is 95 percent pure alcohol (190 proof). Into the process goes whatever grain is available at a cheap price and tank loads of corn syrup or other sources of sugars or starches. Out the other end come *grain neutral spirits,* a clear liquid that is essentially tasteless (except for the strong alcohol taste), which might be sold in small quantities as Everclear or for use in medicine or research. More often, it is processed in bulk in various ways. For example, large quantities of grain neutral spirits are added to gasoline to produce a less polluting fuel, which also helps out the American farmer. Besides other industrial uses for ethyl alcohol, such as in cleaners and solvents, bulk grain neutral spirits are also used in making various beverages, including blended Scotch whiskies. One of the first beverages to be made from straight grain neutral spirits was gin. By filtering the distillate through juniper berries and then diluting it with water, a medicinal-tasting drink was produced. First called "jenever" by the Dutch and "genievre" by the French, the British shortened the name first to "geneva" and then to "gin." Gin became a popular beverage in England and now forms the basis for many an American martini.

Another major use for bulk grain neutral spirits is in the production of *vodka.* American vodkas, and most vodkas from other countries, are simply a mixture of grain neutral spirits and water, adjusted to the desired proof.

The proof at which distillation is carried out influences the taste and other characteristics of the liquor. When alcohol is formed, other related substances, known as **congeners,** are also formed. These may include alcohols other than ethanol, oils, and other organic matter. Luckily they are present only in small amounts, because some of them are quite toxic. Grain neutral spirits contain relatively few congeners and none of the flavor of the grains used in the mash. Whiskey is usually distilled at a lower proof, not more than 160, and thus the distillate contains more congeners and some of the flavor of the grain used. If 51 percent or more of the grain used was rye, then the product is labeled straight *rye whiskey.* When corn

constitutes more than 51 percent of the grain in the mash, the liquor is called *bourbon.* (To be called *corn whiskey* requires that the mash be 80 percent or more corn.) Both rye and bourbon are then diluted to 120 to 125 proof and aged in new, charred oak barrels for at least two years, and usually longer. Whiskey accumulates congeners during aging, at least for the first five years, and the congeners and the grain used provide the variation in taste among whiskeys.

Until Prohibition almost all whiskey consumed in the United States was straight rye or bourbon manufactured in the United States. Prohibition introduced smuggled Canadian and Scotch whisky to American drinkers, and they liked them. World War II sent American men around the world, further exposing them to this different type of liquor. Scotch and Canadian whiskys are lighter than American whiskey, which means lighter in color and less heavy in taste. They are lighter because Canadian and Scotch whiskys are typically *blended* whiskies, made from about two-thirds straight whisky and one-third grain neutral spirits. After World War II, U.S. manufacturers began selling more blended whiskey. Seagram's 7-Crown has been one of the most popular blended American whiskeys.

Liqueurs, or cordials, are similar in some ways to the fortified wines. Originally the cordials were made from brandy mixed with flavorings derived from herbs, berries, or nuts. After dilution with sugar and water, the beverages are highly flavored, sweet, and usually about 20 to 25 percent alcohol. Some of the old recipes are still closely guarded secrets of a particular group of European monks. The late 20th century saw an increase in popularity for these drinks, which are usually consumed in small amounts and have only about half the alcohol content of vodka or whiskey. Many new types were introduced, from Bailey's Irish Cream to varieties of schnapps. Modern American peppermint, peach, and other types of schnapps are made from grain neutral spirits, which are diluted, sweetened, and flavored with artificial or natural flavorings.

Alcohol Use and "The Alcohol Problem"

Historians seem to agree that, at the time of America's revolution against the English in the late 1700s, most Americans drank alcoholic beverages and most people favored these beverages compared with drinking water, which was often contaminated. The per capita consumption of alcohol was apparently much greater than current levels, and little public concern was expressed. Even the early Puritan ministers, who were moralistic about all kinds of behavior, referred to alcoholic drink as "the Good Creature of God." They denounced drunkenness as a sinful misuse of the "Good Creature" but clearly placed the blame on the sinner, not on alcohol itself.[2]

A new view of alcohol as the *cause* of serious problems began to emerge in America soon after the Revolution. That view took root and still exists as a major influence in American culture today. It is so pervasive that some people have a hard time understanding what is meant by the "demonization" of alcohol (viewing alcohol as a demon, or devil). The concept is important, partly because alcohol was the first psychoactive substance to become demonized in American culture, leading the way for similar views of cocaine, heroin, and marijuana in this century. We are referring to a tendency to view a substance as an *active* (sometimes almost purposeful) source of *evil,* damaging everything it touches. Whenever harmful consequences result from the use of something (firearms and nuclear energy are other possible examples), some people find it easiest to simply view that thing as "bad" and seek to eliminate it.

The Temperance Movement in America

The first writings indicating a negative view of alcohol itself are attributed to a prominent Philadelphia physician named Benjamin Rush, one of the signers of the Declaration of Independence. Rush's 1784 pamphlet, "An Inquiry into the Effects of Ardent Spirits on the Mind and Body," was aimed particularly at distilled spirits (*ardent* means "burning," "fiery"), not at the weaker beverages, such as beer and wine. As a physician, Rush had noticed a relationship between heavy drinking and jaundice (an indicator of liver disease), "madness" (perhaps the delirium tremens of withdrawal, or perhaps what we now call Korsakoff's psychosis), and "epilepsy" (probably the seizures seen during withdrawal). All of those are currently accepted and well-documented consequences of heavy alcohol use. However, Rush also concluded that hard liquor damaged the drinker's morality, leading to a variety of antisocial, immoral, and criminal behaviors. Although the correlation between these types of behavior and alcohol use had been documented many times, Rush believed that this was a direct toxic action of distilled spirits on the part of the brain responsible for morality. Rush then introduced for the first time the concept of *addiction* to a psychoactive substance, describing the uncontrollable and overwhelming desires for alcohol experienced by some of his patients. For the first time this condition was referred to as a *disease* (caused by alcohol), and he recommended total abstinence from alcohol for those who were dependent.[2]

Other physicians readily recognized these symptoms in their own patients, and physicians became the first leaders of the **temperance** movement. What Rush proposed, and most early followers supported, was that everyone should avoid distilled spirits entirely, because they were considered to be toxic, and should consume beer and wine in a *temperate,* or moderate, manner. Temperance societies were formed in many parts of the country, at first among the upper classes of physicians, ministers, and businesspeople. In

---

congeners (*con* je nurz): other alcohols and oils contained in alcoholic beverages.

temperance (temp a rance): the idea that people should drink beer or wine in moderation but drink no hard liquor.

the early 1800s, it became fashionable for the middle classes to join the elite in this movement, and hundreds of thousands of American businesspeople, farmers, lawyers, teachers, and their families "took the pledge" to avoid spirits and to be temperate in their use of beer or wine.

In the second half of the 19th century, things changed. Up to this time there had been little consumption of commercial beer in the United States. It was only with the advent of artificial refrigeration and the addition of hops, which helped preserve the beer, that the number of breweries increased. The waves of immigrants who entered the country in this period provided the necessary beer-drinking consumers. At first, encouraged by temperance groups that preferred beer consumption to the use of liquor, breweries were constructed everywhere. However, alcohol-related problems did not disappear. Instead, disruptive, drunken behavior became increasingly associated in the public's mind with the new wave of immigrants—Irish, Italians, and eastern Europeans, more often Catholic than Protestant—and they drank beer and wine. Temperance workers now advocated total abstinence from all alcoholic beverages, and pressure grew to prohibit the sale of alcohol altogether.

Prohibition

The first state prohibition period began in 1851 when Maine passed its prohibition law. Between 1851 and 1855, 13 states passed statewide prohibition laws, but by 1868 9 had repealed them. The National Prohibition Party, organized in 1874, provided the impetus for the second wave of statewide prohibition, which developed in the 1880s. From 1880 to 1889 seven states adopted prohibition laws, but by 1896 four had repealed them.

In 1899, a group of educators, lawyers, and clergymen described the saloon as the "working-man's club, in which many of his leisure hours are spent, and in which he finds more of the things that approximate luxury than in his home. . . ." They went on to say: "It is a centre of learning, books, papers, and lecture hall to them. It is the clearinghouse for common intelligence, the place where their philosophy of life is worked out, and their political and social beliefs take their beginnings."[3] Truth lay somewhere between those statements and the sentiments expressed in a sermon:

> The liquor traffic is the most fiendish, corrupt and hell-soaked institution that ever crawled out of the slime of the eternal pit. It is the open sore of this land. . . . It takes the kind, loving husband and father, smothers every spark of love in his bosom, and transforms him into a heartless wretch, and makes him steal the shoes from his starving babe's feet to find the price for a glass of liquor. It takes your sweet innocent daughter, robs her of her virtue and transforms her into a brazen, wanton harlot. . . .
>
> The open saloon as an institution has its origin in hell, and it is manufacturing subjects to be sent back to hell.[4]

Prohibition was not just a matter of "wets" versus "drys" or a matter of political conviction or health concerns. Intricately interwoven with these factors was a middle-class, rural, Protestant, evangelical concern that the good and true life was being undermined by ethnic groups with a different religion and a lower standard of living and morality. One way to strike back at these groups was through prohibition.

Between 1907 and 1919, 34 states enacted legislation enforcing statewide prohibition, whereas only 2 states repealed their prohibition laws. By 1917, 64 percent of the population lived in dry territory, and between 1908 and 1917 over 100,000 licensed bars were closed.

But a state prohibition law did not mean that the residents did not drink. They did, both legally and illegally. They drank illegally in speakeasies and other private clubs. They drank legally from a variety of the many patent medicines that were freely available. A few of the more interesting ones were Whisko, "a non-intoxicating stimulant" at 55 proof; Golden's Liquid Beef Tonic, "recommended for treatment of alcohol habit" with 53 proof; and Kaufman's

Sulfur Bitters, which "contains no alcohol" but was in fact 20 percent alcohol (40 proof) and contained no sulfur.

In August 1917, the U.S. Senate adopted a resolution, authored by Andrew Volstead, that submitted the national prohibition amendment to the states. The U.S. House of Representatives concurred in December, and 21 days later, on January 8, 1918, Mississippi became the first state to ratify the 18th Amendment. A year later, January 16, 1919, Nebraska was the 36th state to ratify the amendment, and the deed was done.

As stated in the amendment, a year after the 36th state ratified it, national **Prohibition** came into effect—on January 16, 1920. The amendment was simple, with only two operational parts:

> Section 1. After one year from the ratification of this article the manufacture, sale or transportation of intoxicating liquors within, the importation thereof into, or the exportation thereof from the United States and all territory subject to the jurisdiction thereof for beverage purposes is hereby prohibited.
> Section 2. The Congress and the several States shall have concurrent power to enforce this article by appropriate legislation.

The beginning of Prohibition was hailed in a radio sermon by popular preacher Billy Sunday:

> The reign of tears is over. The slums will soon be a memory. We will turn our prisons into factories and our jails into storehouses and corncribs. Men will walk upright now, women will smile, and the children will laugh. Hell will be forever for rent.[2]

The law did not result in an alcohol-free society, and this came as quite a surprise to many people. Apparently the assumption was that prohibition would be so widely accepted that little enforcement would be necessary. Along with saloons, breweries, and distilleries, hospitals that had specialized in the treatment of alcohol dependence closed their doors, presumably because there would no longer be a need for them.

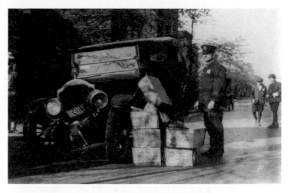

Prohibition laws were frequently violated, and enforcement was an ongoing problem.

It soon became clear that people were buying and selling alcohol illegally and that enforcement was not going to be easy. The majority of the population might have supported the idea of Prohibition, but such a large minority insisted on continuing to drink that *speakeasies, hip flasks,* and *bathtub gin* became household words. Organized crime became both more organized and vastly more profitable as a result of Prohibition.

The popular conception is that Prohibition was a total failure, leading to its repeal. That is not the whole picture. Prohibition did have the apparent effect of reducing overall alcohol intake. Hospital admissions for alcohol dependence and deaths from alcohol declined sharply at the beginning of Prohibition. During the 1920s, it appears that the prohibition laws were increasingly violated, particularly in large eastern cities, such as New York, and the rates of alcohol dependence and alcohol-related deaths began to increase.[5] But even toward the end of the "noble experiment," as Prohibition was called by its detractors, alcohol dependence and alcohol-related deaths were still lower than before Prohibition.

Prohibition: laws prohibiting all sales of alcoholic beverages in the United States from 1920 to 1933.

If Prohibition did reduce alcohol-related problems, why was it repealed? In 1926, the Association Against Prohibition was founded by a small group of America's wealthiest men, including the heads of many of the largest corporations in America. Their primary concern seems to have been the income taxes they were paying. Historically, taxes on alcohol had been one of the primary sources of revenue for the federal government. The federal government relied heavily on alcohol taxes before the income tax was initiated in 1913. A major hope of the repeal supporters was that income taxes could be reduced. There was also fear that the widespread and highly publicized disrespect for the Prohibition law encouraged a sense of "lawlessness," not just among the bootleggers and gangsters but also in the public at large. The Great Depression, which began in 1929, not only made more people consider the value of tax revenues but also increased fears of a generalized revolt. If Prohibition weakened respect for law and order, it had to go.[2]

The 18th Amendment was repealed by the 21st Amendment, proposed in Congress on February 20, 1933, and ratified by 36 states by December 5 of that year. So ended an era. The 21st Amendment was also short and sweet:

> Section 1. The eighteenth article of amendment of the Constitution of the United States is hereby repealed.
>   Section 2. The transportation or importation into any State, Territory, or possession of the United States for delivery or use therein of intoxicating liquors, in violation of the laws thereof, is hereby prohibited.

When national Prohibition ended, America did not return overnight to the pre-1920s levels of alcohol consumption. Sales increased until after World War II, at which point per capita consumption was approximately what it had been before Prohibition. Thus, the prohibition of alcohol, much like the current prohibitions of marijuana and heroin, did work in that it reduced alcohol availability, alcohol use, and related problems. On the other hand, even at its best it did not allow us to close all the jails and mental hospitals, and it encouraged organized crime and created expensive enforcement efforts.

Regulation after 1933

After national Prohibition, control over alcohol was returned to the states. Each state has since had its own means of regulating alcohol. Although a few states remained dry after national Prohibition, most allowed at least beer sales. Thus, the temperance sentiment that beer was a safer beverage continued to influence policy. In many cases, beer containing no more than 3.2 percent alcohol by weight was allowed as a "nonintoxicating" beverage.

Over the years the general trend was for a relaxation of laws: States that did not allow sales of liquor became fewer until in 1966 the last dry state, Mississippi, became wet. The minimum age to purchase alcoholic beverages was set at 21 in all states except New York and Louisiana before 1970, when the national voting age was lowered to 18. During the 1970s, 30 states lowered the drinking age to 18 or 19. Per capita consumption rates, which were relatively stable during the 1950s, increased steadily from 1965 through 1980. However, times have changed; pushed by concerns over young people dying in alcohol-related traffic accidents, in the 1980s Congress authorized the Transportation Department to withhold a portion of the federal highway funds for any state that did not raise its minimum drinking age to 21. In 1988, the final state raised its drinking age, making 21 the uniform drinking age all across the United States.

Taxation

Federal taxes on alcoholic beverages are a significant means of gathering money for the federal government. Although most of the federal revenue comes from individual income taxes, taxes on alcohol produce about 1 percent of the total collections by the Internal Revenue

Service ($8.5 billion in 2003). The states also collect almost $4 billion each year in excise taxes and license fees for alcoholic beverages. When all these are added up, more than half the consumer's cost for an average bottle of distilled spirits is taxes. In 1991, after hearing arguments that taxes on alcoholic beverages had not kept up with inflation, Congress initiated a significant tax increase: The beer tax doubled to $18 per barrel, the tax on bottled wine increased sixfold to about 22 cents per bottle, and the tax on distilled spirits rose less than 10 percent to $13.50 per gallon of 100-proof liquor. There was some controversy about how much such an increase would affect sales, especially because at the same time most producers increased their own prices by about 5 percent. The total increase in cost to the consumer (averaging about 10 percent more) did result in about a 2 percent decrease in sales of beer and liquor during the first half of the year. Domestic wine sales decreased even more, almost 9 percent. That such large price increases resulted in fairly modest declines in purchases might indicate that very large tax increases would be needed if part of the goal were to reduce alcohol intake significantly.

Who Drinks? And Why?

Cultural Influences on Drinking

Comparing alcohol use in various cultures around the world allows us to look at ethnic and social factors that lead to differences in patterns of alcohol use. For example, both the Irish and the Russian cultures are associated with heavy drinking, especially of distilled spirits. This has been attributed to several factors, including early invasions by the hard-drinking Vikings at a time when each of these regions was beginning to develop a national identity. Americans of Irish descent have been studied and found to have higher rates of alcohol-related problems than other ethnic groups. A comparison of Irish-Americans with Italian-Americans is of interest: The Irish forbid children and adolescents from learning to drink, but they seem to expect adult men to drink large quantities. They value hard liquor more than beer and promote drinking in pubs, away from family influences. By contrast, Italian families give their children wine from an early age in a family setting but disapprove of intoxication at any age.[6]

The French drink primarily wine and consume it in the family setting and with meals, so it might be expected that they would not have many heavy drinkers or drinking-related problems. Unfortunately, the French consume more alcohol per capita than any other nation and have the highest rates of alcohol dependence, suicide, and deaths from cirrhosis of the liver. The French associate wine drinking with virility, and French working men traditionally consumed large amounts of wine during the work day (it was not unusual for a French laborer to consume a liter of wine with lunch). In today's postindustrial society, fewer farm and factory workers translates to a drop in the consumption of lower-quality wines. That, combined with a greater tendency to stay home and watch television instead of going to a bistro in the evenings, has led to a decrease in wine consumption in France, but it is still high relative to most other countries. (Italy is a close second.) The Czechs are the world's leading beer drinkers, averaging 162 liters (about 45 gallons) per capita in 2003.[7] They are followed by Ireland, at 146 liters, and then Germany and Austria.

Trends in U.S. Alcohol Consumption

Figure 9.1 shows trends in apparent alcohol consumption in the U.S. over more than two decades. This graph is based on the taxed sale of beer, wine, and spirits.[8] For comparison purposes, each beverage is calculated in terms of the amount of pure alcohol consumed. The figure shows that overall alcohol consumption, which had been rising through most of the 1970s, peaked in 1981. Remember from Chapter 1 that this is about the same time that

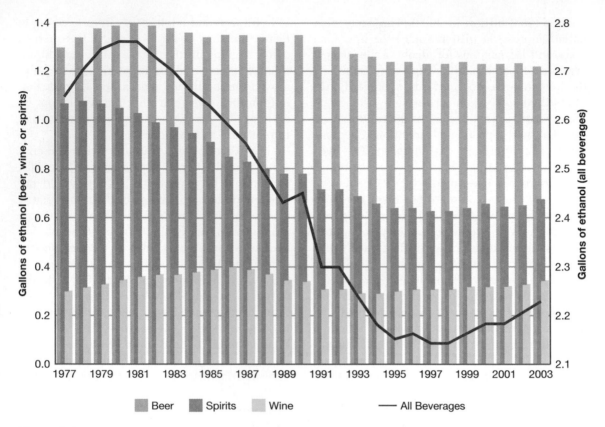

Figure 9.1 Per Capita Ethanol Consumption by Beverage Type for the United States, 1977–2003

SOURCE: Data from *NIAAA Surveillance Report #73,* 2005.

reported use of illicit drugs also reached a peak. Americans drink most of their alcohol in the form of beer. Just over 25 gallons of beer per person per year translates to more than 1 gallon of alcohol per person in that beer. The population consists of those age 14 and older, reflecting the long-known fact that the "drinking" population includes quite a few people who are not legally able to purchase alcohol. Although beer consumption has declined since 1981, the most obvious change has been the decline in the consumption of spirits. Americans now consume just under two-thirds of a gallon of pure alcohol in the form of spirits, and about one-third of a gallon of alcohol per year in the form of wine, for a total from all three beverage types of a little over 2 gallons of pure alcohol per person per year, down more than half a gallon from the 1981 peak.

Regional Differences in the United States

In the United States, about one-third of the adult population label themselves as abstainers. The two-thirds who use alcohol consume an amount that averages out to about three drinks per day. Most don't drink anything near that amount—in fact, another consistent finding is that half the alcohol is consumed by about 10 percent of the drinkers.

Whites are more likely to drink than blacks, northerners more than southerners, younger adults more than older, Catholics and Jews more than Protestants, nonreligious more

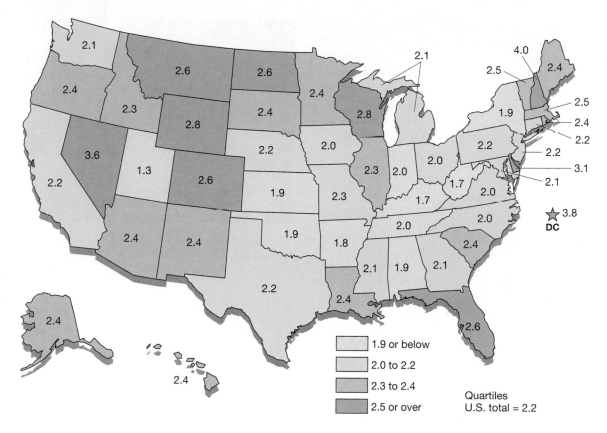

Figure 9.2 Total Estimated U.S. Per Capita Ethanol Consumption in Gallons Per Year by State, 2003, Based on Sales
Source: Data from NIAAA, 2005.

than religious, urban more than rural, large-city dwellers more than small-city residents, and college-educated people more than those with only a high school or grade school education.

Figure 9.2 shows estimated overall alcohol consumption combining beer, wine, and distilled spirits (about half the total U.S. alcohol consumption comes from beer) for each state, based on sales.[8] Nevada and New Hampshire have the highest per capita sales, along with the District of Columbia. The District of Columbia is the leader in consumption of wine, whereas Nevada consumes the most beer. Note the generally low consumption in the southern states and the generally higher consumption in the western states, with the notable exception of Utah, which has a large Mormon population.

These differences in per capita sales reflect differences in the proportion of drinkers in various parts of the country.

One theory about heavy drinking proposes that the populations of people who experience a great deal of social stress and tension (as in cities) and who approve of the use of alcohol to release tension and stress drink more and have more drinking problems. One study compared the various states with regard to such stress indicators as business failures, unemployment, divorces, abortions, disasters, percentage of new residents, and high school dropout rates. On the overall state stress index, Nevada and Alaska scored the highest, Iowa and Nebraska the lowest. Alcohol norms were rated based on the percentage of fundamentalist or

Mormon church members, the percentage of dry areas in the state, the number of liquor outlets per capita, and the number of hours per week allowed for drinking in bars. On this scale Mississippi and Utah were the most restricted, Nevada and Wisconsin the least. Overall, both the stress index and the drinking norms were significantly correlated with indicators of heavy drinking and alcohol-related arrests.[9]

Gender Differences

It will surprise no one that males are somewhat more likely to drink alcohol than females. The difference in proportions of those who have drunk alcohol in their lifetimes is not great, but almost 60 percent of males and fewer than 45 percent of females report current (past month) drinking. These results from the National Survey on Drug Use and Health are based on the U.S. population age 12 and older.[10] When "binge" drinking is defined as having five or more drinks on the same occasion, males are more likely than females to report binge drinking within the past 30 days (22 percent of males versus 17 percent of females). About 8 percent of males and 4 percent of females report "heavy" drinking, defined as binge drinking on five or more separate days during the past month. So, as we look at those who drink the most, as opposed to those who drink only occasionally, we find an increasing proportion of males among the heaviest drinkers.

Drinking Among College Students

The college years have traditionally been associated with alcohol use, and in 2005 the proportion of drinkers was about 6 percent higher among 18-to-22-year-old college students than among others of that age (e.g., about 62 percent of college students reported drinking within the past month, compared with about 56 percent of other 18-to-22-year-olds in the National Survey on Drug Use and Health).[10] Many campuses have banned the sale or ad-

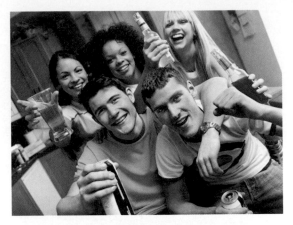

Alcohol abuse by college students usually occurs through binge drinking, which is defined as having five or more drinks in a row.

vertising of alcohol. Many fraternities have banned keg parties and the use of alcohol during "rush," partly out of concern for legal liability for the consequences if a guest becomes intoxicated and has an accident. Despite the changes in laws and rules, drinking behavior itself has not changed much in the past few years. In fact, some evidence shows among college drinkers, a slightly increased incidence of some alcohol-related problems, such as fighting, vandalism, poor grades, trouble with the police, and missing class because of hangovers.[11] These adverse consequences might result from more students drinking off campus in less controlled and less friendly environments. One ray of hope is that today's college students are less likely than those of the early 1980s to drive after drinking.

Alcohol Pharmacology

Absorption

Some alcohol is absorbed from the stomach, but the small intestine is responsible for most absorption. In an empty stomach, the overall rate of absorption depends primarily on the concentration of alcohol. Alcohol taken with or after a meal is absorbed more slowly because the food remains in the stomach for digestive

Table 9.2
Relationships Among Gender, Weight, Alcohol Consumption, and Blood Alcohol
Concentration

Absolute Alcohol (ounces)	Beverage Intake*	BLOOD ALCOHOL CONCENTRATIONS (g/100 ml)					
		Female (100 lb)	Male (100 lb)	Female (150 lb)	Male (150 lb)	Female (200 lb)	Male (200 lb)
1/2	1 oz spirits† 1 glass wine 1 can beer	0.045	0.037	0.03	0.025	0.022	0.019
1	2 oz spirits† 2 glasses wine 2 cans beer	0.090	0.075	0.06	0.050	0.045	0.037
2	4 oz spirits† 4 glasses wine 4 cans beer	0.180	0.150	0.12	0.100	0.090	0.070
3	6 oz spirits† 6 glasses wine 6 cans beer	0.270	0.220	0.18	0.150	0.130	0.110
4	8 oz spirits† 8 glasses wine 8 cans beer	0.360	0.300	0.24	0.200	0.180	0.150
5	10 oz spirits† 10 glasses wine 10 cans beer	0.450	0.370	0.30	0.250	0.220	0.180

*In one hour
†100-proof

action, and the protein in the food retains the alcohol with it in the stomach. Plain water, by decreasing the concentration, slows the absorption of alcohol, but carbonated liquids speed it up. The carbon dioxide acts to move everything quite rapidly through the stomach to the small intestine. It is because of this emptying of the stomach and the more rapid absorption of alcohol in the intestine that champagne has a faster onset of action than noncarbonated wine.

Distribution

The relationship between blood alcohol concentration (BAC) and alcohol intake is rela-

tively simple and reasonably well understood. When taken into the body, alcohol is distributed throughout the body fluids, including the blood. However, alcohol does not distribute much into fatty tissues, so a 180-pound lean person will have a lower BAC than a 180-pound fat person who drinks the same amount of alcohol.

Table 9.2 demonstrates the relationships among alcohol intake, BAC, and body weight for hypothetical, *average* females and males. The chart distinguishes between the sexes because the average female has a higher proportion of body fat and therefore, for a given weight, has less volume in which to distribute the

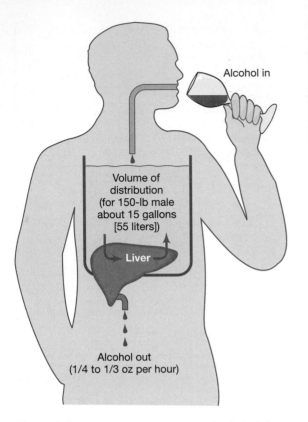

Alcohol in

Volume of
distribution
(for 150-lb male
about 15 gallons
[55 liters])

Liver

Alcohol out
(1/4 to 1/3 oz per hour)

Table 9.3 Blood Alcohol Concentration and Behavioral Effects	
Percent BAC	**Behavioral Effects**
0.05	Lowered alertness, usually good feeling, release of inhibitions, impaired judgment
0.10	Slower reaction times and impaired motor function, less caution
0.15	Large, consistent increases in reaction time
0.20	Marked depression in sensory and motor capability, intoxication
0.25	Severe motor disturbance, staggering, sensory perceptions, great impairment
0.30	Stuporous but conscious—no comprehension of what's going on
0.35	Surgical anesthesia; about LD_1, minimal level causing death
0.40	About LD_{50}

Figure 9.3 The Relationship Between Blood Alcohol Concentration and Alcohol Intake

alcohol. Understanding this table and trying one of the blood alcohol calculators on the Internet (see the Targeting Prevention on page 211) could reveal how much you can probably drink to avoid going above a specified BAC.

Table 9.2 makes the simplifying assumption that all of the alcohol is absorbed quickly so that there is little opportunity for metabolism. If the 150-pound female had a tank of water weighing about 100 pounds (12.5 gallons, or 45 liters) and just dumped 1 ounce (28.3 g) into it and stirred it, the concentration would be about 0.6 g/liter, or 0.06 g/100 ml (0.06 percent). Figure 9.3 shows a schematic of such a tank. The 150-pound average male has a tank with more water in it, so his alcohol concentration after 1 ounce is about 0.05 percent. The major factor determining individual

differences in BAC is the volume of distribution, so find your own weight on Table 9.2 and estimate how many drinks could be poured into your tank to obtain a BAC of 0.05 percent.

Notice that several beverages are equated to 0.5 ounce of absolute alcohol. A 12-ounce can or bottle of beer at about 4 percent alcohol contains $12 \times 0.04 = 0.48$ ounce of alcohol. The same amount is found in a glass containing about 4 ounces of wine at 12 percent alcohol, 1 ounce of 100-proof spirits, or 1.25 ounces of 80-proof spirits. Each of these can be equated as a standard "drink."

We have not yet considered metabolism, but we can do so with one more simple calculation. Alcohol is removed by the liver at a constant rate of 0.25 to 0.30 ounce of ethanol per hour. Most people fall within this range no matter what their body size or drinking experience, unless they have consumed so

Targeting Prevention

Estimating Blood Alcohol Calculations

Table 9.2 is one way to estimate blood alcohol level based on gender, weight, and number of drinks. However, several more dynamic blood alcohol calculators are now available on the Internet. An Internet search for "blood alcohol calculator" turns up several. Whether or not you consume alcohol yourself, it is instructive to understand how your own body (and brain) will respond to various numbers of alcoholic drinks. Try a few of the Internet calculators to see how their results compare with each other and to Table 9.2. An important thing for you to learn is how many drinks it is likely to take to bring your BAC to 0.08, which is the legal limit for driving in all of the United States.

much alcohol that the liver is damaged. To be on the safe side, estimate that you can metabolize about 0.25 ounce per hour, and note that this is one-half of one of our standard drinks (1 beer, 1 shot, or 1 glass of wine). Over the course of an evening, if your rate of intake equals your rate of metabolism, you will maintain a stable BAC. If you drink faster than one drink every two hours, your BAC will climb.

Compared with men, women absorb a greater proportion of the alcohol they drink. Some metabolism of alcohol actually occurs in the stomach, where the enzyme alcohol dehydrogenase is present. Because this stomach enzyme is more active, on the average, in men than in women, women might be more susceptible to the effects of alcohol.[12]

Metabolism

Once absorbed, alcohol remains in the bloodstream and other body fluids until it is metabolized, and more than 90 percent of this metabolism occurs in the liver. A small amount of alcohol, less than 2 percent, is normally

excreted unchanged—some in the breath, some through the skin, and some in the urine.

The primary metabolic system is a simple one: the enzyme *alcohol dehydrogenase* converts alcohol to *acetaldehyde.* Acetaldehyde is then converted fairly rapidly by aldehyde dehydrogenase to acetic acid. With most drugs a constant *proportion* of the drug is removed in a given amount of time, so that with a high blood level the amount metabolized is high. With alcohol, the *amount* that can be metabolized is constant at about 0.25 to 0.30 ounces per hour, regardless of the blood alcohol concentration (BAC). The major factor determining the rate of alcohol metabolism is the activity of the enzyme alcohol dehydrogenase. Exercise, coffee consumption, and so on have no effect on this enzyme, so the sobering-up process is essentially a matter of waiting for this enzyme to do its job at its own speed.

Acetaldehyde might be more than just an intermediate step in the oxidation of alcohol. Acetaldehyde is quite toxic; though its blood levels are only one-thousandth of those of alcohol, this substance might cause some of the physiological effects now attributed to alcohol. One danger in heavy alcohol use might be in the higher blood levels of acetaldehyde.

The liver responds to chronic intake of alcohol by increasing the activity of metabolic enzymes (see Chapter 5). This gives rise to some interesting situations. In a person who drinks alcohol heavily over a long period, the activity of the metabolic enzymes increases. As long as there is alcohol in the system, alcohol gets preferential treatment and the metabolism of other drugs is *slower* than normal. When heavy alcohol use stops and the alcohol has disappeared from the body, the high activity level of the enzymes continues for four to eight weeks. During this time other drugs are metabolized more *rapidly.* To obtain therapeutic levels of other drugs metabolized by this enzyme system (e.g., the benzodiazepines), it is necessary to administer less drug to a chronic heavy drinker and more drug to one who has recently stopped drinking. Thus, alcohol increases the activity of one of the two enzyme systems responsible for its own oxidation. The increased activity of this enzyme is a partial basis for the tolerance to alcohol that is shown by heavy users of alcohol.

Mechanism(s) of Action

Alcohol is like any other general anesthetic: It depresses the CNS. It was used as an anesthetic until the late 19th century, when nitrous oxide, ether, and chloroform became more widely used. However, it was not just new compounds that decreased alcohol's use as an anesthetic; alcohol itself has some major disadvantages. In contrast to the gaseous anesthetics, alcohol metabolizes slowly. This gives alcohol a long duration of action that cannot be controlled. A second disadvantage is that the dose effective in surgical anesthesia is not much lower than the dose that causes respiratory arrest and death. Finally, alcohol makes blood slower to clot.

The exact mechanism for the CNS effect of alcohol is not clear. Until the mid-1980s, the most widely accepted theory was that alcohol acted on all neural membranes, perhaps altering their electrical excitability. However, with increased understanding of the role of the GABA receptor complex in the actions of other depressant drugs (see Chapter 7), researchers began to study the effects of alcohol on GABA receptors. As with the barbiturates and benzodiazepines, alcohol enhances the inhibitory effects of GABA at the GABA-A receptor. This would explain the similarity of behavioral effects among these three different kinds of chemicals. But alcohol has many other effects in the brain, so it has been very difficult to pin down a single mechanism. No matter what neurotransmitter or receptor or transporter is examined, alcohol appears to alter its function in some way. Because alcohol's ability to enhance GABA inhibition at the GABA-A receptor occurs at very low doses, this mechanism probably has special importance. Remember that GABA is a very widespread inhibitory neurotransmitter, so alcohol tends to have widespread inhibitory effects on neurons in the brain. At higher doses alcohol also blocks the effects of the excitatory transmitter glutamate at some of its receptors, so this may enhance its overall inhibitory actions.

Alcohol also produces a variety of effects on dopamine, serotonin, and acetylcholine neurons, and researchers continue to explore these various actions with an eye to understanding not only the acute intoxicating effects of alcohol, but also the long-term changes that occur when the brain is exposed to alcohol on a chronic basis. One of the oldest and chemically simplest psychoactive drugs also seems to have the most complicated set of effects on the nervous system.

Behavioral Effects

At the lowest effective blood levels, complex, abstract, and poorly learned behaviors are disrupted. As the alcohol dose increases, better learned and simpler behaviors are also affected. Inhibitions can be reduced, with the result that the overall amount of behavior increases under certain conditions. Even though alcohol can result in an increase in activity, most scientists would not call alcohol a stimulant. Rather, the increased behavioral output is usually attributed to decreased inhibition of behavior.

If the alcohol intake is "just right," most people experience euphoria, a happy feeling. Below a certain **blood alcohol concentration** (BAC) there are no mood changes, but at some point we become uninhibited enough to enjoy our own "charming selves" and uncritical enough to accept the "clods" around us. We become witty, clever, and quite sophisticated, or at least it seems we are.

Another factor contributing to the feeling of well-being is the reduction in anxieties as a result of the disruption of normal critical thinking. The reduction in concern and judgment can range from not worrying about who'll pay the bar bill to being sure that you can take that next curve at 60 mph.

Drugs in Depth

Alcohol without Liquid

In 2005, news reports began to appear in some locations around the country about bars that had installed "AWOL" machines, short for "alcohol without liquid" (but making a play on the military term "absent without leave)." These devices mix oxygen with alcohol vapor, which is then inhaled through a mask placed over the face. Early reports from users of these machines indicate that they are probably a slow and inefficient method of absorbing alcohol, requiring about 20 minutes of constant inhalation through the mask to obtain an effect similar to one drink. Fears were immediately raised by medical experts about the potential for harmful drying effects on the lung tissue of breathing alcohol vapor in high concentrations. For once, groups like Mothers Against Drunk Driving were on the same side as the liquor manufacturers and distributors in raising fears about the safety of such devices, and legislation to ban them was introduced in several states. HR 613, calling for a ban on such devices unless they are approved by the FDA, was submitted in the U.S. Congress in 2005, but did not make it out of committee.

It is too early to tell whether AWOL devices will increase in popularity and whether research will ultimately find clear evidence of lung damage or other health-related problems in those who do use them frequently.

These effects depend on the BAC—also called blood alcohol level (BAL). BAC is reported as the number of grams of alcohol in 100 ml of blood and is expressed as a percentage. For example, 100 g in 100 ml is 100 percent, and 100 mg of alcohol in 100 ml of blood is reported as 0.10 percent.

Before suggesting relationships between BAC and behavioral change, two factors must be mentioned. One is that the rate at which the BAC rises is a factor in determining behavioral effects. The more rapid the increase, the greater the behavioral effects. Second, a higher BAC is necessary to impair the performance of a chronic, heavy drinker than to impair a moderate drinker's performance.

Performance differences might reflect only the extent to which experienced drinkers have learned to overcome the disruption of nervous system functioning. Another explanation might be that the CNS in the regular drinker develops a tolerance to alcohol. It is established that neural tissue becomes tolerant to alcohol, and tolerance can apparently develop even when the alcohol intake is well spaced over time.

Table 9.3 describes some general behavioral effects of increasing doses of alcohol. These relationships are approximately correct for moderate drinkers. There are some reports that changes in nervous system function have been obtained at concentrations as low as 0.03 to 0.04 percent.

The surgical anesthesia level and the minimum lethal level are perhaps the two least precise points in the table. In any case, they are quite close, and the safety margin is less than 0.1 percent blood alcohol. Death resulting from acute alcohol intoxication usually is the result of respiratory failure when the medulla is depressed.

The relationship between BAC and behavior is similarly, but more enjoyably, described in the following:

At less than 0.03 percent, the individual is dull and dignified.

At 0.05 percent, he is dashing and debonair.

At 0.10 percent, he may become dangerous and devilish.

At 0.20 percent, he is likely to be dizzy and disturbing.

At 0.25 percent, he may be disgusting and disheveled.

blood alcohol concentration; also called blood alcohol level: a measure of the concentration of alcohol in blood, expressed in grams per 100 ml (percentage).

At 0.30 percent, he is delirious and disoriented and surely drunk.

At 0.35 percent, he is dead drunk.

At 0.60 percent, the chances are that he is dead.[5]

Scientific study of the behavioral effects of alcohol is made difficult by the importance of placebo effects. With a substance as pervasive as alcohol, we have a long history of learning about what to expect from this substance, even before taking a drink (and even for those who never drink). Culture passes along a rich set of ideas about how alcohol is supposed to affect people, and we need to be sure which of the many behavioral changes we see after people drink are actually due to the pharmacological effects of having alcohol in the system. A number of laboratory studies have focused on alcohol effects using the *balanced placebo* design. Half the study participants are given mixed drinks that contain alcohol, while the other half get similar-tasting drinks without alcohol. Each of those groups is divided in half, with some being told they are getting alcohol (whether they are or not) and others being told they are testing a nonalcohol drink. By analyzing the behavioral effects seen in the four conditions, it is possible to determine which effects are actually produced by alcohol and which by the belief that one has consumed alcohol (alcohol expectancy effects). Many of the effects on social behavior (increased laughter, talkativeness, flirtation) are strongly influenced by expectancy even when no alcohol has been consumed, whereas such things as impairment in reaction times and driving simulators result from actual alcohol consumption even when the participant is not aware of the alcohol in the drink. Clearly such studies are limited to the effects of fairly low doses, because if enough alcohol is consumed the participants can detect its effects.

Time-out and Alcohol Myopia

Many of the effects experienced by drinkers are based on what they expect to happen, which interacts somewhat with the pharmacological effects of alcohol. One important component of alcohol use is that drinking serves as a social signal, to the drinker and others, indicating a "time-out" from responsibilities, work, and seriousness. Sitting down with a drink indicates "I'm off duty now" and "Don't take anything I say too seriously." Steele and Josephs have proposed that alcohol induces a kind of social and behavioral myopia, or nearsightedness.[13] After drinking, people tend to focus more on the here and now and to pay less attention to peripheral people and activities, and to long-term consequences. That might be why some people are more violent after drinking, whereas others become more helpful even if there is personal risk or cost involved. The idea is that alcohol releases people from their inhibitions, largely because the inhibitions represent concerns about what might happen, whereas the intoxicated individual focuses on the immediate irritant or the person who needs help right now.

Driving Under the Influence

Attention was focused in the early 1980s on the large number of traffic fatalities involving alcohol. The total number of traffic fatalities in 1980 was over 50,000, but by 1983 that had dropped to nearer 40,000, where it has remained since.[14] It is difficult to estimate exactly how many of those fatalities are *caused* by alcohol, but we can obtain some relevant information. Many states mandate that the coroner measure blood alcohol in all fatally injured drivers. Based on those measurements, estimates have been made of the number of alcohol-related traffic crash fatalities. From the peak of over 42 percent in 1982, by 2003 the percentage had declined to about 30 percent (see Figure 9.4).[15]

Several studies have demonstrated that the danger of combining alcohol with automobiles is dose-related. At a BAC of 0.08 percent the relative risk of being involved in a fatal crash is about three times as great as for a sober driver. A British study on younger, less experienced

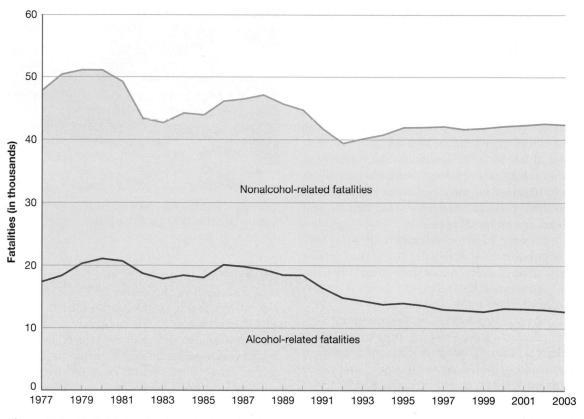

Figure 9.4 Alcohol-Related and Nonalcohol-Related Traffic Crash Fatalities for the United States, 1977–2003

drivers (and drinkers) found that the relative risk at 0.08 percent was about five times as great. The risk rises sharply for all drivers with a BAC above 0.10. Similarly, the risk of involvement in a personal injury crash increases with BAC, as does the risk of involvement in a fatal pedestrian accident.

Other interesting facts have emerged from studies of alcohol and accidents. Alcohol-related traffic fatalities are not a random sample of all fatalities. Single-vehicle fatalities are more likely to involve alcohol than are multiple-vehicle fatalities. Alcohol-related fatalities are a greater proportion of the fatalities occurring during dark hours than of those occurring in daylight and are a greater proportion of fatalities occurring on the weekend than of those occurring during the week. Fatally injured drivers in accidents occurring between midnight and

3 AM are 10 times as likely to have a BAC above 0.08 percent as drivers in accidents occurring between 9 AM and noon.[14]

When you hear that about 85 percent of all the fatally injured drivers who had been drinking were male, that sounds like a big difference, and it is. But it is important to remember that 70 percent of all fatally injured drivers are male, whether or not drinking is involved. That men are more likely to be involved in alcohol-related traffic fatalities reflects three important facts: Any given car is more likely to have a male than a female driver, men might take more chances when driving even when they're sober, and male drivers are more likely than female drivers to have been drinking.

Who is responsible for all these alcohol-related traffic accidents? One question is whether there are certain individuals, such as problem drinkers, responsible for much of the drunk driving. Problem drinkers, although a relatively small fraction of the drinking population, are more likely on a given day to be driving around with a high BAC. On the other hand, almost 90 percent of the intoxicated drivers involved in fatal crashes have never been convicted of DUI in the past. Therefore, whereas individual problem drinkers cause more than their share of traffic accidents, the majority of alcohol-related traffic accidents are caused by individuals who have not been identified as problem drinkers. Anyone who drinks and drives is a potential threat.

Younger drivers have more than their share of alcohol-related accidents. In 2001, persons aged 16 to 24 made up 14 percent of U.S. drivers yet were involved in 27 percent of the alcohol-related traffic accidents.[15]

What can be done about this problem? Current efforts focus mainly on three fronts: identifying repeat offenders and keeping them off the roads, publicizing in the mass media the dangers of drinking and driving, and targeting younger drinkers for special prevention efforts. Although it is impossible to determine the effectiveness of any one of these measures, Figure 9.4 indicates that the total effort has worked to reduce alcohol-related fatalities. In 2000, the U.S. Congress passed legislation requiring states to reduce the BAC for DUI conviction from 0.10 to 0.08.

What's a safe BAC? If you are going to drink and want to remain in reasonable control of your faculties, you should probably stay below 0.05 percent. Individuals differ considerably in their sensitivities to alcohol, however, so the best rule is to learn about your own sensitivity and not to feel compelled to keep up with anyone else's drinking. Alcohol-induced impairment is dose-related and depends on what you're trying to do. Carrying on bar conversation places fewer demands on your nervous system than driving on a crowded freeway during rush hour, where any alcohol at all might interfere.

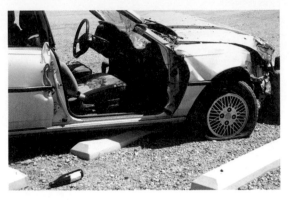

The risk of crashes rises with increasing BAC, with a sharp increase at BACs above 0.10.

BAC gives a good estimate of the alcohol concentration in the brain, and the concentration of alcohol in the breath gives a good estimate of the alcohol concentration in the blood. The concentration in the blood is almost 2,100 times the concentration in air expired from the lungs, making breath samples accurate indicators of BAC. Such breath samples are easily collected by police and can be the basis for conviction as a drunk driver in most states.

Sexual Behavior

No psychoactive substance has been as closely linked to sexuality as alcohol. Movies tell us that a romantic occasion is enhanced with wine or champagne, and the use of sexual attraction in beer ads on television is so common we are barely aware of it. The association has been noted for generations—400 years ago Shakespeare wrote about alcohol in Macbeth: "Lechery, sir, it provokes and unprovokes; it provokes the desire, but it takes away the performance."

Was Shakespeare right? It certainly seems that alcohol does make people less inhibited, and more likely to desire sex, but can we demonstrate that this is a real effect? If so, how much of the enhancement of sexual interest after drinking is really due to the pharmacological effects of the alcohol, and how much is a placebo response based on our expectancies about alcohol's effects? The importance of understanding alcohol's ability to provoke desire is enormous. On one hand, many people of both sexes for many generations and across many cultures have viewed alcohol's ability to enhance sexual interest and pleasure as a great benefit, and many will continue to do so. On the other hand, the use of alcohol is linked with risky sexual behavior (early sexual experience; unprotected sex) as well as with increased likelihood of sexual assault. The analogy to "playing with fire" is an apt one—under the right circumstances both fire and alcohol are beneficial, but both are risky and can lead to destructive outcomes.

And what about the other half of Shakespeare's statement, that alcohol takes away the performance? Anecdotal evidence shows that men with high BACs are unable to attain or maintain an erection, and there is clinical evidence that chronic alcohol abuse can lead to more permanent impotence in men. But are these effects consistent, and are they limited to high doses or long-term exposure?

Human sexual response is complex, but we can somewhat artificially divide our questions about sexuality into psychological effects (ratings of sexual arousal or interest) versus physiological effects (measurements of penile tumescence or vaginal blood volume; measurements of time to orgasm). Also, we should assume that men and women may differ considerably with respect to both dimensions of sexuality and alcohol's effects on them.

A review of the available literature on alcohol and sex points out some still unresolved questions, but also some reliable findings reported by different sets of researchers.[16] First, both men and women tend to agree with the expectancy statements that alcohol enhances or disinhibits sexuality. In balanced-placebo laboratory experiments, men who had stronger expectancies that alcohol would enhance sexuality also reported experiencing more arousal after being given a placebo drink. Therefore, at

least some of the subjective arousal that men experience after drinking is a psychological reaction to the belief that alcohol enhances sexuality. There have been fewer such experiments with women, and the results have been inconsistent.

When men and women have been given alcohol in a laboratory setting and then exposed to erotic films, both sexes report more sexual arousal after alcohol, and there is a correlation between their ratings of feeling intoxicated and their self-reported arousal. These studies have not usually explored BACs above 0.15 percent, and most have used lower BACs. In men, physiological measures of penile tumescence are correlated with self-reports of arousal, whereas in women there is no consistent relation between self-reported arousal and vaginal blood volume.

Many studies have reported that alcohol reduces penile tumescence in men, sometimes even at fairly low doses. The long-standing assumption has been that this is a direct pharmacological effect on the physiological mechanisms responsible for penile erection. However, several studies have found no effect on this measure, even at fairly high doses. Studies on animals and on nocturnal penile tumescence in men who are asleep have generally not found that alcohol suppresses erection. Therefore, attention is now shifting to the idea that when men become less aroused at higher BACs it might be due to impaired attention to or processing of erotic information. Alcohol can also impair the ability to suppress an erection when men are instructed to avoid becoming aroused.

Several studies have reported that when men believe that a woman has been drinking, they rate her as being more interested in sex and more sexually available. A similar finding has been reported for women's perceptions of men who have been drinking.

Surveys typically find that people are more likely to have sex on a date (including first dates) when they drink on that date. With respect to risky sex, both men and women given alcohol in laboratory situations report more willingness to engage in unprotected sex, and more agreement with justifications for not using condoms.

We know that alcohol is a frequent presence in sexual assaults, and laboratory studies on college students have reported some related findings. When a date rape scene is described to either men or women, less blame is assigned to the perpetrator if he has been described as drinking before the rape, and more blame is assigned to the victim if she has been described as drinking. Men are generally more aroused by nonviolent erotic films than by erotic films that contain violence, but after consuming alcohol in the laboratory, they were less discriminating and more likely to be aroused by the violent films.

Many of these effects of alcohol on sexual behavior are consistent with the alcohol myopia theory mentioned previously—alcohol impairs information processing in such a way that people are more likely to attend to what's right in front of them at the time. In a conflicting sexual situation, the person affected by alcohol will be more likely to tend toward immediate gratification and less likely to be inhibited by concerns about outcomes that are uncertain or delayed.

Blackouts

Alcohol-induced blackouts are periods during alcohol use in which the drinking individual appears to function normally but later, when the individual is sober, he or she cannot recall any events that occurred during that period. The drinker might drive home or dance all night, interacting in the usual way with others. When the individual cannot remember the activities, the people, or anything else, that's a blackout. Most authorities include it as one of the danger signs suggesting excessive use of alcohol. The limited amount of recent research on this topic is probably related to ethical concerns about giving such high doses of alcohol to experimental subjects. An article

from 1884 titled "Alcoholic Trance" referred to the syndrome:

> This trance state is a common condition in inebriety, where . . . a profound suspension of memory and consciousness and literal paralysis of certain brain-functions follow.
>
> This trance state may last from a few moments to several days, during which the person may appear and act rationally, and yet be actually a mere automaton, without consciousness or memory of his actual condition.[17]

Crime and Violence

Homicide The correlation between alcohol use and homicides is well known to police and judicial systems around the world. Based on several studies of police and court records, the proportion of murderers who had been drinking before the crime ranged from 36 percent in Baltimore to 70 percent in Sweden.[18] Across all these studies, about 50 percent of the murder victims had been drinking. These data certainly imply that homicide is more likely to occur in situations in which drinking also occurs, but they leave open the question as to whether alcohol plays a causal role in homicides.

Assault and Other Crimes of Violence As with homicide, studies of assault, spousal abuse, and child abuse reveal correlations with drinking: Heavier drinkers are more likely to engage in such behaviors, and self-reports by offenders indicate a high likelihood that they had been consuming alcohol before the violent act. However, scientists are still cautious in trying to determine how much of a causal role alcohol plays in such activity. For example, if fights are likely to occur when men get together in groups at night and drinking is likely to occur when men get together in groups at night, how much of a role does alcohol itself play in increasing the chances of violence? Similarly, if both heavy drinking and violent arguments are characteristics of dysfunctional family situations, how much of the ensuing family violence can be blamed on the use of alcohol? Unfortunately, it has proven difficult to perform controlled experimental studies on these complex problems, so the answers remain unclear.

Suicide Most studies show that alcohol is involved in about one-third of all suicides. Suicide *attempts* seem to have a different background than successful suicides, but alcohol abuse is second only to depression as the diagnosis in suicide attempters. The relationship between alcohol abuse and depression is a strong one and has been the subject of many studies. One interesting finding is that people who abused alcohol first and probably became depressed as a result of their repeated failures and shortcomings have a better prognosis than those who showed clear signs of clinical depression before they became abusers of alcohol.[19]

Physiological Effects

Peripheral Circulation One effect of alcohol on the CNS is the dilation of the peripheral blood vessels. This increases heat loss from the body but makes the drinker feel warm. The heat loss and cooling of the interior of the body are enough to cause a slowdown in some biochemical processes. This dilation of the peripheral vessels argues against giving alcohol to individuals in shock or extreme cold. Under these conditions blood is needed in the central parts of the body, and heat loss must be diminished if the person is to survive.

Fluid Balance One action of alcohol on the brain is to decrease the output of the antidiuretic hormone (ADH, also called vasopressin) responsible for retaining fluid in the body. It is this effect, rather than the actual fluid consumption, that increases the urine flow in response to alcohol. This diuretic effect can lower blood pressure in some individuals.

Hormonal Effects Even single doses of alcohol can produce measurable effects on a variety of hormonal systems: Adrenal corticosteroids are released, as are catecholamines from the adrenal medulla, and the production of the male sex hormone testosterone is suppressed. It is not known what significance, if any, these effects have for occasional, moderate drinkers. However, chronic abusers of alcohol can develop a variety of hormone-related disorders, including testicular atrophy and impotence in men and impaired reproductive functioning in women.

Alcohol Toxicity

Alcohol consumption can result in toxicity, both acute and chronic. We have already discussed the problem of alcohol-related traffic accidents, which we would consider to be examples of acute behavioral toxicity. In a similar vein are other alcohol-related accidents and adverse effects, such as falls, drowning, cycling and boating accidents, and accidents associated with operating machinery. The Centers for Disease Control estimate that acute alcohol-related problems cause more than 20,000 deaths annually in the United States (about 13,000 from automobile accidents).[20]

Acute physiological toxicity in the form of alcohol overdose occurs quite often if you include people who drink enough to become physically ill and/or to experience hangovers. In addition, more than 1,000 people die in the United States each year from accidental alcohol poisoning (high blood alcohol level). As the DAWN data in Chapter 2 revealed, many drug-related deaths include alcohol in combination with some other substance, so it is difficult to know exactly how many overdose deaths are primarily due to alcohol versus another drug, or to the specific combination. Three well-publicized drinking deaths of young college students occurred in the fall of 2004. All of these students had been drinking for many hours before their deaths, and as a result colleges and universities began re-examining their alcohol-use policies. Two pieces of advice are worth mentioning: (1) If one of your friends drinks enough to pass out, DO NOT simply leave her or him alone to sleep it off. The person should be placed on his or

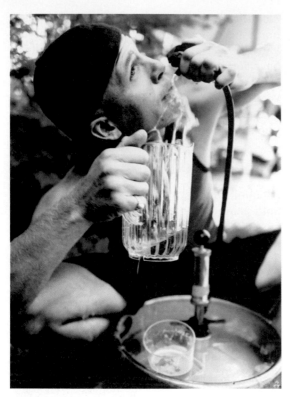

Rapid consumption of alcohol can lead to acute toxicity.

her side so that any vomit is less likely to be aspirated, and someone who is sober needs to monitor the person's breathing until he or she can be aroused and begins to move. If this is not possible, take the victim to the emergency room. Don't worry about getting in trouble for helping out a friend—the alternative can be much worse. (2) It is particularly dangerous to drink to the point of vomiting and then begin drinking again after vomiting. The vomiting reflex is triggered by rapidly rising BAC, usually above 0.12 percent. But the vomiting reflex is inhibited when the BAC rises above 0.20 or so, and it is then possible to continue drinking and reach lethal concentrations.

Hangover

The Germans call it "wailing of cats" *(Katzenjammer)*, the Italians "out of tune" *(stonato)*, the French "woody mouth" *(gueule de boise)*, the Norwegians "workmen in my head" *(jeg har tommeermenn)*, and the Swedes "pain in the roots of the hair" *(hont i haret)*. Hangovers aren't much fun. And they aren't very well understood, either. Even moderate drinkers who only occasionally overindulge are well acquainted with the symptoms: upset stomach, fatigue, headache, thirst, depression, anxiety, and general malaise.

Some authorities believe that the symptoms of a hangover are the symptoms of withdrawal from a short- or long-term dependence on alcohol. The pattern certainly fits. Some people report continuing to drink just to escape the pain of the hangover. This behavior is not unknown to moderate drinkers, either: Many believe that the only cure for a hangover is some of "the hair of the dog that bit you"— alcohol. And it might work to minimize symptoms, because it spreads them out over a longer time. There is no evidence that any of the "surefire-this'll-fix-you-up" remedies are effective. The only known cures are an analgesic for the headache, rest, and time.

Some hangover symptoms are probably reactions to congeners. Congeners are natural products of the fermentation and preparation process, some of which are quite toxic. Congeners make the various alcoholic beverages different in smell, taste, color, and, possibly, hangover potential.

Still other factors contribute to the trials and tribulations of the "morning after the night before." Thirst means that the body has excreted more fluid than was taken in with the alcoholic beverages. However, this does not seem to be the only basis for the thirst experienced the next day. Another cause might be that alcohol causes fluid inside cells to move outside the cells. This cellular dehydration, without a decrease in total body fluid, is known to be related to, and might be the basis of, an increase in thirst.

The nausea and upset stomach typically experienced can most likely be attributed to the fact that alcohol is a gastric irritant. Consuming even moderate amounts causes local irritation of the mucosa lining the stomach. It has been suggested that the accumulation of acetaldehyde, which is quite toxic even in small quantities, contributes to the nausea and headache. The headache can also be a reaction to fatigue. Fatigue sometimes results from a higher than normal level of activity while drinking. Increased activity frequently accompanies a decrease in inhibitions, a readily available source of energy, and a high blood sugar level. One effect of alcohol intake is to increase the blood sugar level for about an hour after ingestion. This can be followed several hours later by a low blood sugar level and an increased feeling of fatigue.

Recently several products that are supposed to prevent hangovers have been advertised on TV and through the Internet, and sold in bars, liquor stores, and convenience stores. Although one of these products claims to have been tested in a placebo-controlled study, the study has not been published in a scientific journal and the product's ingredients, including a small amount of activated charcoal meant to absorb congeners, seems unlikely to have much real effect. The best way to avoid a hangover is still to drink in moderation, regardless of the beverage.

Chronic Disease States

The relationship of alcohol use to many diseases has been studied extensively. As a general rule, heavy alcohol use, either directly or indirectly, affects every organ system in the body. The alcohol or its primary metabolite, acetaldehyde, can irritate and damage tissue directly. Because alcohol provides empty calories, many heavy drinkers do not eat well, and chronic malnutrition leads to tissue damage. Separating the effects of alcohol exposure from those of malnutrition relies to a great extent on experiments with animals. Some animals can be fed adequate diets and exposed to high concentrations of alcohol, whereas other animals are fed diets deficient in certain vitamins or other nutrients.

Brain Damage

Perhaps the biggest concern is the damage to brain tissue that is seen in chronic alcohol abusers. It has been reported for years that the brains of deceased heavy drinkers demonstrate an obvious overall loss of brain tissue: the ventricles (internal spaces) in the brain are enlarged, and the fissures (sulci) in the cortex are widened. Modern imaging techniques have revealed this tissue loss in living alcohol abusers as well. This generalized loss of brain tissue is probably a result of direct alcohol toxicity rather than malnutrition and is associated with *alcoholic dementia,* a global decline of intellect. Patients with this type of organic brain syndrome might have difficulty swallowing in addition to impaired problem solving, difficulty in manipulating objects, and abnormal electroencephalograms. Another classical alcohol-related organic brain syndrome has two parts, which so often go together that the disorder is referred to as **Wernicke-Korsakoff syndrome.** *Wernicke's disease* is associated with a deficiency of thiamine (vitamin B_1) and can sometimes be corrected nutritionally. The symptoms include confusion, ataxia (impaired coordination while walking), and abnormal eye movements. Most patients with Wernicke's disease also exhibit *Korsakoff's psychosis,* characterized by an inability to remember recent events or to learn new information. Korsakoff's psychosis can appear by itself in patients who maintain adequate nutrition, and it appears to be mostly irreversible. There has been great controversy about the specific brain areas that are damaged in Wernicke-Korsakoff syndrome, as well as about the relationship between the two parts of the disorder.

Important practical questions include the following. Exactly how much alcohol exposure is required before behavioral and/or anatomical

---

Wernicke-Korsakoff syndrome (*wer* nick ee core sa kof): chronic mental impairments produced by heavy alcohol use over a long period of time.

evidence can be found indicating brain damage? And how much of the cognitive deficit seen in alcoholic dementia can be reversed when drinking is stopped and adequate nutrition is given? Both have been the subject of several experiments. There is no definitive answer for the first question. Some of the studies on moderate drinkers have included individuals who consume up to 10 drinks per day! Most studies with lower cutoffs for moderate drinking have not found consistent evidence for anatomical changes in the brain. As for recovery, several studies have reported both behavioral improvement and apparent regrowth of brain size in chronic alcohol abusers after some months of abstinence. However, not all such studies find improvement, and some have found improvement in some types of mental tasks but not in others.

Liver Disorders

Fatty acids are the usual fuel for the liver. When present, alcohol has higher priority and is used as fuel instead. As a result, fatty acids (lipids) accumulate in the liver and are stored as small droplets in liver cells. This condition is known as alcohol-related *fatty liver,* which for most drinkers is not a serious problem. If alcohol input ceases, the liver uses the stored fatty acids for energy. Sometimes the droplets increase in size until they rupture the cell membrane, causing death of the liver cells. Before the liver cells die, a fatty liver is completely reversible and usually of minor medical concern.

Sometimes, with prolonged or high-level alcohol intake, another phase of liver damage is observed. Alcoholic hepatitis is a serious disease and includes both inflammation and impairment of liver function. Usually this occurs in areas of the liver where cells are dead and dying, but it is not known if an increasingly fatty liver leads to alcoholic hepatitis. Alcoholic hepatitis does exist in the absence of a fatty liver, so this form of tissue damage might be due to direct toxic effects of alcohol.

Cirrhosis is the liver disease everyone knows is related to high and prolonged levels of alcohol consumption. It's not easy to get cirrhosis from drinking alcohol—you have to work at it. Usually it takes about 10 years of steady drinking of the equivalent of a pint or more of whiskey a day. Not all cirrhosis is alcohol-related, but a high percentage is, and cirrhosis is the seventh leading cause of death in the United States. In large urban areas it is the fourth or fifth leading cause of death in men ages 25 to 65. In cirrhosis, liver cells are replaced by fibrous tissue (collagen), which changes the structure of the liver (see Figure 9.5). These changes decrease blood flow and, along with the loss of cells, result in a decreased ability of the liver to function. When the liver does not function properly, fluid accumulates in the body, jaundice develops, and other infections or cancers have a better opportunity to establish themselves in the liver. Cirrhosis is not reversible, but stopping the intake of alcohol will retard its development and decrease the serious medical effects.

In drinkers with severely damaged livers, liver transplants have been quite successful—a 64 percent survival rate after two years. Most of these recipients do not resume drinking after the transplant.

Heart Disease

Another area of concern is the effect of alcohol on the heart and circulation. Heavy alcohol use is associated with increased mortality resulting from heart disease. Much of this is due to damage to the heart muscle (cardiomyopathy), but the risk of the more typical heart attack resulting from coronary artery disease also increases. Heavy drinkers are also more likely to suffer from high blood pressure and strokes. An interesting twist to this story is that several studies have found a *lower* incidence of heart attacks in moderate drinkers than in abstainers, and for several years this protective effect of moderate alcohol consumption and the possible

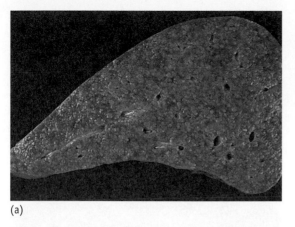
(a)

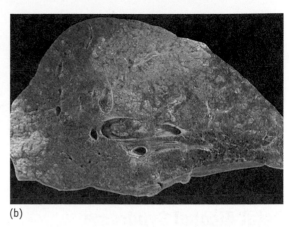
(b)

Figure 9.5   (a) Normal Liver; (b) Cirrhotic Liver

mechanism for it have been discussed. It has been pointed out that the abstainers in such studies might include both abstaining alcohol abusers who once drank heavily and others who quit on their doctor's advice because of poor health. However, one study separated those who never drank from the "quitters" and still reported fewer heart attacks and lower overall mortality in moderate drinkers, with increased mortality for both abstainers and heavy drinkers.[19] It has been proposed that alcohol increases high-density lipoproteins (HDL, sometimes called "good cholesterol"), some of which seem to protect against high blood pressure. The reduced blood clotting produced by alcohol could also play a role. There has been some speculation that red wine might have better effects than other forms of alcohol due to the presence of antioxidants in the grapes from which the wine is made. But the scientific evidence supports only a beneficial effect of alcohol on heart attacks, with an optimal effect occurring at about one drink per day.[21]

Cancer

Alcohol use is associated with cancers of the mouth, tongue, pharynx, larynx, esophagus, stomach, liver, lung, pancreas, colon, and rec-

tum. There are many possible mechanisms for this, from direct tissue irritation to nutritional deficiencies to the induction of enzymes that activate other carcinogens. A particularly nasty interaction with cigarette smoking increases the incidence of cancers of the oral cavity, pharynx, and larynx. Also, suppression of the immune system by alcohol, which occurs to some extent every time intoxicating doses are used, probably increases the rate of tumor growth.

The Immune System

The immune deficits seen in chronic alcohol abusers are associated with at least some increase in the frequency of various infectious diseases, including tuberculosis, pneumonia, yellow fever, cholera, and hepatitis B. Alcohol use might be a factor in AIDS, for several reasons: Loss of behavioral inhibitions probably increases the likelihood of engaging in unprotected sex; alcohol could increase the risk of HIV infection in exposed individuals; and alcohol could suppress the immune system and therefore increase the chances of developing

cirrhosis (sir *oh* sis): an irreversible, frequently deadly liver disorder associated with heavy alcohol use.

full-blown AIDS once an HIV infection is established. Although one epidemiological study did not find an acceleration of HIV-related disease in infected individuals who drank, heavy alcohol use is probably not a good idea for anyone who is HIV-positive.

There is no evidence that the occasional consumption of one or two drinks has overall negative effects on the physical health of most individuals. An important exception to this statement might be drinking during pregnancy.

Fetal Alcohol Syndrome

The unfortunate condition of infants born to alcohol-abusing mothers was noted in an 1834 report to the British Parliament: They have a "starved, shriveled, and imperfect look." Until fairly recently most scientists and physicians believed that any effects on the offspring of heavy alcohol users were the result of poor nutrition or poor prenatal care. Those beliefs changed, however, when a 1973 article reported the following:

> Eight unrelated children of three different ethnic groups, all born to mothers who were chronic alcoholics, have a pattern of craniofacial, limb, and cardiovascular defects associated with prenatal-onset growth deficiency and developmental delay. This seems to be the first reported association between maternal alcoholism and aberrant morphogenesis in the offspring.[22]

That publication signaled the recognition of **fetal alcohol syndrome** (FAS), a collection of physical and behavioral abnormalities that seems to be caused by the presence of alcohol during development of the fetus (see Figure 9.6). There are three primary criteria for diagnosing FAS, at least one of which *must* be present:

1. Growth retardation occurring before and/or after birth.
2. A pattern of abnormal features of the face and head, including small head circumference, small eyes, or evidence of retarded formation of the midfacial area, including a

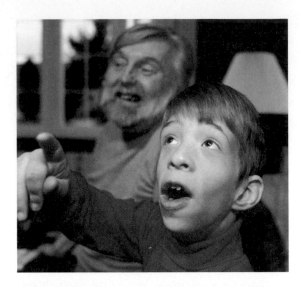

Figure 9.6 This boy shows typical features of fetal alcohol syndrome, including small eyes, flattened bridge of the nose, and flattening of the vertical groove between the nose and mouth.

flattened bridge and short length of the nose and flattening of the vertical groove between the nose and mouth (the philtrum).
3. Evidence of CNS abnormality, including abnormal neonatal behavior, mental retardation, or other evidence of abnormal neurobehavioral development.

Each of these features can be seen in the absence of alcohol exposure, and other features might also be present in FAS, such as eye and ear defects, heart murmurs, undescended testicles, birthmarks, and abnormal fingerprints or palmar creases. Research also found a high frequency of various abnormalities of the eyes, often associated with poor vision. Thus, the diagnosis of FAS is a matter of judgment, based on several symptoms and often on the physician's knowledge of the mother's drinking history.

Many animal studies have been done in a variety of species, and they indicate that FAS is related to peak BAC and to duration of alcohol exposure, even when malnutrition is not an issue. In mice and other animal models, increasing amounts of alcohol yield an increase in mortality, a decrease in infant weight, and increased frequency of soft-tissue malformation. The various components of the complete FAS reflect damage occurring at different developmental stages, so heavy alcohol exposure throughout pregnancy is the most damaging situation, followed by intermittent high-level exposure designed to imitate binge drinking.

Not all infants born to drinking mothers show abnormal development. If they did, it would not have taken so long to recognize FAS as a problem. Estimates of the prevalence of FAS in the overall population range from 0.2 per 1,000 births to 1.5 per 1,000.[22] Estimating the prevalence among problem drinkers or alcohol abusers is more of a problem. There is the difficulty not only of diagnosing FAS but also of diagnosing alcohol abuse. If the physician knows that the mother is a heavy drinker, this can increase the probability of noticing or diagnosing FAS, thus inflating the prevalence statistics among drinking mothers. FAS seems to occur in 23 to 29 per 1,000 births among women who are problem drinkers. If all alcohol-related birth defects (referred to as **fetal alcohol effect,** or FAE) are counted, the rate among heavy-drinking women is higher, from 80 to a few hundred per 1,000. Maternal alcohol abuse might be the most frequent known environmental cause of mental retardation in the Western world.

In addition to the risk of FAS, the fetus of a mother who drinks heavily has a risk of not being born at all. Spontaneous abortion early in pregnancy is perhaps twice as likely among the 5 percent of women who are the heaviest drinkers. The data on later pregnancy loss (stillbirths) are not as clearly related to alcohol for either animals or humans.

An important question, and one that can never be answered in absolute terms, is whether there is an acceptable level of alcohol consumption for pregnant women (see the Taking Sides). The data on drinking during pregnancy rely on self-reports by the mothers, who are assumed to be at least as likely as everyone else to underreport their drinking. In addition,

almost every study has used different definitions of heavy drinking, alcohol abuse, and problem drinking. The heaviest drinkers in each study are the most at risk for alcohol-related problems with their children, but we don't really know if the large number of light or moderate drinkers are causing significant risks. Based on the dose-related nature of birth problems in animal studies, one might argue that any alcohol use at all produces some risk, but at low levels the increased risk is too small to be revealed except in a large-scale study. In 1981, the U.S. surgeon general recommended that "pregnant women should drink absolutely no alcohol because they may be endangering the health of their unborn children." Maybe that went a bit too far. The bottom line is this: Scientific data do not demonstrate that occasional consumption of one or two drinks definitely causes FAS or other alcohol-related birth defects. On the other hand, neither do the data prove that low-level alcohol use is safe nor do they indicate a safe level of use. Remember from Chapter 5 that it is not within the realm of science to declare something totally safe, so it will be impossible to ever set a safe limit on alcohol use. Most women decrease their alcohol use once they have become pregnant, and many decrease it further as pregnancy progresses.

Alcohol Dependence

Withdrawal Syndrome

The physical dependence associated with prolonged heavy use of alcohol is revealed when alcohol intake is stopped. *The abstinence*

---

fetal alcohol syndrome: facial and developmental abnormalities associated with the mother's alcohol use during pregnancy.
fetal alcohol effect: individual developmental abnormalities associated with the mother's alcohol use during pregnancy.

Taking Sides

Protecting the Unborn from Alcohol

Increased concern about fetal alcohol syndrome has led to some significant changes in the status of pregnant women, at least in certain instances and locations. Waiters have refused to serve wine to pregnant women, women have been arrested and charged with child abuse for being heavily intoxicated while pregnant, and others have been charged with endangerment for breastfeeding while drunk. These social interventions represent concerns for the welfare of the child. However, to women already concerned about their own rights because of the issue of government regulation of abortion, such actions seem to be yet another infringement, yet another signal that the woman's rights are secondary to the child's.

We know that heavy alcohol consumption during pregnancy does increase the risk to the child of permanent disfigurement and mental retardation. We also know that, even among the heaviest drinkers, the odds still favor a normal-appearing baby (less than 10 percent of the babies born to the heaviest-drinking 5 percent of mothers exhibit full-blown FAS).

Do you think that men are more likely than women to support limiting the rights of pregnant women to drink while they are pregnant? You might ask a group of both men and women to give you answers to the following questions.

How strongly do you agree (5 = strong agreement, 1 = strong disagreement) with the following statements?

1. Women who repeatedly get drunk while they are pregnant should be kept in jail if necessary until the baby is born.
2. All bartenders should be trained not to serve any drinks at all to a woman who is obviously pregnant.
3. If a man and a pregnant woman are drinking together and both become intoxicated, both the man and the woman should be arrested for child abuse.

syndrome that develops is medically more severe and more likely to cause death than withdrawal from opioid drugs. In untreated advanced cases, mortality can be as high as one in seven. For that reason it has long been recommended that the initial period of **detoxification** (allowing the body to rid itself of the alcohol) be carried out in an inpatient medical setting, especially for people who have been drinking very heavily or have other medical complications.

The progression of withdrawal, the abstinence syndrome, has been described in the following way:

- Stage 1: tremors, excessively rapid heartbeat, hypertension, heavy sweating, loss of appetite, and insomnia.
- Stage 2: hallucinations—auditory, visual, tactile, or a combination of these; and, rarely, olfactory signs.

- Stage 3: delusions, disorientation, delirium, sometimes intermittent and usually followed by amnesia.
- Stage 4: seizure activity.

Medical treatment is usually sought in stage 1 or 2, and rapid intervention with a sedative drug, such as diazepam, will prevent stage 3 or 4 from occurring. The old term **delirium tremens** is used to refer to severe cases including at least stage 3.

Tremors are one of the most common physical changes associated with alcohol withdrawal and can persist for a long period after alcohol intake has stopped. Anxiety, insomnia, feelings of unreality, nausea, vomiting, and many other symptoms can also occur.

The withdrawal symptoms do not develop all at the same time or immediately after abstinence begins. The initial signs (tremors, anxiety) might develop within a few hours, but the individual is relatively rational. Over the next day or two, hallucinations appear and gradually become more terrifying and real to the individual. Huckleberry Finn described these in his father quite vividly:

> Pap took the jug, and said he had enough whisky there for two drunks and one delirium tremens. He drank and drank. . . .
>
> I don't know how long I was asleep, but . . . there was an awful scream and I was up. There was pap looking wild, and skipping around every which way and yelling about snakes. He said they was crawling up on his legs; and then he would give a jump and scream, and say one had bit him on the cheek—but I couldn't see no snakes. He started and run round . . . hollering "Take him off! he's biting me on the neck!" I never see a man look so wild in the eyes. Pretty soon he was all fagged out, and fell down panting; then he rolled over . . . kicking things every which way, and striking and grabbing at the air with his hands, and screaming . . . there was devils a-hold of him. He wore out by and by. . . . He says . . .
>
> "Tramp-tramp-tramp; that's the dead; tramp-tramp-tramp; they're coming after me; but I won't go. Oh, they're here; don't touch me—don't! hands off—they're cold; let go. . . ."
>
> Then he went down on all fours and crawled off, begging them to let him alone. . . .
>
> By and by he . . . jumped up on his feet looking wild . . . and went for me. He chased me round and round the place with a claspknife, calling me the Angel of Death, and saying he would kill me, and then I wouldn't come for him no more. . . . Pretty soon he was all tired out . . . and said he would rest for a minute and then kill me.[23]

The sensation of snakes or bugs crawling on the skin should ring a bell—this also occurs after high doses of stimulant drugs. In the context of alcohol withdrawal, it is an indication that the nervous system is rebounding from constant inhibition and is hyperexcitable.

Optimal treatment of patients during the early stages involves the administration of a benzodiazepine, such as chlordiazepoxide or diazepam (see Chapter 7). Because of the high degree of cross-dependence between alcohol

and chlordiazepoxide, one drug can be substituted for the other and withdrawal continued at a safer rate.[24]

Some withdrawal symptoms can last for up to several weeks. Unstable blood pressure, irregular breathing, anxiety, panic attacks, insomnia, and depression are all reported during this period. These phenomena have been referred to as a protracted withdrawal syndrome, and they can trigger intense cravings for alcohol. Thus, some chronic drinkers might benefit from residential or in-patient treatment for up to six weeks, simply to prevent relapse during this critical period. Preventing relapse for longer periods is a difficult task that is discussed in Chapter 17.

Dependent Behaviors

Probably the most significant influence on American attitudes about alcohol dependence was a 60-year-old book called *Alcoholics Anonymous*. This book described the experiences of a small group of people who formed a society whose "only requirement for membership is a desire to stop drinking." That society has now grown to include more than 1.5 million members in over a hundred countries. A central part of their belief system is that alcohol dependence is a progressive disease characterized by a loss of control over drinking and that the disease can never be cured. People who do not have the disease might drink and even become intoxicated, but they do not "lose control over alcohol." There is a suspicion that the dependent drinker is different even before the first drink is taken. The only treatment is to arrest the disease by abstaining from drinking. This *disease model* of alcohol dependence has

detoxification: an early treatment stage, in which the body eliminates the alcohol or other substance.
delirium tremens (de *leer* ee um *tree* mens): an alcohol withdrawal syndrome that includes hallucinations and tremors.

Mind / Body Connection

Is Alcoholics Anonymous a Religion?

For many young adults, occasional bouts of alcohol abuse appear to be symbolic of their freedom from the constraints and values imposed by their parents. For some, part of the separation from parental authority includes less involvement in the religious practices traditional to the family. And for some whose abuse of alcohol eventually begins to interfere significantly in their lives, getting sober may also involve "getting religion" back into their lives. One good example of this type of change is President George W. Bush, who in 1986 decided to quit drinking and who also became much more involved in religion, both without any direct involvement with Alcoholics Anonymous.

The original founders of Alcoholics Anonymous (AA) were strongly influenced by the Oxford Group, a Christian religious movement that involved reflecting on your own shortcomings (sins), admitting them to another, and helping others as a way of improving yourself. These became the central ideas behind AA, and certainly its first members were expected to

"accept Jesus Christ as your Lord and Savior." But how does that history relate to AA as practiced today and all over the world? Is it essentially a religion?

Most AA members would say no. AA is not intended to replace anyone's church or other religious practices, and the 12 steps (see p. 437 in Chapter 18) include the phrases "God as we understood Him," and "a Power greater than ourselves." For many AA members, this means the traditional Christian view of God, but adherents of Judaism and Islam also find their religions to be compatible with AA's beliefs. Many who are quite firm adherents of AA are even agnostics or atheists, and they are able to interpret this "Power greater than ourselves" in terms of the power of the 12-step program, or the power of the group. For them, taking a "moral inventory" (step 4), confessing their shortcomings to another individual (step 5), and then helping others to maintain sobriety represent their "spiritual awakening," implying perhaps a change of focus from being self-centered to being more responsible to others and for others.

received support from many medical practitioners and has been endorsed by the American Medical Association and other professional groups. In one sense, this description of alcohol dependence as a disease is a reaction against long-held notions that excessive drinking is only a symptom of some other underlying pathology, such as depression, or some type of personality defect. Traditional psychoanalysts practicing many years ago might have treated alcohol abusers by trying to discover the unconscious conflicts or personality deficiencies that caused the person to drink. One important consequence of defining alcohol dependence as a *primary* disease is to recognize that the drinking itself might be the problem and that treatment and prevention should be aimed directly at alcohol abuse/dependence.

However, there are many scientific critics of the disease concept. If alcohol dependence is a disease, what is its cause? How are alcohol

abusers different from others, except that they tend to drink a lot and have many alcohol-related problems? Although sequential stages have been described for this "progressive disease," most individual drinkers don't seem to fit any single set of descriptors. Some don't drink alone, some don't drink in the morning, some don't go on binges, some don't drink every day, and some don't report strong cravings for alcohol. Experiments have shown that alcohol-dependent individuals do retain considerable control over their drinking, even while drinking—it's not that they completely lose control when they start drinking, but they might have either less ability or less desire to limit their drinking because they do drink excessively. Although an "alcoholic personality" has been defined that characterizes many drinkers who enter treatment, the current belief is that these personality factors (impulsive, anxious, depressed, passive, dependent) reflect the years of intoxication and the critical events that led to the decision to enter treatment rather than preexisting abnormalities that caused the problem drinking.

The American Psychiatric Association's *Diagnostic and Statistical Manual of Mental Disorders,* Text Revision,[25] is probably the closest thing there is to a single official, widely accepted set of labels for behavioral disorders, including substance abuse and dependence (see Chapter 2). The *DSM-IV-TR* does not separately define these for alcohol but includes alcohol as one of the psychoactive substances. This manual defines *alcohol abuse,* which is defined in psychosocial terms (a maladaptive pattern of use indicated by continued use despite knowledge of having persistent problems caused by alcohol, and *alcohol dependence,* which involves more serious psychosocial characteristics and includes the physiological factors of tolerance and withdrawal among the possible symptoms.

Why are some people able to drink in moderation all their lives, whereas others repeatedly become intoxicated, suffer from alcohol-related problems, and continue to drink excessively? So far, no single factor and no combination of multiple factors has been presented that allows us to predict which individuals will become alcohol abusers. Multiple theories exist, including biochemical, psychoanalytic, and cultural approaches. At this period of scientific history, probably the most attention is being focused on understanding two types of factors: cognitive and genetic. The importance of cognitive factors with regard to alcohol's effects is perhaps best demonstrated by a series of experiments conducted by Marlatt and his colleagues on loss of control in alcohol abusers and social drinkers.[26] These studies employed the balanced placebo design. Both alcohol-dependent drinkers and social drinkers report more intoxication and consume more drinks when they are told the drinks have alcohol, regardless of the actual alcohol content. It is important that alcohol-dependent people actually given small amounts of alcohol

(equivalent to one or two drinks) do not report becoming intoxicated and do not increase their drinking if they are led to expect that the drink contains no alcohol. Therefore, it would seem that, if alcohol abusers do lose control when they begin drinking, it might be because they have come to *believe* that they will lose control if they drink (this is sometimes referred to as the *abstinence violation effect*). These balanced placebo experiments have been replicated several times by others. The most obvious interpretation of such results is that alcohol use provides a social excuse for behaving in ways that would otherwise be considered inappropriate, and it is enough for one to believe that one has drunk alcohol for such behaviors to be released.

Considerable evidence supports the idea that some degree of vulnerability to alcohol dependence might be inherited. Alcohol dependence does tend to run in families, but some of that could be due to similar expectancies developed through similar cultural influences and children learning from their parents. Studies on twins provide one way around this problem. Monozygotic (one-egg, or identical) twins share the same genetic material, whereas dizygotic (two-egg, or fraternal) twins are no more genetically related than any two nontwin siblings. Both types of twins are likely to share very similar cultural and family learning experiences. If one adult twin is diagnosed as alcohol dependent, what is the likelihood that the other twin will also receive that diagnosis (are the twins concordant for the trait of alcohol dependence)? Almost all such studies report the concordance rate for monozygotic twins is higher than that for dizygotic twins, and in some studies it is as high as 50 percent. These results imply that inheritance plays a strong role but is far from a complete determinant of alcohol dependence. Another important type of study looks at adopted sons whose biological fathers were alcohol dependent. These reports consistently find that such adoptees have a much greater than average chance of becoming alcohol dependent, even though they are raised by "normal" parents. Although these studies again provide clear evidence for a genetic influence, most children of alcohol abusers do not become alcohol dependent—they simply have a statistically greater risk of doing so. For example, in one study, 18 percent of the adopted-away sons of alcohol-dependent drinkers became dependent on alcohol, compared with 5 percent of the adopted-away sons whose parents had not received the diagnosis.

Alcohol dependence is a complicated feature of human behavior, and even if genetic influences are critical, more than one genetic factor could be involved. Probably it is too much to hope that a single genetic marker will ever be found to be a reliable indicator of alcohol dependence in all individuals.

Summary

- Alcohol is made by yeasts in a process called fermentation. Distillation is used to increase the alcohol content of a beverage.
- Reformers first proposed temperate use of alcoholic beverages, and it was not until the late 1800s that alcohol sales were prohibited in several states.
- National Prohibition of alcohol was successful in reducing alcohol consumption and alcohol-related problems, but also led to increased law-breaking and a loss of alcohol taxes.
- Alcohol use has decreased since 1980, and consumption varies widely among different cultural groups and in different regions of the United States.
- Men are more likely than women to be heavy drinkers, and college students are more likely to drink than others of the same age.
- Alcohol is metabolized by the liver at a constant rate, which is not much influenced by body size.
- The exact mechanism(s) by which alcohol exerts its effects in the central nervous

system is not known, but probably its interactions with the GABA receptor are important.

- Knowing a person's weight, gender, and the amount of alcohol consumed, it is possible to estimate the blood alcohol content (BAC), and from that to estimate the typical effects on behavior.
- The balanced placebo design has helped to separate the pharmacological effects of alcohol from the effects of alcohol expectancies.
- Alcohol tends to increase the user's focus on the "here and now," a kind of alcohol myopia.
- Alcohol-related traffic fatalities have decreased considerably since 1980, but there are still thousands every year in the United States.
- Alcohol appears to enhance interest in sex, but to impair physiological arousal in both sexes.
- Alcohol use is statistically associated with homicide, assault, family violence, and suicide.
- Chronic heavy drinking can lead to neurological damage, as well as damage to the heart and liver. However, light drinking has been associated with a decrease in heart attacks.
- Fetal alcohol syndrome is seen in about 3 percent of babies whose mothers drink heavily.
- Withdrawal from heavy alcohol use can be life-threatening when seizures develop.
- The notion that alcohol dependence is a disease in its own right goes back at least to the 1700s, but did not become popular until Alcoholics Anonymous began to have a major influence in the 1940s and 1950s.
- Although many studies have indicated a likely genetic influence on susceptibility to alcohol dependence, the exact nature and extent of this genetic link is not known.

Review Questions

1. What is the maximum percentage of alcohol obtainable through fermentation alone? What would that be in "proof"?
2. Did Prohibition reduce alcohol abuse?
3. In about what year did apparent consumption of alcohol reach its peak in the United States?
4. About how much more likely are men than women to engage in frequent heavy drinking?
5. About how many standard drinks can the typical human metabolize each hour?
6. For your own gender and weight, about how many standard drinks are required for you to reach the legal BAC limit for driving under the influence?
7. Alcohol enhances the action of which neurotransmitter at its receptors?
8. What is the typical behavior of a person with a BAC of 0.20 percent?
9. Describe the four groups in the balanced placebo design.
10. What term is used to describe the fact that drinkers tend to focus on the "here and now"?
11. About what proportion of U.S. traffic fatalities are considered to be alcohol related?
12. What is the role of expectancy in males' increased interest in sex after drinking?
13. If alcohol did not actually increase violent tendencies, how might we explain the statistical correlation between alcohol and such things as assault and homicide?
14. Why is it dangerous to drink alcohol to "stay warm" in the winter?
15. If someone you know has drunk enough alcohol to pass out, what are two things you can do to prevent a lethal outcome?
16. Can brain damage be reversed if someone has been drinking heavily for many years?
17. About what percentage of the heaviest-drinking women will have children diagnosed with FAS?
18. What is the most dangerous withdrawal symptom from alcohol?
19. Did the early founders of AA view alcohol dependence as a disease?
20. If one identical twin is diagnosed with alcohol dependence, what is the likelihood that the other twin will also receive this diagnosis?

References

1. "Craft Beer Sales Soar." Realbeer.com/news, accessed March 16, 2006.
2. "The Alcohol Problem in America: From Temperance to Alcoholism." *British Addiction* 79, pp. 109–19.
3. Koren, J. *Economic Aspects of the Liquor Problem.* New York: Houghton Mifflin, 1899.
4. Clark, N.H. *The Dry Years: Prohibition and Social Change in Washington.* Seattle: University of Washington Press, 1965.
5. Emerson, H. *Alcohol and Man.* New York: Macmillan, 1932, reprinted 1981, New York: Arno Press.
6. Vaillant, G. *Cultural Factors in the Etiology of Alcoholism: A Prospective Study.* In T.F. Babor, ed. *Alcohol and Culture: Comparative Perspectives from Europe and America.* New York: New York Academy of Sciences, 1986.
7. "Czechs Still No. 1." Realbeer.com/news, accessed January 14, 2004.
8. Nephew, T.W., and others. *NIAAA Surveillance Report #73: Apparent Per Capita Alcohol Consumption: National, State and Regional Trends, 1977–2003.* Bethesda, MD: National Institute on Alcohol Abuse and Alcoholism, 2005.
9. Linsky, A.S., and others. "Social Stress, Normative Constraints and Alcohol Problems in American States." *Social Science and Medicine* 24 (1987), pp. 875–883.
10. Substance Abuse and Mental Health Services Administration. (2005). *Overview of Findings from the 2004 National Survey on Drug Use and Health* (Office of Applied Studies, NSDUH Series H-27, DHHS Publication No. SMA 05-4061). Rockville, MD.
11. "Wet or Dry: Schools Ponder Variety of Strategies to Curb Alcohol Problems." *The Bottom Line* 18, no. 3 (1997), pp. 68–72.
12. Frezza, M., and others. "High Blood Alcohol Levels in Women: The Role of Decreased Gastric Alcohol Dehydrogenase Activity and First-Pass Metabolism." *New England Journal of Medicine* 322 (1990), p. 95.
13. Steele, C. M., & R.A. Josephs. "Alcohol Myopia." *American Psychologist* 45 (1990), pp. 921–33.
14. *Fatality Facts 2004: Alcohol.* Insurance Institute for Highway Safety, Washington, DC: 2006.
15. Yi, H.Y., and others. *NIAAA Surveillance Report #71: Trends in Alcohol-Related Traffic Fatalities in the United States, 1977–2003.* Bethesda, MD: USPHS, 2005.
16. George, W.H., & S.A. Stoner. "Understanding Acute Alcohol Effects on Sexual Behavior." *Annual Review of Sex Research* 11 (2000), pp. 1053–2528.
17. Crothers, T.D. "Alcoholic Trance." *Popular Science* 26 (1884), pp. 189, 191.

18. Pernanen, K. *Alcohol in Human Violence.* New York: Guilford Press, 1991.

19. *Eighth Special Report on Alcohol and Health,* NIH Publication Number 94-3699. Washington, DC: U.S. Public Health Service, 1993.

20. Centers for Disease Control and Prevention. "Alcohol-Attributable Deaths and Years of Potential Life Lost—United States, 2001." *Morbidity and Mortality Weekly Report* 53 (2004), pp. 866–70.

21. "Alcohol and the Heart: Consensus Emerges." *Harvard Health Letter* 6, no. 5 (1996).

22. Floyd, R.J., & J.S. Sidhu. "Monitoring Prenatal Alcohol Exposure." *American Journal of Medical Genetics Part C (Seminars in Medical Genetics)* 127C (2004), pp. 3–9.

23. Twain, M. *The Adventures of Huckleberry Finn,* 1885.

24. Mayo-Smith, M.E. "Pharmacological Management of Alcohol Withdrawal: A Meta-analysis and Evidence-based Practice Guideline," *Journal of the American Medical Association* 278 (1997), pp. 144–51.

25. American Psychiatric Association. *Diagnostic and Statistical Manual of Mental Disorders,* 4th ed., text revision. Washington, DC: American Psychiatric Association, 2000.

26. Wilson, G.T. "Cognitive Studies in Alcoholism." *Journal of Consulting and Clinical Psychology* 55 (1987), pp. 325–31.

Check Yourself

How Can You Tell Whether You Have a Drinking Problem?

Many self-tests have been published for people to use to determine if they are alcoholics or if they have a drinking problem. None of them should be taken as an absolute test or as a definite answer to that question, because in most cases it is a complex, subjective judgment as to whether someone should seek help. One of the best popularly printed self-tests appeared in a "Dear Abby" column, and it is offered here as a possible guide. If these questions seem to indicate that you or a friend need to seek help, we recommend a visit to a counselor, psychologist, or physician who is experienced in the assessment of chemical dependence. An assessment would probably include the use of a more professional questionnaire, such as the Michigan Alcoholism Screening Test (MAST) or the Alcohol Dependency Scale (ADS).

Check those that apply to you:

_____ 1. Have you ever decided to stop drinking for a week or so but lasted for only a couple of days?

_____ 2. Do you wish people would stop nagging you about your drinking?

_____ 3. Have you ever switched from one kind of drink to another in the hope that this would keep you from getting drunk?

_____ 4. Have you had a drink in the morning in the past year?

_____ 5. Do you envy people who can drink without getting into trouble?

_____ 6. Have you had problems connected with drinking during the past year?

_____ 7. Has your drinking caused problems at home?

_____ 8. Do you ever try to get "extra" drinks at a party because you did not get enough to drink?

_____ 9. Do you tell yourself you can stop drinking anytime you want to, even though you keep getting drunk when you don't mean to?

_____ 10. Have you missed days at work (or school) because of drinking?

_____ 11. Do you have "blackouts"?

_____ 12. Have you ever felt that your life would be better if you did not drink?

If you checked four or more of these, it would be a good idea to seek the guidance of a specialist in chemical dependence or to seek help directly through Alcoholics Anonymous or a similar organization. It's perfectly acceptable to go to an open AA meeting, listen to what is being said, and decide for yourself if the program would be useful to you.

Familiar Drugs

Some drugs are seen so often that they don't seem to be drugs at all, at least not in the same sense as cocaine or marijuana. However, tobacco and its ingredient nicotine, as well as caffeine in its various forms, are psychoactive drugs meeting any reasonable definition of the term *drug*. Certainly the drugs sold over the counter (OTC) in pharmacies are drugs, and many of them have their primary effects on the brain and behavior. In Section Five, we learn about the psychological effects of all these familiar drugs, partly because they are so commonly used. Also, they provide several interesting points for comparison with the less well-known, more frightening drugs.

10 Tobacco
Why do people smoke, and why do they have such a hard time quitting?

11 Caffeine
How much of an effect does caffeine really produce? What are the relative strengths of coffee, tea, and soft drinks?

12 Dietary Supplements and Over-the-Counter Drugs
Which of the common drugstore drugs are psychoactive?

10

Tobacco

Objectives

When you have finished this chapter, you should be able to:

- **Describe how Europeans spread tobacco around the world.**

- **Explain the historical importance of tobacco to America.**

- **Describe the history of anti-tobacco efforts and the tobacco companies' responses.**

- **Explain the difficulties in marketing "safer" cigarettes as related to FDA regulation.**

- **Describe the most important adverse health consequences of smoking and the total annual smoking-attributable mortality in the U.S.**

- **Understand the controversy over secondhand smoke as both a social issue and a public health issue.**

- **Describe the effects of cigarette smoking on the developing fetus and the newborn.**

- **Explain why smoking is not immediately lethal, in spite of nicotine's powerful toxicity.**

- **Describe how nicotine affects cholinergic receptors in the brain and throughout the body.**

- **Describe the most common physiological and behavioral effects of nicotine.**

- **Describe the roles of counseling, nicotine replacement therapy, and bupropion in smoking cessation.**

The selling and using of tobacco products has always generated controversy, but never greater than today. Tobacco is an interesting social dilemma—a product that is legal for adults to use, and that a significant proportion of adults enjoy using and expect to continue using, yet a substance that is responsible for more adverse health consequences and death than any other. This chapter examines how we arrived at tobacco's current status, and what changes lie on the horizon for this agricultural commodity, dependence-producing substance, and topic for policy discussions from local city councils to Congress.

Tobacco History

Long before Christopher Columbus stumbled onto the Western Hemisphere, the Indians here were using tobacco. It was one of many contributions the New World made to Europe: tobacco, corn, sweet potatoes, white potatoes, chocolate, and—so you could lie back and enjoy it all—the hammock. Columbus recorded that the natives of San Salvador presented him with tobacco leaves on October 12, 1492, a fitting birthday present.

In 1497, a monk who had accompanied Columbus on his second trip wrote a book on

Online Learning Center Resources

www.mhhe.com/ksir12e

Visit our Online Learning Center (OLC) for access to these study aids and additional resources.

- Learning objectives
- Glossary flashcards
- Web activities and links
- Self-scoring chapter quiz
- Audio chapter summaries

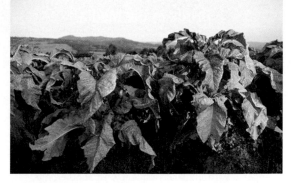

Tobacco was in use by Native Americans long before it was introduced into Europe.

native customs that contained the first printed report of tobacco smoking. It wasn't called tobacco, and it wasn't called smoking. Inhaling smoke was called drinking. In that period you either "took" (used snuff) or "drank" (smoked) tobacco.

The word *tobacco* came from one of two sources. *Tobacco* referred to a two-pronged tube used by natives to take snuff. But some early reports confused the issue by applying the name to the plant they incorrectly thought was being used. Another idea is that the word developed its current usage from the province of Tobacos in Mexico, where everyone used the herb. In 1598, an Italian-English dictionary published in London translated the Italian *Nicosiana* as the herb tobacco, and that spelling and usage gradually became dominant.

One member of Columbus's party, Rodrigo de Jerez, was the poor fellow who introduced tobacco drinking to Europe. When he returned with his habit to Portugal, his friends were convinced the devil had possessed him as they saw the smoke coming out his mouth and nose. The priest agreed, and Rodrigo spent the next several years in jail, only to find on his release that people were doing the same thing for which he had been jailed.

Early Medical Uses

Tobacco was formally introduced to Europe as an herb useful for treating almost everything. A 1529 report indicated tobacco was used for "persistant headaches," "cold or catarrh," and "abscesses and sores on the head."[1] Between 1537 and 1559, 14 books mentioned the medicinal value of tobacco.

The French physician Jean Nicot became enamored with the medical uses of tobacco. He tried it on enough people to convince himself of its value and sent glowing reports of the herb's effectiveness to the French court. He was successful in "curing" the migraine headaches of Catherine de Medicis, queen of Henry II of France, which made tobacco use very much "in." It was called the *herbe sainte,* "holy plant," and *the herbe à tous les maux,* "the plant against all evils." The French loved it and, although tobacco had been introduced earlier to Paris, Nicot received the credit. By 1565, the plant had been called nicotiane, and Linnaeus sanctified it in 1753 by naming the genus *Nicotiana.* When a pair of French chemists isolated the active ingredient in 1828, they acted like true nationalists and called it nicotine.

In the 16th century, Sir Anthony Chute summarized much of the available information and said, "Anything that harms a man inwardly from his girdle upward might be removed by a moderate use of the herb." Others, however, felt differently: "If taken after meals the herb would infect the brain and liver," and "Tobacco should be avoided by (among others) women with child and husbands who desired to have children."[1]

Drugs in the Media

Cigarette Smoking in the Movies

In 1989, U.S. tobacco companies voluntarily agreed to halt a long-standing practice, directly paying film producers for what is known as "product placement" in popular films. All sorts of companies do this, and at times, the practice is fairly obvious once you know about it. For example, you might notice that in one movie a particular brand of new automobile appears with unusual frequency. In another, one type of soft drink can or billboard (and never a competing brand) might be seen in the background of several shots. Despite all the efforts to control more explicit advertising of cigarettes to young people, this practice is especially insidious because research indicates that tobacco use by an adolescent's favorite actor does influence the adolescent's smoking behavior. Thus, this type of product placement is likely to be a very potent form of advertising for cigarette manufacturers. Did the 1989 voluntary ban work?

Apparently not, according to a study reported in the medical journal *The Lancet* in 2001.[2] Researchers from Dartmouth College studied the top 25 U.S. films each year for 10 years (1988–1997, a total of 250 films). The first three of those years should have reflected pre-ban film production, compared with the later seven years. They found that 85 percent of the films portrayed tobacco use. Specific brands were identified in 28 percent of the films. Neither of these statistics varied from before to after the voluntary ban on direct payments for product placement. Films considered suitable for adolescent audiences (those with PG or PG-13 ratings) contained as many brand appearances as films for adult audiences.

One important difference noted was an increase, rather than a decrease, in the frequency of use of an identified brand by an actor, as opposed to the appearance of a package or billboard in the background. This suggests that this effective form of hidden advertising in movies is actually increasing rather than decreasing. Ironically, in the 2005 film "Thank You for Smoking," about a tobacco company spokesman, there are no scenes of actual smoking behavior.

In 1617, Dr. William Vaughn phrased the last thought a little more poetically:

Tobacco that outlandish weede
It spends the braine and spoiles the seede
It dulls the spirite, it dims the sight
It robs a woman of her right.[3]

Dr. Vaughn may have been ahead of his time: Current research verifies tobacco's adverse effects on reproductive functioning in both men and women (see page 250).

Special note must be made of a series of experiments reported in 1805 by Dr. D. Legare, because his work pushed back the boundaries of ignorance and clearly disproved an old folk remedy. Beyond the shadow of a doubt, Dr. Legare personally proved that, contrary to general opinion, blowing tobacco smoke into the intestinal canal did *not* resuscitate drowned animals or people.[4] The slow advance of medical science through the 18th and 19th centuries gradually removed tobacco from the doctor's black bag, and nicotine was dropped from *The United States Pharmacopoeia* in the 1890s.

The Spread of Tobacco Use

There are more than 60 species of *Nicotiana*, but only two major ones. **Nicotiana tobacum,** the major species grown today in more than a hundred countries, is a large-leaf species. *Tobacum* was indigenous only to South America, so the Spanish had a monopoly on its production for over a hundred years. **Nicotiana rustica** is a small-leaf species and was the plant existing in the West Indies and eastern North America when Columbus arrived.

The Spanish monopoly on tobacco sales to Europe was a thorn in the side of the British. When settlers returned to England in 1586 after failing to colonize Virginia, they took with them seeds of the *rustica* species and planted them in England, but this never grew well. The English crown again attempted to establish a tobacco colony in Virginia in 1610, when John Rolfe arrived as leader of a group. From 1610 to 1612, Rolfe tried to cultivate *rustica,* but the small-leaf plant was weak and poor in flavor, and it had a sharp taste.

In 1612, Rolfe somehow got some seeds of the Spanish *tobacum* species. This species grew beautifully and sold well. The colony was saved, and every available plot of land was planted with *tobacum.* By 1619, as much Virginia tobacco as Spanish tobacco was sold in London. That was also the year that King James prohibited the cultivation of any tobacco in England and declared the tobacco trade a royal monopoly.

Tobacco became one of the major exports of the American colonies to England. The 30 Years' War spread smoking throughout central Europe, and nothing stopped its use. Measures such as one in Bavaria in 1652 probably slowed tobacco use, but only momentarily. This law said that "tobacco-drinking was strictly forbidden to the peasants and other common people" and made tobacco available to others only on a doctor's prescription from a druggist.[4]

Snuff

During the 18th century, smoking gradually diminished, but the use of tobacco did not. Snuff replaced the pipe in England. At the beginning of that century, the upper class was already committed to snuff. The middle and lower classes only gradually changed over, but by 1770 very few people were smoking. The reign of King George III (1760–1820) was the time of the big snuff. His wife, Charlotte, was such a heavy user of the powder that she was called "Snuffy Charlotte," although for obvious reasons not to her face. On the continent, Napoleon had tried smoking once, gagged horribly, and returned to his seven pounds of snuff per month.

Tobacco in Early America

Trouble developed in the colonies, which made the richest man in Virginia (perhaps the richest in the colonies) commander in chief of the Revolutionary Army. In 1776, George Washington said in one of his appeals, "If you can't send money, send tobacco."[5] Tobacco played an important role in the Revolutionary War; it was one of the major products for which France would lend the colonies money. Knowing the importance of tobacco to the colonies, one of Cornwallis's major campaign goals in 1780 and 1781 was the destruction of the Virginia tobacco plantations.

After the war, ordinary Americans rejoiced and rejected snuff as well as tea and all other things British. The aristocrats who organized the republic were not as emotional, though, and installed a communal snuff box for members of Congress. However, to emphasize the fact that snuff was a nonessential, the new Congress put a luxury tax on it in 1794.

Chewing Tobacco

If you don't smoke and you don't snuff
How can you possibly get enough?

You can get enough by chewing, which gradually increased in the United States. Chewing was a suitable activity for a country on the go; it freed the hands, and the wide-open spaces made an adequate spittoon. There were also other considerations: Boston, for example, passed an ordinance in 1798 forbidding anyone from possessing a lighted pipe or "segar" in public streets. The original impetus was a concern for the fire hazard involved in smoking, not the individual's health, and the ordinance was finally repealed in 1880. Today it is difficult to appreciate how much of a chewing country we were in the 19th century. In 1860, only 7 of 348 tobacco factories in Virginia and

Nicotiana tobacum (ni co she *ann* a toe *back* um): the species of tobacco widely cultivated for smoking and chewing products.
Nicotiana rustica (*russ* tick a): the less desirable species of tobacco, which is not widely grown in the United States.

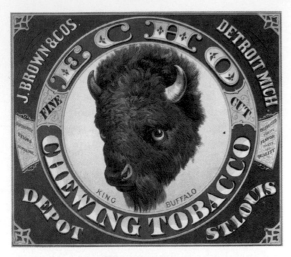

Most tobacco produced in the nineteenth century was chewing tobacco.

North Carolina manufactured smoking tobacco. The amount of tobacco for smoking did not equal the amount for chewing until 1911 and did not surpass it until the 1920s.

The high level of chewing-tobacco production during the Industrial Age led to occasional accidents, as suggested by a quote from a 1918 decision of the Mississippi Supreme Court:

> We can imagine no reason why, with ordinary care, human toes could not be left out of chewing tobacco, and if toes were found in chewing tobacco, it seems to us that somebody has been very careless.[6]

The start of the 20th century was the approximate high point for chewing tobacco, the sales of which slowly declined through the early part of that century, as other tobacco products became more popular. In 1945, cuspidors were removed from all federal buildings.

Cigars

The transition from chewing to cigarettes had a middle point, a combination of both smoking and chewing: cigars. Cigarette smoking was coming, and the cigar manufacturers did their best to keep cigarettes under control. They sug-gested that cigarettes were drugged with opium, so one could not stop using them and that the paper was bleached with arsenic and, thus, was harmful. They had some help from Thomas Edison in 1914:

> The injurious agent in Cigarettes comes princi-pally from the burning paper wrapper. . . . It has a violent action in the nerve centers, pro-ducing degeneration of the cells of the brain, which is quite rapid among boys. Unlike most narcotics, this degeneration is permanent and uncontrollable. I employ no person who smokes cigarettes.[6]

The efforts of the cigar manufacturers worked for a while, and cigar sales reached their high-est level in 1920, when 8 billion were sold. As sales increased, though, so did the cost of the product. Lower cost and changing styles led to the emergence of cigarettes as the leading form of tobacco use.

Cigarettes

Thin reeds filled with tobacco had been seen by the Spanish in Yucatan in 1518. In 1844, the French were using them, and the Crimean War circulated the cigarette habit throughout Europe. The first British cigarette factory was started in 1856 by a returning veteran of the Crimean War, and in the late 1850s an English tobacco merchant, Philip Morris, began pro-ducing handmade cigarettes. On the continent the use of this new dose form must have devel-oped fairly rapidly. One company in Austria began making double cigarettes in 1865—both ends had a mouthpiece, and the consumer cut them in two—and sold 16 million in 1866.

In the United States, cigarettes were being produced during the same period (14 million in 1870), but their popularity increased rapidly in the 1880s. The date of the first patent on a cigarette-making machine was 1881, and by 1885 more than a billion cigarettes a year were being sold. Not even that great he-man, boxer John L. Sullivan, could stem the tide, though in 1905 his opinion of cigarette smokers was pretty clear:

Smoke cigarettes? Not on your tut-tut. . . . You can't suck coffin-nails and be a ring-champion. . . . You never heard of . . . a bank burglar using a cigarette, did you? They couldn't do it and attend to biz. Why, even drunkards don't use the things. . . . Who smokes 'em? Dudes and college stiffs—fellows who'd be wiped out by a single jab or a quick undercut. It isn't natural to smoke cigarettes. An American ought to smoke cigars. . . . It's the Dutchmen, Italians, Russians, Turks and Egyptians who smoke cigarettes and they're no good anyhow.[6]

At the start of the 20th century, there was a preference for cigarettes with an aromatic component—that is, Turkish tobacco. Camels, a new cigarette in 1913, capitalized on the lure of the Near East while rejecting it in actuality. The Camel brand contained just a hint of Turkish tobacco. Eliminating most of the imported tobacco made the price lower. Low price was combined with a big advertising campaign: "The Camels are coming. Tomorrow there'll be more CAMELS in town than in all of Asia and Africa combined." In 1918, Camels had 40 percent of the market and stayed in front until after World War II.

The first ad showing a woman smoking appeared in 1919. To make the ad easier to accept, the woman was pictured as Asian and the ad was for a Turkish type of cigarette. King-size cigarettes appeared in 1939 in the form of Pall Mall, which became the top seller. Filter cigarettes as filter cigarettes, not cigarettes that happen to have filters along with a mouthpiece, appeared in 1954 with Winston, which rapidly took over the market and continued to be number one until the mid-1970s. Filter cigarettes captured an increasing share of the market and now constitute over 90 percent of all U.S. cigarette sales.

Tobacco Under Attack

As with every other psychoactive substance, use by some raises concerns on the part of others, and many efforts have been made over the years to regulate tobacco use. In 1604, King

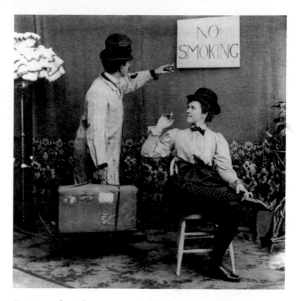

Some early tobacco control efforts focused on women, associating tobacco use with immoral behavior.

James of England (the same one who had the Bible translated) wrote and published a strong antitobacco pamphlet stating that tobacco was "harmefull to the braine, dangerous to the lungs." Never one to let morality or health concerns interfere with business, he also supported the growing of tobacco in Virginia in 1610, and when the crop prospered, he declared the tobacco trade a royal monopoly.

New York City made it illegal in 1908 for a woman to use tobacco in public, and in the Roaring Twenties women were expelled from schools and dismissed from jobs for smoking. These concerns were partly for society and partly to "protect women from themselves." Those sensitive to feminist issues will find an analogy to current reactions to drug and alcohol use by pregnant women in this quote from the 1920s:

Smoking by women and even young girls must be considered from a far different standpoint than smoking by men, for not only is the female organism by virtue of its much more frail structure and its more delicate tissues much less able to resist the poisonous action of tobacco than that of men, and thus, like many a delicate flower, apt to fade and wither more quickly in consequence, but the fecundity of woman is greatly impaired by it. Authorities cannot be expected to look on unmoved while a generation of sterile women, rendered incapable of fulfilling their sublime function of motherhood, is being produced on account of the immoderate smoking of foolish young girls.[7]

And those familiar with the 1930s "Reefer Madness" arguments might find it interesting that earlier in the same decade a weed other than marijuana was blamed for various social ills:

> Fifty percent of our insanity is inherited from parents who were users of tobacco. . . . Thirty-three percent of insanity cases are caused direct from cigarette smoking and the use of tobacco. . . .
>
> Judge Gimmill, of the court of Domestic Relations of Chicago, declared that, without exception, every boy appearing before him that had lost the faculty of blushing was a cigarette fiend. The poison in cigarettes has the same effect upon girls: it perverts the morals and deadens the sense of shame and refinement. . . .
>
> The bathing beaches have become resorts for women smokers, where they go to show off with a cigarette in their mouths. The bathing apparel in the last ten years has been reduced from knee skirts to a thin tight-fitting veil that scarcely covers two-thirds of their hips. Many of the girl bathers never put their feet in the water, but sit on the shore, show their legs and smoke cigarettes.[8]

The long and slowly-developing attack on tobacco as a major health problem had its seeds in reports in the 1930s and 1940s indicating a possible link between smoking and cancer. A 1952 article in *Readers' Digest* called "Cancer by the Carton" drew public attention to the issue, and led to a temporary decline in cigarette sales. The major U.S. tobacco companies recognized the threat and responded vigorously in two important ways. One was the formation of the supposedly independent Council for Tobacco Research to look into the health claims (later investigations revealed this council was not independent of tobacco company

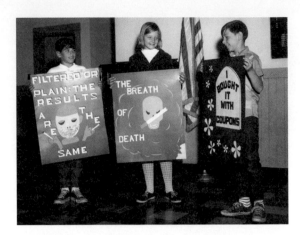

Evidence about the health dangers of tobacco accumulated slowly over time.

influence and served largely to try to undermine any scientific evidence demonstrating the negative health consequences of tobacco use). The other response was the mass marketing of filter cigarettes and cigarettes with lowered tar and nicotine content. The public apparently had faith in these "less hazardous" cigarettes, because cigarette sales again began to climb. In the early 1960s, the U.S. Surgeon General's office formed an Advisory Committee on Smoking and Health. Its first official report, released in 1964, stated clearly that cigarette smoking was a cause for increased lung cancer in men (at the time, the evidence for women was less extensive). Per capita sales of cigarettes began a decline that continued over the next 40 years (see Figure 10.1). In 1965, Congress required cigarette packages to include the surgeon general's warning. All television and radio advertising of cigarettes was banned in 1971, and smoking was banned on interstate buses and domestic airline flights in 1990.[9] The list of state and local laws prohibiting smoking in public buildings, offices, restaurants, and even bars grows every year. Clearly, momentum is behind efforts to restrict smoking and exposure to secondhand smoke.

The original laws regulating drugs had specifically excluded tobacco products, reflect-

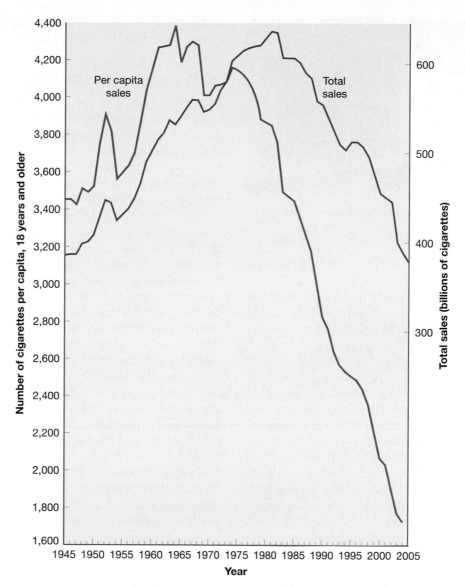

Figure 10.1   Trends in Cigarette Sales Since 1945

SOURCE: USDA Economic Research Service, Tobacco Briefing Room (http://www.ers.usda.gov/Briefing/Tobacco)

ing their status as an agricultural commodity, their widespread use among the social elite, and the economic importance of tobacco to the U.S. economy. In 1995, the Food and Drug Administration announced plans to regulate tobacco. After a year of discussion, rules were proposed that further limited advertising on billboards and other public displays, sponsorship of sporting events, promotional giveaways of caps and T-shirts, and advertising in magazines with significant youth readership. In 2004, further FDA regulation of tobacco products was under discussion by Congress (see following).

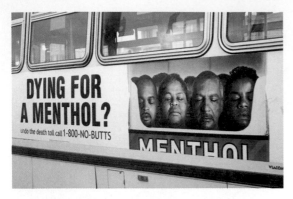

Just as smoking ads have targeted specific groups, so do current antismoking campaigns. Rates of menthol cigarette use are highest among African Americans.

One important attack on tobacco has come from lawsuits seeking compensation for the health consequences of smoking. For years the tobacco companies had succeeded in winning such lawsuits, based on the idea that smokers had a significant share of the responsibility for their smoking-related illnesses. But changing legal climate combined with the disclosure of internal tobacco company documents demonstrating both the companies' knowledge of the adverse health consequences of smoking and their efforts to hide that knowledge from customers. A group of attorneys, representing individual clients, several state governments seeking compensation for increased Medicaid costs due to cigarette smoking, and eventually the federal government, reached a 1997 settlement with the major U.S. tobacco producers that included $368 billion in payments as well as agreeing to the previously proposed FDA advertising regulations and a federally-supported program to enforce laws prohibiting sales to minors. In exchange, the companies received a cap on certain aspects of their legal liability, which otherwise threatened to bankrupt the industry.[10]

The 1997 settlement seemed to empower both state governments and the U.S. Congress, and further regulations have been proposed at all levels. It is not clear what will become of tobacco as a product and of smoking as a regulated behavior in the years to come.

The Quest for "Safer" Cigarettes

Nicotine appears to be the constituent in tobacco that keeps smokers coming back for more—if the nicotine content of cigarettes is varied, people tend to adjust their smoking behavior, taking more puffs and inhaling more deeply when given low-nicotine cigarettes, and reporting no satisfaction if all the nicotine is removed.[11] Another complex product of burning tobacco is something called tar, the sticky brown stuff that can be seen on the filter after a cigarette is smoked. Beginning in the mid-1950s with the mass marketing of filter cigarettes, the tobacco companies began to promote the idea of a "safer" cigarette, without actually admitting that there was anything unsafe about their older products. Because the companies were advertising their cigarettes as being lower in tar and nicotine, for many years the Federal Trade Commission (with industry support and cooperation) monitored the tar and nicotine yields of the various cigarette brands and made those results public. The U.S. Congress and the National Cancer Institute promoted research to develop safer cigarettes. The public listened to all this talk about safer cigarettes and bought in—sales of filter cigarettes took off, and by the 1980s low tar and nicotine cigarettes dominated the market.

The problem with all this is that "safer" doesn't mean "safe," and it wasn't at all clear how much safer these low tar and nicotine cigarettes actually are for people over a lifetime of smoking. Some early studies had indicated that those who had smoked lower-yield cigarettes for years were at less risk for cancer and heart disease than those who smoked high-yield brands. But other studies seemed to show that if a smoker switched from a high-yield to a low-yield cigarette, changes in puff rate and depth of inhalation would compensate for the lower yield per puff, and there might be no advantage to switching. The tobacco industry was caught in an ironic position, as evidenced by the plight of Liggett (former manufacturers of Chesterfield, L&M, and Lark, now selling Eve and other brands). During the 1960s, Liggett developed a cigarette which in the laboratory significantly reduced tumors in mice compared to the company's standard brand. Lawyers advised Liggett against reporting these results because the data would confirm that the standard brand was hazardous. Liggett suppressed the information and did not market the "safer" cigarette, a fact that was revealed in a lawsuit during the 1980s.[12]

The "safer" cigarette controversy arose again in 1988 when Reynolds attempted to market Premier, a sort of noncigarette cigarette. Although packaged like cigarettes and having the appearance of a plastic cigarette, the product contained catalytic crystals coated with a tobacco extract but no obvious tobacco. When "lit" with a flame, these cigarettes produced no smoke, but inhaling through them allowed the user to absorb some nicotine. The FDA couldn't accept that this was the traditional agricultural product rather than a nicotine "delivery device," something it would have to regulate as a drug. How would Reynolds get this approved as a drug—what was its indicated medical use? Perhaps the company could have tested and marketed it as a nicotine replacement to help smokers who wanted to quit, but that wasn't its goal. Raising the issue led some to suggest that the FDA should review all cigarettes as if they were drugs. It's hard to imagine how such a product could get approved, with demonstrated toxicity and dependence potential and no indicated medical use. After investing a lot of money in Premier, Reynolds was unable to find a legal way to sell the product and was forced to drop it. But the company did not give up. In 2004, Reynolds marketed Eclipse, another high-tech "cigarette" that it was said "may present less risk," and produces up to 80 percent less smoke than a regular cigarette. This one contains tobacco, but it is not burned. Instead, the user lights a carbon element that heats a small aluminum tube that in turn heats the tobacco, releasing vapors and a small amount of

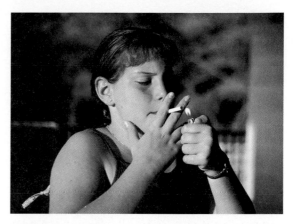

Despite antismoking education, one in five young people still becomes a regular smoker.

smoke. Several health-promoting groups have petitioned the FDA to regulate this product, but a decision has not yet been made.[13]

Current Cigarette Use

The Monitoring the Future study found that among the high school senior class of 2005, 25 percent of the boys and 21 percent of the girls reported smoking cigarettes within the past 30 days. The recent trend in these figures has been downward—about 36 percent of seniors reported smoking in the class of 1997.[14] This downward trend is reflected in overall per capita sales of cigarettes (see Figure 10.1) as well as in the annual household survey of drug use and health.[15] In the 2004 survey, 44 percent of 18- to 25-year-old males reported past month cigarette use, compared to 36 percent of females in this age group. Education does make a difference: 24 percent of 18- to 22-year-old college students reported smoking cigarettes in the past month, compared to 37 percent of 18- to 22-year-olds not enrolled in college. Among older adults, fewer college graduates smoke than those who only completed high school.

Smokeless Tobacco

In the early 1970s, many cigarette smokers apparently began to look for alternatives that would reduce the risk of lung cancer. Pipe and cigar smoking enjoyed a brief, small increase, followed by a long period of decline. Sales of **smokeless tobacco** products—specifically, different kinds of chewing tobacco—began to increase. Once limited to western movies and the baseball field in terms of public awareness, smokeless tobacco use grew to become a matter of public concern.

The most common types of oral smokeless tobacco in the United States are loose-leaf (Red Man, Levi Garrett, Beech Nut), which is sold in a pouch, and **moist snuff** (Copenhagen, Skoal), which is sold in a can. When you see a baseball player on TV with a big wad in his cheek, it is probably composed of loose-leaf tobacco. Sales of loose-leaf tobacco, growing from a traditional base in the Southeast and Midwest, increased by about 50 percent during the 1970s and then declined through the 1980s and 1990s. Moist snuff is not "snuffed" into the nose in the European manner; a small pinch is dipped out of the can and placed beside the gum, often behind the lower lip. One form of moist snuff also comes in a little teabag type of packet, so that loose tobacco fragments don't stray out onto the teeth. Moist snuff, which has its traditional popularity base in the rural West, continued to show sales gains through the 1980s, until a federal excise tax was imposed. With all forms of oral smokeless tobacco, nicotine is absorbed through the mucous membranes of the mouth into the bloodstream, and users achieve blood nicotine levels comparable to those of smokers.

Smokeless tobacco enjoys many advantages over smoking. First, it is unlikely to cause lung cancer. Smokeless tobacco is less expensive than cigarettes, with an average user spending only a few dollars a week. Despite the Marlboro advertisements, a cowboy or anyone else who is working outdoors finds it more convenient to keep some tobacco in the mouth than to try to light cigarettes in the wind and then have ashes blowing in the face. And chewing might be more socially acceptable than smoking under most circumstances. After all, the user doesn't blow smoke all around,

and most people don't even notice when someone is chewing, unless the chewer has a huge wad in the mouth or spits frequently. Many users can control the amount of tobacco they put in their mouths so that they don't have to spit very often. What they do with the leftover **quid** of tobacco is a different story and often not a pretty sight.

The use of chewing tobacco had never completely died out in rural areas, and its resurgence was strongest there. The high school senior class of 2005 reported that 13 percent of the boys and about 2 percent of the girls were using smokeless tobacco in the past month, down from 19 percent of boys and 2 percent of girls in 1993.[14]

Chewing tobacco might not be as unhealthy as smoking it. However, smokeless tobacco is not without its hazards. Of most concern is the increased risk of cancer of the mouth, pharynx, and esophagus. Snuff and chewing tobacco do contain potent carcinogens, including high levels of tobacco-specific **nitrosamines**. Many users experience tissue changes in the mouth, with **leukoplakia** (a whitening, thickening, and hardening of the tissue) a relatively frequent finding. Leukoplakia is considered to be a precancerous lesion (a tissue change that can develop into cancer). The irritation of the gums can cause them to become inflamed or to recede, exposing the teeth to disease. The enamel of the teeth can also be worn down by the abrasive action of the tobacco. Dentists are also becoming more aware of the destructive effects of oral tobacco.

Concerns about these oral diseases led the surgeon general's office to sponsor a conference and produce a 1986 report, *The Health Consequences of Using Smokeless Tobacco*.[16] This report went into some depth in reviewing epidemiological, experimental, and clinical data and concluded "the oral use of smokeless tobacco represents a significant health risk. It is not a safe substitute for smoking cigarettes. It can cause cancer and a number of noncancerous oral conditions and can lead to nicotine addiction and dependence." Packages of smoke-

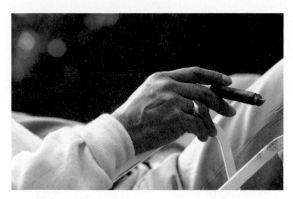

Expensive cigars have become trendy, with "cigar bars," smoke-ins, and magazines devoted to the aficionado.

less tobacco now carry a series of rotating warning labels describing these dangers.

Are Cigars Back?

After many years of declining popularity, cigar smoking reappeared on the cultural scene in the mid-1990s. Yuppies, businesspeople, and celebrities of both sexes began lighting up large, expensive cigars, many of which are made in Florida from tobacco supposedly grown using Cuban seeds. Magazines devoted to cigars, "cigar bars," and radio talk–show discussions of the merits of specific brands all helped to spread the habit. In the 2002 household survey, 5 percent of 18- to 25-year-olds reported smoking cigars in the past month.

Hookahs

In the early 2000s, an ancient form of tobacco use has increased somewhat in popularity. *Hookahs* are large, ornate water pipes, imported to the United States from Egypt and other Arab countries where their use has never completely gone out of style. Burning charcoal is put into the pipe bowl, and a piece of prepared flavored tobacco *(shisha)* is placed on a screen over the charcoal. The smoke is drawn down through a tube into a water reservoir by drawing on mouthpieces connected to tubes that enter the hookah above the water. The water-filtered smoke is milder, and the social nature of smoking in this manner has led to some bars providing hookahs for their customers' use (in cities that do not outlaw smoking in bars). Hookahs and shisha are being sold over the Internet and in tobacco shops, but it is not clear how widespread the habit has become.

Causes for Concern

Although the first clear scientific evidence linking smoking and lung cancer appeared in the 1950s, acceptance of the evidence was slow to come. Each decade brought clearer evidence and more forceful warnings from the surgeon general. The tobacco industry fought back by establishing in 1954 the Council for Tobacco Research to provide funds to independent scientists to study the health effects of tobacco use. A 1993 exposé in *The Wall Street Journal*[17] detailed the manipulation of this "independent" research by tobacco industry lawyers, who arranged direct funding for research casting doubt on smoking-related health problems and who suppressed the publication of findings that threatened the industry. Despite tobacco industry efforts, it is abundantly clear that tobacco is America's true "killer weed" and is a bigger public health threat than all the other drug substances combined, including alcohol. It was not until the late 1990s, however, that a tobacco manufacturer finally admitted in public that cigarettes have seriously adverse effects on health.

smokeless tobacco: a term used for chewing tobacco during the 1980s.
moist snuff: finely chopped tobacco, held in the mouth rather than snuffed into the nose.
quid: a piece of chewing tobacco.
nitrosamines (nye *troh* sa meens): a type of chemical that is carcinogenic; several are found in tobacco.
leukoplakia (luke o *plake* ee ah): a whitening and thickening of the mucous tissue in the mouth, considered to be a precancerous tissue change.

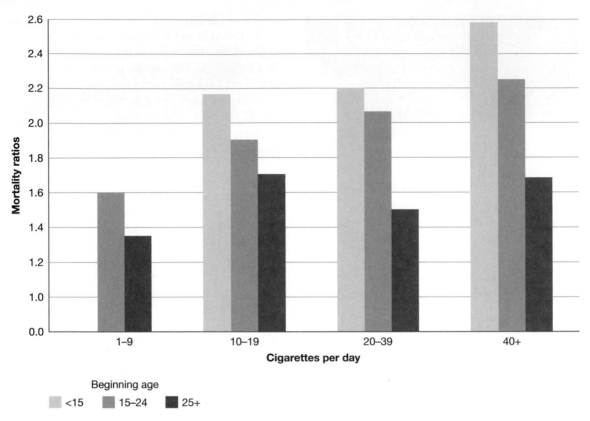

Figure 10.2   Mortality Ratios (total deaths, mean ages, 55 to 64) as a Function of the Age at which Smoking Started and the Number of Cigarettes Smoked per Day

Adverse Health Effects

The smoke has now cleared after many government and other reports detailing the health hazards of tobacco use, and we can see the overall picture. Although lung cancer is not common, about 85 percent of all lung cancers occur in smokers. Among deaths resulting from all types of cancer, smoking is estimated to be related to 30 percent, or about 160,000 premature deaths per year. However, cancer is only the second leading cause of death in the United States. It now appears that smoking is also related to about 30 percent of deaths from the leading killer, cardiovascular disease, or about 140,000 premature deaths per year. In addition, cigarette smoking is the cause of 80 to 90 percent of deaths resulting from chronic obstructive lung disease—another 90,000 cigarette-related premature deaths per year. The total "smoking attributable mortality" is more than 440,000 premature deaths per year in the United States, representing about 20 percent of all U.S. deaths.[18] No wonder these reports keep saying that "cigarette smoking is the chief, single, avoidable cause of death in our society and the most important public health issue of our time."

Think of anything related to good physical health; the research says that cigarette smoking will impair it. The earlier the age at which you start smoking, the more smoking you do, and the longer you do it, the greater the impairment (see Figure 10.2). Smoking doesn't do any part of the body any good, at any time, under any conditions (see Figure 10.3).

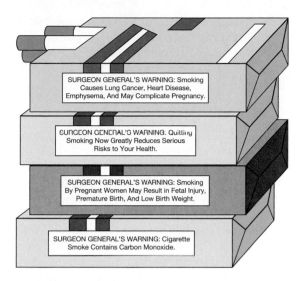

Figure 10.3 Cigarette Packages and Advertisements Are Required to Rotate among Different Warning Labels

Passive Smoking

A great deal has been said and written about **passive smoking**—that is, the inhaling of cigarette smoke from the environment by nonsmokers. The importance of this issue can best be demonstrated by a couple of court cases. In 1976, the Superior Court of New Jersey ruled in favor of a Mrs. Shimp, a telephone company employee who was allergic to cigarette smoke and who worked in a small office along with some smokers. The judge's opinion established several principles:

> The evidence is clear and overwhelming. Cigarette smoke contaminates and pollutes the air creating a health hazard not merely to the smoker but to all those around her who must rely upon the same air supply. The right of an individual to risk his or her own health does not include the right to jeopardize the health of those who must remain around him or her in order to properly perform the duties of their jobs. The portion of the population which is especially sensitive to cigarette smoke is so significant that it is reasonable to expect an employer to foresee health consequences and to impose upon him a duty to abate the hazard which causes the discomfort.

In determining the extent to which smoking must be restricted, the rights and interests of smoking and nonsmoking employees alike must be considered. The employees' rights to a safe working environment makes it clear that smoking must be forbidden in the work area. The employee who desires to smoke on his own time, during coffee breaks and lunch hours should have a reasonably accessible area in which to smoke.[19]

It is obvious that cigarette smoke can be irritating to others, but is it damaging? Besides the cases of individuals who have lung disorders or are allergic to smoke, is there evidence that cigarette smoke is harmful to exposed non-smokers? Research is complicated; the smoke rising from the ash of the cigarette (**sidestream smoke**) is higher in many carcinogens than is the mainstream smoke delivered to the smoker's lungs. Of course, it is also more diluted. How many smokers are in the room? How much do they smoke? How good is the ventilation? How much time does the nonsmoker spend in this room? These variables have made definitive research difficult, but enough studies have produced consistent enough findings that the Environmental Protection Agency in 1993 declared secondhand smoke to be a known carcinogen and estimated that passive smoking is responsible for several thousand lung cancer deaths each year. The tobacco companies countered with full-page newspaper ads attacking the methods used by the EPA, but a review of the issue by an independent consumer group found that the EPA had used accepted techniques and that the tobacco company objections were based on the opinions of a few industry-funded scientists.[20]

Concerns about the effects of secondhand smoke have led to many more restrictions on

---

passive smoking: the inhalation of tobacco smoke by individuals other than the smoker.
sidestream smoke: smoke arising from the ash of the cigarette or cigar.

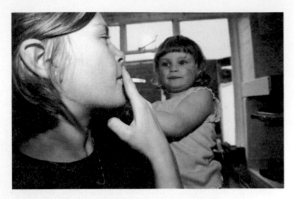

Breathing passive smoke subjects infants and children to dangerous carcinogens.

smoking in the workplace and in public. Most states and municipalities now have laws prohibiting smoking in public conveyances and requiring the establishment of smoking and nonsmoking areas in public buildings and restaurants, and some communities have banned smoking in all restaurants. A few employers have gone so far as to either encourage or attempt to force their employees to quit smoking both on the job and elsewhere, citing health statistics indicating more sick days and greater health insurance costs associated with smoking. This conflict between smoker and nonsmoker seems destined to get worse before it gets better. Although to some this battle might seem silly, it represents a very basic conflict between individual freedom and public health.

Smoking and Health in Other Countries

Cigarette smoking is a social and medical problem worldwide. An international report estimated that, worldwide, smoking is killing 3 million people a year and that by the year 2020 the rate might be as high as 10 million per year.[21] In recent years, as sales declined in developed countries, advertising and promotions in Third World countries (touting cigarettes as delivering "the great taste of America") resulted in large increases in exports of American cigarettes. Asians, in particular, seemed to want American cigarettes, and one of the major efforts was to open Japanese, Taiwanese, Korean, and Chinese cigarette markets to U.S. imports.

Smoking and Pregnancy

The nicotine, hydrogen cyanide, and carbon monoxide in a smoking mother's blood also reach the developing fetus and have significant negative consequences there. On the average, infants born to smokers are about half a pound lighter than infants born to nonsmokers. This basic fact has been known for almost 30 years and has been confirmed in numerous studies. There is a dose-response relationship: the more the woman smokes during pregnancy, the greater the reduction in birth weight. Is the reduced birth weight the result of an increased frequency of premature births or of retarded growth of the fetus? Smoking shortens the gestation period by an average of only two days, and when gestation length is accounted for, the smokers still have smaller infants. Ultrasonic measurements taken at various intervals during pregnancy show smaller fetuses in smoking women for at least the last two months of pregnancy. The infants of smokers are normally proportioned, are shorter and smaller than the infants of nonsmokers, and have smaller head circumference. The reduced birth weight of infants of women smokers is not related to how much weight the mother gains during pregnancy, and the consensus is that a reduced availability of oxygen is responsible for the diminished growth rate. Women who give up smoking early in pregnancy (by the fourth month) have infants with weights similar to those of nonsmokers.

Besides the developmental effects evident at birth, several studies indicate small but consistent differences in body size, neurological problems, reading and mathematical skills, and hyperactivity at various ages. It therefore appears that smoking during pregnancy can

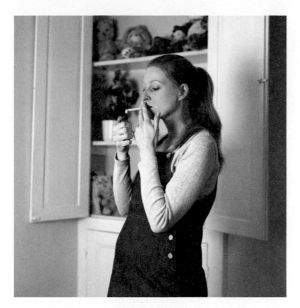

Smoking during pregnancy is associated with miscarriage, low birth weight, smaller head circumference, and later effects on the physical and intellectual development of the child.

have long-lasting effects on both the intellectual and physical development of the child. The increased perinatal (close to the time of birth) smoking-attributable mortality associated with sudden infant death syndrome (SIDS), low birthweight, and respiratory difficulties adds up to about 10,000 infant deaths per year in the United States.[18]

So far we have been talking about normal deliveries of babies. Spontaneous abortion (miscarriage) has also been studied many times in relation to smoking and with consistent results: Smokers have more spontaneous abortions than nonsmokers (perhaps 1.5 to 2 times as many). As for congenital malformations, the evidence for a relationship to maternal smoking is not as clear. If there is a small effect here, it could be either related to or obscured by the fact that many smokers also drink alcohol and coffee. One study indicated an increased risk of facial malformations associated with the father's smoking. Several studies have

also found an increased risk of SIDS if the mother smokes, but it is not clear if this is related more to the mother's smoking during pregnancy or to passive smoking (the infant's breathing smoke) after birth.

The overall message is very clear. Definite, serious risks are associated with smoking during pregnancy. In fact, the demonstrated effects of cigarette smoking on the developing child are of the same magnitude and type as those reported for "crack babies," and many more pregnant women are smoking cigarettes than using cocaine. If a woman smoker discovers herself to be pregnant, that should signal to her to quit smoking.

Pharmacology of Nicotine

Nicotine is a naturally occurring liquid alkaloid that is colorless and volatile. On oxidation it turns brown and smells much like burning tobacco. Tolerance to its effects develops, along with the dependency that led Mark Twain to remark how easy it was to stop smoking—he'd done it several times!

Nicotine was isolated in 1828 and has been studied extensively since then. The structure of nicotine is shown in Figure 10.4; there are both *d* and *l* forms, but they are equipotent. It is of some importance that nicotine in smoke has two forms, one with a positive charge and one

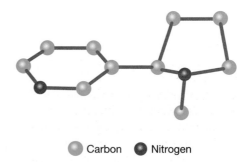

⬤ Carbon   ⬤ Nitrogen

Figure 10.4   Nicotine (1-methyl-2 [3-pyridyl] pyrrolidone)

that is electrically neutral. The neutral form is more easily absorbed through the mucous membranes of the mouth, nose, and lungs.

Absorption and Metabolism

Inhalation is a very effective drug-delivery system; 90 percent of inhaled nicotine is absorbed. The physiological effects of smoking one cigarette have been mimicked by injecting about 1 mg of nicotine intravenously.

Acting with almost as much speed as cyanide, nicotine is well established as one of the most toxic drugs known. In humans, 60 mg is a lethal dose, and death follows intake within a few minutes. A cigar contains enough nicotine for two lethal doses (who needs to take a second one?), but not all of the nicotine is delivered to the smoker or absorbed in a short enough time period to kill a person.

Nicotine is primarily deactivated in the liver, with 80 to 90 percent being modified before excretion through the kidneys. Part of the tolerance that develops to nicotine might result from the fact that either nicotine or the tars increase the activity of the liver microsomal enzymes that are responsible for the deactivation of drugs. These enzymes increase the rate of deactivation and thus decrease the clinical effects of the benzodiazepines and some antidepressants and analgesics. The final step in eliminating deactivated nicotine from the body may be somewhat slowed by nicotine itself, since it acts on the hypothalamus to cause a release of the hormone that acts to reduce the loss of body fluids.

Physiological Effects

The effect of nicotine on areas outside the central nervous system has been studied extensively. Nicotine mimics acetylcholine by acting at several nicotinic subtypes of cholinergic receptor site. Nicotine is not rapidly deactivated, and continued occupation of the receptor prevents incoming impulses from having an effect, thereby blocking the transmission of

Drugs in Depth

Possible New Painkiller?

One of the early uses of tobacco was as a painkiller. Nicotine itself does have some analgesic properties, but its toxicity limits its usefulness for this. The discovery of a substance in the skin of Ecuadorian "poison-arrow" frogs that binds strongly to nicotinis acetylcholine receptors led in 1997 to the development of a synthetic analgesic with a novel mechanism. Animal testing with ABT-594 indicated that it may be a potent pain reliever with fewer side effects and less abuse potential than morphine and other opiate analgesics. The drug was in clinical trials with humans, but side effects such as nausea and dizziness have been a problem. It remains to be seen whether this or a related drug will someday be available for pain relief.

information at the synapse. Thus, nicotine first stimulates and then blocks the receptor. These effects at cholinergic synapses are responsible for some of nicotine's effects, but others seem to be the result of an indirect action.

Nicotine also causes a release of adrenaline from the adrenal glands and other sympathetic sites and thus has, in part, a sympathomimetic action. Additionally, it stimulates and then blocks some sensory receptors, including the chemical receptors found in some large arteries and the thermal pain receptors found in the skin and tongue.

The symptoms of low-level nicotine poisoning are well known to beginning smokers and small children behind barns and in alleys: nausea, dizziness, and a general weakness. In acute poisoning, nicotine causes tremors, which develop into convulsions, terminated frequently by death. The cause of death is suffocation resulting from paralysis of the muscles used in respiration. This paralysis stems from the blocking effect of nicotine on the cholinergic system that normally activates the muscles. With lower doses respiration rate actually increases because the nicotine stimulates oxygen-need receptors in the carotid artery. At these lower doses of 6 to 8 mg there is also a considerable effect on the cardiovascular system as a result of the release of adrenaline. Such release leads to an increase in coronary blood flow, along with vasoconstriction in the skin and increased heart rate and blood pressure. The increased heart rate and blood pressure raise the oxygen need of the heart but not the oxygen supply. Another action of nicotine with negative health effects is that it increases platelet adhesiveness, which increases the tendency to clot. Within the CNS, nicotine seems to act at the level of the cortex to increase somewhat the frequency of the electrical activity, that is, to shift the EEG toward an arousal pattern.

Many effects of nicotine are easily discernible in the smoking individual. The heat releases the nicotine from the tobacco into the smoke. Inhaling while smoking one cigarette has been shown to inhibit hunger contractions of the stomach for up to an hour. That finding, along with a very slight increase in blood sugar level and a deadening of the taste buds, might be the basis for a decrease in hunger after smoking.

In line with the last possibility, it has long been folklore that a person who stops smoking begins to nibble food and thus gains weight. Carbohydrate-rich snack foods appear to be even more appealing when smokers are deprived of nicotine.[22] In addition, there is evidence that smoking increases metabolism rate, so that a weight gain on quitting might be partially due to a decreasing metabolism rate or less energy utilization by the body.

In a regular smoker, smoking results in a constriction of the blood vessels in the skin, along with a decrease in skin temperature and an increase in blood pressure. The blood supply to the skeletal muscles does not change with smoking, but in regular smokers the amount of carboxyhemoglobin in the blood is usually abnormally high (up to 10 percent of all hemoglobin). All smoke contains carbon monoxide; cigarette smoke is about 1 percent carbon monoxide, pipe smoke 2 percent, and cigar smoke 6 percent. The carbon monoxide combines with the hemoglobin in the blood, so that it can no longer carry oxygen. This effect of smoking, a decrease in the oxygen-carrying ability of the blood, probably explains the shortness of breath smokers experience when they exert themselves.

The decrease in oxygen-carrying ability of the blood and the decrease in placental blood flow probably are related to the many results showing that pregnant women who smoke greatly endanger their unborn children.

Behavioral Effects

Despite all the protests and cautionary statements, the evidence is overwhelming that nicotine is the primary, if not the only, reinforcing substance in tobacco. Monkeys will work very hard when their only reward consists of regular intravenous injections of nicotine. The more nicotine in a cigarette, the lower the level of smoking. Intravenous injections and oral administration of nicotine will decrease smoking under some conditions—but not all.

An ongoing debate—among smokers as well as researchers—is whether nicotine acts to arouse and activate the smoker or whether it calms and tranquilizes the user. Smokers report seeking both effects, and experimental results are heavily influenced by the smoker's history and the situation.[23]

Most people smoke in a fairly consistent way, averaging one to two puffs per minute, with each puff lasting about two seconds with a volume of 25 ml. This rate delivers to the individual about 1 to 2 μg of nicotine per kg of body weight with each puff. Smokers could increase the dose by increasing the volume of smoke with each puff or puffing more often, but this dose appears to be optimal for producing stimulation of the cerebral cortex.

Several studies have shown that smokers are able to sustain their attention to a task requiring rapid processing of information from a computer screen much better if they are allowed to smoke before beginning the task. This

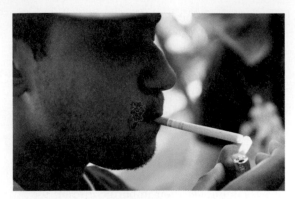

Nicotine is a dependence-producing substance, and users typically have a difficult time quitting.

could be either because the nicotine produces a beneficial effect on this performance or because when the smokers are not allowed to smoke they suffer from some sort of withdrawal symptom.

Nicotine Dependence

Evidence that nicotine is a reinforcing substance in nonhumans, that most people who smoke want to stop and can't, that when people do stop smoking they gain weight and exhibit other withdrawal signs, and that people who chew tobacco also have trouble stopping led to a need for a thorough look at the dependence-producing properties of nicotine. A 1988 surgeon general's report provided it, in the form of a 600-page tome.[24] This had been a traditionally difficult subject: Not many years ago, psychiatrists were arguing that smoking fulfilled unmet needs for oral gratification and therefore represented a personality defect. It has come to light that the cigarette manufacturing company Philip Morris obtained evidence of the dependence-producing nature of nicotine with rats in the early 1980s, but, instead of publishing the results, it fired the researchers and closed the laboratory.[25] Industry executives in 1994 congressional hearings unanimously testified that nicotine was not "addicting," still arguing that smoking was simply a matter of

personal choice and that many people have been able to quit. One can theoretically choose to stop using a drug but one has a very difficult time doing so because of the potent reinforcing properties of the substance. That is the case with nicotine. The following conclusions of the surgeon general's report were pretty strong:

1. Cigarettes and other forms of tobacco are addicting.
2. Nicotine is the drug in tobacco that causes addiction.
3. The pharmacological and behavioral processes that determine tobacco addiction are similar to those that determine addiction to drugs such as heroin and cocaine.

That message met with predictably negative reactions from the tobacco industry and from some tobacco-state politicians, and the debate continued until the late 1990s. Successful lawsuits by former smokers or their survivors finally convinced the tobacco companies that they were going to have to take seriously the issues of toxicity and dependence. In 1998, one company even faced criminal charges for growing a high-nicotine strain of tobacco with the presumed intent of manipulating nicotine levels to "hook" more smokers.

For the past several years, research into the mechanism of nicotine dependence has focused on the fact that nicotine affects dopamine in the nucleus accumbens, a major target of the mesolimbic dopamine system, described in Chapter 4.[26] The brains of chronic nicotine smokers also show a large reduction in one type of monoamine oxidase (MAO), the enzyme that breaks down dopamine and some other neurotransmitters.[27] This slowing of the breakdown of dopamine in chronic smokers might therefore enhance the effect of the dopamine released by each acute dose of nicotine, perhaps contributing to the strength of the dependence on nicotine experienced by most smokers.

The past decade has seen a great deal of research into the different subtypes of nicotinic

Mind/Body Connection

The Hidden Costs of Smoking

Have you ever started to hug a smoker and then involuntarily reacted to the strong smell of smoke in his or her hair and clothing? Or have you ever wanted to kiss someone but held back because you had just smoked a cigarette and thought you needed to brush your teeth first? Smoking erects barriers between people. Some nonsmokers are adamant about not wanting people they care about to smoke. They don't want to breathe in smoke themselves, and they want to protect their children from the dangers of passive and sidestream smoke. When the smoker is a relative or friend, it's difficult to feel close to someone who's doing something you strongly disapprove of, such as smoking. And, from the smoker's viewpoint, it's hard to feel comfortable with someone who acts superior and doesn't accept you as you are.

Imagine a family celebration where a smoker would like to have a cigarette after dinner, in the living room, where everyone else is gathered. The nonsmokers, however, tell the smoker to go outside to smoke. What do the children think about all this? Does a "good" relative smoke? If smoking is bad, as a little boy hears often at school, why does his favorite uncle smoke? Is the family celebration marred by the tension?

The physical cost of smoking is obvious when a young smoker has to step out of a basketball game because he's out of breath or coughing. A smoker may find it embarrassing that she can't keep up on an "easy" hike and needs a break after only 10 minutes. No one wants to feel out of shape and limited in ability.

At work, smoking has become politically incorrect. Many companies have a no-smoking policy or allow smoking in designated areas only. Have you ever seen a group of smokers huddled outside a large office building or factory, "dragging" on their cigarettes? Once again, smokers are isolated and feeling the judgment of others about their "weakness."

Smoking takes a physical toll, but it also extracts a psychological cost. How does it feel to be unaccepted by much of society? to be the outsider? Why does the smoker have to miss part of a special occasion to go smoke a cigarette? Why must the smoker bow out of a fun outdoor activity—or slow down the rest of the group—because of lack of stamina? Why does the smoker have to feel the resentment of co-workers because he or she takes a smoking break every hour? It's not easy to quit smoking, and many smokers make several attempts before they stick with it. Many who have stopped say they thought about more than their physical health before they tossed that last pack.

---

cholinergic receptors, and several companies are developing new drugs targeted more specifically to certain subtypes. The three main potential uses for these drugs would be in treating Alzheimer's disease and other cognitive disorders of aging, controlling pain, and possibly in treating ADHD.[28] Although several such drugs are being tested in human trials, none is yet on the market.

How to Stop Smoking

When you're young and healthy, it's difficult, if not impossible, to imagine dying, being chronically ill, or having **emphysema** so that you can't get enough oxygen to walk across the room without having to stop to catch your breath. By the time you're old enough to worry about those things, it's difficult to change your health habits.

Many people want to stop smoking. A lot of people have already stopped. Are there ways to efficiently and effectively help those individuals who want to stop smoking to stop? With any form of pleasurable drug use, it is easier to

> **emphysema (em fah *see* mah):** a chronic lung disease characterized by difficulty breathing and shortness of breath.

keep people from starting to use the drug than it is to get them to stop once they have started. All the educational programs have had an effect on our society and on our behavior. There are now more than 40 million former smokers in the United States, and about 90 percent of them report that they quit smoking without formal treatment programs. There is some indication that those who have quit on their own do better than those who have been in a treatment program, but then those who quit on their own also tend not to have been smoking as much or for as long.

One reason it is so hard for people to stop is that a pack-a-day smoker puffs at least 50,000 times a year. That's a lot of individual nicotine "hits" reinforcing the smoking behavior. A variety of behavioral treatment approaches are available to assist smokers who want to quit, and hundreds of research articles have been published on them. Although most of these programs are able to get almost everyone to quit for a few days, by six months 70 to 80 percent of participants are smoking again.

If nicotine is the critical thing, why not provide nicotine without the tars and carbon monoxide? Prescription nicotine chewing gum became available in 1984, after carefully controlled studies showed it to be a useful adjunct to smoking cessation programs. This gum is now available over the counter. In 1991, several companies marketed nicotine skin patches that allow slow release of nicotine to be absorbed through the wearer's skin. Nicotine lozenges are now available over the counter, and smokers can also get a prescription for a nicotine inhaler or nasal spray. Also, the prescription drug bupropion (Zyban) has been shown to help many people.[28]

There is money to be made helping people quit smoking, especially if it can apparently be done painlessly with a substitute. The controlled studies done to demonstrate the usefulness of gum or skin patches have been carried out under fairly strict conditions, with a prescribed quitting period, several visits to the clinic to assess progress, and the usual trappings

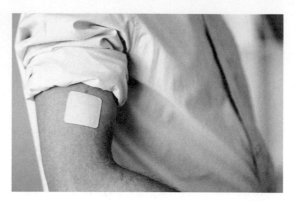

Nicotine replacement therapy—in the form of gum, patch, lozenge, inhaler, or nasal spray—helps some smokers quit.

of a clinical research study, often including the collection of saliva or other samples to detect tobacco use. That's a far cry from buying nicotine gum and a patch off the shelf, with no plan for quitting, no follow-up interviews, and no monitoring. No wonder that some people have found themselves, despite warnings, wearing a nicotine patch and smoking at the same time.

Is there an effective nondrug program for quitting smoking? Yes and no. The effect of any program varies—some people do very well, some very poorly—and if one program won't work for an individual, maybe another one will. Combining counseling and pharmacological treatments increases the odds of quitting.[29] We don't yet know which program will be best for any particular individual. If you want to stop smoking, keep trying programs; odds are you'll find one that works—eventually.

Summary

- Tobacco was introduced to Europe and the East after Columbus's voyage to the Americas.

- As with most other "new" drugs, Europeans either loved tobacco and prescribed it for all ailments or hated it and considered it responsible for many ills.

- The predominant style of tobacco use went from pipes to snuff to chewing to cigars to cigarettes.

- The typical modern cigarette is about half as strong in tar and nicotine content as a cigarette of 50 years ago.

- Cigarette smoking has declined considerably since the 1960s, but about 20 percent of young people still become regular smokers.

- The use of smokeless tobacco increased during the 1980s, causing concerns about increases in oral cancer.

- Although tobacco continues to be an important economic factor in American society, it is also responsible for more annual deaths than all other drugs combined, including alcohol.

- Cigarette smoking is clearly linked to increased risk of heart disease, lung and other cancers, emphysema, and stroke.

- There is increased concern about the health consequences of passive smoking.

- Smoking cessation leads to immediate improvements in mortality statistics, and new products, including different types of nicotine replacement therapy, are being widely used by those who wish to quit.

Review Questions

1. Why was nicotine named after Jean Nicot?
2. Which was the desired species of tobacco that saved the English colonies in Virginia?
3. What techniques have been used to produce "safer" cigarettes?
4. About what proportion of 18- to 25-year-olds are smokers in the United States?
5. What is the significance of tobacco-specific nitrosamines?
6. What are the major causes of death associated with cigarette smoking?
7. What evidence is there that passive smoking can harm nonsmokers?
8. What are the effects of smoking during pregnancy?

9. Nicotine acts through which neurotransmitter in the brain? How does it interact with this neurotransmitter?
10. What is the evidence as to why cigarette smoking produces such strong dependence?

References

1. Stewart, G.G. "A History of the Medicinal Use of Tobacco, 1492–1860." *Medical History* 11 (1967), pp. 228–68.
2. Sargent, J.D., and others. "Brand Appearances in Contemporary Cinema Films and Contribution to Global Marketing of Cigarettes." *The Lancet,* 357 (2001), pp. 29–32.
3. Vaughn, W. Quoted in Dunphy, E.B. "Alcohol and Tobacco Amblyopia: A Historical Survey." *American Journal of Ophthalmology* 68 (1969), p. 573.
4. Corti, E.C. *A History of Smoking.* London: George G. Harrap, 1931.
5. Heimann, R.K. *Tobacco and Americans.* New York: McGraw-Hill, 1960.
6. Brooks, J.E. *The Mighty Leaf.* Boston: Little, Brown, 1952.
7. Lorand, A. *Life Shortening Habits and Rejuvenation.* Philadelphia: F.A. Davis, 1927.
8. Eaglin, J. *The CC Cough-fin Brand Cigarettes.* Cincinnati: Raisbeck, 1931.
9. CNN. "A Brief History of Tobacco." www.cnn.com/US/9705/tobacco/history/ (November, 2004).
10. "Highlights of the Tobacco Settlement." *Facts on File World News Digest,* June 26, 1997.
11. Sherer, G. "Smoking Behavior and Compensation: A Review of the Literature." *Psychopharmacology* 145 (1999), pp. 1–20.
12. Fairchild, A., & J. Colgrove. "Out of the Ashes: The Life, Death, and Rebirth of the "Safer" Cigarette in the United States." *American Journal of Public Health* 94 (2004), pp. 192–205.
13. National Center for Tobacco-Free Kids and others. "Petition for Regulation of R.J. Reynolds' Eclipse Product." Food and Drug Administration, 2001. Available at news.findlaw.com/hdocs/docs/tobacco/eclipsefda121801pet.pdf (November, 2004).
14. Johnston, L.D., P.M. O'Malley, J.G. Bachman, and J.E. Schulenberg. *"Decline in Teen Smoking Appears to Be Nearing Its End."* University of Michigan News and Information Services: Ann Arbor, MI. www.monitoringthefuture.org (December 19, 2005).
15. Substance Abuse and Mental Health Services Administration. *Overview of Findings from the 2004 National Survey on Drug Use and Health:* (NHSDA Series H-27, DHHS Publication No. SMA 05-4061). Rockville, MD: Office of Applied Studies, 2005.
16. *The Health Consequences of Using Smokeless Tobacco: A Report of the Advisory Committee to the Surgeon General.* (NIH Pub. No. 86-2874). Washington, DC: U.S. Government Printing Office, 1986.
17. Smoke and mirrors: How cigarette makers keep health question "open" year after year, *Wall Street Journal,* Feb 11, 1993.
18. Centers for Disease Control. "Annual Smoking-Attributable Mortality, Years of Potential Life Lost, and Economic

Costs—United States, 1997–2001." *Morbidity and Mortality Weekly Report* 54 (2005).

19.   *Shimp v. New Jersey Bell Telephone Company,* Superior Court of New Jersey, Chancery Division, Salem County, Docket No. C-2904-75, filed December 22, 1976.

20.   "Secondhand Smoke: Is It a Hazard?" *Consumer Reports,* January 1995.

21.   *Mortality from Smoking in Developed Countries.* Geneva: World Health Organization, 1994.

22.   Spring, B., and others. "Altered Reward Value of Carbohydrate Snacks for Female Smokers Withdrawn from Nicotine." *Pharmacology, Biochemistry & Behavior* 76 (2003), pp. 351–60.

23.   Kalman, D. "The Subjective Effects of Nicotine: Methodological Issues, a Review of Experimental Studies, and Recommendations for Future Research." *Nicotine & Tobacco Research* 4 (2002), pp. 25–71.

24.   *The Health Consequences of Smoking: Nicotine Addiction, a Report of the Surgeon General.* DHHS Pub. No. (CDC) 88-8406. Washington, DC: U.S. Government Printing Office, 1988.

25.   Kessler, D. *A Question of Intent.* New York: Public Affairs, 2001, pp. 113–39.

26.   Hart, C., & C. Ksir. "Nicotine Effects on Dopamine Clearance in Rat Nucleus Accumbens." *Journal of Neurochemistry* 66: (1996), pp. 216–21.

27.   Fowler, J.S., and others. "Inhibition of Monoamine Oxidase B in the Brains of Smokers." *Nature* 379 (1996), p. 733.

28.   Buccafusco, J.J. "Neuronal Nicotinic Receptor Subtypes: Defining Therapeutic Targets." *Molecular Interventions* 4 (2004), pp. 285–95.

29.   Lamburg, L. "Patients Need More Help to Stop Smoking.: *JAMA* 292 (2004), p. 1286.

Check Yourself

Test Your Tobacco Awareness

Whether you smoke, chew, or don't use tobacco at all, tobacco is an important economic and political issue in virtually every community and in every country. See how well you do with these questions about tobacco's place in the United States and the world:

1. About what proportion of adults in the United States are smokers?
2. About how many Americans die each day from tobacco-related illnesses?
3. What two tobacco-related health problems account for most deaths among smokers?
4. Which country produces the most cigarettes?

Answers

1. About one-third (Most people tend to overestimate the proportion of smokers, which makes smoking seem to be a typical behavior, when in fact, it's not.)
2. About 1,200 per day, representing about 20 percent of all deaths in the United States.
3. Smoking-related heart disease kills about 140,000 in the United States each year, along with about 160,000 smoking-related lung cancer deaths.
4. China produces about 30 percent of the world's cigarettes, with the United States a distant second. Most of the cigarettes produced in China are consumed in China.

11

Caffeine

Objectives

When you have finished this chapter, you should be able to:

- Describe the early history of coffee, tea, and chocolate use.

- Name the xanthines found in coffee, tea, and chocolate.

- Describe the methods for removing caffeine from coffee.

- Name the one plant from which hundreds of varieties of tea are produced.

- Distinguish among the terms cacao, cocoa, and coca.

- Describe the origin of Coca-Cola in relation to cocaine, caffeine, and FDA regulations.

- Explain the caffeine content of "energy drinks" in relation to colas and coffee.

- Describe the caffeine content of drugs like No-Doz and Vivarin.

- Explain how caffeine exerts its actions on the brain.

- Describe the time course of caffeine's effects after ingestion.

- Describe caffeine's withdrawal symptoms.

- Discuss the circumstances in which caffeine appears to enhance mental performance and those in which it does not.

- Describe the concerns about high caffeine consumption during pregnancy.

Caffeine: The World's Most Common Psychostimulant

On a daily basis, more people use caffeine than any other psychoactive drug. Many use it regularly, and there is evidence for dependence and some evidence that regular use can interfere with the very activities people believe that it helps them with. It is now so domesticated that most modern kitchens contain a specialized device for extracting the chemical from plant products (a coffeemaker), but Western societies were not always so accepting of this drug.

How many drugs can lay claim to divine intervention in their introduction to humankind? The xanthines, of which caffeine is the best known, have three such legends, and that fact alone tells you this has been an important class of drugs throughout the ages.

Coffee

The legends surrounding the origin of coffee are at least geographically correct. The best one concerns an Arabian goatherd named Kaldi who couldn't understand why his goats were bounding around the hillside so playfully. One

Online Learning Center Resources

www.mhhe.com/ksir12e

Visit our Online Learning Center (OLC) for access to these study aids and additional resources.

- Learning objectives
- Glossary flashcards
- Web activities and links
- Self-scoring chapter quiz
- Audio chapter summaries

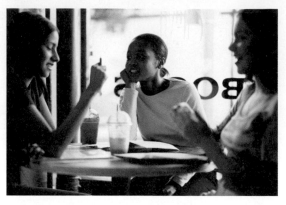

Younger coffee drinkers are a growing customer base for espresso bars and coffeehouses.

day he followed them up the mountain and ate some of the red berries the goats were munching. "The results were amazing. Kaldi became a happy goatherd. Whenever his goats danced, he danced and whirled and leaped and rolled about on the ground." Kaldi had taken the first human coffee trip! A holy man took in the scene, and "that night he danced with Kaldi and the goats." The legend continues with Muhammad telling the holy man to boil the berries in water and have the brothers in the monastery drink the liquid so they could keep awake and continue their prayers.[1]

Around AD 900, an Arabian medical book suggested that coffee was good for almost everything, including measles and lust reduction. Once something gets into the literature, it's very difficult to change people's minds about it. Women in England argued against the use of coffee more than 700 years later, in a 1674 pamphlet titled "The Women's Petition Against Coffee, representing to public consideration the grand inconveniences accruing to their sex from the excessive use of the drying and enfeebling liquor." The women claimed men used too much coffee, and as a result the men were as "unfruitful as those *Desarts* whence that unhappy *Berry* is said to be brought." The women were *really* unhappy, and the pamphlet continued:

> Our Countrymens pallates are become as *Fanatical* as their Brains; how else is't possible they should *Apostatize* from the good old primitive

way of Ale-drinking, to run a *Whoreing* after such variety of distructive Foreign Liquors, to trifle away their time, scald their *Chops*, and spend their *Money*, all for a little *base, black, thick, nasty bitter stinking, nauseous* Puddle water.[2]

Some men probably sat long hours in one of the many coffeehouses composing "The Men's Answer to the Women's Petition Against Coffee," which said in part:

> Why must innocent COFFEE be the object of your Spleen? That harmless and healing Liquor, which Indulgent Providence first sent amongst us. . . . Tis not this incomparable fettle Brain that shortens Natures standard, or makes us less Active in the Sports of Venus, and we wonder you should take these Exceptions.[2]

We can all rest easier today and discuss over a cup of coffee the fact that gradually became clear: There is no truth to the idea that coffee diminishes sexual excitability or reduces lust. It is doubtful that the Arabians believed it, either, because the use of coffee spread throughout the Muslim world. In Mecca, people spent so much time in coffeehouses that the use of coffee was outlawed and all coffee bean supplies were burned. Prohibition rarely works, and coffee speakeasies began to open. Wiser heads prevailed, and the prohibition was lifted.

Drugs in the Media

Fancy Coffee Drinks and Humor

During the past 30 years, coffee has experienced a renaissance in the United States. Although overall coffee consumption is flat, specialty coffee is booming, driven by 18-to-24-year-olds. In its 2000 survey of coffee trends, the National Coffee Association found that 45 percent of this market segment had drunk cappuccino in the past year, 24 percent had drunk espresso, 21 percent latte, 29 percent café mocha, and 36 percent iced or ice-blended coffees. Espresso bars and coffee shops continue to proliferate. Starbucks alone had over 10,000 outlets worldwide, as of February, 2006. As specialty coffees have enjoyed this phenomenal growth, their effect on our popular culture has been reflected in the media.

Coffee bars often are settings for social encounters on television and in the movies. Coffee bars are appealing backdrops in popular TV situation comedies. An interesting phenomenon is how humorous we seem to find all the complicated coffee drinks. Cartoons, jokes, and witty references are common. In these jokes the espresso sophisticate ordering a "half-caf skinny latte, grande" or a "tall cap with three shots" is often contrasted with some plain folks wanting a regular old cup of coffee. The high price of these upscale specialty drinks compared with just plain coffee is another point of some of the humor.

Why do we find this funny? In some ways the humor may be an indirect attempt to poke fun at social-class differences or generational differences using an issue that seems harmless. Another possible way to look at this is to remember from Chapter 1 that an informal method of dealing with social deviance is to make light of it by making it a joke. As a new behavior permeates the social system, its newness and strangeness make it seem somewhat deviant—not yet completely fitting into what we think of as everyday life. These coffee bars and their associated lingo are now becoming so commonplace, however, that they may soon lose their power to provoke a chuckle.

The middle of the 17th century saw the same play enacted but with a new cast of characters and a different locale. Coffeehouses began appearing in England (1650) and France (1671), and a new era began. Coffeehouses were all things to all people: a place to relax, to learn the news of the day, to seal bargains, and to plot. This last possibility made Charles II of England so nervous that he outlawed coffeehouses, labeling them "hotbeds of seditious talk and slanderous attacks upon persons in high stations." King Charles was no more successful than the women's petition had been. In only 11 days the ruling was withdrawn, and the coffeehouses developed into the "penny universities" of the early 18th century. For a penny a cup people could listen to and learn from most of the great literary and political figures of the period. Lloyds of London, an insurance house, started in Edward Lloyd's coffeehouse around 1700.

Across the channel, cheap wine made the need for another social drink less essential in France than in England, but French coffeehouses made at least one contribution to Western culture—the cancan.

Across the Atlantic, coffee drinking increased in the English colonies, although tea was still preferred. Cheaper and more available than coffee, tea had everything, including, beginning in 1765, a 3-pence-a-pound tax on its importation.

The British Act that taxed tea helped fan the fire that lit the musket that fired the shot heard around the world. That story is better told in connection with tea, but the final outcome was that to be a tea drinker was to be a Tory, so coffee became the new country's national drink.

Coffee use expanded as the West was won, and per capita consumption steadily increased in the early 1900s. Some experts became worried about the increase, which some believed was caused by the widespread prohibition of alcohol.

But even after Prohibition went away, coffee consumption continued to rise. In 1946, annual per capita coffee consumption reached an all-time high of 20 pounds. The overall trend has been basically downhill since then, despite an upsurge of interest in espresso and specialty coffees in the late 1990s.

Some of the decrease in coffee consumption can be attributed to changing lifestyles—sun and fun and convenient canned drinks seem to fit together better, and soft drinks seem to go with fast food. In 1970, Americans still drank more gallons of coffee per capita than of any other nonalcoholic beverage product, but by 2003 Americans were consuming almost 50 gallons of soft drinks per person, compared with about 24 gallons of coffee.[3]

If the national drink is not as national as it once was, neither is it as simple. Kaldi and his friends were content to simply munch on the coffee beans or put them in hot water. Somewhere in the dark past the Middle East discovered that roasting the green coffee bean improved the flavor, aroma, and color of the drink made from the bean. For years housewives, storekeepers, and coffeehouse owners bought the green bean, then roasted and ground it just before use. Commercial roasting started in 1790 in New York City, and the process gradually spread through the country. However, although the green bean can be stored indefinitely, the roasted bean deteriorates seriously within a month. Ground coffee can be maintained at its peak level in the home only for a week or two, and then only if it is in a closed container and refrigerated. Vacuum packing of ground coffee was introduced in 1900, a process that maintains the quality until the seal is broken.

Coffee growing spread worldwide when the Dutch began cultivation in the East Indies in 1696. Latin America had an ideal climate for coffee growing, and with the world's greatest coffee-drinking nation just up the road several thousand miles, it became the world's largest producer. Different varieties of the coffee tree and different growing and processing conditions

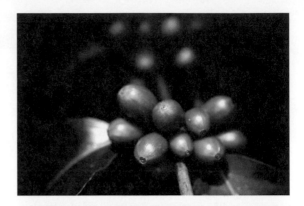

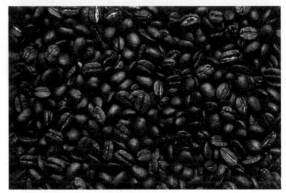

Green coffee beans are roasted to improve the color and flavor of the drink made from the beans.

provide many opportunities for varying the characteristics of coffee.

No one went commercial with a combination of different coffee beans until J. O. Cheek developed a blend in 1892 and introduced it through a famous Nashville hotel: Maxwell House. The coffee was so well received that the hotel owners let the coffee be named after the hotel.

In the early 1950s, about 94 percent of American coffee was from Latin America, but that percentage has steadily declined; today less than half is grown in this hemisphere. Mexico, Brazil, and Colombia are the largest exporters to the United States. These countries grow *arabica,* which has a caffeine content of about 1 percent. *Robusta,* with a caffeine level at 2 percent, is the variety imported from Vietnam, Indonesia, and Thailand, and is usually of a lower grade and price.

The economics of coffee (it is number two in international trade, far behind oil) have as much to do with coffee consumption as does our changing lifestyle. A price increase in the early 1950s—to a dollar a pound—shifted us from being a 40-cups-per-pound nation to being a 60-cups-per-pound nation. This dilution reduced the cost but also the quality of the beverage. Two things happen when prices go up: the quality of the coffee decreases and people drink less coffee.

Instant coffee has been around since before the start of the 20th century, but sales began their marked increase in the hustle and bustle after World War II: another decrease in the quality of the beverage but an increase in the convenience. Interestingly, Brazilians import many inexpensive African coffee beans to use in manufacturing instant coffee because they believe that their coffee is too good to be used in that way.

Over the past 20 years, health-conscious Americans began to drink more decaffeinated coffee and less regular coffee. There are several ways of removing caffeine from the coffee bean. In the process used by most American companies, the unroasted beans are soaked in an organic solvent, raising concerns about residues of the solvent remaining in the coffee. The most widely used solvent has been methylene chloride, and studies have shown that high doses of that solvent can cause cancer in laboratory mice. In 1985, the FDA banned the use of methylene chloride in hair sprays, which can be inhaled during use, but allowed the solvent to be used in decaffeination as long as residues did not exceed 10 parts per million. Because the solvent residue evaporates during roasting, decaffeinated coffees contain considerably lower amounts than that, so the assumption is that the risk is minimal. The Swiss water process, which is not used on a large commercial scale in the United States, removes more of the coffee's flavor. The caffeine that is taken out of the coffee is used mostly in soft drinks. One of the largest decaffeinating companies is owned by Coca-Cola.

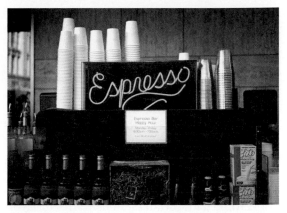

Specialty coffee drinks are expected to continue to gain popularity.

Today's supermarket shelves are filled with an amazing variety of products derived from this simple bean—pure Colombian, French Roast, decaf, half-caf, flavored coffees, instants, mixes, and even cold coffee beverages. The competition for the consumer's coffee dollar has never been greater, it seems. And Americans are lining up in record numbers at espresso bars to buy cappuccinos, lattes, and other exotic-sounding mixtures of strong coffee, milk, and flavorings. The number of these specialty coffee shops increased from fewer than 200 in 1989 to more than 15,000 in 2004.[4] They are found in small towns, shopping malls, and on practically every corner in cities.

Tea

Tea and coffee are not like day and night, but their differences are reflected in the legends surrounding their origins. The bouncing goatherd of Arabia suggests that coffee is a boisterous, blue-collar drink. Tea is a different story: much softer, quieter, more delicate. According to one legend, Daruma, the founder of Zen Buddhism, fell asleep one day while meditating. Resolving that it would never happen again, he cut off both eyelids. From the spot where his eyelids touched the earth grew a new plant. From its leaves a brew could be made that would keep a person awake. Appropriately, the tea tree, *Thea sinensis* (now classed as *Camellia sinensis*), is an evergreen, and *sinensis* is the Latin word for "Chinese."

The first report of tea that seems reliable is in a Chinese manuscript from around AD 350, when it was primarily seen as a medicinal plant. The nonmedical use of tea is suggested by an AD 780 book on the cultivation of tea, but the real proof that it was in wide use in China is that a tax was levied on it in the same year. Before this time Buddhist monks had carried the cultivation and use of tea to Japan.

Europe had to wait eight centuries to savor the herb that was "good for tumors or abscesses that come from the head, or for ailments of the bladder . . . it quenches thirst. It lessens the desire for sleep. It gladdens and cheers the heart." The first European record of tea, in 1559, says, "One or two cups of this decoction taken on an empty stomach removes fever, headache, stomach-ache, pain in the side or in the joints. . . ." Fifty years later, in 1610, the Dutch delivered the first tea to the continent of Europe.

An event that occurred 10 years before had tremendous impact on the history of the world and on present patterns of drug use. In 1600, the English East India Company was formed, and Queen Elizabeth gave the company a monopoly on everything from the east coast of Africa across the Pacific to the west coast of South America. In this period the primary imports from the Far East were spices, and the company prospered. A major conflict developed between Dutch and English trade interests over who belonged where in the East. In 1623, a resolution gave the Dutch East India Company the islands (the Dutch East Indies), and the English East India Company had to be content with India and other countries on the continent.

The English East India Company concentrated on importing spices, so the first tea was taken to England by the Dutch. As the market for tea increased, the English East India Company expanded its imports of tea from China. Coffee had arrived first, so most tea was sold in coffeehouses. Even as tea's use as a popular

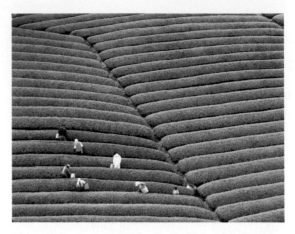

Most tea is grown in Sri Lanka, India, and Indonesia. The leaves are harvested by hand, with only the top few leaves of new growth harvested every 6–10 days.

social drink expanded in Europe, there were some prophets of doom. A 1635 publication by a physician claimed that, at the very least, using tea would speed the death of those over 40 years old. The use of tea was not slowed, however, and by 1657 tea was being sold to the public in England. This was no more than 10 years after the English had developed the present word for it: *tea*. Although spelled *tea,* it was pronounced tay until the 19th century. Before this period the Chinese name *ch'a* had been used, anglicized to either *chia* or *chaw*.

With the patrons of taverns off at coffeehouses living it up with tea, coffee, and chocolate, tax revenues from alcoholic beverages declined. To offset this loss, coffeehouses were licensed, and a tax of eight pence was levied on each gallon of tea and chocolate sold. To keep at home the profits from the expanding tea trade, Britain banned Dutch imports of tea in 1669, which gave the English East India Company a monopoly. Profit from the China tea trade colonized India, brought about the Opium Wars between China and Britain, and induced the English to switch from coffee to tea. In the last half of the 18th century, the East India Company conducted a "Drink Tea" campaign unlike anything ever seen. Advertising, patriotism, low cost on tea, and high taxes on alcohol made Britain a nation of tea drinkers.

That same profit motive led to the American Revolution. Because the English East India Company had a monopoly on importing tea to England and thence to the American colonies, the British government imposed high duties on tea when it was taken from warehouses and offered for sale. But, as frequently happens, when taxes went up, smuggling increased. Eventually, more smuggled tea than legal tea was being consumed in Britain. The American colonies, ever loyal to the king, had become big tea drinkers, which helped the king and the East India Company stay solvent. The Stamp Act of 1765, which included a tax on tea, changed everything. Even though the Stamp Act was repealed in 1766, it was replaced by the Trade and Revenue Act of 1767, which did the same thing.

These measures made the colonists unhappy over paying taxes they had not helped formulate (taxation without representation), and in 1767 this resulted in a general boycott on the consumption of English tea. Coffee use increased, but the primary increase was in the smuggling of tea. The drop in legal tea sales filled the tea warehouses and put the East India Company in financial trouble. To save the company, in 1773 Parliament gave the East India Company the right to sell tea in the American colonies without paying the tea taxes. The company was also allowed to sell the tea through its own agents, thus eliminating the profits of the merchants in the colonies.

Several boatloads of this tea, which would be sold cheaper than any before, sailed toward various ports in the colonies. The American merchants, who would not have made any profit on this tea, were the primary ones who rebelled at the cheap tea. Some ships were turned away from port, but the beginning of the end came with the 342 chests of tea that turned the Boston harbor into a teapot on the night of December 16, 1773.

The revolution in America and the colonists' rejection of tea helped tea sales in Great Britain—to be a tea drinker was to be loyal to the Crown. Many factors contributed to

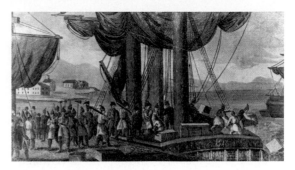

The Boston Tea Party contributed to the English preference for tea over coffee.

change the English from coffee drinkers to tea drinkers, and the preference for tea persists today. Although their use of coffee increases yearly and that of tea declines, the English are still tea drinkers. The annual per capita consumption of tea in the United Kingdom is about 5.5 pounds, second in the world only to Ireland. In comparison, Americans consume about one pound of tea per person per year.

About 70 percent of the tea that comes to America starts life on a four- to five-foot bush high in the mountains of Sri Lanka (Ceylon), India, or Indonesia. Unpruned, the bush would grow into a 15-to-30-foot tree, which would be difficult to pluck, as picking tea leaves is called. The pluckers select only the bud-leaf and the first two leaves at each new growth. The bud-leaf is called flowering orange pekoe, the second leaf is larger and called orange pekoe, and the third and largest is pekoe (pekoe is pronounced "peck-ho," not "peak-o"). Thus, orange pekoe is not a variety of tea plant but, rather, a size and quality of tea leaf; generally the bud-leaf is of the highest quality and the third leaf is the lowest quality.

In one day a plucker will pluck enough leaves to make 10 pounds of tea as sold in the grocery store. Plucking is done every 6 to 10 days in warm weather as new growth develops on the many branches. The leaves are dried, rolled to crush the cells in the leaf, and placed in a cool, damp place for fermentation (oxidation) to occur. This oxidation turns the green leaves to a bright copper color. Nonoxidized leaves are packaged and sold as green tea, sales of which have seen large increases in recent years. Oxidized tea is called black tea and accounts for about 98 percent of the tea Americans consume. Oolong tea is greenish-brown, consisting of partially oxidized leaves.

Until 1904, the only choices available were sugar, cream, and lemon with your hot tea. At the Louisiana Purchase Exposition in St. Louis in 1904, iced tea was sold for the first time. It now accounts for 75 percent of all tea consumed in America. Tea lovers found 1904 to be a very good year. Fifteen hundred miles east of the fair, a New York City tea merchant decided to send out his samples in handsewn silk bags rather than tin containers. Back came the orders—send us tea, and send it in the same little bags you used to send the samples. From that inauspicious beginning evolved the modern tea bag machinery, which cuts the filter paper, weighs the tea, and attaches the tag—all this at a rate of 150 to 180 tea bags per minute.

Pound for pound, loose black tea contains a higher concentration of caffeine than coffee beans. However, because about 200 cups of tea can be made from each pound of dry tea leaves, compared with 50 or 60 cups of coffee per pound, a typical cup of tea has less caffeine than a typical cup of coffee. The caffeine content of teas varies widely, depending on brand and the strength of the brew. Most teas have 40 to 60 mg of caffeine per cup.

The market has been flooded with a variety of tea products. Most tea is sold in tea bags these days, but instant teas, some containing flavorings and sweeteners, are popular for convenience. Flavored teas—which contain mint, spices, or other substances along with tea—offer other options. The biggest boom in recent years has been in so-called herbal teas, which mostly contain no real "tea." These teas are made up of mixtures of other plant leaves and flowers for both flavor and color and have become quite popular among people who avoid caffeine.

The largest seller of tea in America is a company named after a man, born in Scotland of Irish parents, who emigrated to America,

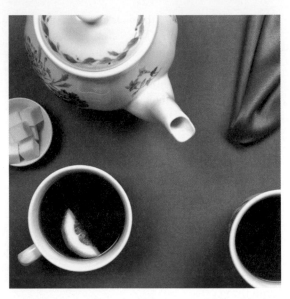

A wide variety of tea products is available—black, oolong, green, flavored, and herbal teas. A pound of dry tea leaves makes about 200 cups of tea.

became rich and famous in England, and believed in ships with sails right up to the end: Sir Thomas Lipton (1850–1931).

Although tea contains another chemical that derived its name from the tea plant, **theophylline** ("divine leaf") is present only in very small, nonpharmacological amounts in the beverage. Theophylline is very effective at relaxing the bronchial passages and is widely prescribed for use by asthmatics.

Chocolate

Now we come to the third legend, concerning the origin of the third xanthine-containing plant. Long before Columbus landed on San Salvador, Quetzalcoatl, Aztec god of the air, gave humans a gift from paradise: the chocolate tree. Linnaeus was to remember this legend when he named the cocoa tree *Theobroma*, "food of the gods." The Aztecs treated it as such, and the cacao bean was an important part of their economy, with the cacao bush being cultivated widely. Montezuma, emperor of Mexico in the early 16th century, is said to have consumed nothing other than 50 goblets of *chocolatl* every day. The *chocolatl*—from the Mayan words *choco* ("warm") and *latl* ("beverage")—was flavored with vanilla but was far from the chocolate of today. It was a thick liquid, like honey, that was sometimes frothy and had to be eaten with a spoon. The major difference was that it was bitter; the Aztecs didn't know about sugarcane.

Cortez introduced sugarcane plantations to Mexico in the early 1520s and supported the continued cultivation of the *Theobroma cacao* bush. When he returned to Spain in 1528, Cortez carried with him cakes of processed cocoa. The cakes were eaten, as well as being ground up and mixed with water for a drink. Although chocolate was introduced to Europe almost a century before coffee and tea, its use spread very slowly. Primarily this was because the Spanish kept the method of preparing chocolate from the cacao bean a secret until the early 17th century. When knowledge of the technique spread, so did the use of chocolate.

During the 17th century, chocolate drinking reached all parts of Europe, primarily among the wealthy. Maria Theresa, wife of France's Louis XIV, had a "thing" about chocolate, and this furthered its use among the wealthy and fashionable. Gradually it became more of a social drink, and by the 1650s chocolate houses were open in England, although usually chocolate was sold alongside coffee and tea in the established coffeehouses.

In the early 18th century, health warnings were issued in England against the use of chocolate, but use expanded. Its use and importance are well reflected in a 1783 proposal in the U.S. Congress that the United States raise revenue by taxing chocolate as well as coffee, tea, liquor, sugar, molasses, and pepper.

Although the cultivation of chocolate never became a matter to fight over, it, too, has spread around the world. The New World plantations were almost destroyed by disease at the

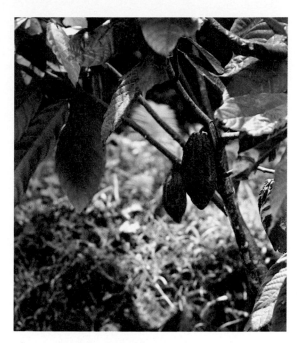

The genus of the chocolate (cacao) tree, *Theobroma*, is Latin for "food of the gods."

beginning of the 18th century, but cultivation had already begun in Asia, and today a large part of the crop comes from Africa.

Until 1828, all chocolate sold was a relatively indigestible substance obtained by grinding the cacao kernels after processing. The preparation had become more refined over the years, but it still followed the Aztec procedure of letting the pods dry in the sun, then roasting them before removing the husks to get to the kernel of the plant. The result of grinding the kernels is a thick liquid called chocolate liquor. This is baking chocolate. In 1828, a Dutch patent was issued for the manufacture of "chocolate powder" by removing about two thirds of the fat from the chocolate liquor.

The fat that was removed, cocoa butter, became important when someone found that, if it was mixed with sugar and some of the

theophylline (thee *off* a lin): a xanthine found in tea.

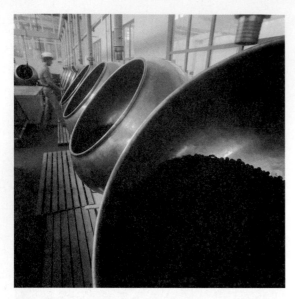

Chocolate candy is made by mixing cocoa butter, sugar, and chocolate powder.

Table 11.1
Caffeine in Beverages and Foods

Item	CAFFEINE (MG) Average	Range
Coffee (5 oz cup)		
Brewed, drip method	115	60–180
Brewed, percolator	80	40–170
Instant	65	30–120
Decaffeinated, brewed	3	2–5
Decaffeinated, instant	2	1–5
Tea (5 oz cup)		
Brewed, major U.S. brands	40	20–90
Brewed, imported brands	60	25–110
Instant	30	25–50
Iced (12 oz glass)	70	67–76
Cocoa beverage (5 oz cup)	4	2–20
Chocolate milk beverage (8 oz glass)	5	2–7
Milk chocolate (1 oz)	6	1–15
Dark chocolate, semisweet (1 oz)	20	5–35
Baker's chocolate (1 oz)	26	26
Chocolate-flavored syrup (1 oz)	4	4

chocolate powder, it could easily be formed into slabs or bars. In 1847, the first chocolate bars appeared, but it was not until 1876 that the Swiss made their contribution to the chocolate industry by inventing milk chocolate, which was first sold under the Nestlé label. By FDA standards, milk chocolate today must contain at least 12 percent milk solids, although better grades contain almost twice that amount.

You can check whether your piece of chocolate is all chocolate and properly manufactured by putting it on your tongue: It should melt at body temperature. But be careful! One chocolate lover has said, "Each of us has known such moments of orgastic anticipation, our senses focused at their finest, when control is irrevocably abandoned. Then the tongue possesses, is possessed by, what it most desires; the warm, liquid melting of thick, dark chocolate."[5]

The unique xanthine in chocolate is **theobromine.** Its physiological actions closely parallel those of caffeine, but it is much less potent in its effects on the central nervous system. The average cup of cocoa contains about 200 mg of theobromine but only 4 mg of caffeine. Table 11.1 compares the caffeine contents of various forms of coffee, tea, and chocolate.

Other Sources of Caffeine
Soft Drinks

The early history of cola drinks is not shrouded in the mists that veil the origins of the other xanthine drinks, so there is no problem in selecting the correct legend. And that's what the story of Coca-Cola is: a true legend in our time. From a green nerve tonic in 1886 in Atlanta, Georgia, that did not sell well at all, Coca-Cola has grown into "the real thing," providing "the pause that refreshes," selling almost 3 billion cases a year and operating in more than 200 countries.

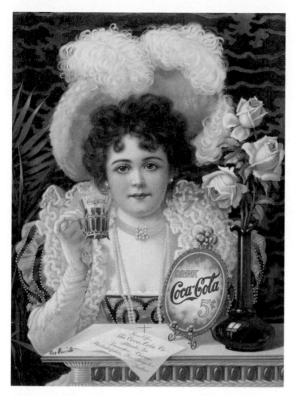

When introduced in the late 1800s, Coca-Cola was marketed as a tonic and named for two flavoring ingredients with tonic properties—coca leaves and cola (kola) nuts. The coca leaves used in Coca-Cola today have had the cocaine extracted.

Dr. J. C. Pemberton's green nerve tonic in the late 1800s contained caramel, fruit flavoring, phosphoric acid, caffeine, and a secret mixture called Merchandise No. 5. A friend of Dr. Pemberton, F. M. Robinson, suggested the name by which it is still known: Coca-Cola. The unique character of Coca-Cola and its later imitators comes from a blend of fruit flavors that makes it impossible to identify any of its parts. An early ad for Coca-Cola suggested its varied uses:

> The "INTELLECTUAL BEVERAGE" and TEMPERANCE DRINK contains the valuable TONIC and NERVE STIMULANT properties of the Coca plant and Cola (or Kola) nuts, and makes not only a delicious, exhilarating, refreshing and invigorating Beverage, (dispensed from the soda

water fountain or in other carbonated beverages), but a valuable Brain Tonic, and a cure for all nervous affections—SICK HEADACHE, NEURALGIA, HYSTERIA, MELANCHOLY, &c.[6]

Coca-Cola was touted as "the new and popular fountain drink, containing the tonic properties of the wonderful coca plant and the famous cola nut." This was the period of Sherlock Holmes, Sigmund Freud, and patent medicine—all saying very good things about the product of the coca plant: cocaine. In 1903, the company admitted its beverage contained small amounts of cocaine, but soon after that it quietly removed all the cocaine; a government analysis of Coca-Cola in 1906 did not find any.

The name *Coca-Cola* was originally conceived to indicate the nature of its two ingredients with tonic properties. The suggestion of the presence of extracts of coca leaves and cola (kola) nuts in the beverage was supposed to be furthered by the use on each bottle of a pictorial representation of the leaves and nuts. Unfortunately, the artist-glass blower didn't know that the coca and cacao plants were different, so the bottle had kola leaves and cacao pods. In 1909, the FDA seized a supply of Coca-Cola syrup and made two charges against the company. One was that the syrup was misbranded because it contained "no coca and little if any cola" and, second, that it contained an "added poisonous ingredient," caffeine.

Before a 1911 trial in Chattanooga, Tennessee, the company paid for research into the physiological effects of caffeine, and when all the information was in the company won. The government appealed the decision. In 1916, the U.S. Supreme Court upheld the lower court by rejecting the charge of misbranding, stating that the company had repeatedly said that "certain extracts from the leaves of the coca shrub and the nut kernels of the cola tree were used for the purpose of obtaining a flavor" and that "the

theobromine (thee oh *broh* meen): a xanthine found in chocolate.

ingredients containing these extracts," with the cocaine eliminated, was called Merchandise No. 5. Today, coca leaves are imported by a pharmaceutical company in New Jersey. The cocaine is extracted for medical use and the decocainized leaves are shipped to the Coca-Cola plant in Atlanta, where Merchandise No. 5 is produced. A 1931 report indicated that Merchandise No. 5 contained an extract of three parts coca leaves and one part cola nuts, but to this day it remains a secret formula.

In 1981, the FDA changed its rules, so that a cola no longer has to contain caffeine. If it does contain caffeine, it may not be more than 0.02 percent, which is 0.2 mg/ml, or a little less than 6 mg per ounce. Some consumer and scientist groups believe that all cola manufacturers should indicate on the label the amount of caffeine the beverage contains. This has not happened, even though soft drinks, as with other food products, must now list nutrition information, such as calories, fat, sodium, and protein content.

Table 11.2 lists the caffeine content in a 12-ounce serving of popular soft drinks. Diet soft drinks, most now sweetened with aspartame, and caffeine-free colas are commanding a larger share of the market, but regular colas are still the single most popular type of soft drink. As with beers and some other products, the modern marketing strategy seems to be for each company to try to offer products of every type, in order to cover the market. Also as with beers, the large companies are buying up their competitors: in 2001, the Coca-Cola and PepsiCo companies represented more than 75 percent of total shipments. Coca-Cola Classic remains the most popular single brand, with almost 20 percent of the total market. Soft drinks have become increasingly popular. Per capita consumption of soft drinks has continued to edge upward and is now about 50 gallons per year.

"Energy" Drinks

Some consumers have always preferred to obtain their caffeine from soft drinks instead of

Table 11.2
Caffeine in Popular Soft Drinks

Brand	Caffeine* (mg)
Jolt	71
RC Edge (Royal Crown)	70
Diet Sun Drop	69
Sun Drop Regular	63
Kick	58
Mountain Dew	55
Diet Mountain Dew	55
Pepsi One	55
KMX	53
Mello Yello	51
Diet Mello Yello	51
Surge	51
Nehi Wild Red Soda	50
Diet Coke	45
Royal Crown	43
Pepsi Cola	38
Diet Pepsi	36
Coca-Cola Classic	34

*Per 12-oz serving.

Source: Data from National Soft Drink Association, 2003.

from coffee. This led to the development and promotion of Jolt cola, which had the maximum allowable caffeine content per ounce, or almost 72 mg in a 12-ounce can. This might be a lot for a soft drink, but it isn't a great deal when compared to 100 mg in the "standard" four-ounce cup of coffee. Mountain Dew's hugely successful television marketing campaign links its product with heavy-metal music and extreme skiing, snowboarding, and similar high-energy activities. The parent company, PepsiCo, says on the Mountain Dew Web site that "Doing the 'Dew' is like no other soft drink experience because of its daring, high-energy, high-intensity, active, extreme citrus taste," but most of its users know its caffeine content is higher than the major brands of colas (but still

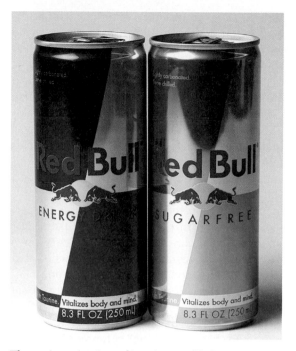

The main active ingredient in so-called energy drinks is caffeine.

Table 11.3 Caffeine Content of Nonprescription Drugs	
Drug	**Caffeine (mg)**
Stimulants	
No Doz	100.0
Vivarin	200.0
Analgesics	
Anacin	32.0
Excedrin	65.0
Goody's Headache Powders	32.5
Midol	32.4
Vanquish	33.0
Diuretics	
Aqua-Ban	100.0
Maximum-Strength Aqua-Ban Plus	200.0

not high compared with brewed coffee). Then along came the Austrian sensation in a small can, Red Bull. Touted as an "energy drink," the main active ingredient in this expensive drink is caffeine, at 80 mg per 8.3-ounce can (still less than a cup of coffee). The original marketers seemed to be aiming the product at people who exercise and want to "build" their bodies by including some ingredients found in dietary supplements sold to athletes, such as the amino acid taurine. Although rumors abound about Red Bull, the product does not appear to have any unique properties, and there is no evidence that the ingredients besides caffeine and sugar have any particular effect, either psychologically or in helping one to gain strength. Because Red Bull has also become a popular mixer with alcohol, there have been some concerns that taurine might intensify alcohol's effect, but careful animal studies have found no interaction between taurine and the behavioral effects of alcohol.[7]

Much of the explosion in soft drink varieties has been aimed at this "high-energy" market. (The hype has been pretty high energy, even if the products are nothing special, urging consumers to "feed the rush," or "blow your mind" using the drink.) The list of Mountain Dew competitors includes Kick and Surge, while Red Bull imitators have names like Stallion, Whoopass, Adrenaline Rush, Monster, and Rockstar.

Over-the-Counter Drugs

Few people realize that many nonprescription drugs also include caffeine, some in quite large amounts. Table 11.3 lists the caffeine content of some of these drugs. Presumably many people who buy "alertness tablets," such as No Doz, are aware that they are buying caffeine. But many buyers of such things as Excedrin might not realize how much caffeine they are getting. Imagine the condition of someone who took a nonprescription water-loss pill and a headache tablet containing caffeine, who then drank a couple of cups of coffee.

Considering all the various sources of caffeine, it is estimated that 80 percent of

Americans regularly use caffeine in some form, and that the average intake is 200 to 250 mg per day.[8] As with other psychoactive substances, this "average" takes in a wide range, with some users regularly consuming 1,000 mg or more each day.

Caffeine Pharmacology

Xanthines are the oldest stimulants known. *Xanthine* is a Greek word meaning "yellow," the color of the residue that remains after xanthines are heated with nitric acid until dry. The three xanthines of primary importance are caffeine, theophylline, and theobromine. These three chemicals are methylated xanthines and are closely related alkaloids. Most alkaloids are insoluble in water, but these are unique, because they are slightly water soluble.

These three xanthines have similar effects on the body. Caffeine has the greatest effect. Theobromine has almost no stimulant effect on the central nervous system and the skeletal muscles. Theophylline is the most potent, and caffeine the least potent, agent on the cardiovascular system. Caffeine, so named because it was isolated from coffee in 1820, has been the most extensively studied and, unless otherwise indicated, is the drug under discussion here.

Time Course

In humans, the absorption of caffeine is rapid after oral intake; peak blood levels are reached 30 minutes after ingestion. Although maximal CNS effects are not reached for about two hours, the onset of effects can begin within half an hour after intake. The half-life of caffeine in humans is about three hours, and no more than 10 percent is excreted unchanged.

Cross-tolerance exists among the methylated xanthines; loss of tolerance can take more than two months of abstinence. The tolerance, however, is low grade, and by increasing the dose two to four times an effect can be obtained even in the tolerant individual. There is less tolerance to the CNS stimulation effect of caffeine than to most of its other effects. The direct action on the kidneys, to increase urine output, and the increase of salivary flow do show tolerance.

Dependence on caffeine is real (see the Taking Sides). People who are not coffee drinkers or who have been drinking only decaffeinated coffee often report unpleasant effects (nervousness, anxiety) after being given caffeinated coffee, but those who regularly consume caffeine report mostly pleasant mood states after drinking coffee. Various experiments have reported on the reinforcing properties of caffeine in regular coffee drinkers; one of the most clear-cut allowed patients on a research ward to choose between two coded instant coffees, identical except that one contained caffeine. Participants had to choose at the beginning of each day which coffee they would drink for the rest of that day. People who had been drinking caffeine-containing coffee before this experiment almost always chose the caffeine-containing coffee.[10] Thus, the reinforcing effect of caffeine probably contributes to psychological dependence.

There has long been clear evidence of physical dependence on caffeine as well. The most reliable withdrawal sign is a headache, which occurs an average of 18 to 19 hours after the most recent caffeine intake. Other symptoms include increased fatigue and decreased sense of vigor. These withdrawal symptoms are strongest during the first two days of withdrawal, then decline over the next five or six days.[11]

Mechanism of Action

For years no one really knew the mechanism whereby the methylxanthines had their effects on the CNS. In the early 1980s, evidence was presented that caffeine and the other xanthines block the brain's receptors for a substance known as **adenosine,** which is a neurotransmitter or neuromodulator. Adenosine normally acts in several areas of the brain to produce behavioral sedation by inhibiting the release of

Taking Sides

Caffeine-Dependence Syndrome?

As reviewed in Chapter 3, the American Psychiatric Association's *DSM-IV-TR* lists the criteria for substance abuse, substance dependence, substance withdrawal, and substance intoxication. The team that developed the latest revision did not include caffeine among the substances that would be considered to produce substance dependence. However, in 1994 a group of researchers reported the cases of 16 individuals who they considered to meet the general criteria for a *DSM-IV-TR* diagnosis of substance disorder.[9]

Of 99 subjects who responded to newspaper notices asking for volunteers who believed they were psychologically or physically dependent on caffeine, 27 were asked to undergo further testing, which included a psychiatric interview to assess caffeine dependence. Although the *DSM-IV-TR* requires that only three of seven criteria be met for a diagnosis of dependence, this study was more conservative in requiring three of the four most serious criteria (tolerance, withdrawal, persistent desire or efforts to cut down, and continued use despite knowledge of a persistent or recurrent problem caused by use). Sixteen of the twenty-seven were diagnosed as having caffeine dependence using these criteria. Of those 16, 11 agreed to participate in a double-blind caffeine withdrawal experiment. All were placed on a restricted diet during two two-day study periods and were given capsules to take at various times of the day to match their normal caffeine intake. During one of the two sessions, each volunteer was given caffeine, and during the other session the capsules contained a placebo. Neither the participants nor the interviewers were told on which session they were getting the caffeine. Withdrawal symptoms found during the placebo session included headaches, fatigue, decreased vigor, and increased depression scores. Several of the subjects were unable to go to or stay at work, went to bed several hours early, or needed their spouse to take over child-care responsibilities.

A decision to accept caffeine-dependence syndrome as an official diagnosis would have several implications—some feel that it would trivialize the diagnosis for "serious" drug dependence or complicate questions of insurance payment for treatment of substance dependence. Others feel that this syndrome could be a serious dependence disorder for some coffee drinkers and deserves to be recognized as such.

other neurotransmitters. Caffeine's stimulant action results from blocking the receptors for this inhibitory effect.[12] Now that this mechanism is understood, it may lead to the development of new chemicals having similar but perhaps more potent effects.

Physiological Effects

The pharmacological effects on the CNS and the skeletal muscles are probably the basis for the wide use of caffeine-containing beverages. With two cups of coffee taken close together (about 200 mg of caffeine), the cortex is activated, the EEG shows an arousal pattern, and drowsiness and fatigue decrease. This CNS stimulation is also the basis for "coffee nerves," which can occur at low doses in sensitive individuals and in others when they have consumed large amounts of caffeine. In the absence of tolerance, even 200 mg will increase the time it takes to fall asleep and will cause sleep disturbances. There is a strong relationship between the mood-elevating effect of caffeine and the extent to which it will keep the individual awake.

xanthines (*zan* theens): the class of chemicals to which caffeine belongs.
adenosine (a *den* o sen): an inhibitory neurotransmitter through which caffeine acts.

Mind/Body Connection

Caffeine and the "Geek" Culture: Buying a Dream

Considerable mythology surrounds the supposed ability of caffeine to support sustained, high-level mental effort. For example, the famous mathematician Paul Erdos once said, "A mathematician is a device for turning coffee into theorems." This mythology of caffeine as brain fuel has been adopted by the so-called geek culture that grew so rapidly during the dot.com era of the late 1990s and remains strong among programmers and systems engineers and those who identify with them. ThinkGeek.com, purveyors of all kinds of gadgets and supplies related to geek culture, sells an amazing variety of caffeine-based products in addition to coffee and tea, including candies, syrups, gum, and even ShowerShock, a caffeinated soap that is supposed to help you get going even before you get to the coffee cup (this is probably not an effective delivery method for caffeine; see www.erowid.org/ask/ask.cgi?ID=3010).

One has to ask whether those people who believe they can't work effectively without their coffee are more dependent on the caffeine or on the idea that caffeine helps them work harder or smarter. The evidence reviewed in this textbook indicates that once a person has developed a tolerance to higher levels of daily caffeine consumption, the caffeine probably does little good. However, stopping use at that point will likely lead to a lack of energy and headaches, interfering with work production.

In this competitive world, we'd all like to think that there's a magic substance that could give us "smarts" and energy, and it's that mythical dream that helps sell everything from ShowerShock to Red Bull.

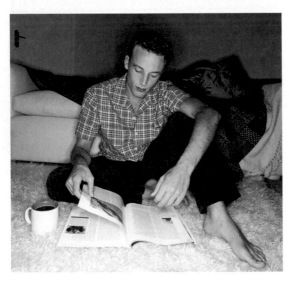

People can develop dependence on caffeine and experience withdrawal symptoms such as headaches if they discontinue caffeine intake.

Higher dose levels (about 500 mg) are needed to affect the autonomic centers of the brain, and heart rate and respiration can in-crease at this dose. The direct effect on the cardiovascular system is in opposition to the effects mediated by the autonomic centers. Caffeine acts directly on the vascular muscles to cause dilation, whereas stimulation of the autonomic centers results in constriction of blood vessels. Usually dilation occurs, but in the brain the blood vessels are constricted, and this constriction might be the basis for caffeine's ability to reduce migraine headaches.

The opposing effects of caffeine, directly on the heart and indirectly through effects on the medulla, make it very difficult to predict the results of normal (that is, less than 500 mg) caffeine intake. At higher levels, the heart rate increases, and continued use of large amounts of caffeine can produce an irregular heartbeat in some individuals.

The basal metabolic rate might be increased slightly (10 percent) in chronic caffeine users, because 500 mg has frequently been shown to have this effect. This action probably combines with the stimulant effects on skeletal muscles to increase physical work output and decrease fatigue after the use of caffeine.

Behavioral Effects

Stimulation A hundred years ago, French essayist Balzac spoke with feeling when describing the effects of coffee:

> It causes an admirable fever. It enters the brain like a bacchante. Upon its attack, imagination runs wild, bares itself, twists like a pythoness and in this paroxysm a poet enjoys the supreme possession of his faculties; but this is a drunkenness of thought as wine brings about a drunkenness of the body.[13]

In the original French, the description is even more stimulating and erotic. Unfortunately it does not refer to the effect most people receive from their morning cup of coffee. The hard research data are not so uniformly positive—the effects of caffeine depend on the difficulty of the task, the time of day, and to a great extent on how much caffeine the subject normally consumes. When regular users of high amounts of caffeine (more than 300 mg/day, the equivalent of three cups of brewed coffee) were tested on a variety of study-related mental tasks without caffeine, they performed more poorly than did users of low amounts, perhaps because of withdrawal effects. Although their performance was improved after being given caffeine, they still performed more poorly on several of the tasks than did users of low amounts. It seems as though the beneficial short-term effects can be offset by the effects of tolerance and dependence in regular users.[15] High levels of caffeine consumption among college students have been associated with lower academic performance.[16]

There is considerable evidence that 200 to 300 mg of caffeine will partially offset fatigue-induced decrement in the performance of motor tasks. Like the amphetamines, but to a much smaller degree, caffeine prolongs the amount of time an individual can perform physically exhausting work.

Headache Caffeine's vasoconstricitve effects are considered to be responsible for the drug's ability to relieve migraine headaches. However, a study of nonmigraine headache pain found that

Drugs in Depth

Caffeine and Panic Attacks

The National Institute of Mental Health (NIMH) has reported that caffeine can precipitate full-blown *panic attacks* in some people.[14] Panic attacks are not common but can be very debilitating for those who suffer them. They consist of sudden, irrational feelings of doom, sometimes accompanied by choking, sweating, heart palpitations, and other symptoms.

In an experiment conducted at NIMH laboratories in Maryland, a group of people who had previously suffered panic attacks were given 480 mg caffeine, equivalent to about five cups of brewed coffee. Panic attacks were precipitated in almost half of those people. In a group of 14 people who had never before experienced a panic attack, two suffered an attack after receiving 720 mg caffeine.

The results are interesting from a scientific point of view not only because they reveal individual differences in susceptibility to panic but also because of the possible implications for an understanding of the biochemistry of panic disorders. The experiment may also have more immediate and practical implications in that, if a person does experience a panic attack, caffeine consumption should be looked at as a possible cause.

caffeine reduced headache pain, even in individuals who normally consumed little or no caffeine (in other words, not only headaches resulting from caffeine withdrawal).[17] As for migraine headaches, in 1998, the FDA allowed the relabeling of extra-strength Excedrine, which contains 65 mg caffeine, for over-the-counter use as "Excedrine Migraine."

Hyperactivity Many studies have looked at the effect of caffeine on the behavior of children diagnosed with attention deficit hyperactivity disorder, and the results have been inconsistent. There is some indication that relatively high doses of caffeine may decrease hyperactivity, though not as well as methylphenidate[18] (see Chapter 6).

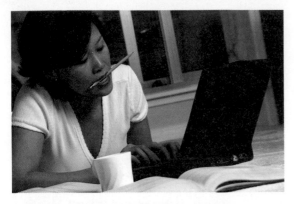

The primary behavioral effect of caffeine is stimulation, although high levels of caffeine consumption among college students have been associated with lower academic performance.

Sobering Up The television ads tell you—make coffee that "one last drink for the road," but little evidence supports the value of this. Caffeine will not lower blood alcohol concentration, but it might arouse the drinker. As they say—put coffee in a sleepy drunk and you get a wide-awake drunk. This might be more dangerous than if the drunk had been left to sleep it off.

Causes for Concern

Caffeine is one of those drugs that seem to always be in trouble. It's always suspected of doing bad things. Because it is probably the most widely used psychoactive drug in the world (it's acceptable to those in most Judeo-Christian as well as Islamic traditions), it is understandable that it would elicit both good and bad reports. Although there is not yet clear evidence that moderate caffeine consumption is dangerous, the scientific literature has investigated the possible effects of caffeine in cancer, benign breast disease, reproduction, and heart disease. Part of the problem in knowing for certain about some of these things is that epidemiological research on caffeine consumption is difficult to do well, because of the many sources of caffeine and the variability of caffeine content in coffee. Coffee drinkers also tend to smoke more, for example, so the statistics have to correct for smoking behavior.

Cancer

In the early 1980s, an increased risk of pancreatic cancers was reported among coffee drinkers. However, studies since then have criticized procedural flaws in that report and have found no evidence of such a link. The 1984 American Cancer Society nutritional guidelines indicated there is no reason to consider caffeine a risk factor in human cancer.

Reproductive Effects

Although studies in pregnant mice have indicated that large doses of caffeine can produce skeletal abnormalities in the pups, studies on humans have not found a relationship between caffeine and birth defects. However, studies do strongly suggest that consumption of more than 300 mg of caffeine per day by a woman can reduce her chances of becoming pregnant, increase the chances of spontaneous abortion (miscarriage), and slow the growth of the fetus so that the baby weighs less than normal at birth.[19] The most controversial of these findings has been the reported increase in spontaneous abortion, which is found in some studies, but not in others. The best advice for a woman who wants to become pregnant, stay pregnant, and produce a strong, healthy baby is to avoid caffeine, alcohol, tobacco, and any other drug that is not absolutely necessary for her health.

Heart Disease

There are many reasons for believing that caffeine might increase the risk of heart attacks, including the fact that it increases heart rate and blood pressure. Until recently, about as many studies found no relationship between caffeine use and heart attacks as did studies that found such a relationship. One very interesting report used an unusual approach. Rather than ask people who had just had heart attacks about their prior caffeine consumption and compare them with people who were hospitalized for another ailment (the typical retrospective study), this study began in 1948 to track male medical students enrolled in the Johns Hopkins Medical School.[20] More than 1,000 of these students were followed for 20 years or more after graduation and were periodically asked about various habits, including drinking, smoking, and coffee consumption. Thus, this was a prospective study, to see which of these habits might predict future health problems. Those who drank five or more cups per day were about 2.5 times as likely as nondrinkers to suffer from coronary heart disease. This result and recent indications that coffee drinking can increase blood cholesterol levels stimulated more research, including a large-scale retrospective study, which reported that the incidence of nonfatal heart attacks in men under 55 years old was directly related to the amount of coffee consumed, among both smokers and nonsmokers. Those drinking five or more cups per day were about twice as likely to suffer a heart attack as those who drank no coffee.[21]

The best research, then, gives a strong suggestion that caffeine can increase the risk of heart attacks. This is of special concern to those with other risk factors (e.g., smoking, family history of heart disease, obesity, high blood pressure, and high cholesterol levels).

Caffeinism

Caffeine is not terribly toxic, and overdose deaths are extremely rare. An estimated 10 g (equivalent to 100 cups of coffee) would be required to cause death from oral caffeine taken by mouth. Death is produced by convulsions, which lead to respiratory arrest.

However, **caffeinism** (excessive use of caffeine) can cause a variety of unpleasant symptoms, and because of caffeine's domesticated social status it might be overlooked as the cause. For example, nervousness, irritability, tremulousness, muscle twitching, insomnia, flushed appearance, and elevated temperature

can all result from excessive caffeine use. There can also be palpitations, heart arrhythmias, and gastrointestinal disturbances. In several cases in which serious disease has been suspected, the symptoms have miraculously improved when coffee was restricted.

Summary

- The ancient plants coffee, tea, and cacao contain caffeine and two related xanthines.
- Caffeine is also contained in soft drinks and nonprescription medicines.
- Caffeine has a longer-lasting effect than many people realize.
- Caffeine exerts a stimulating action in several brain regions by blocking inhibitory receptors for adenosine.
- In regular caffeine users, headache, fatigue, or depression can develop if caffeine use is stopped.
- Caffeine is capable of reversing the effects of fatigue on both mental and physical tasks, but it might not be able to improve the performance of a well-rested individual, particularly on complex tasks.
- Heavy caffeine use during pregnancy is not advisable.
- Daily use of large amounts of caffeine increases the risk of heart attack.
- Excessive caffeine consumption, referred to as caffeinism, can produce a panic reaction.

Review Questions

1. What role did the American Revolution and alcohol prohibition play in influencing American coffee consumption?
2. What are the differences among black tea, green tea, and oolong?

caffeinism: excessive use of caffeine.

3. What are the two xanthines contained in tea and chocolate, besides caffeine?

4. Rank the caffeine content of a cup of brewed coffee, a cup of tea, a chocolate bar, and a 12-ounce serving of Coca-Cola.

5. How does caffeine interact with adenosine receptors?

6. What are some of the behavioral and physiological effects of excessive caffeine consumption?

7. Describe the effects of caffeine on migraine headaches, caffeine-withdrawal headaches, and other headaches.

8. What are the typical symptoms associated with caffeine withdrawal?

9. What are three possible ways in which caffeine use by a woman might interfere with reproduction?

10. What is the relationship between caffeine and panic attacks?

References

1. Uribe Compuzano, A. *Brown Gold.* New York: Random House, 1954.

2. Meyer, H. *Old English Coffee Houses.* Emmaus, PA: Rodale Press, 1954.

3. U.S. Department of Commerce: *Statistical Abstract of the United States.* Washington, DC: U.S. Government Printing Office, 2006.

4. Pressler, M.W. "Another Cup? Coffee Bars Just Keep Spilling Across the Landscape." *Washington Post,* May 23, 2004.

5. Prial, F.J. "Secrets of a Chocoholic." *The New York Times,* May 16, 1979.

6. Huisking, C.L. *Herbs to Hormones.* Essex, CT: Pequot Press, 1968.

7. Quertemont, E., & K.A. Grant. "Discriminative Stimulus Effects of Ethanol: Lack of Interaction with Taurine." *Behavioural Pharmacology* 15 (2004), pp. 495–501.

8. Patton, C., & D. Beer. "Caffeine: The Forgotten Variable." *International Journal of Psychiatry in Clinical Practice* 5 (2001), pp. 231–36.

9. Juliano, L.M., & R.R. Griffiths. "A Critical Review of Caffeine Withdrawal: Empirical Validation of Symptoms and Signs, Incidence, Severity, and Associated Features." *Psychopharmacology* 176 (2004), pp. 1–29.

10. Griffiths, R.R., and others. "Human Coffee Drinking: Reinforcing and Physical Dependence Producing Effects of Caffeine." *J Pharmacol Exp Ther* 239 (1986), pp. 416–25.

11. Hughes, J.R., and others. "Should Caffeine Abuse, Dependence, or Withdrawal Be Added to DSM-IV and ICD-10?" *American Journal of Psychiatry* 149 (1992), p. 33.

12. Julien, R.M. *A Primer of Drug Action,* 10th ed. New York: Worth, 2005.

13. Mickel, E.J. *The Artificial Paradises in French Literature.* Chapel Hill, NC: University of North Carolina Press, 1969 (Free translation from French) 1969.

14. Stewart, S.A. "Caffeine Can Push the Panic Button." *USA Today,* October 23, 1985.

15. Mitchell, P.J., & J.R. Redman. "Effects of Caffeine, Time of Day, and User History on Study-Related Performance." *Psychopharmacology (Berl)* 109 (1992), p. 121.

16. Gilliland, K., & D. Andress. "Ad Lib Caffeine Consumption, Symptoms of Caffeinism, and Academic Performance." *American Journal of Psychiatry* 138, no. 4 (1981), pp. 512–14.

17. Ward, N., and others. "The Analgesic Effects of Caffeine in Headache." *Pain* 44 (1991), pp. 151–55.

18. Leon, M.R. "Effects of Caffeine on Cognitive, Psychomotor, and Affective Performance of Children with Attention Deficit/Hyperactivity Disorder." *Journal of Attention Disorders* 4 (2000), pp. 27–47.

19. "Statement on the reproductive effects of caffeine." UK Food Standards Agency, 2001. Retrieved from www.food.gov.uk/science/ouradvisors/toxicity/statements/cotstatements2001/caffeine (November, 2004).

20. LaCroix, A.Z., and others. "Coffee Consumption and the Incidence of Coronary Heart Disease." *New England Journal of Medicine* 315 (1986), pp. 977–82.

21. Rosenberg, L., and others. "Coffee Drinking and Nonfatal Myocardial Infarction in Men Under 55 Years of Age." *American Journal of Epidemiology* 128 (1988), pp. 570–78.

Check Yourself

How Much Caffeine Do You Consume?

How many different products do you use that contain caffeine (Review Tables 11.1 to 11.3)? Keep a complete record of your own intake of coffee, tea, soft drinks, and so on for a typical three-day period (72 hours). From that record, estimate as closely as you can your total caffeine intake in milligrams. If you regularly consume 300 mg or more per day, you might ask yourself if caffeine is interfering with your sleep, work, or studying.

12 Dietary Supplements and Over-the-Counter Drugs

Objectives

When you have finished this chapter, you should be able to:

- **Explain the legal distinction between drugs and dietary supplements, particularly with regard to health-related claims.**

- **Understand the implications of the 1994 Dietary Supplement Health and Education Act.**

- **Recognize Saint-John's-wort, SAMe, and ginkgo biloba as dietary supplements intended to have psychoactive effects.**

- **Explain the concepts behind the terms GRAS and GRAE.**

- **Name the only active ingredient allowed in OTC stimulants.**

- **Explain the risks of PPA and ephedra and describe how their removal from the market impacted OTC products promoted for weight loss.**

- **Name the primary ingredient in OTC sleep aids.**

- **Describe the benefits and dangers of aspirin.**

- **Explain what is meant by NSAID and give some examples.**

- **Name the four types of ingredients found in many OTC cold and allergy drugs and give a common example of each type.**

Dietary Supplements

When does "food" become a "drug"? When we think of typical food items, such as a loaf of bread or an apple, it seems unlikely that we would confuse those with drugs, such as a prescription antibiotic or illicit heroin. Both contain chemicals that interact with the body's ongoing physiology, in one case to provide nutrients, in the other to alter functioning in some way desired by the user. But a huge class of pills, capsules, liquids, and powders that look like drugs, and that many consumers think of and use in the same way as drugs, is legally classified as food products. This is very important to the consumer because of substantial differences in the way foods and drugs are regulated by the Food and Drug Administration (FDA). This distinction has been at the heart of an ongoing conflict between the FDA and various manufacturers of these "dietary supplements" over health-related claims.

To make the food versus drug issue more concrete, let's think about Saint-John's-wort (*Hypericum*). The plant is a perennial shrub with yellow flowers and, like many plants, a history of use as a folk remedy. An Internet search will find numerous references to Saint-John's-wort as a "natural remedy for depression," or "nature's Prozac," and suggestions that it can improve mood, reduce anxiety, and aid sleep. Many people take tablets or capsules

Online Learning Center Resources

www.mhhe.com/ksir12e

Visit our Online Learning Center (OLC) for access to these study aids and additional resources.

- Learning objectives
- Glossary flashcards
- Web activities and links
- Self-scoring chapter quiz
- Audio chapter summaries

containing Saint-John's-wort for these purposes. Food or drug? Sure sounds like a drug, right? But both the manufacturers of these products and the FDA have agreed that these products are not drugs, but foods, even though people take them not when they're hungry, but when they're seeking relief from depression, anxiety, or insomnia.

The Food, Drug and Cosmetic Act under which the FDA operates says a product "intended for use in the diagnosis, cure, mitigation, treatment or prevention of disease in man" is a drug. So, if the users and sellers of Saint-John's-wort intend it to be used to mitigate or treat depression, shouldn't it be considered a drug? Chapter 3 reported that when this whole process of regulating patent medicines began in 1906, the FDA was concerned about purity of the products and accurate *labeling* so that consumers would know what they were buying. Later, when issues of the accuracy of health claims arose, the FDA's primary focus was on the claims made on the label affixed to the product. A bottle of Saint-John's-wort tablets may look like a drug bottle, and the tablets may say "300 mg" and look like drug tablets, but if it was sold in the United States its label will include terms you don't expect to see on a drug product, such as "nutrition information" and "serving size," the kind of information you see on breakfast cereal packages. Also, the label will not claim that the product is good for treating depression or insomnia. If it did, it would legally be a drug and subject to FDA regulation.

Remember also from Chapter 3 that drug manufacturers have to demonstrate to the FDA, before marketing the drug, that the drug is (1) *safe* when used as intended, and (2) *effective* for its intended use. Since 1906, the FDA has also been concerned about the purity and safety of food products and ingredients, but not with efficacy. Food products contain some ingredients with known nutritional value, but other ingredients that may enhance flavor or simply provide bulk. Processed foods also contain ingredients that are simply preservatives—included to keep the product from going bad, but having no nutritional value. For many years, people have also taken "dietary supplements," such as vitamins and minerals, meant to ensure sufficient intake of these important chemicals in case they are insufficient in the diet. Ongoing controversy about how much of each vitamin is needed and how much is too much has led to the establishment of "recommended daily allowances," which are sometimes adjusted in response to industry pressure to raise them or medical research suggesting a need to limit them. Saint-John's-wort and a wide variety of other products are now sold as dietary supplements. Under this category, they need to be pure and they need to be safe, but the manufacturer doesn't have to show to the FDA or to anyone else that they provide any benefit, either nutritionally or as a treatment for disease.

If the "300 mg" tablet of Saint-John's-wort contains some amount of the plant, then it's accurately labeled. With a drug, we'd expect to know exactly how much of the active ingredient it contains, but with a dietary supplement derived from a plant (an "herbal" supplement), we might not even know what the active ingredient is, let alone how much is in the 300 mg tablet. It's possible that no amount of Saint-John's-wort is really effective (the research evidence on this is mixed, see below and Chapter 8), and also possible that the amount contained in a given pill is too small in any case. That's legal because the seller isn't directly making a health claim, so it doesn't have to demonstrate effectiveness.

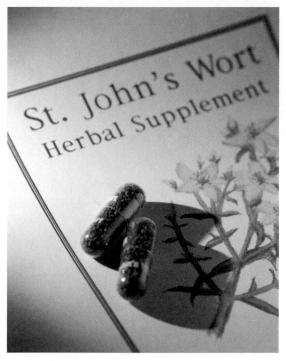

Dietary supplements such as St.-John's-wort are not regulated as over-the-counter drugs. They do not have to be shown to be effective, and the amount of presumed active ingredient varies widely.

In the early 1990s, the FDA had become concerned about two things. One was claims such as "heart healthy" being put on food products, and the other was the rapidly growing market in dietary supplements, fueled partly by Americans interested in healthful nutrition to prevent disease and partly by the emergence of several aggressive multilevel marketing organizations that recruited individuals to become distributors, offering both "wholesale" prices for their own products and the potential of high profits on sales to their friends and neighbors. In 1993 the FDA took two important actions. One was the approval, after careful study, of seven health claims that food manufacturers could use if their products met certain requirements (for example, foods high in calcium can say they reduce the risk of osteoporosis, and foods low in sodium can say

they reduce the risk of high blood pressure). In doing so, the FDA also made it clear it was not going to allow other unapproved health claims on foods. The second important action in 1993 was the release of the publication "Unsubstantiated Claims and Documented Health Hazards in the Dietary Supplement Marketplace." This document, as well as specific enforcement actions against products the FDA considered were violating the existing law, led to a rapid and strong reaction on the part of the nutritional supplement industry. Raising fears among customers that the federal government would soon require them to get a doctor's prescription before they could purchase nutritional supplements, and using the multilevel marketing networks to generate a widespread grass-roots campaign, the dietary supplement industry pressured Congress to clarify the FDA's role. In 1994, both houses of Congress unanimously passed the Dietary Supplement Health and Education Act (DSHEA).

The DSHEA made several important changes. First, it redefined dietary supplements to include a variety of substances such as herbs, amino acids, and concentrates and extracts of herbs. Previously, the FDA had only allowed "essential nutrients," such as vitamins and minerals that were known to be required in a healthy diet, to be sold as dietary supplements in tablet, capsule, or liquid form. Second, the definition of safety was altered so that the FDA could declare a product to be "adulterated" only if it presents "a significant or unreasonable risk of illness or injury." Any ingredient being sold at the time the DSHEA was passed was presumed not to meet this criterion unless the FDA could demonstrate its risk. Any new ingredient introduced after 1994 would need to be accompanied by some evidence that it would not present a significant or unreasonable risk. Previously, an ingredient was not supposed to be sold until after the FDA reviewed it and allowed it to be included on the "generally recognized as safe" list. Third, while a dietary supplement still cannot claim to be a cure or treatment for a disorder, statements can be made indicating the supplement has a beneficial effect on some structure or function of the body, or on "well being." The sellers do not have to prove these claims, as they would for a drug, but they have to provide supporting evidence that the claims are not false or misleading. In other words, if there is some indication that the statement is possibly true, and some that it might not be true, then the information can be included because the evidence does not indicate the statement is clearly false and misleading. Finally, products running such statements must also include the following: "This statement has not been evaluated by the Food and Drug Administration. This product is not intended to diagnose, treat, cure, or prevent any disease."

The result of this 1994 law was that dietary supplement manufacturers were now free to market a wide variety of products without fear that the FDA would consider them to be drugs, requiring solid premarketing evidence of both safety and effectiveness. The already growing dietary supplement market expanded rapidly from an estimated total of $3.5 billion in 1992 to $11 billion in 1995, and by 2003 it was estimated at $19 billion, about the same size as the market for over-the-counter (OTC) drugs such as aspirin and cough and cold remedies.[1]

Was the DSHEA a boon or a threat to consumers? On one hand, consumers now had available a wider variety of products. However, critics say more regulation is needed. In 1994, the FDA first publicized serious concerns about products containing *ephedra* (see Chapter 6). Many of these products were used by people seeking to control their weight. Ten years later, in 2004, after the widely publicized death of baseball pitcher Steve Bechler, the FDA declared that products containing *ephedra* did pose significant and unreasonable risk and therefore were not to be sold. That it took 10 years to accomplish this action and that it was up to the FDA to compile evidence supporting the risks are indicators that the burden of proof might have swung too far away from the sellers

and onto the FDA. In late 2003, Senate hearings were held on whether the FDA needed more authority or simply needed more resources to implement the authority allowed it under the DSHEA, but no action was taken.

Consumer Reports magazine has published a list of dietary supplements that it considers to be potentially dangerous to consumers (see Table 12.1). The FDA has taken regulatory action against some of these (shown in the table), but most remain on the market unless or until the FDA can develop clear evidence that they present "a significant or unreasonable risk of illness or injury."

Some Psychoactive Dietary Supplements

Saint-John's-wort

Saint-John's-wort (botanical name *Hypericum perforatum*) has been used for centuries and was once known as "the devil's scourge" because it was supposed to prevent possession by demons. In recent years its psychoactive uses have included the treatment of both anxiety and depression. There is limited evidence on the effectiveness of Saint-John's-wort in the treatment of anxiety, but several studies have indicated some usefulness in treating depression. One summary analysis of 23 clinical trials with daily *Hypericum* doses from 300 to 1,000 mg found it to be superior to a placebo and about as effective as tricyclic antidepressants.[2] However, a careful large-scale study reported in 2001 found no benefit in using Saint-John's-wort to treat depression.[3]

The FDA has raised concerns about Saint-John's-wort interacting with various prescription drugs (see Chapter 5), so people using it should notify their physicians.

SAMe

S-adenosyl-L-methionine is a naturally occurring substance found in the body. It is an active

Table 12.1
Twelve Supplements to Avoid

Name (Also known as)	Dangers	Regulatory Actions
DEFINITELY HAZARDOUS *Documented Organ Failure and Known Carcinogenic Properties*		
Aristolochic acid (*Aristolochia,* birthwort, snakeroot, snakeweed, sangree root, sangrel, serpentary, serpentaria; *asarum canadense,* wild ginger). Can be an ingredient in Chinese herbal products labeled fang ji, mu tong, ma dou ling, and mu xiang. Can be an unlabeled substitute for other herbs, including akebia, asarum, clematis, cocculus, stephania, and vladimiria species.	Potent human carcinogen; kidney failure, sometimes requiring transplant; deaths reported.	FDA warning to consumers and industry and import alert, in April 2001. Banned in 7 European countries and Egypt, Japan, and Venezuela.
VERY LIKELY HAZARDOUS *Banned in Other Countries, FDA Warning, or Adverse Effects in Studies*		
Comfrey (*Symphytum* officinale, ass ear, black root, blackwort, bruisewort, consolidae radix, consound, gum plant, healing herb, knitback, knitbone, salsify, slippery root, symphytum radix, wallwort)	Abnormal liver function or damage, often irreversible; deaths reported.	FDA advised industry to remove from market in July 2001.
Androstenedione (*4-androstene-3,* 17-dione, andro, androstene)	Increased cancer risk, decrease in HDL cholesterol.	FDA warned 23 companies to stop manufacturing, marketing, and distributing in March 2004. Banned by athletic associations.
Chaparral (*Larrea divaricata,* creosote bush, greasewood, hediondilla, jarilla, larreastat)	Abnormal liver function or damage, often irreversible; deaths reported.	FDA warning to consumers in December 1992.
Germander (*Teucrium chamaedrys,* wall germander, wild germander)	Abnormal liver function or damage, often irreversible; deaths reported.	Banned in France and Germany.
Kava (*Piper methysticum,* ava, awa, gea, gi, intoxicating pepper, kao, kavain, kawa-pfeffer, kew, long pepper, malohu, maluk, meruk, milik, rauschpfeffer, sakau, tonga, wurzelstock, yagona, yangona)	Abnormal liver function or damage, occasionally irreversible; deaths reported.	FDA warning to consumers in March 2002. Banned in Canada, Germany, Singapore, South Africa, and Switzerland.

continued

form of the amino acid methionine, and it acts as a "methyl donor" in a variety of biochemical pathways. (A methyl group consists of one carbon and three hydrogen atoms.) As long ago as the 1970s, SAMe was tested in Italy for its effectiveness as an antidepressant, and a recent summary analysis found that SAMe was more effective than a placebo, and apparently it is no less effective than tricyclic antidepressants.[4] Less research is available on SAMe for this use than for Saint-John's-wort. Researchers continue to investigate the possibility that, by combining SAMe with approved antidepressants, a more rapid remission of symptoms can be achieved.

Table 12.1
Twelve Supplements to Avoid—*concluded*

Name (Also known as)	Dangers	Regulatory Actions
LIKELY HAZARDOUS *Adverse-Event Reports or Theoretical Risks*		
Bitter orange (*Citrus aurantium,* green orange, kijitsu, neroli oil, Seville orange, shangzhou zhiqiao, sour orange, zhi oiao, zhi xhi)	High blood pressure; increased risk of heart arrythmias, heart attack, stroke.	None
Organ/glandular extracts (brain/adrenal/pituitary/placenta/other gland "substance" or "concentrate")	Theoretical risk of mad cow disease, particularly from brain extracts.	FDA banned high-risk bovine materials from older cows in foods and supplements in January 2004. (High-risk parts from cows under 30 months still permitted.) Banned in France and Switzerland.
Lobelia (*Lobelia inflata,* asthma weed, bladderpod, emetic herb, gagroot, lobelie, indian tobacco, pukeweed, vomit wort, wild tobacco)	Breathing difficulty, rapid heartbeat, low blood pressure, diarrhea, dizziness, tremors; possible deaths reported.	Banned in Bangladesh and Italy.
Pennyroyal oil (*Hedeoma pulegioides,* lurk-in-the-ditch, mosquito plant, piliolerial, pudding grass, pulegium, run-by-the-ground, squaw balm, squawmint, stinking balm, tickweed)	Liver and kidney failure, nerve damage, convulsions, abdominal tenderness, burning of the throat; deaths reported.	None
Scullcap (*Scutellaria lateriflora,* blue pimpernel, helmet flower, hoodwort, mad weed, mad-dog herb, mad-dog weed, quaker bonnet, scutelluria, skullcap)	Abnormal liver function or damage.	None
Yohimbe (*Pausinystalia yohimbe,* johimbi, yohimbehe, yohimbine)	Change in blood pressure, heart arrythmias, respiratory depression, heart attack: deaths reported.	None

Source: "Dietary Supplements" © 2004 by Consumers Union of U.S., Inc. Yonkers, NY 10703-1057, a nonprofit organization. Reprinted with permission from the May 2005 posting of ConsumerReports.org® for educational purposes only.

No commercial use or reproduction permitted. www.ConsumerReports.org®.

Ginkgo Biloba

Extracts from the leaves of the ginkgo biloba tree have a long history of medical use in China. It is not clear which of the identified ingredients in ginkgo are the active agents, and it is not completely clear how effective it is for a variety of uses for which it has been proposed. The substance does reduce blood clotting, so it has been proposed as a blood thinner, which improves circulation. However, combining ginkgo with aspirin, which also reduces clotting, could be dangerous. The most interesting suggestion is that ginkgo biloba extract might

Drugs in the Media

Natural Male Enhancement?

Television ads for Enzyte or some other brand of "natural male enhancement" don't explain exactly what that means, but the not-so-subtle implication is that the guy who takes this is going to improve his sex life. Following on the success of prescription erectile-dysfunction drugs such as Viagra and Cialis, the makers of these "male enhancement" pills are perhaps hoping that consumers will think that their products are nonprescription versions of the same thing. An unwary shopper might even confuse the term *enhancement* with *enlargement*. Enzyte's Web site (www.enzyte.com) explains that the product will not alter the size or shape of the penis, but that it contains a mixture of ingredients "designed to improve the quality of men's erections." Notice that it doesn't actually claim to be effective in doing so, only that it was designed to do that. The pills contain small amounts of several plant extracts, most notably *Tribulus terrestris, Panax ginseng,* and *ginkgo biloba.* Controlled clinical studies provide limited evidence

that *ginseng* (widely available in many products) might be helpful in treating men with erectile dysfunction, though it is not clear what value this would have for men with otherwise normal penile function. The clinical results for *ginkgo* have been mixed, but the only controlled study showed no effect. Controlled clinical studies have not been done with *Tribulus terrestris,* which proponents claim will enhance the production of the steroid DHEA, a form of andosterone.[6] In other words, the existing evidence would be far from enough to allow the FDA to approve this product as a drug to treat any type of sexual dysfunction.

This is just one example of the kinds of products sold as *dietary supplements.* These tablets and capsules are treated by the FDA more like foods than drugs, and as such there is no requirement that the manufacturer demonstrate the effectiveness of the products. The label for Enzyte includes the standard disclaimer that "these statements have not been evaluated by the Food and Drug Administration."

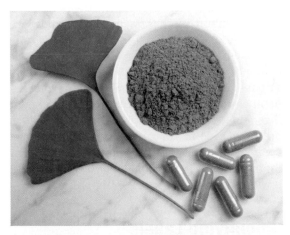

Evidence suggests that a compound in ginkgo acts as a blood thinner; it may be dangerous for people to take ginkgo supplements in combination with aspirin or other drugs that also reduce clotting.

ginkgo in both normal and memory-impaired older adults. Overall, the results have found slight improvements for some people, but not a reliable effect that would be really useful.[5]

Over-the-Counter Drugs

Over-the-counter drugs are those that are self-prescribed and self-administered for the relief of symptoms of self-diagnosed illnesses. The FDA estimates that consumers self-treat four times more health problems than doctors treat, often using OTC drugs.

Americans spend over $18 billion a year on OTC products.[1] That's not as much as we spend on prescription drugs, alcohol, cigarettes, or illicit cocaine, but it's enough to keep several OTC drug manufacturers locked in fierce competition for those sales. The two biggest markets are for aspirinlike analgesics and for the collection of cough, cold, and flu products.

improve memory in Alzheimer's patients, due to its presumed ability to increase blood circulation in the brain. Several studies have tested

Do we really need all these nonprescription tablets, capsules, liquids, and creams? How much of what we buy is based on advertising hype, and how much is based on sound decisions about our health? How are we as consumers to know the difference? The FDA is trying to help us with these decisions.

FDA Regulation of OTC Products

The 1962 Kefauver-Harris amendment required that all drugs be evaluated for both safety and efficacy. The FDA was not only to set up criteria for new drugs entering the market but also to establish a procedure for reviewing all the OTC drugs already on the market. At first glance this seemed an impossible task, because there were between 250,000 and 300,000 products already being sold (no one knew for sure how many). In addition, each product was likely to change its ingredients without warning. The FDA made the decision not to study individual products but to review each active ingredient. Many competing brands contain the same ingredients, so there are many fewer ingredients than products. The FDA divided OTC products into 26 classes and appointed an advisory panel for each class. Each panel was to look at the active ingredients contained in the products in its class, decide whether evidence indicated each ingredient was safe and effective for its purpose, and determine what claims could be made for that ingredient on the label. Several of the 26 classes of OTC drugs to be reviewed by the FDA included psychoactive ingredients: sedatives and sleep aids, analgesics, cold remedies and antitussives, antihistamines and allergy products, and stimulants.

Before the panel could begin work, some rules had to be laid down about what was meant by such terms as *safe* and *effective,* keeping in mind that no drug is entirely safe and that many might have only limited effectiveness. The FDA uses the acronym **GRAS** ("generally recognized as safe") to mean that, given the currently available information, people who are informed and qualified would agree that

the ingredient should be considered safe. "Safe" means "a low incidence of adverse reactions or significant side effects under adequate directions for use and warnings against unsafe use as well as low potential for harm which may result from abuse." Similar acronyms are used for two other important concepts: GRAE ("generally recognized as effective") and GRAHL ("generally recognized as honestly labeled").

> Effectiveness means a reasonable expectation that, in a significant proportion of the target population, the pharmacological effect of the drug, when used under adequate directions for use and warnings against unsafe use, will provide clinically significant relief of the type claimed.

The advisory panel was to rule on each active ingredient and decide whether the evidence indicates that the ingredient is both GRAS and GRAE, or failed on one or both criteria, or if further information was needed.

The overall result of this procedure can be seen by taking a trip to your neighborhood drugstore and looking at the lists of ingredients on medications of a given type. All the competing brands contain much the same few ingredients. In some classes, there might be only one approved active ingredient, meaning that all competing brands are essentially identical. The differences among them often are in the long list of other (inactive) ingredients (colorings, flavorings, etc.). The exact number of OTC products on the market is not known because they still come and go and change, but we do know that there are more than 100,000, and they contain fewer than 1,000 total active ingredients.

Simplifying Labels

Both the safety and effectiveness of OTC drugs depend greatly on consumers using them according to the directions and warnings on the label. To reduce confusion and make it more likely that consumers will be able to understand the labels, the FDA moved in 1997 to create uniform standards for labels, with minimum

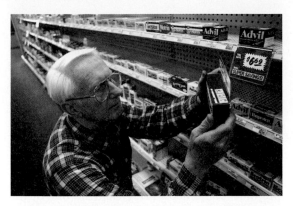

A shopper reads the label on an OTC medication.

print size, topics in a consistent order (active ingredients, directions for use, warnings), and bold, bulleted headings. One important change was to make the language clearer and more concise, avoiding medical terminology (e.g., "pulmonary" replaced by "lung"). This new, consistent approach to labeling has made it easier to compare products and their ingredients.

Over-the-Counter versus Prescription Drugs

The 1938 Food, Drug, and Cosmetic Act established a classification of drugs that would be available only by prescription. A drug is supposed to be permitted for OTC sale unless, because of potential toxicity or for other reasons (e.g., if it must be injected), it may be safely sold and used only under a prescription.

Sometimes the only difference between an OTC product and a prescription product is the greater amount of active ingredient in each prescription dose. More often, however, prescription drugs are chemicals that are unavailable OTC. Until the FDA began its OTC Drug Review process, once a new drug was approved for prescription sale it almost never became available OTC. Neither the FDA nor the manufacturers seemed to have much interest in switching drugs to OTC status. However, the FDA advisory panels that reviewed products in a given OTC category sometimes did more than

was required of them. In some cases, they recommended that higher doses be allowed in OTC preparations—and as a result we can now buy higher-strength OTC antihistamines. And in several cases the suggestion was that previous prescription-only ingredients, such as ibuprofen, be sold OTC.

Between 1972 and 1992, 20 ingredients were switched to OTC status. Then the FDA established the Nonprescription Drug Advisory Committee, which has an advisory role regarding all the drug categories and has helped move many more drugs from prescription to OTC. Drugs recently switched to OTC status include nicotine lozenges and the antihistamine loratadine.[7]

Some Psychoactive OTC Products

Stimulants

Stimulants, one of the original FDA categories, is one of the simplest categories. The FDA allows stimulants to be sold to "help restore mental alertness or wakefulness when experiencing fatigue or drowsiness." If it sounds like caffeine could do this, you're right! No Doz, a well-known product that has been around for years, has the tried-and-true formula: 100 mg of caffeine (about the equivalent of an average cup of brewed coffee). The recommended dose is two tablets initially, then one every three hours. Another well-known product, Vivarin, contains 200 mg of caffeine, and the initial dose is one tablet. Thus, although the packages look different and different companies make them, a smart consumer would choose between these two based on the price per milligram of caffeine. Or he or she could choose a less expensive store brand, or buy coffee (usually more expensive), or just get enough rest and save money. The labels warn against using these caffeine tablets with coffee, tea, or cola

GRAS: "generally recognized as safe."

drinks. The only active ingredient the FDA allows in OTC stimulants is caffeine.[8]

There is a reasonably brisk business in the semilegal field of selling caffeine tablets or capsules resembling prescription stimulants, such as the amphetamines. Many street purchases of speed turn out to contain caffeine as their major ingredient. It is, however, a violation of the controlled substances act to sell something that is represented to be a controlled substance. The FDA has ruled that products labeled as stimulants that contain anything other than caffeine as an active ingredient cannot be sold OTC. The FDA also outlawed OTC products, labeled for any purpose, that contained combinations of caffeine and ephedrine and has taken legal action against several mail-order distributors of such combination products.

Weight-Control Products

The original FDA list of OTC drug categories did not include appetite suppressants or a similar term. Apparently the FDA didn't think it would be dealing with such a product, because, at the time, the use of the prescription amphetamines for this purpose was under widespread attack. However, data were presented indicating that **phenylpropanolamine (PPA)** was safe and effective, and by the late 1970s several products were being sold that contained PPA as their only active ingredient. Some studies indicated that caffeine could potentiate the appetite-suppressing effect of PPA, and for a brief period during the early 1980s several of the products included both PPA and caffeine. After the 1983 FDA ruling prohibiting such combinations on the grounds that they might not be safe, all products returned to PPA only. The recommended dose for appetite suppression was 75 mg per day. There was some concern about the safety even of 75 mg doses, with the threat being increased blood pressure resulting from sympathetic stimulation. There was also some controversy about the effectiveness of PPA, given that its effect, as with most appetite suppressant drugs, is small and rather short-lived.

In November 2000, the FDA issued a Public Health Advisory on the safety of PPA, based on a new study showing that women taking PPA had an increased risk of hemorrhagic stroke (bleeding into the brain, usually a result of elevated blood pressure). The FDA requested that all drug companies discontinue marketing products containing PPA and that consumers not use any products containing PPA. Manufacturers and retailers responded quickly, and by early 2001 no remaining weight-control products contained PPA. Dexatrim, one of the most widely sold products previously based on PPA, was marketing a "natural" (dietary supplement) version containing various herbal products, including a small amount of *ma huang* (ephedra). Ephedra was found in several weight-control products until its ban in 2004. The current Dexatrim formula relies on "green tea extract." There are currently no approved OTC weight-control drugs, but many dietary supplements of dubious value.

The FDA has reviewed and ruled against several other products that have been advertised for weight control. Benzocaine-containing candies and gums were supposed to numb the tongue, reducing the sense of taste, but it was never shown that this was an effective way to reduce food intake. Starch blockers, which were supposed to interfere with the absorption of carbohydrates from starchy foods, have never been proved to do so. The FDA asked for all sales to stop until safety and effectiveness could be established, and the government seized the products after promoters failed to comply. Cholecystokinin (CCK) is a hormone that does decrease food intake when injected directly into the brains of experimental animals, but the chemical is quickly destroyed in the digestive tract if taken by mouth. Nevertheless, products claiming to include CCK have been advertised and sold, and the FDA has ordered this practice discontinued. Other unapproved products for weight reduction that have come under FDA scrutiny in recent years include DHEA, arginine and ornithine, spirulina, and glucomannan. None of these products has been demonstrated to be effective in weight loss, despite claims of "burning fat," "natural" weight loss, "Oriental weight-loss secret," and so on.

Sedatives and Sleep Aids

A few years ago the shelves contained a number of OTC sedative, or "calmative," preparations, including Quiet World and Compoz, which contained very small amounts of the acetylcholine receptor blocker *scopolamine* combined with the **antihistamine** methapyrilene. At the same time, sleep aids, such as Sleep-Eze and Sominex, contained just a bit more of the same two ingredients. The rationale for the scopolamine, particularly at these low doses, was under FDA investigation, but scopolamine had traditionally been included in many such medications in the past. Some antihistamines do produce a kind of sedated state and might produce drowsiness. The FDA advisory panel accepted methapyrilene but eventually rejected scopolamine. For a while all of these medications contained only methapyrilene. Then in 1979, it was reported that methapyrilene caused cancer in laboratory animals, so it was no longer GRAS. Next came pyrilamine maleate, then doxylamine succinate, and then *diphenhydramine,* all antihistamines. If you bought the same brand from one year to the next, you would get a different formulation each time. But if you bought several different brands at the same time, you stood a good chance of getting the same formulation in all of them.

The sedative category no longer exists for OTC products. One product, Miles Nervine, which went from being a sedative containing bromide salts to a calmative containing whatever they all contained each year, is now Miles Nervine Nighttime Sleep-Aid, containing 25 mg of diphenhydramine. Nytol is also a nighttime sleep aid containing the same ingredient. Sominex and Sleep-Eze are still around, and both contain diphenhydramine.

As we saw in Chapter 7, insomnia is perceived to be a bigger problem than it actually is for most people, and it is rare that medication

Targeting Prevention

The Medicine Chest

The family medicine chest is often a treasure trove of old tablets, capsules, liquids, and lozenges. Start digging around and see how many different OTC drugs you can find in yours. How old do you think some of them are? If any of them have expiration dates, have the dates passed?

Because formulations change from year to year, there's a good chance the medicines you now have are not the same as the ones being sold in the drugstore. Write down the formulations for a few of your medicine chest drugs. Then go to the drugstore and compare them with the current formulation for the same brand of product. Do you wonder if some of the old ingredients were removed because the FDA no longer considers them safe?

is really required. Antihistamines can induce drowsiness, but not very quickly. If you do feel the need to use these to get you to sleep more rapidly, take them at least 20 minutes before retiring. Their sedative effects are potentiated by alcohol, so it is not a good idea to take them after drinking.

Analgesics
People and Pain

Pain is such a little word for such a big experience. Most people have experienced pain of varying intensities, from mild to moderate to severe to excruciating. Two major classes of drugs are used to reduce pain or the awareness of pain, anesthetics and analgesics. Anesthetics (meaning "without sensibility") have this

phenylpropanolamine (PPA) (fen il pro pa *nole* a meen): until 2000, an active ingredient in OTC weight-control products.

antihistamine: the active ingredient in OTC sleep aids and cough/cold products.

effect by reducing all types of sensation or by blocking consciousness completely. The local anesthetics used in dentistry and the general anesthetics used in major surgery are examples of this class of agent. The other major class, the analgesics (meaning "without pain"), are compounds that reduce pain selectively without causing a loss of other sensations. The analgesics are divided into two groups. Opioids (see Chapter 13) are one group of analgesics, but this chapter primarily discusses the OTC internal analgesics, such as aspirin, acetaminophen, and ibuprofen.

Although pain itself is a complex psychological phenomenon, there have been attempts to classify different types of pain to develop a rational approach to its treatment. One classification divides pain into two types, depending on its place of origin. Visceral pain, such as intestinal cramps, arises from nonskeletal portions of the body; opioids are effective in reducing pain of this type. Somatic pain, arising from muscle or bone and typified by sprains, headaches, and arthritis, is reduced by salicylates (aspirin) and related products.

Pain is unlike other sensations in many ways, mostly because of nonspecific factors. The experience of pain varies with personality, gender, and time of day and is increased with fatigue, anxiety, fear, boredom, and anticipation of more pain. Because pain is very susceptible to nonspecific factors, studies have shown that about 35 percent of patients will receive satisfactory pain relief from a placebo.

Aspirin

More than 2,400 years ago the Greeks used extracts of willow and poplar bark in the treatment of pain, gout, and other illnesses. Aristotle commented on some of the clinical effects of similar preparations, and Galen made good use of these formulations. These remedies fell into disrepute, however, when St. Augustine declared that all diseases of Christians were the work of demons and thus a punishment from God. American Indians, unhampered by this enlightened attitude, used a tea brewed from willow bark to reduce fever. This remedy was not rediscovered in Europe until about 200 years ago, when an Englishman, the Reverend Edward Stone, prepared an extract of the bark and gave the same dose to 50 patients with varying illnesses and found the results to be "uniformly excellent." In the 19th century, the active ingredient in these preparations was isolated and identified as salicylic acid. In 1838, salicylic acid was synthesized, and in 1859 procedures were developed that made bulk production feasible. Salicylic acid and sodium salicylate were then used for many ills, especially arthritis.

In the giant Bayer Laboratories in Germany in the 1890s worked a chemist named Hoffmann. His father had a severe case of rheumatoid arthritis, and only salicylic acid seemed to help. The major difficulty then, as today, was that the drug caused great gastric discomfort. So great was the stomach upset and nausea that Hoffmann's father frequently preferred the pain of the arthritis. Hoffmann studied the salicylates to see if he could find one with the same therapeutic effect as salicylic acid but without the side effects.

In 1898, he synthesized **acetylsalicylic acid** and tried it on his father, who reported relief from pain without stomach upset. The compound was tested, patented, and released for sale in 1899 as *Aspirin*. Aspirin was a trademark name derived from the name *acetyl* and *spiralic acid* (the old name for salicylic acid).

The two famous compounds that the Bayer Laboratories in Germany were instrumental in introducing to the world are rapidly transformed in the body to their original form after absorption. Both heroin and aspirin were first synthesized in the Bayer Laboratories. Aspirin, either in the gastrointestinal tract or in the bloodstream, is converted to salicylic acid. Taken orally, aspirin is a more potent analgesic than salicylic acid, because aspirin irritates the stomach less and is thus absorbed more rapidly.

Aspirin was marketed for physicians and sold as a white powder in individual dosage

Taking Sides

Should There Be a Class of "Pharmacist-Recommended" Drugs?

Professional pharmacists may feel that they "get no respect" from some drug purchasers. Pharmacists are trained to be familiar with not only the prescription orders they fill but also with the ingredients and indications for OTC products. Most feel that consumers should take advantage of their advice on decisions to purchase and use OTC drugs. However, increasing numbers of people are purchasing their OTC medications in grocery and convenience stores, rather than in pharmacies. In addition, there is concern that, as more and more former prescription products are allowed for OTC sale, many people will simply assume that the drugs are safe and will use them carelessly. Pharmacists' organizations have proposed the establishment of "pharmacist-legend" drugs in the United States, similar to programs that have been used in England and Australia and that are being studied in Canada. Ibuprofen is one drug that Australian pharmacists keep "behind the counter"—no physician's prescription is required, but the pharmacist will dispense it only after giving some advice on its safe use. With such a system, perhaps other drugs (including oral contraceptives?) could become available without a physician's order.

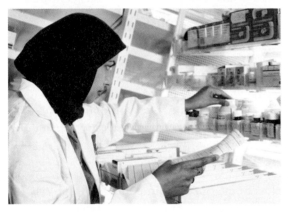

Should some over-the-counter drugs be kept behind the counter, where they can be dispensed only after a pharmacist has advised the consumer about safe use?

packets, available only by prescription. It was immediately popular worldwide, and the U.S. market became large enough that it was very soon manufactured in this country. In 1915, the 5 grain (325 mg) white tablet stamped "Bayer" first appeared, and, for the first time, aspirin became a nonprescription item. The Bayer Company was on its way. It had an effective drug that could be sold to the public and was known by one name—Aspirin—and the name was trademarked. Before February 1917, when the patent on Aspirin was to expire, Bayer started an advertising campaign to make it clear that there was only one Aspirin, and its first name was Bayer. Several companies started manufacturing and selling Aspirin as aspirin, and Bayer sued. What happened after this is a long story, but Bayer obviously lost, and aspirin is now a generic name.

Therapeutic Use Aspirin is truly a magnificent drug. It is also a drug with some serious side effects. Aspirin has three effects that are the primary basis for its clinical use. It is an analgesic that effectively blocks somatic pain in the mild-to-moderate range. Aspirin is also **antipyretic:** it reduces fever. Last but not least, aspirin is an **anti-inflammatory** agent: It reduces the swelling, inflammation, and soreness in an injured area. Its anti-inflammatory action is the basis for its extensive use in arthritis. It is difficult to find another drug that has this span of effects coupled with a relatively low toxicity. It

acetylsalicylic acid (a *see* **till sal i** *sill* **ick):** the chemical known as aspirin.
antipyretic (an tee pie *reh* **tick):** fever-reducing.
anti-inflammatory: reducing swelling and inflammation.

does, however, have side effects that pose problems for some people.

Aspirin is readily absorbed from the stomach but even faster from the intestine. Thus, anything that delays movement of the aspirin from the stomach should affect absorption time. The evidence is mixed on whether taking aspirin with a meal, which delays emptying of the stomach, increases the time before onset of action. It should, however, reduce the stomach irritation that sometimes accompanies aspirin use.

The *therapeutic* dose for aspirin is generally considered to be in the range of 600 to 1,000 mg. Most reports suggest that 300 mg is usually more effective than a placebo, whereas 600 mg is clearly even more effective. Many studies indicate that increasing the dose above that level does not increase aspirin's analgesic action, but some research indicates that 1,200 mg of aspirin provides greater relief than 600 mg. The maximum pain relief is experienced about one hour after taking aspirin, and the effect lasts for up to four hours.

At therapeutic doses, aspirin has analgesic actions that are fairly specific. First, and in marked contrast to narcotic analgesics, aspirin does not affect the impact of the anticipation of pain. It seems probable also that aspirin has its primary effect on the ability to withstand continuing pain. This, no doubt, is the basis for much of the self-medication with aspirin, because moderate, protracted pain is fairly common. Aspirin is especially effective against headache and musculoskeletal aches and pains, less effective for toothache and sore throat, and only slightly better than placebo in visceral pain, as well as in traumatic (acute) pain.

The antipyretic (fever-reducing) action of aspirin does not lower temperature in an individual with normal body temperature. It has this effect only if the person has a fever. The mechanism by which aspirin decreases body temperature is fairly well understood. It acts on the temperature-regulating area of the hypothalamus to increase heat loss through peripheral mechanisms. Heat loss is primarily increased by vasodilation of peripheral blood vessels and by increased perspiration. Heat production is not changed, but heat loss is facilitated so that body temperature can go down.

More aspirin has probably been used for its third major therapeutic use than for either of the other two. The anti-inflammatory action of the salicylates is the major basis for its use after muscle strains and in rheumatoid arthritis.

Most tablets, including aspirin, develop a harder external shell the longer they sit. This hardening effect does not change the amount of the active ingredient, but it does make the active ingredient less effective because disintegration time is increased by the hard exterior coating. Along the same line, moisture and heat speed the decomposition of acetylsalicylic acid into two other compounds: salicylic acid, which causes gastric distress, and acetic acid—vinegar. When the smell of vinegar is strong in your aspirin bottle, discard it.

Effects: Adverse and Otherwise *Aspirin increases bleeding time by inhibiting blood platelet aggregation.* This is not an insignificant effect. Two or three aspirins can double bleeding time, the time it takes for blood to clot, and the effect can last four to seven days. There's good and bad in the anticoagulant effect of aspirin. Its use before surgery can help prevent blood clots from appearing in patients at high risk for clot formation. For many surgical patients, however, facilitation of blood clotting is desirable, and the general rule is no aspirin for 7 to 10 days before surgery.

Aspirin will induce gastrointestinal bleeding in about 70 percent of normal subjects. In most cases, this is only about 5 ml per day, but that is five times the normal loss. In some people the blood loss can be great enough to cause anemia. The basis for this effect is not clear but is believed to be a direct eroding by the aspirin tablets of the gastric mucosa. Aspirin can be deadly with severe stomach ulcers. For the rest of us, the rule is clear: drink lots of water when you take aspirin or, better yet, crush the tablets and drink them in orange juice or other liquid.

The anticoagulant effect of aspirin has a potentially beneficial effect in preventing heart attacks and strokes. Either can be brought on by a blood clot becoming lodged in a narrowed or hardened blood vessel. Several studies have demonstrated that patients who are at high risk for these problems can help to prevent both strokes and heart attacks by taking a small dose of aspirin daily. Many doctors are recommending that all their patients over a certain age begin taking low-dose aspirin (82 mg is typical) regularly, even though the available research doesn't provide clear evidence for any benefit for low-risk patients.[9]

In the early 1980s, concern increased about the relationship of aspirin use to *Reye's syndrome,* a rare disease (fewer than 200 cases per year in the United States). Almost all of the cases occur in people under the age of 20, usually after they have had a viral infection, such as influenza or chicken pox. The children begin vomiting continuously; then they might become disoriented, undergo personality changes, shout, or become lethargic. Some enter comas, and some of those either die or suffer permanent brain damage. The overall mortality rate from Reye's syndrome is about 25 percent.

No one knows what causes Reye's, and it isn't believed to be caused by aspirin. However, data suggest the disease is more likely to occur in children who have been given aspirin during a preceding illness. In late 1984, the results of a Centers for Disease Control and Prevention pilot study were released, indicating that the use of aspirin can increase the risk of Reye's syndrome as much as 25 times. In 1985, makers of all aspirin products were asked to put warning labels on their packages. These labels recommend that you consult a physician before giving aspirin to children or teenagers with chicken pox or flu.

In early 1986, it was reported that fewer parents in Michigan were giving aspirin to children for colds and influenza, and the incidence of Reye's syndrome had also decreased in Michigan. The Michigan study lends further strength to the relationship between aspirin use and Reye's syndrome. No one under the age of 20 should use aspirin in treating chicken pox, influenza, or even what might be suspected to be a common cold.

Aspirin has long been associated with a large number of accidental poisonings of children, as well as with suicide attempts. It has now been joined on the DAWN lists (see Chapter 2) by its relatives acetaminophen and ibuprofen. Together, these drugs were mentioned in 750 drug-related deaths in the 2003 DAWN data.

Mechanism of Action Aspirin is now believed to have both a central and a peripheral analgesic effect. The central effect is not clear, but the peripheral effect is well on its way to being understood; it is now known that aspirin modifies the *cause* of pain.

Prostaglandins are local hormones that are manufactured and released when cell membranes are distorted or damaged—that is, injured. The prostaglandins then act on the endings of the neurons that mediate pain in the injured areas. The prostaglandins sensitize the neurons to mechanical stimulation and to stimulation by two other local hormones, histamine and bradykinin, which are more slowly released from the damaged tissue. Aspirin blocks the synthesis of the prostaglandins by inhibiting two forms of the cyclooxygenase enzyme (COX-1 and COX-2).

The antipyretic action has also been spelled out: a specific prostaglandin acts on the anterior hypothalamus to decrease heat dissipation through the normal procedures of sweating and dilation of peripheral blood vessels. Aspirin blocks the synthesis of this prostaglandin in the anterior hypothalamus, and this is followed by increased heat loss.

Acetaminophen

There are two related analgesic compounds: *phenacetin* and **acetaminophen.** Phenacetin was

> **acetaminophen (a seet a min o fen):** an aspirinlike analgesic and antipyretic.

sold for many years in combination with aspirin and caffeine in the "APC" tablets that fought headache pain "three ways." Phenacetin has been around since 1887 and had long been suspected of causing kidney lesions and dysfunction. In 1964, the FDA required a warning on all products containing phenacetin, which limited their use to 10 days because the phenacetin might damage the kidneys. Phenacetin has now gone to the land of dead drugs: The review panel considered it not to be GRAS.

The only real question is why all these drugs took so long to get off the market. Phenacetin was known to be rapidly converted to acetaminophen, which was the primary active agent. Acetaminophen is equipotent with aspirin in its analgesic and antipyretic effects. Acetaminophen causes less gastric bleeding than aspirin, but it is also less useful as an anti-inflammatory drug for arthritis.

Acetaminophen has been marketed as an OTC analgesic since 1955, but it was the big advertising pushes in the 1970s for two brand-name products, Tylenol and Datril, that brought acetaminophen into the big time. Acetaminophen was advertised as having most of the good points of "that other pain reliever" and many fewer disadvantages. To a degree this is probably true: if only analgesia and fever reduction are desired, acetaminophen might be safer than aspirin *as long as dosage limits are carefully observed.* Overuse of acetaminophen can cause serious liver disorders. Acetaminophen has now surpassed aspirin for both drug-related emergency room visits and drug-related deaths, according to the DAWN statistics (see Chapter 2). The FDA doesn't want to advertise on the package that acetaminophen can be lethal, for fear of attracting suicide attempts. So it requires a warning against overdose and includes the statement "Prompt medical attention is critical for adults as well as for children even if you do not notice any signs or symptoms." This statement reflects the fact that damage to the liver might not be noticed until 24 to 48 hours later, when the symptoms of impaired liver function finally emerge. You

Drugs in Depth

The Vioxx Controversy

In 2004, the NSAID drug Vioxx, widely used as an anti-inflammatory drug by arthritis sufferers, was pulled from the market because it increased risk of heart attacks. As a selective COX-2 inhibitor it produced only half as many gastric ulcers as the nonspecific inhibitors such as aspirin. COX-2 is not involved in regulating blood platelets, so gastrointestinal bleeding is much less than when COX-1 is also inhibited. Early studies indicated a somewhat higher rate of heart attacks in patients on Vioxx compared to nonselective COX inhibitors, but at first this was interpreted to mean that the nonselective inhibitors were protecting against clotting and therefore heart attacks, and Vioxx was simply not providing this preventive effect. But eventually it became clear that Vioxx actually increased the risk relative to placebo, and the drug was discontinued.

This has led to controversy about whether the manufacturer was ignoring early warning signs and whether the FDA had done its job, particularly in enforcing postmarketing studies and the reporting of adverse side effects. The FDA is likely to make some organizational changes to strengthen its postmarketing research on newly introduced drugs.

should remember that acetaminophen is not necessarily safer than aspirin, especially if the recommended dose is exceeded.

Ibuprofen and Other NSAIDs

Since the discovery that aspirin and similar drugs work by inhibiting the two COX enzymes, the drug companies have used that information to design new and sometimes more potent analgesics, which were introduced as prescription products. **Ibuprofen,** which originally was available only by prescription, is now found in several OTC analgesics. In addition to its analgesic potency, ibuprofen is a potent anti-inflammatory and has received wide use in the treatment of arthritis. The most common side effects of ibuprofen are gastrointestinal:

Table 12.2
Ingredients in OTC Analgesics (mg)

Brand	Aspirin	Acetaminophen	Ibuprofen	Naproxen	Caffeine	Other
Aleve	—	—	—	200	—	—
Anacin	400	—	—		32	—
Advil	—	—	200		—	—
Bufferin	325	—	—		—	Magnesium carbonate, calcium carbonate, magnesium oxide
Empirin	325	—	—		—	—
Excedrin	250	250	—		65	—
Mediprin	—	—	200		—	—
Nuprin	—	—	200		—	—
Vanquish	227	194	—		33	Magnesium hydroxide, aluminum hydroxide gel

nausea, stomach pain, and cramping. There have been reports of fatal liver damage with overdoses of ibuprofen, so again it is wise not to exceed the recommended dose.

Ibuprofen was the first of several new drugs that are now collectively referred to as "nonsteroidal anti-inflammatory drugs" (**NSAIDs**). Naproxen is also available OTC.

One product that luckily did not make the switch to OTC was vofecoxib (Vioxx), which was pulled from the market in 2004 after it was clear that it increased the risk of heart attacks.

Table 12.2 lists several OTC internal analgesics along with the amounts of each ingredient they contain. The FDA has been discussing whether or not to exclude products that contain both aspirin and acetaminophen. Products containing ibuprofen warn against combining them with aspirin, because that mixture hasn't been thoroughly studied.

Cold and Allergy Products

The All-Too-Common Cold

There has to be something good about an illness that Charles Dickens could be lyrical about:

I am at this moment
Deaf in the ears,
Hoarse in the throat,
Red in the nose,
Green in the gills,
Damp in the eyes,
Twitchy in the joints,
And fractious in temper
From a most intolerable
And oppressive cold.[10]

The common cold is caused by viruses: more than a hundred have been identified. But in 40 to 60 percent of individuals with colds, researchers cannot connect the infection to a specific virus. That makes it tough to find a cure. Two groups of viruses are known to be associated with colds—the *rhinoviruses* and the more recently identified *coronaviruses*. These viruses are clearly distinct from those that cause influenza, measles, and pneumonia.

ibuprofen (eye bu *pro* fen): an aspirinlike analgesic and anti-inflammatory.
NSAIDs: nonsteroidal anti-inflammatory drugs, such as ibuprofen.

Success in developing vaccines against other diseases has made some experts optimistic about finding a vaccine for the common cold. Others are pessimistic because of the great variety of viruses and the fact that the rhinoviruses can apparently change their immunologic reactivity very readily.

Viruses damage or kill the cells they attack. The rhinoviruses zero in on the upper respiratory tract, at first causing irritation, which can lead to reflex coughing and sneezing. Increased irritation inflames the tissue and is followed by soreness and swelling of the mucous membranes. As a defense against infection, the mucous membranes release considerable fluid, which causes the runny nose and the postnasal drip that irritates the throat.

Although the incubation period for a cold can be a week in some cases, the more common interval between infection and respiratory tract symptoms is two to four days. Before the onset of respiratory symptoms, the individual might just feel bad and develop joint aches and headaches. When fever does occur, it almost always develops early in the cold.

Most of us grew up believing that colds are passed by airborne particles jet-propelled usually through unobstructed sneezing. ("Cover your mouth! Cover your face!") The old folklore—and the scientists—were wrong. You need to know four things so you can avoid the cold viruses of others—and avoid reinfecting yourself:

1. Up to 100 times as many viruses are produced and shed from the nasal mucosa as from the throat.
2. There are few viruses in the saliva of a person with a cold, probably no viruses at all in about half of these individuals.
3. Dried viruses survive on dry skin and nonporous surfaces—plastic, wood, and so on—for over three hours.
4. Most cold viruses enter the body through the nostrils and eyes.

Usually colds start by the fingers picking up viruses and then the individual rubs the eyes

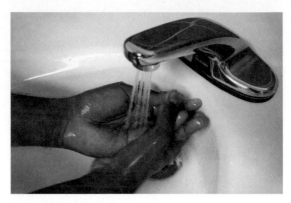

Frequent handwashing is a good strategy to reduce the risk of contracting a cold.

or picks the nose. In one study of adults with colds, 40 percent had viruses on their hands but only 8 percent expelled viruses in coughs or sneezes.[11] The moral of the story is clear. To avoid colds, wash your hands frequently, and you may kiss but not hold hands with your cold-infected sweetheart. You don't have to worry about your pets—only humans and some apes are susceptible to colds.

The experimental animal of choice for studying colds has to be the human. In many studies with human volunteers, three types of findings seem to recur. First, not all who are directly exposed to a cold virus develop cold symptoms. In fact, only about 50 percent do. Second, in individuals with already existing antibodies to the virus, there might be only preliminary signs of a developing cold. These signs might last for a brief period (12 to 24 hours) and then disappear. Finally, it doesn't seem to matter whether people are subjected to "chilling" treatment (e.g., sitting in a draft in a wet bathing suit). *Being* cold has nothing to do with *catching* a cold.

Treatment of Cold Symptoms

There's no practical way to prevent colds and no way to cure the infection once it starts. So why do Americans spend billions each year on cold "remedies"? Apparently, it's in an effort to

Table 12.3
Ingredients* in Selected Brand-Name OTC Cold and Allergy Products

Brand	Sympathomimetic	Antihistamine	Analgesic	Cough suppressant	Other
Night Comtrex	30 pseudoephedrine HCl	2 chlorpheniramine maleate	500 acetaminophen	15 dextromethorphan	—
Dristan	5 phenylephrine HCl	2 chlorpheniramine maleate	325 acetaminophen	—	—
Drixoral Cold and Allergy	120 pseudoephedrine	6 dexbrompheniramine maleate	—	—	—
Tylenol Cold	30 pseudoephedrine HCl	2 chlorpheniramine maleate	325 acetaminophen	15 dextromethorphan	—
Theraflu Severe Cold	60 pseudoephedrine	4 chlorpheniramine maleate	1000 acetaminophen	30 dextromethorphan	—

*mg/tablet

reduce those miserable symptoms described by Dickens. Cold symptoms are fairly complex, so most cold remedies have traditionally included several active ingredients, each aimed at a particular type of symptom. In some ways, the FDA's Cold, Cough, Allergy, Bronchodilator, and Antiasthmatic Advisory Review Panel probably had the most difficult job: multiple symptoms, many ingredients for each symptom, and rapid changes in scientific evidence during the time it studied these products. In the preliminary report, issued in 1976, the panel approved less than half of the 119 ingredients it reviewed. Modern cold remedies contain three common types of ingredients: *antihistamines,* for the temporary relief of runny nose and sneezing; *nasal decongestants,* for the temporary relief of swollen membranes in the nasal passages; and *analgesic-antipyretics,* for the temporary relief of aches and pains and fever reduction. The most common antihistamine to be found on the shelves is **chlorpheniramine maleate.** The most common nasal decongestant in cold remedies is now pseudoephedrine. The analgesic-antipyretic is usually acetaminophen.

Table 12.3 gives recent formulations for five popular OTC cold remedies. Note that three of them also contain the cough suppressant **dextromethorphan,** which is the most common active ingredient in OTC cough medicines.

It is ironic that the one type of ingredient found in almost every cold remedy before the FDA began its review continues to be under attack. The FDA advisory panel had serious questions about the data supporting the effectiveness of antihistamines in treating colds. Although some studies have since reported that chlorpheniramine maleate is better than placebo at reducing runny noses, prompting the FDA to approve several antihistamines, more recent controlled experiments have not found any benefit. A 1987 symposium of specialists concluded

chlorpheniramine maleate (clor fen *eer* a meen mal i ate): a common antihistamine in cold products.
dextromethorphan (dex tro meh *thor* fan): an OTC antitussive (cough control) ingredient.

Mind/Body Connection

Abuse of OTC Dextromethorphan

High school and college students have been "getting high" with large doses of OTC cough suppressants containing dextromethorphan (DM). Possibly, students first came on the effects of DM by drinking large quantities of Robitussin or similar cough syrups containing alcohol. However, the effects reported by those using 4 to 8 ounces of Robitussin (up to 720 mg DM) could not be due to the less than one-half ounce of alcohol in them and include visual and auditory hallucinations.[12] The altered psychological state may last for several hours. The few cases reported in the literature and individual reports from college students indicate that habitual use (e.g., twice per week or more) is common.

DM has been the standard ingredient in OTC cough suppressants for many years and was originally developed as a nonopiate relative to codeine. DM is not an opioid-like narcotic, produces no pain relief, and does not produce an opioid-like abstinence syndrome. More recent evidence indicates that it may interact with a specific receptor from the opioid family known as the sigma receptor. This apparently safe and simple drug, which is contained in more than 50 OTC products, has more complicated effects when taken in the large doses by recreational users.

It's not clear how recent this phenomenon really is. The Swedish government restricted DM to prescription-only use in 1986 as a result of abuse of OTC preparations, and there were two later reports of DM-caused fatalities in Sweden. In the United States, this has remained a mostly underground activity, apparently spread by word of mouth.

A posting to the alt.psychoactives newsgroup on the Internet described a user's first DM experience, after taking 20 capsules of an OTC cough remedy (600 mg DM):

> . . . 45 minutes worth of itching and for ten seconds it stopped. During one of the most weirdest and stupidest visions, I flew quickly over a mountain. As I did this in that second the itching seemed to go away and it seemed like I wasn't in my body anymore. I flew from one side of a rainbow to another. Then I was flying quickly towards the head of an ostrich and when I got close it only showed the silhouette of the head and I flew into the black nothingness. All that craziness in ten seconds made me laugh out loud as I tried to look at it all soberly. Then the itching came back into my body. No matter how hard I tried the itching never went away.

The itching feeling has been reported by others, along with nausea and other unpleasant side effects. Despite such unpleasantness, some users find it difficult to stop using DM once they have tried it a few times.

---

that "antihistamines do not have a place in the management of upper respiratory infection, though they continue to be useful for allergy." Still more studies have been done that question the effectiveness of antihistamines, and congressional hearings were held in 1992, asking why the FDA still allowed antihistamines in cough and cold remedies. They're still there.

Allergy and Sinus Medications

There are other related products on your pharmacy shelves. In addition to the cough medicines, there are *allergy* relief pills, which rely mainly on an antihistamine, to slow down the runny nose. Sinus medicines use one of the sympathomimetic nasal decongestants (pseudoephedrine), often combined with an analgesic, to reduce swollen sinus passages and to treat sinus headache.

Choosing An OTC Product

By now you should be getting the idea that, thanks to the FDA's decision to review ingredients rather than individual formulations, you as a consumer can now review and choose from among the great variety of products by knowing just a few ingredients and what they

Table 12.4
Common OTC Ingredients

Ingredient	Action	Source
Acetylsalicylic acid (ASA; aspirin)	Analgesic-antipyretic	Headache remedies, arthritis formulas, cold and sinus remedies
Acetaminophen	Analgesic-antipyretic	Headache remedies, cold and sinus remedies
Caffeine	Stimulant	"Alertness" medications
Chlorpheniramine maleate	Antihistamine	Cold remedies, allergy products
Dextromethorphan	Antitussive	Cough suppressants, cold remedies
Diphenhydramine	Antihistamine	Sleep aids, some cold remedies
Pseudoephedrine	Sympathomimetic	Cold and sinus remedies

are intended to accomplish. Table 12.4 lists only seven ingredients. Those seven are the major active ingredients to be found in different combinations in OTC stimulants, sleep aids, weight-control products, analgesics, cold, cough, allergy, and sinus medications.

Do you want to treat your cold without buying a combination cold remedy? If you have aches and pains, take your favorite analgesic. For the vast majority of colds, the slight elevation in temperature should probably not be treated, because it is not dangerous and can even help fight the infection. Unless body temperature remains at 103°F or above or reaches 105°F, fever is not considered dangerous. If you have a runny nose, you might or might not get relief from an antihistamine. Generic chlorpheniramine maleate or a store-brand allergy tablet is an inexpensive source. These will probably give you a dry mouth and might produce some sedation or drowsiness (which, of course, is why some of the more sedating antihistamines are used in sleep aids). Do you have a stuffed-up nose? Pseudoephedrine nose drops will shrink swollen membranes for a time. Although oral sympathomimetics will work, nose drops are more effective. You can find these ingredients in sinus and allergy preparations. However, these sympathomimetics should be used cautiously. There is a rapid tolerance to their effects, and, if they are used repeatedly, a

rebound stuffiness can develop when they are stopped. Do you have a cough? Dextromethorphan can be obtained in cough medications.

Why not buy all this in one tablet or capsule? That's a common approach. But why treat symptoms you don't have? During the course of a cold, a runny nose might occur at one time, congestion at another, and coughing not at all. By using just the ingredients you need, when you need them, you might save money, and you would have the satisfaction of being a connoisseur of colds. Then again, given the state of research on the effectiveness of these "remedies," why buy them at all? It's easy for a skeptic to conclude that there's little or no real value in cold remedies. The experts say to rest and drink fluids. But when they actually have a cold, most people are less inclined to be skeptical and more inclined to be hopeful that something will help.

Summary

- In contrast to FDA-approved OTC drugs, dietary supplements do not have to be proven effective. Also, the burden of proof for safety concerns is on the FDA as opposed to the manufacturer.

- Saint-John's-wort and SAMe have been proposed to treat depression, but the effectiveness of either is not clear from the available research.

- A drug can be sold over the counter only if a panel of experts agrees it can be used safely when following the label directions.

- For a given category of OTC drug, most of the various brands all contain the same few ingredients.

- OTC stimulants are based on caffeine.

- OTC sleep aids are based on antihistamines.

- There are no approved OTC weight-control drugs.

- Aspirin has analgesic, antipyretic, and anti-inflammatory actions. Acetaminophen, ibuprofen, and other NSAIDs have related effects.

- Cold remedies usually contain an antihistamine, an analgesic, and a decongestant.

- An informed consumer can understand a large fraction of OTC medicines by knowing only seven ingredients.

Review Questions

1. What is the main difference between OTC drugs and dietary supplements?
2. What do the acronyms GRAS and GRAE stand for?
3. What are the criteria for deciding whether a drug should be sold OTC or by prescription?
4. What is the main ingredient found in OTC stimulants?
5. How safe and effective are OTC weight-control products, according to the FDA?
6. Diphenhydramine is found in what three brand-name sleep aids?
7. What effect of aspirin might be involved in its use to prevent TIAs and heart attacks in men?

8. What are the differences in the therapeutic effects of acetaminophen and ibuprofen?
9. What is the most common route for a cold virus to enter a person's system?
10. Which cold symptoms are supposed to be relieved by chlorpheniramine maleate and which by pseudoephedrine?

References

1. National Council on Patient Information and Education. *Fact Sheet: The Use of Over-the-Counter Medicines,* September 2003.
2. Linde, K., and others. "St. John's Wort for Depression: An Overview and Meta-analysis of Randomized Clinical Trials." *British Medical Journal* 313 (1996), p. 253.
3. Shelton, R.C. "Effectiveness of St. John's Wort in Major Depression: A Randomized Controlled Trial." *Journal of the American Medical Association* 285 (2001), pp. 1978–86.
4. Bressa, G.M. "S-adenosyl-l-methionine (SAMe) as Antidepressant: Meta-analysis of Clinical Studies." *Acta Neurol Scand Suppl* 154 (1994), pp. 7–14.
5. Evans, J.G., and others. "Evidence-Based Pharmacotherapy of Alzheimer's Disease." *International Journal of Neuropsychopharmacology* 3 (2004), pp. 351–69.
6. MacKay, D. "Nutrients and Botanicals for Erectile Dysfunction: Examining the Evidence." *Alternative Medicine Review* 9 (2004), pp. 4–16.
7. Consumer Healthcare Products Association. "Ingredients and Dosages Transferred from Rx to OTC Status by the Food and Drug Administration." Retrieved from www.chpa.org, March 2006.
8. FDA. "OTC Stimulant Drug Products, Final Monograph." *Federal Register,* February 29, 1988.
9. Boltri, M., and others. "Aspirin Prophylaxis in Patients at Low Risk for Cardiovascular Disease: A Systematic Review of All-cause Mortality." *Journal of Family Practice* 51 (2002), pp. 700–05.
10. Dickens, C. *The Collected Letters of Charles Dickens.* Chapman & Hall, 1880.
11. Klumpp, T.G. "The Common Cold—New Concepts of Transmission and Prevention." *Medical Times* 108, no. 11 (1980), pp. 98, 1s–3s.
12. Price, L. H., & J. Lebel. "Dextromethorphan-Induced Psychosis." *American Journal of Psychiatry* 157 (2000), p. 304.

Check Yourself

Can You Guess What These OTC Products Are Used For?

The following mock product labels include the actual list of ingredients from some OTC products. Your job is to figure out what each product is used for (hint: none of them is a laxative, acne medication, or contraceptive).

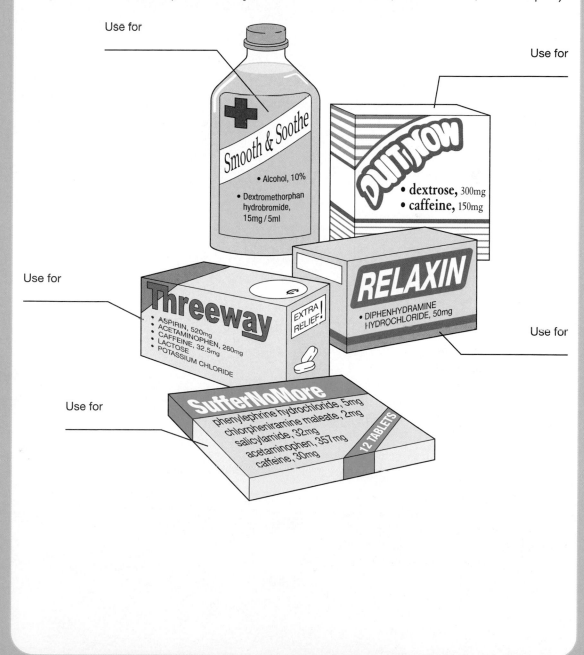

Use for

Smooth & Soothe
- Alcohol, 10%
- Dextromethorphan hydrobromide, 15mg / 5ml

Use for

QUIT NOW
- **dextrose,** 300mg
- **caffeine,** 150mg

Use for

Threeway EXTRA RELIEF!
- ASPIRIN, 520mg
- ACETAMINOPHEN, 260mg
- CAFFEINE, 32.5mg
- LACTOSE
- POTASSIUM CHLORIDE

RELAXIN
- DIPHENHYDRAMINE HYDROCHLORIDE, 50mg

Use for

SufferNoMore
phenylephrine hydrochloride, 5mg
chlorpheniramine maleate, 2mg
salicylamide, 32mg
acetaminophen, 357mg
caffeine, 30mg

12 TABLETS

Use for

Restricted Drugs

In contrast to the everyday drugs such as nicotine and caffeine, the drugs discussed in this section include some of the least familiar and most feared substances: heroin, LSD, and marijuana. More recently, the anabolic steroids used by some athletes have also become widely feared by the public, most of whom have no direct contact with the drugs. Along with the stimulants, cocaine, and amphetamines, these substances are commonly viewed as evil, "devil drugs."

13 Opioids
The opioids, or narcotics, include some of the oldest useful medicines. Why did they also become the most important illicit drugs of this century?

14 Hallucinogens
Are some drugs really capable of enhancing intellectual experiences? Of producing madness?

15 Marijuana
Why has a lowly and common weed become such an important symbol of the struggle between lifestyles?

16 Performance-Enhancing Drugs
What improvements can athletes obtain by resorting to drugs? What are the associated dangers?

13

Opioids

Objectives

When you have finished this chapter, you should be able to:

- **Describe how opium is obtained from poppies.**

- **List several historical uses for opium and describe early recreational uses of opium and its derivatives.**

- **Explain the role of the opium trade in the wars between Great Britain and China in the 1800s.**

- **Describe the relationship of morphine and codeine to opium and the relationship of heroin to morphine.**

- **Explain how the "typical" opioid abuser has changed from the early 1900s to the present.**

- **Describe how sources of supply for heroin have changed over the past 30 years and list the current major source countries.**

- **Explain how opioid antagonists block the effects of opioid drugs.**

- **Recognize that endorphins and enkephalins are endogenous opioids (and explain what is meant by "endogenous").**

- **Describe three current medical uses for opioids.**

- **Describe the typical opioid withdrawal syndrome.**

- **Explain how people die from opioid overdose.**

- **Describe the typical method of preparing and injecting illicit heroin.**

And soon they found themselves in the midst of a great meadow of poppies. Now it is well known that when there are many of these flowers together their odor is so powerful that anyone who breathes it falls asleep, and if the sleeper is not carried away from the scent of the flowers he sleeps on and on forever. But Dorothy did not know this, nor could she get away from the bright red flowers that were everywhere about; so presently her eyes grew heavy and she felt she must sit down to rest and to sleep. . . . Her eyes closed in spite of herself and she forgot where she was and fell among the poppies, fast asleep. . . . They carried the sleeping girl to a pretty spot beside the river, far enough from the poppy field to prevent her breathing any more of the poison of the flowers, and here they laid her gently on the soft grass and waited for the fresh breeze to waken her.[1]

From the land of Oz to the streets of San Francisco, the poppy has caused much grief—and much joy. **Opium** is a truly unique substance. This juice from the plant *Papaver somniferum*

Online Learning Center Resources

www.mhhe.com/ksir12e

Visit our Online Learning Center (OLC) for access to these study aids and additional resources.

- Learning objectives
- Glossary flashcards
- Web activities and links
- Self-scoring chapter quiz
- Audio chapter summaries

has a history of medical use perhaps 6,000 years long. Except for the past century and a half, opium has stood alone as the one agent from which physicians could obtain sure results. Compounds containing opium solved several of the recurring problems for medical science wherever used. Opium relieved pain and suffering magnificently. Just as important in the years gone by was its ability to reduce the diarrhea and subsequent dehydration caused by dysentery, which is still a leading cause of death in underdeveloped countries.

Parallel with the medical use of opium was its use as a deliverer of pleasure and relief from anxiety. Because of these effects, extensive recreational use of opium has also occurred throughout history. Through all those years, many of its users experienced dependence.

History of Opioids

Opium

Early History of Opium The most likely origin of opium is in a hot, dry, Middle Eastern country several millennia ago, when someone discovered that for 7 to 10 days of its yearlong life *Papaver somniferum* produced a substance that, when eaten, eased pain and suffering. The opium poppy is an annual plant that grows three to four feet high with large flowers four to five inches in diameter. The flowers can be white, pink, red, purple, or violet.

Opium is produced and available for collection for only a few days of the plant's life, between the time the petals drop and the seedpod matures. Today, as before, opium harvesters move through the fields in the early evening and use a sharp, clawed tool to make shallow cuts into, but not through, the unripe seedpods. During the night a white substance oozes from the cuts, oxidizes to a red-brown color, and becomes gummy. In the morning the resinous substance is carefully scraped from the pod and collected in small balls. This raw opium forms the basis for the opium medicines that have been used throughout history and is the substance from which morphine is extracted and then heroin is derived.

The importance and extent of use of the opium poppy in the early Egyptian and Greek cultures are still under debate, but in the Ebers papyrus (circa 1500 BC) a remedy is mentioned "to prevent the excessive crying of children." Because a later Egyptian remedy for the same purpose clearly contained opium (as well as fly excrement), many writers report the first specific medical use of opium as dating from the Ebers papyrus.

Homer's *Odyssey* (1000 BC) contains a passage that some authors believe refers to the use of opium. A party was about to become a real drag because everyone was sad, thinking about Ulysses and the deaths of their friends, when

> Helen, daughter of Zeus, poured into the wine they were drinking a drug, nepenthes, which gave forgetfulness of evil. Those who had drunk of this mixture did not shed a tear the whole day long, even though their mother or father were dead, even though a brother or beloved son had been killed before their eyes.[2]

The drug could only have been opium.

opium: a raw plant substance containing morphine and codeine.

Drugs in the Media

The Rise and Fall of Heroin "Epidemics"

The term *epidemic* refers to a rapidly spreading outbreak of contagious disease or, by extension, to any rapid spread, growth, or development of a problem. Heroin use has always been restricted to a very small proportion of the U.S. population, and it would be an overstatement to say that heroin use has reached or will reach epidemic proportions, if by that we mean that the problem is widely prevalent. Nevertheless, there are periodic news reports about the most recent "heroin epidemic," amid speculation about its rapid spread.

What usually triggers these reports is the spectacular seizure of a large drug shipment, police reports about new supplies of low-cost heroin, or the arrest of some young heroin users (seen as evidence that a new generation is being affected). Despite these scary news accounts, filled with lurid details and predictions of doom, the predicted epidemic never seems to materialize and fades from memory. Once the epidemic has been forgotten, the television and newspaper reporters are primed to warn us about the next epidemic a few years later.

Seizures of drugs, for example, are a notoriously poor way to measure drug use trends. Researchers estimate that authorities capture only about one-tenth of the drugs on the market, but sometimes they get lucky. The amount of drugs seized, however, doesn't answer the question of whether the seizure is a representative portion of a steady market, a growing portion of a shrinking market, or a smaller portion of a growing market.

News articles in *The New York Times* in 2003, the *Edinburgh Evening News* (Edinburgh, Scotland) in 2004, and the *Brockton Enterprise* (Brockton, Massachusetts) in 2006, all referred to new "heroin epidemics" occurring in those cities. Two of the cities had noticed an increase in overdose deaths, and in New York the statistic that triggered the news article was an increase in admissions to treatment programs. These numbers all tend to fluctuate up and down, but the "up" periods are more likely to trigger sensational news articles.

Keep your eyes and ears open, and it won't be long before you read or hear a news report about an epidemic of heroin use in a part of the United States or in another country (such reports also have appeared in Australia, Ireland, Pakistan, and elsewhere). Does the report cite formal studies that help quantify the problem, or does it vaguely point to "ominous signs" of increasing drug use? These reports really attract attention—and increase sales and advertising revenue—so there's always a market for the stories. As we have seen before, most of this kind of illicit drug use is better viewed as occurring in localized areas, taking on more of the character of a fad than of an epidemic.

Opium was important in Greek medicine. Galen, the last of the great Greek physicians, emphasized caution in the use of opium but felt that it was almost a cure-all, saying that it

> resists poison and venomous bites, cures chronic headache, vertigo, deafness, epilepsy, apoplexy, dimness of sight, loss of voice, asthma, coughs of all kinds, spitting of blood, tightness of breath, colic, the iliac poison, jaundice, hardness of the spleen, stone, urinary complaints, fevers, dropsies, leprosies, the troubles to which women are subject, melancholy and all pestilences.[2]

Recreational use even then must have been extensive. Galen also commented on the opium cakes and candies that were being sold everywhere in the streets.

Greek and Roman knowledge of opium use in medicine languished during the Dark Ages and thus had little influence on the world's use of opium for the next thousand years. The Arabic world, however, clutched opium to its breast. Because the Koran forbade the use of alcohol in any form, opium and hashish became the primary social drugs wherever the Islamic culture moved, and it did move. While Europe rested through the Dark Ages, the Arabian world reached out and made contact with India and China. Opium was one of the products they traded, but they also sold the seeds of the opium poppy, and cultivation began in these countries. By the 10th century AD, opium had been referred to in Chinese medical writings.

During this period when the Arabic civilization flourished, two Arabic physicians made substantial contributions to medicine and to the history of opium. Shortly after AD 1000, Biruni composed a pharmacology book. His descriptions of opium contained what some believe to be the first written description of **opioid** dependence.[3] In the same period the best-known Arabic physician, Avicenna, was using opium preparations very effectively and extensively in his medical practice. His writings, along with those of Galen, formed the basis of medical education in Europe as the Renaissance dawned, and thus the glories of opium were advanced. (Avicenna, a knowledgeable physician and a believer in the tenets of Islam, died as a result of drinking too much of a mixture of opium and wine.)

Early in the 16th century lived a European medical phenomenon. Paracelsus apparently was a successful clinician and accomplished some wondrous cures for the day. One of his secrets was an opium extract called laudanum. Paracelsus was one of the early Renaissance supporters of opium as a panacea and referred to it as the "stone of immortality."

Due to Paracelsus and his followers, awareness increased of the broad effectiveness of opium, and new opium preparations were developed in the 16th, 17th, and 18th centuries. One of these was laudanum as prepared by Dr. Thomas Sydenham, the father of clinical medicine. Sydenham's general contributions to English medicine are so great that he has been called the English Hippocrates. He spoke more highly of opium than did Paracelsus, saying that "without opium the healing art would cease to exist." His laudanum contained two ounces of strained opium, one ounce of saffron, a dram of cinnamon, and a dram of cloves dissolved in one pint of Canary wine, taken in small quantities.

Writers and Opium: The Keys to Paradise In a momentous year for opium, 1805, Thomas De Quincey, a 20-year-old English man who had run away from home at 17, purchased some laudanum for a toothache and received change for his shilling from the apothecary. Here is his description of his response to this dose:

> I took it: and in an hour, O heavens! what a revulsion! what a resurrection, from its lowest depths, of the inner spirit! what an apocalypse of the world within me! That my pains had vanished was now a trifle in my eyes; this negative effect was swallowed up in the immensity of those positive effects which had opened before me, in the abyss of divine enjoyment thus suddenly revealed. Here was a panacea . . . for all human woes; here was the secret of happiness, about which philosophers had disputed for so many ages, at once discovered; happiness might now be bought for a penny, and carried in the waistcoat-pocket; portable ecstasies might be had corked up in a pint-bottle; and peace of mind could be sent down by the mail.[4]

For the rest of his life De Quincey used laudanum. He did not try to conceal the extent of his opium use. Rather, his writings are replete with insight into the opium-hazed world, particularly his article "The Confessions of an English Opium-Eater," which was published in 1821 (and in book form in 1823). (Throughout this period, *opium eating* was the phrase generally used to refer to laudanum drinking.)

Several other famous English authors also drank laudanum, including Elizabeth Barrett Browning and Samuel Taylor Coleridge. Coleridge's magnificently beautiful "Kubla Khan" was probably conceived and composed

opioid: a drug derived from opium (e.g., morphine and codeine) or a synthetic drug with opium-like effects (e.g., oxycodone).

in an opium reverie and then written down as best as he could remember it. However, De Quincey is of primary interest here. His emphasis was on understanding the effects that opium has on consciousness, experience, and feeling, and as such he provided some of the most vivid accounts of the power of opium.

Opium does not produce new worlds for the user:

> If a man, "whose talk is of oxen," should become an opium-eater, the probability is, that (if he is not too dull to dream at all)—he will dream about oxen; whereas, in the case before him [De Quincey], the reader will find that the opium-eater boasteth himself to be a philosopher; and accordingly, that the phantasmagoria of his dreams (waking or sleeping, day-dreams or night-dreams) is suitable to one of that character.[5]

Opium does, however, change the way the user perceives the world. For example, "an opium eater is too happy to observe the motion of time."[5]

De Quincey pointed out the sharp contrast between the effects of alcohol and those of opium:

> Crude opium . . . is incapable of producing any state of body at all resembling that which is produced by alcohol. . . . It is not in the quantity of its effects merely, but in the quality, that it differs altogether. The pleasure given by wine is always rapidly mounting, and tending to a crisis, after which as rapidly it declines; that from opium, when once generated, is stationary for eight or ten hours. . . . The one is a flickering flame, the other a steady and equable glow. But the main distinction lies in this—that, whereas wine disorders the mental faculties, opium, on the contrary (if taken in a proper manner), introduces amongst them the most exquisite order, legislation, and harmony. Wine robs a man of his self-possession; opium sustains and reinforces it. Wine unsettles the judgment. . . . Opium, on the contrary, communicates serenity and equipoise to all the faculties.[5]

Despite all the good things De Quincey said about opium and the effects it had on him, he suffered from its use. For long periods in his life he was unable to write as a result of his opium dependence. As with most things, "Opium gives and takes away. It defeats the steady habit of exertion; but it creates spasms of irregular exertion. It ruins the natural power of life; but it develops preternatural paroxysms of intermitting power."[6]

The publication of De Quincey's book in 1823 and its first translation into French in 1828 spurred the French Romantic writers to explore opium and hashish in the 1840s and later. The only associated American article of note in this period, "An Opium-Eater in America,"[7] appeared in an American magazine in 1842.

The Opium Wars   Although opium and the opium poppy had been introduced to China well before the year AD 1000, there was only a moderate level of use there by a select, elite group. Tobacco smoking spread much more rapidly after its introduction. It is not clear when tobacco was introduced to the Chinese, but its use had spread and become so offensive that in 1644 the emperor forbade tobacco smoking in China. The edict did not last long (as is to be expected), but it was in part responsible for the increase in opium smoking.

Up to this period the smoking of tobacco and the eating of opium had existed side by side. The restriction on the use of tobacco and the population's appreciation of the pleasures of smoking led to the combining of opium and tobacco for smoking. Presumably the addition of opium took the edge off the craving for tobacco. The amount of tobacco used was gradually reduced and soon omitted. Although opium eating had never been very attractive to most Chinese, opium smoking spread rapidly, perhaps, partly because smoking opium results in a rapid effect, compared with oral use.

In 1729, China's first law against opium smoking mandated that opium shop owners be strangled. Once opium for nonmedical purposes was outlawed, it was necessary for the drug to be smuggled in from India, where poppy plantations were abundant. Smuggling opium was so profitable for everyone—the

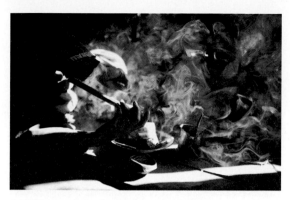

Smoking opium results in rapid effects.

growers, the shippers, and the customs officers—that unofficial rules were gradually developed for the "game."[2] The background to the Opium Wars is lengthy and complex, but the following can help explain why the British went to war so they could continue pouring opium into China against the wishes of the Chinese national government.

Since before 1557, when the Portuguese were allowed to develop the small trading post of Macao, pressure had been increasing on the Chinese emperors to open up the country to trade with the "barbarians from the West." Not only the Portuguese but also the Dutch and the English repeatedly knocked on the closed door of China. Near the end of the 17th century the port of Canton was opened under very strict rules to foreigners. Tea was the major export, and the British shipped out huge amounts. There was little that the Chinese were interested in importing from the "barbarians," but opium could be smuggled so profitably that it soon became the primary import. The profit the British made from selling opium paid for the tea they shipped back to England.[8] In the early 19th century the government of India was actually the British East India Company. As such, it had a monopoly on opium, which was legal in India. However, smuggling it into China was not. The East India Company auctioned chests of opium cakes to private merchants, who gave the chests to selected British firms, which sold them for a commission to Chinese merchants.

In this way the British were able to have the Chinese "smuggle" the opium into China. The number of chests of opium, each with about 120 pounds of smokable opium, imported annually by China increased from 200 in 1729 to about 5,000 at the century's end to 25,000 chests in 1838.

In 1839, the emperor of China made a fatal mistake—he sent an honest man to Canton to suppress the opium smuggling. Commissioner Lin demanded that the barbarians deliver all their opium supplies to him and subjected the dealers to confinement in their houses. After some haggling, the representative of the British government ordered the merchants to deliver the opium—20,000 chests worth about $6 million—which was then destroyed and everyone was set free. Pressures mounted, however, and an incident involving drunken American and British sailors killing a Chinese citizen started the Opium Wars in 1839. The British army arrived 10 months later, and in two years, largely by avoiding land battles and by using the superior artillery of the royal navy ships, they won a victory over a country of more than 350 million citizens. As victors, the British were given the island of Hong Kong, broad trading rights, and $6 million to reimburse the merchants whose opium had been destroyed.

The Chinese opium trade posed a great moral dilemma for Britain. The East India Company protested until its end that it was not smuggling opium into China, and technically it was not. From 1870 to 1893, motions in Parliament to end the extremely profitable opium commerce failed to pass but did cause a decline in the opium trade. In 1893, a moral protest against the trade was supported, but not until 1906 did the government support and pass a bill that eventually ended the opium trade in 1913.

Morphine

In 1805 in London, 20-year-old De Quincey eased a toothache and fell into the abyss of divine enjoyment. In Hanover, Germany, another

20-year-old worked on experiments that were to have great impact on science, medicine, and the pleasure seekers. In 1806, this German, Frederich Sertürner, published his report of more than 50 experiments, which clearly showed that he had isolated the primary active ingredient in opium. The active agent was 10 times as potent as opium. Sertürner named it *morphium* after Morpheus, the god of dreams. Use of the new agent developed slowly, but by 1831 the implications of his chemical work and the medical value of **morphine** had become so overwhelming that this pharmacist's assistant was given the French equivalent of the Nobel Prize. Later work into the mysteries of opium found more than 30 different alkaloids, with the second most important one being isolated in 1832 and named **codeine,** the Greek word for "poppy head."

The availability of a clinically useful, pure chemical of known potency is always capitalized on in medicine. The major increase in the use of morphine came as a result of two non-drug developments, one technological and one political. The technological development was the perfection of the hypodermic syringe in 1853 by Dr. Alexander Wood. This made it possible to deliver morphine directly into the blood or tissue rather than by the much slower process of eating opium or morphine and waiting for absorption to occur from the gastrointestinal tract. A further advantage of injecting morphine was thought to exist. Originally it was felt that morphine by injection would not produce the same degree of craving (hunger) for the drug as with oral use. This belief was later found to be false.

The political events that sped the drug of sleep and dreams into the veins of people worldwide were the American Civil War (1861–1865), the Prussian-Austrian War (1866), and the Franco-Prussian War (1870). Military medicine was, and to some extent still is, characterized by the dictum "first provide relief." Morphine given by injection worked rapidly and well, and it was administered regularly in large doses to many soldiers for the reduction

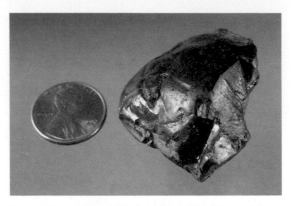

Raw opium is the substance from which morphine is extracted and then heroin is derived.

of pain and relief from dysentery. The percentage of veterans returning from these wars who were dependent on morphine was high enough that the illness was later called "soldier's disease" or the "army disease."

Heroin

Toward the end of the 19th century, a small but important chemical transformation was made to the morphine molecule. In 1874, two acetyl groups were attached to morphine, yielding diacetylmorphine, which was given the brand name Heroin and placed on the market in 1898 by Bayer Laboratories. The chemical change was important because **heroin** is about three times as potent as morphine. The pharmacology of heroin and morphine is identical, except that the two acetyl groups increase the lipid solubility of the heroin molecule, and thus the molecule enters the brain more rapidly. The additional groups are then detached, yielding morphine. Therefore, the effects of morphine and heroin are identical, except that heroin is more potent and acts faster.

Heroin was originally marketed as a non-habit-forming substitute for codeine.[9] It seemed to be the perfect drug, more potent yet less harmful. Although not introduced commercially until 1898, heroin had been studied, and many of its pharmacological actions had been reported in 1890.[10] In January 1900, a comprehensive review article, concluded that tolerance and dependence on heroin were only minor problems.

> Habituation has been noted in a small percentage . . . of the cases. . . . All observers are agreed, however, that none of the patients suffer in any way from this habituation, and that none of the symptoms which are so characteristic of chronic morphinism have ever been observed. On the other hand, a large number of the reports refer to the fact that the same dose may be used for a long time without any habituation.[11]

The basis for the failure to find dependence probably was the fact that heroin was initially used as a substitute for codeine, which meant oral doses of 3 to 5 mg used for brief periods of time. Slowly the situation changed, and a 1905 text, *Pharmacology and Therapeutics,* took a middle ground on heroin by saying that it "is stated not to give rise to habituation. A more extended knowledge of the drug, however, would seem to indicate that the latter assertion is not entirely correct."[12] In a few more years, everyone knew that heroin could produce a powerful dependence when injected in higher doses.

Opioid Abuse Before the Harrison Act

In the second half of the 19th century, three forms of opioid dependence were developing in the United States. The long-useful oral intake of opium, and then morphine, increased greatly as patent medicines became a standard form of self-medication. After 1850, Chinese laborers were imported in large numbers to the West Coast, and they introduced opium smoking to this country. The last form, medically the most dangerous and ultimately the most disruptive socially, was the injection of morphine.

Around the start of the 20th century the percentage (and perhaps the absolute number) of Americans dependent on one of the opioids was probably greater than at any other time before or since. Several authorities, both then and more recently, agree that no less than 1 percent of the population was dependent on opioids, although accurate statistics are not available. Despite the high level of dependence, it was not a major social problem. In this period,

> The public then had an altogether different conception of drug addiction from that which prevails today. The habit was not approved, but neither was it regarded as criminal or monstrous. It was usually looked upon as a vice or personal misfortune, or much as alcoholism is viewed today. Narcotics users were pitied rather than loathed as criminals or degenerates.[13]

The opium smoking the Chinese brought to this country never became widely popular, although about one-fourth of the opium imported was smoking opium at the start of the 20th century. Perhaps it was because the smoking itself occupies only about a minute and is then followed by a state of reverie that can last two or three hours—hardly conducive to a continuation of daily activities or consonant with the outward, active orientation of most Americans in that period. Another reason that opium smoking did not spread was that it originated with Asians, who were scorned by whites.

The growth of the patent medicine industry after the Civil War has been well documented. Everything seemed to be favorable for the industry, and it took advantage of each opportunity. There were few government regulations on the industry, and as a result drugs with a high abuse potential were an important part of many tonics and remedies, although this fact did not have to be indicated on the label.

Patent medicines promised, and in part delivered, the perfect self-medication. They were easily available, not too expensive, socially acceptable, and they worked. The amount of

---

morphine: the primary active agent in opium.
codeine: the secondary active agent in opium.
heroin: diacetylmorphine, a potent derivative of morphine.

alcohol and/or opioids in many of the nostrums was certain to relieve the user's aches, pains, and anxieties.

Gradually some medical concern developed over the number of people who were dependent on opioids, and this concern was a part of the motivation that led to the passage of the 1906 Pure Food and Drugs Act. In 1910, a government expert in this area made clear that this law was only a beginning:

> The thoughtful and foremost medical men have been and are cautioning against the free use of morphine and opium, particularly in recurring pain. The amount they are using is decreasing yearly. Notwithstanding this fact, and the fact that legislation, federal, state and territorial, adverse to the indiscriminate use and sale of opium and morphine, their derivatives and preparations, has been enacted during the past few decades, the amount of opium per capita imported and consumed in the United States has doubled during the last forty years. . . . It is well known that there are many factors at work tending to drug enslavement, among them being the host of soothing syrups, medicated soft drinks containing cocaine, asthma remedies, catarrh remedies, consumption remedies, cough and cold remedies, and the more notorious so-called "drug addiction cures." It is often stated that medical men are frequently the chief factors in causing drug addiction.[14]

Data presented in this paper tended to support the belief that medical use of opioids initiated by a physician was one, if not the, major cause of dependence in this country at that time. A 1918 government report clearly indicted the physician as the major cause of dependence in individuals of "good social standing."

That physicians widely used opioid medications is understandable in light of articles that had been published, such as one in 1889 titled "Advantages of Substituting the Morphia Habit for the Incurably Alcoholic." The author stated:

> In this way I have been able to bring peacefulness and quiet to many disturbed and distracted homes, to keep the head of a family out of the gutter and out of the lock-up, to keep him from

scandalous misbehavior and neglect of his affairs, to keep him from the verges and actualities of delirium tremens horrors, and above all, to save him from committing, as I veritably believe, some terrible crime.[15]

Besides all those good things, a morphine habit was cheap: by one estimate it was 10 times as expensive to be heavy drinker—costing 25 cents a day. The article concluded:

> I might, had I time and space, enlarge by statistics to prove the law-abiding qualities of opium-eating peoples, but of this any one can perceive somewhat for himself, if he carefully watches and reflects on the quiet, introspective gaze of the morphine habitue, and compares it to the riotous, devil-may-care leer of the drunkard.[15]

An 1880 report called opioid dependence a "vice of middle life." The typical opioid user of this period was a 30-to-50-year-old white woman who functioned well and was adjusted to her life as a wife and mother. She bought opium or morphine legally at the local store, used it orally, and caused few, if any, social problems. She might have ordered her "family remedy" through the mail from Sears, Roebuck—two ounces of laudanum for 18 cents or 1½ pints for $2. Of course, there were problems associated with dependence during this period. There are always individuals who are unable to control their drug intake, whether the drug is used for self-medication or recreation. Because of the high opioid content of patent medicines and the ready availability of dependence-producing drugs for drinking and/or injecting, very high levels of drug were frequently used. As a result, the symptoms of withdrawal were very severe—much worse than today—and the only relief to be found was by taking more of the drug.

Abuse After the Harrison Act

The complex reasons for the passage of the 1914 Harrison Act were discussed in detail in Chapter 3. Remember that this was a fairly simple revenue measure. However, as is true of most laws, it is not the law itself that becomes

Taking Sides

Should Heroin Be Made Available for Medical Purposes?

Since the 1920s, heroin has been unavailable to physicians for any purpose. It was the first such drug to be so restricted, and its status has now been codified, along with that of LSD and marijuana, under the status of Schedule I controlled substances—those with "no medical use."

However, heroin has been available all along in most countries as a potent pain reliever. It has repeatedly been proposed over the years that heroin should be moved to Schedule II and thus become available for medical use by prescription. Whether heroin is actually a better pain reliever than morphine has been argued for many years—it is more potent, in that less is required for the same effect, but

since heroin is converted to morphine in the brain, morphine should be just as effective if given in a higher dose. Regardless of the limited amount of evidence on either side, some physicians believe that heroin should be available in the United States for pain relief. Under some of the proposals, heroin would be available only under restricted circumstances, such as the failure of other potent narcotics to control pain.

As the situation now stands, according to one prominent proponent of medical heroin, the drug is more readily available to a 16-year-old kid on the street than it is to a terminally ill cancer patient in constant pain.

important in the ensuing years, but the court decisions and enforcement practices that evolve as the law interacts with the people it affects.

> The passing of the Harrison Act in 1914 left the status of the addict almost completely indeterminate. The act did not make addiction illegal and it neither authorized nor forbade doctors to prescribe drugs regularly for addicts. All that it clearly and unequivocally did require was that whatever drugs addicts obtained were to be secured from physicians registered under the act and that the fact of securing drugs be made a matter of record. While some drug users had obtained supplies from physicians before 1914, it was not necessary for them to do so since drugs were available for purchase in pharmacies and even from mail-order houses.[16]

In 1915, the United States Supreme Court decided that possession of smuggled opioids was a crime, and thus users not obtaining the drug from a physician became criminals with the stroke of a pen. Dependent users could still obtain their supply of drugs on a prescription from a physician, until this avenue was removed by Supreme Court decisions in 1919 and 1922 (see Chapter 3). Even though the

Lindner case in 1925 reversed these earlier decisions and stated that a physician could prescribe drugs to nonhospitalized users just to maintain their dependence, the doctors had been harassed and arrested enough. Even though it was legal again to prescribe drugs to a dependent user, few physicians would do so. Clinics for the treatment of opioid dependence were closed during the 1920s under pressure from federal officials.

The number of oral opioid users began to decline in response to these pressures, and the primary remaining group were those who injected morphine or heroin. By 1922, about the only source of opioids for a nonhospitalized abuser was an illegal dealer. Because heroin was the most potent opioid available, it was the easiest to conceal and therefore became the illegal dealer's choice. The cost through this source was 30 to 50 times the price of the same drug through legitimate sources, which no longer were available to drug-dependent users. Because of this cost, users wanted to be certain to get the most "bang for their buck," so intravenous injection became more and more common. To maintain a supply of the drug in this way was expensive.

Many users resorted to criminal activity, primarily burglary and other crimes against property, to finance their dependence.

During this period, law enforcement agencies and the popular press brought about a change in the attitudes of society toward the drug abusers. Thus, sometime during the 1920s,

> The addict was no longer seen as a victim of drugs, an unfortunate with no place to turn and deserving of society's sympathy and help. He became instead a base, vile, degenerate who was weak and self-indulgent, who contaminated all he came in contact with and who deserved nothing short of condemnation and society's moral outrage and legal sanction. The law enforcement approach was accepted as the only workable solution to the problem of addiction.[17]

The Changing Population of Opioid Users After the Harrison Act, the number of white middle-aged people using opioids orally declined. One paper commented that between World War I and World War II heroin received little publicity and was primarily used by "people in *the life*—show people, entertainers and musicians; racketeers and gangsters; thieves and pickpockets; prostitutes and pimps."

In the early years after World War II, heroin use slowly increased in the lower-class, slum areas of the large cities. Heroin was inexpensive in this period; a dollar would buy enough for a good high for three to six people; $2-a-day habits were not uncommon. As the 1950s passed, heroin use spread. As demand increased, so did both the price and the amount of adulteration.

The 1960s In the 1960s, the use of various drugs skyrocketed. Flower children, hippies, Tim Leary, and LSD received most of the media attention, but within the central core of the large American cities the number of regular and irregular heroin users increased also. Mainstream USA became concerned with the heroin problem of the large cities. The most visible abusers were African-American or Latino and because of the association of heroin use with crime, the white majority expressed little patience or tolerance toward people who were dependent on heroin.

Vietnam The attitude of people in the street toward the relevance of heroin use to their personal lives changed rapidly with the reports that began to filter out of Southeast Asia toward the end of the 1960s. Public anxiety increased dramatically with the possibility that the Vietnam conflict might produce thousands of drug users among the military personnel stationed there.

The Department of Defense established a Task Force on Drug Abuse in 1967; its initial reports emphasized concern over the widespread use of marijuana by troops in combat zones, as well as in rest and rehabilitation areas. In 1970, public and federal concern began to focus on the problem of heroin dependence among service personnel stationed in Southeast Asia.

Heroin was about 95 percent pure and almost openly sold in South Vietnam, whereas purity in the United States was about 5 percent in 1969. Not only was the Southeast Asia heroin undiluted, but it also was inexpensive. Ten dollars would buy about 250 mg, enough for 10 injections, and an amount that would cost more than $500 in the United States. The high purity of the heroin made it possible to obtain psychological effects by smoking or sniffing the drug. This fact, coupled with the fallacious belief that dependence occurs only when the drug is used intravenously, resulted in about 40 percent of the users sniffing, about half smoking, and only 10 percent injecting their heroin.[18]

Some early 1971 reports estimated that 10 to 15 percent of the American troops in Vietnam were dependent on heroin. As a result of the increased magnitude and visibility of the heroin problem, the U.S. government took several rapid steps in mid-1971. One step was to initiate Operation Golden Flow, a urine-testing

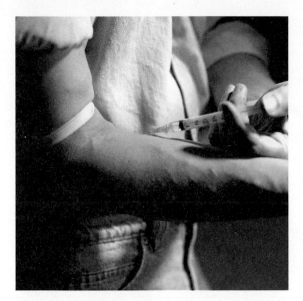

Although heroin dependence is often associated with intravenous use, dependence can also occur among users who smoke or sniff the drug.

program to detect opioids in service personnel ready to leave Vietnam.

In October 1971, the Pentagon released figures for the first three months of testing, which showed that 5.1 percent of the 100,000 personnel tested showed traces of opioids in their urine. Most of the opioid users were in the lower ranks.

In retrospect the Vietnam drug-use situation was "making a mountain out of a molehill," but much was learned. An excellent follow-up study[19] of veterans who returned from Vietnam in September 1971 showed that most of the Vietnam heroin users did not continue heroin use in this country. Only 1 to 2 percent were using opioids 8 to 12 months after returning from Vietnam and being released from the service, approximately the same percentage of individuals found to be using opioids when examined for induction into the service.

One of the important things learned from this experience is that opioid dependence and compulsive use are not inevitable among occasional users. The pattern of drug use in Vietnam also supports the belief that under certain conditions—availability and low cost of the drug, limited sanctions, stress—a relatively high percentage of individuals will use opioids recreationally.

The 1970s and 1980s Beginning in the late 1960s, the federal government made several efforts to estimate the number of heroin users in the United States. This is an impossible task to perform with much accuracy, given that heroin use is conducted in great secrecy and is not uniformly distributed across the country. Nevertheless, several sophisticated statistical techniques were brought to bear, combining various sources of information. Different groups of researchers estimated the number of heroin-dependent individuals from 1970 to the mid-1980s, and the estimates ranged between 400,000 and 500,000.[20] Perhaps because of considerable variability in the estimates, no particular trends or patterns can be seen in these data, and one might argue that heroin dependence didn't really change much over that period.

In 1972, the major source of U.S. heroin was opium grown in Turkey and converted into heroin in southern French port cities, such as Marseilles. This "French connection" accounted for as much as 80 percent of U.S. heroin before 1973. In 1972, Turkey banned all opium cultivation and production in return for $35 million the United States provided to make up for the financial losses to farmers and to help them develop new cash crops. This action, combined with a cooperative effort with the French (also partially funded by the United States), did lead to a reduction in the supply of heroin on the streets of New York in 1973.

This relative shortage did not last for long. In Mexico, opium is processed into morphine by a different process, and the resulting pure heroin has a brown or black color. In 1975, the Drug Enforcement Administration (DEA) estimated that 80 percent or more of all U.S. heroin was from Mexico (depending on its appearance, either called *Mexican brown* or

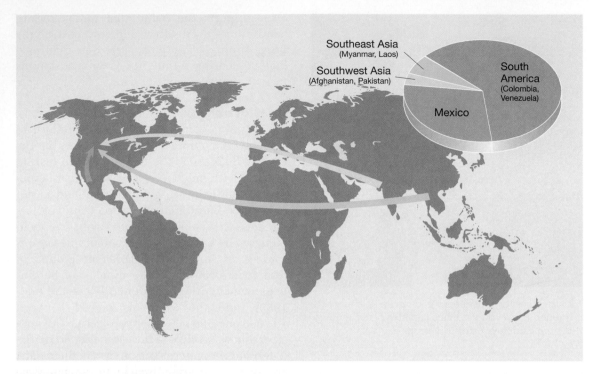

Figure 13.1   Sources of Illicit Heroin for the United States

black tar). The supply was plentiful, the price low, and the purity high. In 1974, the United States began to finance opium eradication programs in Mexico. Although it is hopeless to try to eliminate all such production, these monumental and expensive efforts did slow the importation from Mexico to some extent, and the "epidemic" of the 1970s began to decline.

In the late 20th century, about half of the U.S. heroin supply apparently originated in Southwest Asia (Afghanistan, Pakistan, Iran). Mexico was the next biggest contributor, with the Golden Triangle area of Southeast Asia (Myanmar, Laos, and Thailand) producing about 15 to 20 percent of the total.

Current Use of Heroin   The supply of heroin to the United States has shifted dramatically in recent years, with increased cultivation of opium poppies in South America. The illicit drug cartels that were organized in the 1980s to feed the U.S. demand for cocaine seem to have diversified into heroin production. In the early years of the 21st century, 60 percent of the heroin sold in the United States originates in Colombia or Venezuela, with Mexico continuing to supply about 25 percent of the U.S. market. Southeast Asian heroin accounts for about 10 percent, with only 5 percent now coming from poppies grown in Afghanistan (see Figure 13.1).[21] The Taliban government of Afghanistan had severely restricted opium production, but after the U.S.-led invasion in 2001 toppled that government, opium farming resumed at a high level.

Increased production in South America has resulted in both greater availability and greater purity in the U.S. market. From the mid-1970s through the mid-1980s the average purity varied from 4 to 6 percent heroin (more than 90 percent was something else the dealers used to cut the heroin). However, in the late 1980s, increased shipments of increasingly pure heroin began to arrive, and in 1989 the average street purity was estimated to be 25.2 percent, at least four times as strong as in years past. In 2002, the estimated purity was 27 percent for Mexican heroin and 46 percent for South American heroin. The price of a "bag" has not changed much, so the price per milligram of actual heroin was down considerably.

One change that began in the 1990s was the return of smoking opioids, although in a slightly different form than the old opium den. Piggybacking on the smoking of crack cocaine, inner-city users were either mixing the new high-potency heroin with crack or simply heating the heroin and inhaling the vapors from a crack pipe. The increased purity of available heroin has allowed smoking, as well as snorting, to produce the effects users want, while they avoid the use of needles that might spread AIDS or other diseases.

Heroin use has for many years been restricted to a small fraction of any population studied. For example, in the 2003 National Survey on Drug Use described in Chapter 1, only 1.6 percent of U.S. adults reported ever having used heroin in their lifetimes, with 0.1 percent reporting use in the past year. The Arrestee Drug Monitoring Program mentioned in Chapter 2 found that only about 6 percent of adult arrestees tested positive for opioids in 2003, much lower rates than for cocaine or marijuana.[22] For all the publicity heroin receives, the vast majority of people avoid it.

Abuse of Prescription Opioids

In 2004, about 5 percent of Americans aged 12 and over reported nonmedical use of a prescription pain reliever within the past year.[23] The most popular type appeared to be various brands of hydrocodone (e.g., Vicodin, Lortab). These are mostly taken orally, and there is evidence for both dependence and toxicity resulting from this misuse of prescription opioids. One particular product, Oxycontin (a Schedule II drug), came under scrutiny beginning in 2000 after reports of pharmacy break-ins and rapidly increasing prescription rates were followed by stories of users crushing the time-release capsules to allow the entire dose to be dissolved quickly. Some users were injecting the drug, others simply taking advantage of the higher total doses provided in this time-release product. Both the FDA and the drug's manufacturer have taken steps to reduce the misuse of Oxycontin.[24] In the 2003 Drug Abuse Warning Network data displayed in Table 2.2 (page 31), prescription opioids ranked third among emergency room mentions and first among drug-associated deaths. These controlled substances (Schedules II and III) are advertised for sale through foreign Internet pharmacies, which probably contributes to their increased availability for nonmedical use.

Pharmacology of the Opioids

Chemical Characteristics

Raw opium contains about 10 percent morphine by weight and a smaller amount of codeine. The addition of two acetyl groups to the morphine molecule results in diacetylmorphine, or heroin (Figure 13.2). The acetyl groups allow heroin to penetrate the blood-brain barrier more readily, and heroin is therefore two to three times more potent than morphine.

Medicinal chemists have worked hard over the decades to produce compounds that would be effective painkillers, trying to separate the analgesic effect of the opioids from their dependence-producing effects. Although the two effects could not be separated, the research has resulted in a variety of opioids that are sold as pain relievers (see Table 13.1). Especially interesting among these is fentanyl, which is approximately a hundred times as potent as morphine. Fentanyl is used primarily in conjunction with surgical anesthesia, although both fentanyl and some of its derivatives have also been manufactured illegally and sold on the streets.

black tar: a type of illicit heroin usually imported from Mexico.

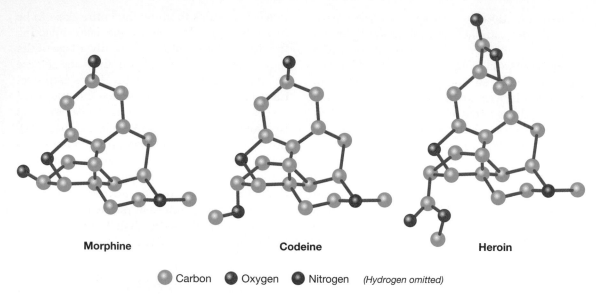

Morphine   **Codeine**   **Heroin**

● Carbon ● Oxygen ● Nitrogen   *(Hydrogen omitted)*

Figure 13.2 Narcotic Agents Isolated or Derived from Opium

In addition to the opioid analgesics, this search for new compounds led to the discovery of **opioid antagonists,** drugs that block the action of morphine, heroin, or other opioid agonists. The administration of a drug such as **naloxone** or *nalorphine* can save a person's life by reversing the depressed respiration resulting from an opioid overdose. If given to an individual who has been taking opioids and who has become physically dependent, these antagonists can precipitate an immediate withdrawal syndrome. Both naloxone and the longer-lasting *naltrexone* have been given to dependent individuals to prevent them from experiencing a high if they then use heroin.

Mechanism of Action

In the early 1970s, techniques were developed that led to the discovery of selective opioid receptors in rat brain tissue. For decades before this, theories of opioid drug action had relied on the concept of an opioid receptor, but the finding that such structures actually exist in the membranes of neurons led to the next question: What are opioid receptors doing in the synapses of the brain—waiting for someone to extract the juice from a poppy? The distribution of these receptors didn't agree with the distribution of any known neurotransmitter substance, so scientists all over the world went to work, looking for a substance in the brain that could serve as the natural activator of these opioid receptors. Groups in England and in Sweden succeeded in 1974: a pair of molecules, leu-enkephalin and met-enkephalin, were isolated from brain extracts. These **enkephalins** acted like morphine and were many times more potent. Next came the discovery of a group of **endorphins** (endogenous morphinelike substances) that are also found in brain tissue and have potent opioid effects. In addition to these two major types of endogenous opioids, dynorphins and other substances have some actions similar to those of morphine. These substances, as well as the natural and synthetic opioid drugs, have actions on at least three types of opioid receptors, the structures of which were discovered in the 1990s. Both mu and kappa opioid receptors play a role in pain perception, while the functions of the delta receptor are not as easily understood.[25] One of the most

Table 13.1
Some Prescription Narcotic Analgesics

Generic Name	Trade Name	Recommended Dose (mg)
Natural Products		
morphine		10–30
codeine		30–60
Semisynthetics		
heroin, diamorph	(Not available in the United States)	5–10
Synthetics		
methadone	Dolophine	2.5–10
meperidine	Demerol	50–150
oxycodone	Percodan, Oxycontin	2.25–4.5
oxymorphone	Numorphan	1–1.5
hydrocodone	Vicodin, Lortab	5–10
hydromorphone	Dilaudid	1–4
dihydrocodeine		32
propoxyphene	Darvon	32–65
pentazocine	Talwin	30
fentanyl	Sublimaze	0.05–0.10

important sites of action may be the midbrain central gray, a region known to be involved in pain perception. However, there are many other sites of interaction between these systems and areas that relate to pain, and pain itself is a complex psychological and neurological phenomenon, so we cannot say that we understand completely how opioids act to reduce pain.

In addition to the presence of these endogenous opioids in the brain, large amounts of endorphins are released from the pituitary gland in response to stress. Also, enkephalins are released from the adrenal gland. The functions of these peptides circulating through the blood as hormones are not understood at this point. They could perhaps reduce pain by acting in the spinal cord, but they are unlikely to produce direct effects in the brain because they probably do not cross the blood-brain barrier. It has been speculated that long-distance runners experience a release of endorphins that might be responsible for the so-called runner's high. Unfortunately, the only evidence in support of this notion was measurements of blood levels of endorphins that seemed to be elevated in some, but not all, runners. These endorphins are presumably from the pituitary and might not be capable of producing a high. It is not known whether exercise alters *brain* levels of these substances.

Beneficial Uses
Pain Relief

The major therapeutic indication for morphine and the other opioids is the reduction of pain. After the administration of an analgesic dose of morphine, some patients report that they are still aware of pain but that the pain is no longer

opioid antagonists: drugs that can block the actions of opioids.
naloxone (nal *ox* own): an opioid antagonist.
enkephalins (en *kef* a lins): morphinelike neurotransmitters found in the brain and adrenals.
endorphins (en *dor* fins): morphinelike neurotransmitters found in the brain and pituitary gland.

aversive. The opioids seem to have their effect in part by diminishing the patient's awareness of and response to the aversive stimulus. Morphine primarily reduces the emotional response to pain (the suffering) and to some extent the knowledge of the pain stimulus.

The effect of opioids is relatively specific to pain. Fewer effects on mental and motor ability accompany analgesic doses of these agents than accompany equipotent doses of other analgesic and depressant drugs. Although one of the characteristics of these drugs is their ability to reduce pain without inducing sleep, drowsiness is not uncommon after a therapeutic dose. (In the user's vernacular, the patient is "on the nod.") The patient is readily awakened if sleeping, and dreams during the sleep period are frequent.

Intestinal Disorders

Opioids have long been valued for their effects on the gastrointestinal system. They quiet colic and save lives by counteracting diarrhea. In years past and today in many underdeveloped countries, contaminated food and water have resulted in severe intestinal infections (dysentery). Particularly in the young and the elderly, diarrhea and resulting dehydration can be a major cause of death.

Opioid drugs decrease the number of peristaltic contractions, which is the type of contraction responsible for moving food through the intestines. Considerable water is absorbed from the intestinal material; this fact, plus the decrease in peristaltic contractions, often results in constipation in patients taking the drugs for pain relief. This side effect is what has saved many lives of dysentery victims. Although modern synthetic opioids are now sold for this purpose, old-fashioned paregoric, an opium solution, is still available for the symptomatic relief of diarrhea.

Cough Suppressants

The opioids also have the effect of decreasing activity in what the advertisers refer to as the cough control center in the medulla. Although coughing is often a useful way of clearing unwanted material from the respiratory passages, at times nonproductive coughing can itself become a problem. Since it was first purified from opium, codeine has been widely used for its *antitussive* properties and is still available in a number of prescription cough remedies. Nonprescription cough remedies contain dextromethorphan, an opioid analogue that is somewhat more selective in its antitussive effects. At high doses, dextromethorphan produces hallucinogenic effects through a different mechanism, by blocking one type of glutamate receptor (see Chapter 14).

Causes for Concern

Dependence Potential

Tolerance Tolerance develops to most of the effects of the opioids, although with different effects tolerance can occur at different rates. If the drug is used chronically for pain relief, for example, it will probably be necessary to increase the dose to maintain a constant effect. The same is true for the euphoria sought by recreational users: Repeated use results in a decreased effect, which can be overcome by increasing the dose. Cross-tolerance exists among all the opioids. Tolerance to one reduces the effectiveness of each of the others. Siegel and others have shown that psychological processes can play an important role in the tolerance to opioids.[26] When a user repeatedly injects an opioid agonist, various physiological effects occur (changes in body temperature, intestinal motility, respiration rate, and so on). With repeated experience the dependent person might unconsciously learn to anticipate those effects and to counteract them. Animal experiments have shown that, after repeated morphine injections, a placebo injection produces changes in body temperature opposite to those originally produced by morphine. Thus, some of the body's tolerance to opioids results from conditioned reflex responses to the stimuli

Table 13.2
Sequence of Appearance of Some of the Abstinence Syndrome Symptoms

Signs	APPROXIMATE HOURS AFTER PREVIOUS DOSE	
	Heroin and/or morphine	Methadone
Craving for drugs, anxiety	6	24
Yawning, perspiration, running nose, teary eyes	14	34–48
Increase in above signs plus pupil dilation, goose bumps (pilorection), tremors (muscle twitches), hot and cold flashes, aching bones and muscles, loss of appetite	16	48–72
Increased intensity of above, plus insomnia; raised blood pressure; increased temperature, pulse rate, respiratory rate and depth; restlessness; nausea	24–36	
Increased intensity of above, plus curled-up position, vomiting, diarrhea, weight loss, spontaneous ejaculation or orgasm, hemoconcentration, increased blood sugar	36–48	

associated with taking the drugs. To demonstrate how important these conditioned protective reflexes can become, Siegel and his colleagues injected rats with heroin every other day in a particular environment. After 15 such injections, the rats were given a much larger dose of heroin, half in the environment previously associated with heroin and half in a different environment. Of the group given the heroin injection in the different environment, most of the rats died. However, of the group given heroin in the environment that had previously predicted heroin, most of the rats lived.[27] Those rats had presumably learned to associate that environment with heroin injections, and conditioned reflexes occurred that counteracted some of the physiological effects of the drug. This is one example of behavioral tolerance.

Physical Dependence Concomitant with the development of tolerance is the establishment of physical dependence: In a person who has used the drug chronically and at high doses, as each dose begins to wear off, certain withdrawal symptoms begin to appear. These symptoms and their approximate timing after opioid use

are listed in Table 13.2. This list of symptoms might have more personal meaning for you if you compare it to a case of the 24-hour, or intestinal, flu. Combine nausea and vomiting with diarrhea, aches, pains, and a general sense of misery, and you have a pretty good idea of what a moderate case of opioid withdrawal is like—rarely life-threatening but most unpleasant. If an individual has been taking a large amount of the drug, then these symptoms can be much worse than those caused by 24-hour flu and can last at least twice as long. Note that **methadone,** a long-lasting synthetic opioid, produces withdrawal symptoms that are usually less severe and that appear later than with heroin but may last longer. Cross-dependence is seen among the opioids. No matter which of them was responsible for producing the initial dependence, withdrawal symptoms can be prevented by an appropriate dose of any opioid agonist. This is the basis for the use of methadone in treating

methadone (*meth* a doan): a long-lasting synthetic opioid.

heroin dependence, because substituting legal methadone prevents withdrawal symptoms for as much as a day.

An interesting clue to the biochemical mechanism of withdrawal symptoms has been the finding that *clonidine,* an alpha-adrenergic agonist that is used to treat high blood pressure, can diminish the severity of withdrawal symptoms. Studies on brain tissue reveal that opioid receptors and alpha-adrenergic receptors are found together in some brain areas, including the norepinephrine-containing cells of the locus ceruleus. Clonidine and morphine produce identical effects on the enzyme activity and neurophysiology of these cells. In other brain areas, opioid receptors are found that are not associated with alpha-adrenergic receptors, which is why clonidine does not produce narcotic-like euphoria and is not a good analgesic.

Psychological Dependence That opioids produce psychological dependence is quite clear; in fact, experiments with opioids were what led to our current understanding of the importance of the reinforcing properties of drugs (see Chapter 2). Animals allowed to self-administer low doses of morphine or heroin intravenously will learn the required behaviors quickly and will perform them for prolonged periods, even if they have never experienced withdrawal symptoms. This is an example of what psychologists refer to as *positive reinforcement:* A behavior is reliably followed by the presentation of a stimulus, leading to an increase in the probability of the behavior and its eventual maintenance at a higher rate than before. Remember that the rapidity with which the reinforcing stimulus follows the behavior is an important factor, which is why fewer experiences are needed with an opioid injected intravenously (fast acting) than with the same drug taken orally (delayed action).

Once physical dependence has developed and withdrawal symptoms are experienced, the conditions are set up for another behavioral mechanism, *negative reinforcement.* In this situation an act (drug taking) is followed by the

removal of withdrawal symptoms, leading to further strengthening of the habit. In heroin dependence, the appearance of early withdrawal symptoms after only a few hours and their rapid alleviation by another injection, typically leads to the development of a more robust dependence in many users. Remember, however, that heroin was prescribed in low doses and taken orally by many patients for several years during which it was believed not to produce dependence. Although heroin is more potent than morphine and may have a higher abuse potential because of its more rapid access to the brain, morphine taken intravenously is more likely to produce dependence than heroin taken orally.

The Needle Habit Each heroin administration is followed by a decrease in discomfort, an increase in pleasure, or both. As a result, the behavior of preparing and injecting the drug and the setting in which it occurs acquire pleasurable, positive associations through learning mechanisms. Because of this conditioning, the process of using heroin also becomes rewarding. One occasional user commented on the ritual of heroin use:

> Once you decide to get off it's very exciting. It really is. Getting some friends together and some money, copping, deciding where you're going to do it, getting the needles out and sterilizing them, cooking up the stuff, tying off, then the whole thing with the needle, booting, and the rush, that's all part of it. . . . Sometimes I think that if I just shot water I'd enjoy it as much.[28]

Though it might seem strange, that last statement is true for some individuals. These users have been called "needle freaks"—at least part of the relief and pleasure they obtain from injecting is a conditioned response to the stimuli (such as needles) associated with heroin use.

Toxicity Potential

Acute Toxicity One specific effect of the opioids is to depress the respiratory centers in the brain, so that respiration slows and becomes shallow. This is perhaps the major side effect of the opioids and one of the most dangerous, because death resulting from respiratory depression can easily follow an excessive dose of these drugs. The basis for this effect is that the respiratory centers become less responsive to carbon dioxide levels in the blood. It is this effect that keeps heroin/morphine near the top of the list of mentioned drugs in DAWN coroners' reports. This respiratory depression is additive with the effects of alcohol or other sedative-hypnotics, and a large fraction of those who die from heroin overdose have elevated blood alcohol concentrations and might better be described as dying from a combination of heroin and alcohol. Opioid overdose can be diagnosed on the basis of the *opioid triad:* coma, depressed respiration, and pinpoint pupils. Emergency medical treatment calls for the use of naloxone (Narcan), which antagonizes the opioid effects within a few minutes.

The behavioral consequences of having morphine-like drugs in the brain are probably less dangerous. Those who inject heroin might nod off into a dream-filled sleep for a few minutes, and opium smokers are famous for their "pipe dreams." It is perhaps not surprising that individuals under the influence of opioids are likely to be less active and less alert than they otherwise would be. A clouding of consciousness makes mental work more difficult. And opioid users not only are less likely to be interested in sex, but men also can suffer primary impotence as a direct effect of the drug.

Opioid agonists also stimulate the brain area controlling nausea and vomiting, which are other frequent side effects. Nausea occurs in about half of ambulatory patients given a 15 mg dose of morphine. Also, nausea and vomiting are a common reaction to heroin injection among street users.

Chronic Toxicity Although early in the 20th century many medical authorities believed that chronic opioid use weakened the user both mentally and physically, there is no scientific evidence that exposure to opioid drugs per se causes long-term damage to any tissue or organ system. Many street users do suffer from sores and abscesses at injection sites, but these can be attributed to the lack of sterile technique. Also, the practice of sharing needles can result in the spread of such blood-borne diseases as serum hepatitis and HIV. Again, this is a result not of the drug but of the technique used to inject it.

Patterns of Abuse

The Life of a Heroin User Only a glimpse of some of the mechanics of a heroin user's life can be presented here. Withdrawal signs might begin about four hours after the previous use of the drug, but many users report that they begin to feel ill six to eight hours after the previous dose. That puts most heroin abusers on a schedule of three or four injections every day. Today's heroin user is not spending a lot of time nodding off in opium dens, as in the "good old days." When you have a very important appointment to keep every six to eight hours, every day of the week, every day of the year, you've got to hustle not to miss one of them. Remember, there are no vacations, no weekends off for the regular user, just 1,200 to 1,400 appointments per year to keep.

And each one costs money. Heroin is frequently sold on the street in "dime" bags: $10 for a small plastic bag containing anybody's guess. The material in a $10 bag might have 3 mg or 30 mg. Of course, you might not get *any* heroin, and you can't complain to the Better Business Bureau. At any rate, your habit can cost you $30 to $100 a day.

The variability is a problem because of the possibility of an overdose. Heroin users should worry about an overdose with each new batch of drug used. A sophisticated user buying from a new or questionable source will initially try a much smaller than normal amount of the powder to evaluate its potency.

Once the user has acquired the drug, he or she prepares it for injection. Usually, the user mixes the powder with unsterile water, heats

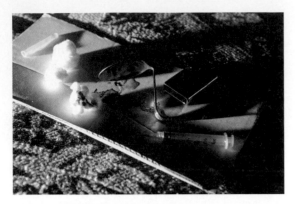

Supplies for shooting up heroin.

the mixture briefly in a spoon or bottle cap with a match or lighter to help the drug dissolve, then draws the heroin into a syringe or eyedropper through cotton, thus filtering out the larger impurities. The heroin is then injected intravenously, often without any attempt at skin cleansing. Under these conditions, infections are not surprising. Some users prefer an eyedropper with a hypodermic needle attached, because the rubber bulb of the dropper is easier to operate than the plunger of a syringe.

The most common form of heroin use by male users is to inject the drug intravenously—that is, to mainline the drug. A convenient site is the left forearm (for right-handed users), and frequent injection leaves the arm marked with scar tissue. If the larger veins of the arm collapse, then other body areas are used. Many beginning users start by "skin-popping"—subcutaneous injections. Skin-popping increases the danger of tetanus but decreases the risk of hepatitis compared with mainlining. Because of the lack of sterility, hepatitis, tetanus, and abscesses at the site of injection are not uncommon in street users who inject drugs.

If the user survives the perils of an overdose, escapes the dangers of contaminated equipment, and avoids being caught, there are still other dangers. Heroin is a potent analgesic, and its regular use can conceal the early symptoms of an illness, such as pneumonia. The user's lack of money for, or interest in, food frequently results in malnutrition. With low resistance from malnutrition and the symptoms of illness going unnoticed as a result of heroin use, the user becomes susceptible to serious disease.

If all these dangers are overcome, the user might continue to use opioids to an advanced age. Sometimes, however, the user who avoids illness, death, or arrest and who does not enter and stay in a rehabilitation program or withdraw him- or herself from the drug might no longer feel the need for the drug and gradually stop using it. This "maturing out" is probably what happens to a large number of heroin abusers. Even if the user lives, the street life of a heroin-dependent individual isn't a rose garden.

Misconceptions and Preconceptions Although heroin users haven't received as much press as methamphetamine users in recent years, most people have strongly held beliefs about heroin, derived from television, magazines, movies, and conversations. Most people, including many professionals, have major misconceptions about nonmedical use and misuse of opioids.

One of the most common misconceptions is that injecting heroin or morphine induces in everyone an intense pleasure unequaled by any other experience. Often it is described as similar to a whole-body orgasm that persists up to five or more minutes. Some users report that they try with every injection to reexperience the extreme euphoria of the first injection, but always have a lesser effect. However, studies, as well as clinical and street reports, show that some people experience only nausea and discomfort after the initial intravenous administration of morphine or heroin. For whatever reasons, some of these users persist and the discomfort decreases—that is, it shows tolerance more rapidly than the euphoric effects. Under these conditions the injections soon result primarily in pleasant effects. To maintain these pleasurable feelings, though, the dose level must gradually be increased.

Another misconception has to do with the development of withdrawal symptoms. The heroin user undergoing withdrawal without medication is always portrayed as being in excruciating pain, truly suffering. It depends. With a large habit, withdrawal without medication is truly hell. The opioid abuse scene is changing too rapidly to be definite about today's user, but many street users use a low daily drug dose. For many such users, the withdrawal symptoms resemble a mild case of intestinal flu (cramps, diarrhea).

Perhaps the most common misconception about heroin is that, after one shot, you are hooked for life. None of the opioids, or any other drug, fits into that fantasized category. Becoming dependent takes time, perhaps a week or more, and persistence on the part of the beginner. Regular use of the drug seems to be more important in establishing physical dependence than the size of the dose used. Becoming physically dependent is possible on a weekend, but it frequently requires a longer period, with three or four injections a day.

There are probably about 500,000 opioid-dependent individuals in the United States. There may be two to three times as many heroin *chippers*—occasional users. Several reports have appeared on the characteristics of these occasional users, but no consistent differences, compared with heroin-dependent persons, have yet been found other than the pattern of use.

Summary

- Opium was used in its raw form for centuries, both medicinally and for pleasure.

- Opium had significant influences on medicine, literature, and world politics through the 1800s.

- Dependence on opioids has been recognized for a long time, but no concerted effort to control dependence was tried until the patent medicine era of the late 1800s, combined with opium smoking by Chinese-Americans, led to federal regulations in the early 1900s.

- The typical opioid abuser changed from being a middle-aged, middle-class woman

using patent medicines by mouth to being a young, lower-class man using heroin by intravenous injection.

- Various synthetic opioids are now available along with the natural products of the opium poppy. These drugs all act at opioid receptors in the brain.

- Opioid receptors are normally acted on by the naturally occurring opioid-like products of the nervous system and endocrine glands, endorphins and enkephalins.

- The opioid overdose triad consists of coma, depressed respiration, and pinpoint pupils. Death occurs because breathing ceases.

- Illicit heroin comes primarily from South America, Mexico, Southeast Asia, and Southwest Asia.

Review Questions

1. What two chemicals are extracted from the opium poppy?
2. What was the significance of De Quincey's writing about opium eating?
3. What were the approximate dates and who were the combatants in the Opium Wars?
4. How is it possible that heroin was at first sold as a nonaddicting pain reliever?
5. How did the typical opioid abuser change from the early 1900s to the 1920s?
6. Why and when did private physicians and public clinics stop maintaining dependent individuals with morphine and other opioids?
7. What were some of the lessons learned about heroin dependence as a result of the Vietnam experience?
8. What two factors were probably responsible for the increase in the smoking of heroin in 1989 and 1990?
9. What is the effect of a narcotic antagonist on someone who has developed a physical dependence on opioids?
10. What are the enkephalins and endorphins, and how do they relate to plant-derived opioids such as morphine?

References

1. Baum, L.F. *The New Wizard of Oz.* New York: Grosset & Dunlap, 1944.
2. Scott, J.M. *The White Poppy: A History of Opium.* New York: Funk & Wagnalls, 1969.
3. Hamarneh, S. "Sources and Development of Arabic Medical Therapy and Pharmacology." *Sudhoffs Archiv fur Geschichte der Medizin und der Naturwissenschaften* 54 (1970), p. 34.
4. De Quincey, T. *Confessions of an English Opium-eater.* New York: EP Dutton, 1907.
5. Turk, M.H. *Selections from De Quincey.* Boston: Ginn & Co., 1902.
6. De Quincey Works, Vol. 206. Quoted in Lowes, J.L. *The Road to Xanadu.* Boston: Houghton Mifflin, 1927.
7. Blair, W. "An Opium-eater in America." *The Knickerbocker* 20 (1842), pp. 47–57.
8. Kramer, J.C. "Opium Rampant: Medical Use, Misuse and Abuse in Britain and the West in the 17th and 18th Centuries." *British Journal of Addiction:* 1979, p. 377.
9. Kramer, J.C. "Heroin in the Treatment of Morphine Addiction." *Journal of Psychedelic Drugs* 9, no. 3 (1977), pp. 193–97.
10. Dott, D.B., & R. Stockman. *Proceedings of the Royal Society of Edinburgh,* 1890, p. 321.
11. Manges, M. "A Second Report on the Therapeutics of Heroine." *New York Medical Journal* 71 (1900), pp. 51, 82–83.
12. Wilcox, R.W. *Pharmacology and Therapeutics,* 6th ed. Philadelphia: P. Blakiston's Son, 1905.
13. Lindesmith, A.R. *Addiction and Opiates.* Chicago: Aldine, 1968.
14. Kebler, L.F. "The Present Status of Drug Addiction in the United States." In *Transactions of the American Therapeutic Society.* Philadelphia: FA Davis, 1910.
15. Black, J.R. "Advantages of Substituting the Morphia Habit for the Incurably Alcoholic." *The Cincinnati Lancet—Clinic* 22 (1889), pp. 538–41.
16. Lindesmith, A.R. *The Addict and the Law.* Bloomington: Indiana University Press, 1965.
17. Smith, R. "Status Politics and the Image of the Addict." *Issues in Criminology* 2, no. 2 (1966), pp. 157–75.
18. *The World Heroin Problem.* Committee Print, House of Representatives, Committee on Foreign Affairs, Ninety-second Congress, First Session, May 27, 1971. Washington, DC: U.S. Government Printing Office, 1971.
19. Robins, L.N. *The Vietnam Drug User Returns.* Special Action Office for Drug Abuse Prevention Monograph, Series A, No. 2, May 1974, Contract No. HSM-42-72-75.
20. Brodsky, M.D. "History of Heroin Prevalence Estimation Techniques." In *Self-Report Methods of Estimating Drug Use,* NIDA Research Monograph No. 57. Washington, DC: U.S. Government Printing Office, 1985.
21. U.S. Office of National Drug Control Policy. *Heroin Fact Sheet.* Washington, DC: The White House, 2004. www.whitehousedrugpolicy.gov/publications/international/factsht/heroin.html.
22. U.S. Office of National Drug Control Policy. *Heroin.* Washington, DC: The White House, 2004. www.whitehousedrugpolicy.gov/drugfact/heroin/index.html#production.
23. Substance Abuse and Mental Health Services Administration. *Results from the 2004 National Survey on Drug Use and Health: National Findings.* Rockville, MD: Office of Applied Studies, NHSDA, 2005.
24. United States General Accounting Office. *Oxycontin Abuse and Diversion and Efforts to Address the Problem.* GAO Publication 04-110, December 2003.
25. Julien, R.M. *A Primer of Drug Action,* 10th ed. New York: Worth, 2005.
26. Siegel, S. "Morphine Analgesic Tolerance: Its Situation Specificity Supports a Pavlovian Conditioning Model." *Science* 193 (1976), pp. 323–25.
27. Siegel, S., and others. "Heroin 'Overdose' Death: Contribution of Drug-Associated Environmental Cues." *Science* 216 (1982), pp. 436–37.
28. Powell, D.H. "A Pilot Study of Occasional Heroin Users." *Arch Gen Psychiatry* 28 (1973), pp. 586–94.

Check Yourself

Draw lines to match these street terms for drugs and related terms (left-hand column) with the appropriate term or definition in the right-hand column:

Black tar	Heroin
Chipper	Fentanyl or a derivative
Smack	Withdrawal symptoms
Dime bag	Occasional heroin user
China white	Injecting equipment (syringe or dropper)
Works	$10 worth of heroin
Jones	A type of ilicit heroin

14 Hallucinogens

Objectives

When you have finished this chapter, you should be able to:

- **Explain why plants with psychoactive effects have been used in religious practices all over the world.**

- **Differentiate phantastica and deleriants and recognize several examples of indole and catechol hallucinogens.**

- **Describe the relationship of LSD to the ergot fungus.**

- **Discuss the early research and evidence on LSD for use in interrogation and in psychotherapy.**

- **Understand what is meant by "hallucinogen persisting perception disorder."**

- **Describe the major active ingredient and some history of use of psilocybe, morning glories, ayahuasca, peyote, San Pedro cactus, *Amanita,* and *Salvia divinorum*.**

- **Understand the chemical relationship among DOM, MDA, and MDMA.**

- **Compare and contrast PCP effects with those of LSD.**

- **Explain how anticholinergic hallucinogens act in the brain.**

- **Compare stories about medieval witches using belladonna to contemporary stories about people using marijuana, LSD, or cocaine.**

From the soft, quiet beauty of the sacred *Psilocybe* mushroom to the angry, mottled appearance of the toxic *Amanita,* from the mountains of Mexico to the streets of Anytown, USA, from before history to the 21st century, humans have searched for the perfect aphrodisiac, spiritual experiences, and other worlds. The plants have been there to help; plants have evolved to produce chemicals that alter the biochemistry of animals. If they make us feel sick, we are unlikely to eat them again, and if they kill us, we are certain not to eat them again. But humans long ago learned to "tame" some of these plants, to use them in just the right ways and in just the right amounts to alter perceptions and emotions without too many unpleasant consequences.

Animism and Religion

Animism, the belief that animals, plants, rocks, streams, and so on derive their special characteristics from a spirit contained within the object, is

Online Learning Center Resources

www.mhhe.com/ksir12e

Visit our Online Learning Center (OLC) for access to these study aids and additional resources.

- Learning objectives
- Glossary flashcards
- Web activities and links
- Self-scoring chapter quiz
- Audio chapter summaries

a common theme in most of the world's religions. Plants that are able to alter our perception of the world and of ourselves fit right into such a view. If the plant contains a spirit, then eating the plant transfers that spirit to the person who eats it, and the spirit of the plant can speak to the consumer, make her feel the plant's joy or provide her with special powers or insights.

In early hunter-gatherer societies, certain individuals became specialists in the ways of these plants, learning when to harvest them and how much to use under what circumstances. These traditions were passed down from one generation to another, and colorful stories were used to teach the principles to apprentices. Our modern term for these individuals is *shaman* or *medicine man/woman* because of their knowledge of drug-containing plants. But because they also were the experts on obtaining power from the spirit world, their function in hunter-gatherer societies had as much to do with the origins of religion as with the origins of modern medicine. These plants and their psychoactive effects were probably important reasons for the development of spiritual and religious traditions and folklore in many societies all over the world.[1]

Terminology and Types

The issue of what to call this group of drugs is an old one. In 1931, Lewin referred to a class of **phantastica,** drugs that can create in our minds a world of fantasy. Peyote, psilocybin, and LSD all produce this type of effect. In the 1960s, these drugs were described by enthusiastic users as allowing them to see into their own minds, and the term **psychedelic** ("mind-viewing") was widely used. The term itself implies a beneficial, visionary type of effect, and there is considerable disagreement over whether such effects are really beneficial. Because the drugs are capable of producing hallucinations and some altered sense of reality, a state that could be called psychotic, they have also been referred to as **psychotomimetic** drugs. This term implies that the drugs produce dangerous effects and a form of mental disorder, which is also a controversial conclusion.

More recently, proponents have popularized newer terms, such as *entheogen* and *entactogen,* to describe these substances. For example, *entheogen* is used to describe substances (e.g., sacred mushrooms) that are thought to create spiritual or religious experiences, whereas *entactogen,* meaning "to produce a touching within," is used to describe substances, such as MDMA, that are said to enhance feelings of empathy.

Is there a descriptive and unbiased term that will allow us to categorize the drugs and then to examine their effects without prejudice? One thing common to these drugs is some tendency to produce hallucinations, so we will refer to them by the name *hallucinogens.*

Phantastica

Although we will call all of these drugs hallucinogens, there are important differences among them. They can be classified according to their chemical structures, their known pharmacological properties, how much loss of awareness occurs under their influence, and how dangerous they are. The first types we will review are the classical phantastica: They are capable of altering perceptions while allowing the person to remain in communication with the present world. The individual under the influence of these drugs will

Drugs in the Media

The Psychedelic 60s—Reflections in Film, Music, and Literature

In a peculiar interaction between a new drug phenomenon (experimenting with perception-altering drugs, such as LSD) and a time of many radical changes in American society (the civil rights movement, the war in Vietnam, the British invasion of popular music led by the Beatles), a cultural mixture was formed that we now call "the psychedelic 60s" (which for most people probably coincided with the decade 1965 to 1975). All you need to do is to look at popular films from that time or at photographs of relatives to see the influence on hairstyles and clothing. But what was psychedelic about this period, and was it in fact important or interesting from a cultural or an artistic perspective?

One can see the transition in the music of the Beatles. Their early work sounded a lot like mainstream rock and roll, but a visit to India and experimentation with various drugs changed the way they sounded, dressed, and talked. And they in turn influenced many others.

What other writers, artists, and musicians are associated with this phenomenon? The Grateful Dead and Jefferson Airplane may have started it all in music, and Ken Kesey may have started it all in literature, but no popular figure could ignore the influence. Perhaps its most obvious presentation can be seen by looking at album covers, the cardboard jackets that contained the long-playing record albums of the era. To say that the art form of these music-album covers flowered during that period would be both a pun and an understatement.

The University of Virginia library supports a virtual exhibition on a Web site, www.lib.virginia.edu/exhibits/sixties/, called The Psychedelic Sixties: Literary Tradition and Social Change. There you can read about the music, the social protests, the literature, and the big events that shaped the period, and you can view enough psychedelic art to satisfy anyone's curiosity.

often be aware of both the fantasy world and the real world at the same time, might talk avidly about what is being experienced, and will be able to remember much of it later. These drugs can be seen as having more purely hallucinogenic effects in that they do not produce much acute physiological toxicity—that is, there is relatively little danger of dying from an overdose of LSD, psilocybin, or mescaline. The two major classes of phantastica, the indole and catechol hallucinogens, are grouped according to their chemical structures.

Indole Hallucinogens

The basic structure of the neurotransmitter serotonin is referred to as an **indole** nucleus. Figure 14.1 illustrates that the hallucinogens LSD and psilocybin also contain this structure. For that reason and the fact that some other chemicals with this structure have similar hallucinogenic effects, we refer to one group of the phantastica as the indoles.

d-Lysergic Acid Diethylamide (LSD) The most potent and notorious of the hallucinogens, and the one that brought these drugs into the public eye in the 1960s, is not found in nature. Although there are naturally occurring compounds that resemble the indole *d*-lysergic acid diethylamide (LSD), their identity as hallucinogens

animism: the belief that objects attain certain characteristics because of spirits.
phantastica (fan *tass* tick a): drugs that create a world of fantasy.
psychedelic (sy ka *dell* ick): "mind-viewing."
psychotomimetic (sy cot o mim *et* ick): mimicking psychosis.
indole (*in* dole): a particular chemical structure found in serotonin and LSD.

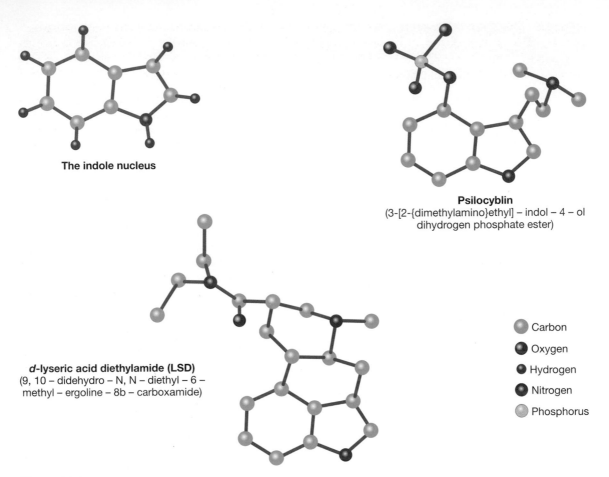

The indole nucleus

Psilocyblin
(3-[2-{dimethylamino}ethyl] – indol – 4 – ol
dihydrogen phosphate ester)

***d*-lyseric acid diethylamide (LSD)**
(9, 10 – didehydro – N, N – diethyl – 6 –
methyl – ergoline – 8b – carboxamide)

- ● Carbon
- ● Oxygen
- ● Hydrogen
- ● Nitrogen
- ● Phosphorus

Figure 14.1   Indole Hallucinogens

was not known until after the discovery of LSD. LSD was originally synthesized from ergot alkaloids extracted from the ergot fungus *Claviceps purpurea.* This mold occasionally grows on grain, especially rye, and eating infected grain results in an illness called *ergotism.*

Saint Anthony's Fire Grain that has been infected with the ergot fungus is readily identified and is usually destroyed. During periods of famine, however, the grain might be used in making bread. In France between AD 945 and 1600, there were at least 20 outbreaks of ergotism, the illness that results from eating infected bread. Although the cause of the illness was established before 1700, only symptomatic treatment exists

even today. There are two forms of the disease. In one, tingling sensations in the skin and muscle spasms develop into convulsions, insomnia, and various disturbances of consciousness and thinking. In the other form, gangrenous ergotism, the limbs become swollen and inflamed, with the individual experiencing "violent burning pains" before the affected part becomes numb. Sometimes the disease moves rapidly, with less than 24 hours between the first sign and the development of gangrene. Gangrene develops because the ergot causes a contraction of the blood vessels, cutting off blood flow to the extremities.

During the 12th century, ergotism became associated with Saint Anthony, although the reason for this is not completely clear. It might be that the hospital for the treatment of ergotism was built near the shrine of Saint Anthony because he had suffered from a minor attack of ergotism. Others believe the illness was called Saint Anthony's fire because those who made the pilgrimage to Egypt, where Saint Anthony had lived, were cured. Those who journeyed to Egypt and those who entered the hospital did lose their symptoms, probably as a result of a diet that did not include ergot-infected rye.

Two interesting articles discussed a possible link between convulsive ergotism and the Salem witch trials of 1692, in which 20 people were executed. The first article built a very strong case that (1) the original symptoms exhibited by the "possessed" eight girls were similar to those seen in convulsive ergotism and (2) the conditions were right for the growth of the ergot fungus on the rye that was the staple cereal.[2] The second article constructed an equally convincing case that ergotism could not have been involved and that the "possession" was psychological.[3] We will never know for sure, but there are enough similarities and lingering doubts that ergotism seems to remain a possible basis for the Salem incident.

LSD Discovery and Early Research In the Sandoz Laboratories in Basel, Switzerland, in 1938, Dr. Albert Hofmann synthesized *lysergsaurediethylamid*, the German word from which *LSD* comes and that names the substance known in English as d-lysergic acid diethylamide. Hofmann was working on a series of compounds derived from ergot alkaloids that had as their basic structure lysergic acid. LSD was synthesized because of its chemical similarity to a known stimulant, nikethamide. It was not until 1943, however, that LSD entered the world of biochemical psychiatry, when Hofmann recorded the following in his laboratory notebook:

> Last Friday, April 16, 1943, I was forced to stop my work in the laboratory in the middle of the afternoon and go home, as I was seized by a peculiar restlessness associated with a sensation of mild dizziness. Having reached home, I lay

down and sank in a kind of drunkenness which was not unpleasant and which was characterized by extreme activity of imagination. As I lay in a dazed condition with my eyes closed (I experienced daylight as disagreeably bright) there surged upon me an uninterrupted stream of fantastic images of extraordinary plasticity and vividness and accompanied by an intense, kaleidoscope-like play of colors. This condition gradually passed off after about two hours.[4]

Hofmann later said, "The first experience was a very weak one, consisting of rather small changes. It had a pleasant, fairy tale—magic theater quality." He was sure that the experience resulted from the accidental absorption, through the skin of his fingers, of the compound with which he was working. The next Monday morning Hofmann prepared what he thought was a very small amount of LSD, 0.25 mg, and made the following record in his notebook:

> April 19, 1943: Preparation of an 0.5% aqueous solution of d-lysergic acid diethylamide tartrate.
> 4:20 P.M.: 0.5 cc (0.25 mg LSD) ingested orally. The solution is tasteless.
> 4:50 P.M.: no trace of any effect.
> 5:00 P.M.: slight dizziness, unrest, difficulty in concentration, visual disturbances, marked desire to laugh.

At this point the laboratory notes are discontinued:

> The last words could only be written with great difficulty. I asked my laboratory assistant to accompany me home as I believed that my condition would be a repetition of the disturbance of the previous Friday. While we were still cycling home, however, it became clear that the symptoms were much stronger than the first time. I had great difficulty in speaking coherently, my field of vision swayed before me, and objects appeared distorted like images in curved mirrors. I had the impression of being unable to move from the spot, although my assistant told me afterwards that we had cycled at a good pace.
> Six hours after ingestion of the LSD-25 my condition had already improved considerably. Only the visual disturbances were still pronounced. Everything seemed to sway and the

proportions were distorted like the reflections in the surface of moving water. Moreover, all objects appeared in unpleasant, constantly changing colors, the predominant shades being sickly green and blue. When I closed my eyes, an unending series of colorful, very realistic and fantastic images surged in upon me. A remarkable feature was the manner in which all acoustic perceptions (e.g., the noise of a passing car) were transformed into optical effects, every sound causing a corresponding colored hallucination constantly changing in shape and color like pictures in a kaleidoscope. At about 1 o'clock I fell asleep and awakened the next morning somewhat tired but otherwise feeling perfectly well.[4]

The amount Albert Hofmann took orally is five to eight times the normal effective dose, and it was the potency of the drug that attracted attention to it. Mescaline had long been known to cause strange experiences, alter consciousness, and lead to a particularly vivid kaleidoscope of colors, but it takes 4,000 times as much mescaline as LSD. LSD is usually active when only 0.05 mg (50 µg) is taken, and in some people a dose of 0.03 mg is effective.

The first report on LSD in the scientific literature came from Zurich in 1947. In 1953, Sandoz applied to the Food and Drug Administration to study LSD as an investigational new drug. Between 1953 and 1966, Sandoz distributed large quantities of LSD to qualified scientists throughout the world. Most of this legal LSD was used in biochemical and animal behavior research.

Besides an interest in trying to develop "model psychoses" in animals and humans so that treatments could be developed, the major thrust of LSD research had to do with its alleged ability to access the "subconscious mind." This notion probably derived from the dreamlike quality of the reports of LSD experiences and the long-held psychoanalytic view that dreams represent subconscious thoughts trying to express themselves. Thus, LSD was widely used as an adjunct to psychotherapy. When a psychiatrist felt that a patient had reached a roadblock and was unable to dredge up repressed memories and motives, LSD might be used for its psychedelic (mind-viewing) properties. Thus, LSD took over as a modern truth serum, replacing sodium pentothal and scopolamine. Whether LSD actually helped these patients in the long run or only seemed helpful to the psychiatrists who believed in it is still being debated.

Two other potentially therapeutic uses were studied: For various theoretical reasons it was believed that LSD might be a good treatment for alcohol dependence, and initial reports of its effectiveness were quite positive. Later, it was hoped that LSD would allow terminal cancer patients to achieve a greater understanding of their own mortality. Thus, many such patients were allowed to explore their feelings while under the influence of this fantasy-producing agent.

In April 1966, the Sandoz Pharmaceutical Company recalled the LSD it had distributed and withdrew its sponsorship for work with LSD. Large quantities of illegally manufactured LSD of uncertain purity were being used in the street, and Sandoz decided to give the responsibility for the legal distribution of LSD to the federal government.

Scientific study of the hallucinogens declined in the 1970s. A 1974 report by a National Institute of Mental Health (NIMH) research task force on hallucinogenic research stated:

> Virtually every psychological test has been used to study persons under the influence of LSD or other such hallucinogens, but the research has contributed little to our understanding of the bizarre and potent effects of this drug.[5]

Partly as a reality-oriented response to this type of evaluation and partly because of the dead ends, the NIMH stopped its in-house LSD research on humans in 1968 and stopped funding university human research on LSD in 1974. The National Cancer Institute and the National Institute on Alcohol Abuse and Alcoholism stopped supporting psychedelic research in 1975 because it was nonproductive. Most of the

LSD research since that time has been conducted on animals in an effort to better understand the mechanism of action at a neural level.

Although interest in the therapeutic properties of LSD has faded, interest in the therapeutic properties of several other types of hallucinogens has continued. This research is often not funded from U.S. government sources, but much of it is supported by interested private donors through organizations such as the Multidisciplinary Association for Psychedelic Studies.

Secret Army/CIA Research with LSD The unveiling of CIA/Army human research programs using hallucinogens began with a June 1975 report by the Rockefeller Commission on the CIA. A 43-year-old biochemist, Frank Olson, had committed suicide on November 28, 1953, less than two weeks after CIA agents had secretly slipped LSD into his after-dinner drink. This drug had caused a panic reaction in Dr. Olson, and he was taken to New York City for psychiatric treatment. After his suicide, his family was told only that he had jumped or fallen from his 10th-story hotel room in Manhattan. In 1975, when the LSD link was uncovered, President Ford quickly apologized to the Olson family at the White House and said the incident was "inexcusable and unforgivable . . . a horrible episode in American history."[6] It was not until October 1976 that enough government red tape was cut through to make it possible to award $750,000 to the Olson family.

Awareness of the Olson death started Congress and journalists digging for more, this time into the military as well. The Army's interest in, and human experiments on, the use of psychedelics for warfare and for interrogation of prisoners and spies was not hidden. It was open knowledge in the scientific and military communities that such research was conducted at Edgewood Arsenal in Maryland, where Dr. Olson was poisoned, and at several major universities in the United States.

It was easy to see how the military and intelligence agencies got involved in this work.

"American military and intelligence officials watched men with glazed eyes pouring out rambling confessions at the Communist purge trials in Eastern Europe after World War II, and for the first time they began to worry about the threat of mind-bending drugs as weapons."[7] They worried enough to repeatedly contact Dr. Hofmann about the feasibility of large-scale production of LSD,[8] and the CIA considered buying 10 kg in 1953 for $240,000. We can all be pleased that they decided against the purchase, which would have provided 100 million doses.

As the information kept pouring out of government files from 1975 to 1976, it became clear that the Army-sponsored research on 585 soldiers and 900 civilians between 1956 and 1967 had been very poorly done. The Army and some of the university scientists had violated many of the ethical codes established as a result of the Nuremberg war crimes trials after World War II. Three failures were especially blatant: Many of the volunteers were not really volunteers, many of the participants could not quit an experiment if they wanted to, and the participants were not told the nature of the experiment.

This horror story could go on almost without end; mention could be made of CIA agents picking up patrons in bars and secretly putting LSD in their drinks or of the administration of LSD to unsuspecting civilians around the world. The inspector general of the Army issued a long report that criticized almost every aspect of the Army's involvement with human LSD research: its conception, its execution, and its productivity.[9] This story should bring home the dangers of giving drugs to persons without their knowledge. These drugs can be mind-breaking when used incautiously.

Recreational Use of LSD The story starts in the summer of 1960 in Mexico, where for the first time a psychologist named Timothy Leary used magic mushrooms containing psilocybin. As he later said, he realized then that the old Timothy Leary was dead; the "Timothy Leary game" was over. Working at Harvard University,

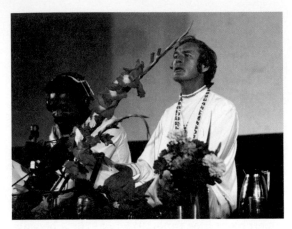

Timothy Leary was a well-known early proponent of the use of LSD.

Leary collaborated with Dr. Richard Alpert and discussed the meaning and implication of this new world with Aldous Huxley.

During the 1960–1961 school year, Leary and Alpert began a series of experiments on Harvard graduate students using pure psilocybin, which they had obtained through a physician. Leary's original work was apparently done under proper scientific controls and with a physician in attendance because drugs were used. The use of a physician was later eliminated, and then other controls were dropped. Leary believed strongly that the experimenter should use the drug along with the subject, in order to be able to communicate with the subject. This practice removes the experimenter from the role of objective observer, and calls into question the scientific value of the research.

Leary's drug taking in the role of experimenter and the apparent abandonment of a scientific approach were questioned by Harvard authorities and other scientists. Some of the major issues were that no physician was present when drugs were administered, undergraduates were used in drug experiments, and drug sessions were conducted outside the laboratory in Leary's home and at other places off campus. As a result of many factors, Alpert and Leary were dismissed from their academic positions in the spring of 1963.[10]

All was reasonably quiet in 1964 and 1965. Alpert, now known as Baba Ram Dass, separated from Leary and lectured on the West Coast, whereas Leary settled at an estate in Millbrook, New York, which was owned by a wealthy supporter of Leary's beliefs. In 1964, Leary announced that drugs were not necessary to rise above and go beyond one's ego. He reiterated this again in 1966 after he was arrested for possession of marijuana at the Millbrook estate.

Also in 1966, Leary started his religion, the League of Spiritual Discovery, with LSD as the sacrament. The league got off to a slow start, and Leary's home base at Millbrook was under attack around the same time. The concern was that Leary would attract "drug addicts to Millbrook. When their money runs out, they will murder, rob and steal, to secure funds with which to satisfy their craving."[11]

Leary was the guru of the age, but his sacrament was already being secularized. Increasing numbers of young people were responding to the motto of the League for Spiritual Discovery: "Turn on, tune in, and drop out." Leary phrased it meaningfully:

> Turning on correctly means to understand the many levels that are brought into focus; it takes years of discipline, training, and discipleship. To turn on on a street corner is a waste. To tune in means you must harness rigorously what you are learning. . . .
>
> To drop out is the oldest message that spiritual teachers have passed on. You can get only by giving up.[12]

These were noble words, perhaps, but street-corner turn-ons were becoming more frequent. A combination of many things increased the use of hallucinogens, and especially LSD, during the early and mid-1960s. LSD's promise of new sensations (which were delivered), of potent aphrodisiac effects (which were not forthcoming), of feelings of kinship with a friendly peer group (which occurred) spread the drug rapidly.

In the summer of 1966, delegates to the annual convention of the American Medical

Association passed a resolution urging greater controls on hallucinogens. They were a little uptight, as was the nation; in part, the resolution stated that

> These drugs can produce uncontrollable violence, overwhelming panic . . . or attempted suicide or homicide, and can result, among the unstable or those with preexisting neurosis or psychosis, in severe illness demanding protracted stays in mental hospitals.[13]

LSD use appears to have peaked in 1967 and 1968, after which it tapered off. Several factors probably contributed to this decline, including widely publicized "bad trips," prolonged psychotic reactions, worries about possible chromosome damage, self-injurious behavior, and "flashbacks." Concerned, many people began to avoid hallucinogens, whereas others shunned the synthetic LSD for the natural experiences produced by psilocybin or mescaline (actually, into the mid-1970s these natural substances were in short supply, and most street samples of either psilocybin or mescaline contained primarily LSD or PCP).

After a series of arrests on drug charges, Timothy Leary was sent to a minimum security prison in 1969, from which he escaped in 1970. After wandering around the world for a couple of years, he surrendered and was sent back to prison. Before his release in 1976, he stated that he was "totally rehabilitated" and would "never, under any circumstances, advocate the use of LSD or any drug." Touring college campuses on the lecture circuit in the early 1980s, Leary talked about "how to use drugs without abusing them."[14]

LSD Pharmacology LSD is odorless, colorless, tasteless, and one of the most potent psychochemicals known. Remember the pharmacological meaning of *potent:* It takes little LSD to produce effects. A drug can be highly potent and yet not produce much in the way of effects. For example, LSD has never been definitely linked to even one human overdose death. In rats, reliable behavioral effects can be produced by 0.04 mg/kg, whereas the LD_{50} is about 16 mg/kg, 400 times the behaviorally effective dose.

Absorption from the gastrointestinal tract is rapid, and most humans take LSD through the mouth. At all postingestion times, the brain contains less LSD than any of the other organs in the body, so it is not selectively taken up by the brain. Half of the LSD in the blood is metabolized every three hours, so blood levels decrease fairly rapidly. LSD is metabolized in the liver and excreted as 2-oxy-lysergic acid diethylamide, which is inactive.

Tolerance develops rapidly, repeated daily doses becoming ineffective in three to four days. Recovery is equally rapid, so weekly use of the same dose of LSD is possible. Cross-tolerance has been shown among LSD, mescaline, and psilocybin, and the psychological effects of each can be blocked with chlorpromazine. Physical dependence to LSD or to any of the hallucinogens has not been shown.

LSD is a sympathomimetic agent, and the autonomic signs are some of the first to appear after LSD is taken. Typical symptoms are dilated pupils, elevated temperature and blood pressure, and an increase in salivation.

The fact that the indole structure of LSD resembles that of serotonin led first to the idea that LSD works by acting at serotonin receptors. Mescaline and other catechol hallucinogens have chemical structures more similar to the neurotransmitters dopamine and norepinephrine than to serotonin. However, they have psychological effects that are very similar to those of LSD. Rats trained to press one lever after an injection of LSD and another lever after a saline (placebo) injection will respond on the LSD lever if given other indole or catechol hallucinogens, but not if given PCP, anticholinergics, stimulants, sedatives, or opiates.[15] Thus, the highly specific "LSD stimulus" in a rat appears to be similar to the stimuli produced by other indole and catechol hallucinogens.

Whereas most of the behavioral effects of LSD and the catechol hallucinogens can be blocked by drugs that act as serotonin-receptor antagonists, others cannot. Add to this that there are several subtypes of serotonin receptors, some of which are excitatory and others inhibitory, and that LSD can act as either an agonist or an antagonist at different serotonin receptors and you can begin to see how complicated this issue becomes. At the present time, the best evidence seems to indicate that LSD and other hallucinogens, including mescaline and psilocybin, act by stimulating the "serotonin-2A" subtype of receptors. Among a large group of hallucinogenic chemicals, there is a high correlation between their potency in binding to this type of receptor from rat brains and their potency in producing hallucinogenic effects in humans.[16]

The LSD Experience Regardless of the chemical mechanism, most scientists feel that the most important effect is the modification of perception, particularly of visual images. Some of the experiences reported, especially after low doses, might best be described as illusions, or perceptual distortions, in which an object that is, in fact, present is seen in a distorted form (brighter than normal, moving, in multiple images). Siegel, who conducted laboratory research on the visual images reported after the ingestion of various drugs, reported that some images can be seen with eyes open or closed and thus are hallucinations rather than illusions.[17] One stage of such hallucinogen-induced imagery consists of form-constants: lattices, honeycomb or chessboard designs, cobwebs, tunnels, alley or cone shapes, and spiral figures. These shapes are generally combined with intense colors and brightness. At another stage, complex images, such as landscapes, remembered faces, or objects, might be combined with the form-constants (e.g., a face might be seen "through" a honeycomb lattice, or multiple images of the face might appear in a honeycomb configuration). Siegel suggested that the perceptual processing mechanisms might be activated at the same time as the sensory inputs are either reduced or impaired, thus allowing vivid perception of images that come from inside, rather than outside, the brain.

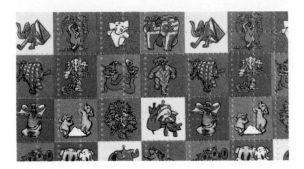

A very small dose of LSD has powerful effects. Liquid LSD solution may be taken orally; it is often applied to blotter paper divided into squares containing single doses.

Besides changes in visual perception, users also report an altered sense of time, changes in the perception of one's own body (perhaps indicating a reduction in somatic sensory input), and some alterations of auditory input. A particularly interesting phenomenon is that of **synesthesia**, a "mixing of senses," in which sounds might appear as visual images (as reported by Dr. Hofmann on the first-ever LSD trip), or the visual picture might alter in rhythm with music.

Altered perception is combined with enhanced emotionality, perhaps related to the arousal of the sympathetic branch of the autonomic nervous system. Thus, one might interpret the images as exceptionally beautiful or awe-inspiring because of an enhanced tendency to react with intense emotion. Alternatively, an object appearing to break apart or move away from or toward the perceiver might be reacted to with intense sadness or fear. This fear can result in a pounding heart and rapid, shallow breathing, which further frightens the tripper and can lead to a full-blown panic reaction.

Part of the wonder of these agents is that they do not give repeat performances. Even though each trip differs, the general type of experience and the sequence of experiences are reasonably well delineated. When an effective dose (30 to 100 µg) is taken orally, the trip will last six to nine hours. It can be greatly attenuated at any time through the administration of chlorpromazine intramuscularly.

The initial effects noticed are autonomic responses, which develop gradually over the first 20 minutes. The individual might feel dizzy or hot and cold; the mouth might be dry. These effects diminish and, in addition, are less and less the focus of attention as alteration in sensations, perceptions, and mood begin to develop over the following 30 to 40 minutes. In one study, after the initial autonomic effects, the sequence of events over the next 20 to 50 minutes consisted of mood changes, abnormal body sensation, decrease in sensory impression, abnormal color perception, space and time disorders, and visual hallucinations. One visual effect was described beautifully:

> The guide asked me how I felt, and I responded, "Good." As I muttered the word "Good," I could see it form visually in the air. It was pink and fluffy like a cloud. The word looked "Good" in its appearance and so it had to be "Good." The word and the thing I was trying to express were one, and "Good" was floating around in the air.[18]

About one hour after taking LSD, the intoxication is in full bloom, but it is not until near the end of the second hour that changes occur in the perception of the self. Usually these changes center around a depersonalization. The individual might feel that the sensations he or she experiences are not from the body or that he or she has no body. Body distortions are common, the sort of thing suggested by the comment of one user: "I felt as if my left big toe were going to vomit!" Not unusual is a loss of self-awareness and loss of control of behavior.

Two frequent types of overall reactions in this stage have been characterized as "expansive" and "constricted." In the expansive reaction (a good trip) the individual can become excited and grandiose and feel that he or she is uncovering secrets of the universe or profundities previously locked within him- or herself. Feelings of creativity are not uncommon: "If I only had the time, I could write the truly great American novel." The other end of the continuum is the constricted reaction, in which the user shows little movement and frequently becomes paranoid and exhibits feelings of per-secution. The prototype individual in this situation is huddled in a corner, fearful that some harm will come to him or her or that the person is being threatened by some aspect of the hallucinations. As the drug effect diminishes, normal psychological controls of sensations, perceptions, and mood return.

Adverse Reactions The adverse reactions to LSD ingestion have been repeatedly emphasized in the popular and scientific literature. Because there is no way of knowing how much illegal LSD is being used or how pure the LSD is that people are taking, there is no possibility of determining the true incidence of adverse reactions to LSD. Adverse reactions to the street use of what is thought to be LSD can result from many factors. Drugs obtained on the street frequently are not what they are claimed to be—in purity, chemical composition, or quantity.

A 1960 study surveyed most of the legal U.S. investigators studying LSD and mescaline effects in humans. Data were collected on 25,000 administrations of the drug to about 5,000 individuals. Doses ranged from 25 to 1,500 μg of LSD and 200 to 1,200 mg of mescaline. In some cases the drug was used in patients undergoing therapy; in other cases the drug was taken in an experimental situation to study the effects of the drug. Only LSD and mescaline used under professional supervision were surveyed.

A 1964 article, "The LSD Controversy," stated:

> It would seem that the incidence statistics better support a statement that the drug is exceptionally safe rather than dangerous. Although no statistics have been compiled for the dangers of psychological therapies, we would not be surprised if the incidence of adverse reactions, such as psychotic or depressive episodes and suicide attempts, were at least as high or higher in any comparable group of psychiatric patients exposed to any active form of therapy.[19]

---

synesthesia (sin ess *thees* ya): the blending of different senses, such as "seeing" sounds.

But it then went on to say:

> It is also important to distinguish between the proper use of this drug in therapeutic or experimental settings and its indiscriminate use and abuse by thrill seekers, "lunatic fringe," and drug addicts. More dangers seem likely for the unstable character who takes the drug for "kicks," curiosity, or to escape reality and responsibility than someone taking the drug for therapeutic reasons under strict medical aegis and supervision.

Panic reactions One type of adverse reaction that can develop during the drug-induced experience is the panic reaction, which is typified in the following case history:

> A 21-year-old woman was admitted to the hospital along with her lover. He had had a number of LSD experiences and had convinced her to take it to make her less constrained sexually. About half an hour after ingestion of approximately 200 microgm., she noticed that the bricks in the wall began to go in and out and that light affected her strangely. She became frightened when she realized that she was unable to distinguish her body from the chair she was sitting on or from her lover's body. Her fear became more marked after she thought that she would not get back into herself. At the time of admission she was hyperactive and laughed inappropriately. Stream of talk was illogical and affect labile. Two days later, this reaction had ceased. However, she was still afraid of the drug and convinced that she would not take it again because of her frightening experience.[20]

Flashbacks More than any other reaction, the recurrence of symptoms weeks or months after an individual has taken LSD brings up thoughts of brain damage and permanent biochemical changes. Flashbacks consist of the recurrence of certain aspects of the drug experience after a period of normalcy and in the absence of any drug use. The frequency and duration of these flashbacks are quite variable and seem to be unpredictable. They are most frequent just before going to sleep, while driving, and in periods of psychological stress. They seem to diminish in frequency and intensity with time if the individual stops using psychoactive drugs.

The term *flashback* has been replaced in the DSM-IV-TR by the more formal term *Hallucinogen Persisting Perception Disorder*. An individual receiving this diagnosis has not used the drug recently, but has re-experienced one or more of the perceptual symptoms experienced while intoxicated, such as geometric hallucinations, false perceptions of movement, flashes of color, intensified color, trails of images of moving objects, and so on. Because these experiences are rare and unpredictable, and vary so much from one person to another, it has been very difficult to develop any kind of scientific understanding of either the cause of the delayed experiences or of the best treatment to reduce or prevent them.[21]

Beliefs About LSD LSD is truly a legend in its own time—actually, there are many legends. People probably have more ideas about what LSD does and does not do than they have about any other drug.

- *Creativity.* One of the most widely occurring beliefs is that these hallucinogenic agents increase creativity or release creativity that our inhibitions keep bottled inside us. Several experiments have attempted to study the effects of LSD on creativity, but there is no good evidence that the drug increases it. In one laboratory study using LSD at doses of 0.0025 or 0.01 mg/kg body weight, "the authors concluded that the administration of LSD-25 to a relatively unselected group of people for the purpose of enhancing their creative ability is not likely to be successful."[22] A double-blind, placebo-controlled study found that psilocybin made remote mental associations more available, which might enhance creativity. On the other hand, the research volunteers were less able to focus on their tasks under the influence of psilocybin.[23]

- *Therapy.* Another belief is that LSD has therapeutic usefulness, particularly in the treatment of alcohol dependence, even though reports of results with LSD in alcohol treatment gradually changed from glowing and enthusiastic to cautious and disappointing. One well-controlled study compared the effectiveness of one dose of 0.6 mg of LSD with 60 mg of dextroamphetamine in reducing drinking. No additional therapy, physical or psychological, was used. The authors found that "LSD produced slightly better results early, but after six months the results were alike for both treatment groups."[24] Some investigators reported considerable success with LSD in reducing the pain and depression of patients with terminal cancer. The LSD experiences were part of a several-day program involving extensive verbal interaction between the therapist and patient. Although not successful in every case, the LSD therapy was followed by a reduction in the use of narcotics, "less worry about the future," and "the appearance of a positive mood state." The authors concluded that they had a treatment "which may be highly promising for patients facing fatal illness if implemented in the context of brief, intensive, and highly specialized psychotherapy catalyzed by a psychedelic drug such as LSD." However, federally funded research of this type ended in the 1970s, when a scientific peer review by NIMH concluded, "Research on the therapeutic use of LSD has shown that it is not a generally useful therapeutic drug as an adjunct to a routine psychotherapeutic approach or as a treatment in and of itself."[25]

Psilocybin The magic mushrooms of Mexico have a long history of religious and ceremonial use. These plants, as well as peyote, dropped from Western sight (but not from native use) for 300 years after the Spanish conquered the Aztecs and systematically destroyed their writings and teachings. The mushrooms were particularly suppressed. The name *teonanacatl* can be translated as "God's flesh" or as "sacred mushroom," and either name was very offensive to the Spanish priests.

It was not until the late 1930s that it was clearly shown that these mushrooms were still being used by natives in southern Mexico and the first of many species was identified. The real breakthrough came in 1955. During that year a New York banker turned ethnobotanist and his wife established rapport with a native group still using mushrooms in religious ceremonies. Gordon Wasson became the first outsider to participate in the ceremony and to eat of the magic mushroom. He wrote of his experiences in a 1957 *Life* magazine article, spreading knowledge of the mushrooms and their psychoactive properties and religious uses.

The most well-known psychoactive mushroom is *Psilocybe mexicana*. The primary active agent in this mushroom is **psilocybin,** an indole that the discoverer of LSD, Albert Hofmann, isolated in 1958 and later synthesized.

Another psilocybin-containing mushroom, *Psilocybe cubensis,* grows on cow dung along the U.S. Gulf Coast. Aside from the obvious questions about eating something found on manure, identifying the correct psilocybin containing mushrooms in the field can be tricky. Most *Psilocybe* species are described as "little brown mushrooms," and there are several toxic look-alikes.

The dried mushrooms are 0.2 to 0.5 percent psilocybin. The hallucinogenic effects of psilocybin are quite similar to those of LSD and the catechol hallucinogen mescaline, and cross-tolerance exists among these three agents.

The psychoactive effects are clearly related to the amount used, with up to 4 mg yielding a pleasant experience, relaxation, and some body sensations. Higher doses cause considerable perceptual and body-image changes, with hallucinations in some individuals. Accompanying these psychic changes are dose-related

psilocybin (sill o *sy* bin): the active chemical in *Psilocybe* mushrooms.

sympathetic arousal symptoms. There is some evidence that psilocybin has its central nervous system effects only after it has been changed in the body to psilocin. Psilocin is present in the mushroom only in trace amounts but is about 1.5 times as potent as psilocybin. Perhaps the greater CNS effect of psilocin is the result of its higher lipid solubility.

One of Timothy Leary's followers used psilocybin in the now-classic Good Friday study. The Good Friday study was designed to investigate the ability of psilocybin to induce meaningful religious experiences in individuals when the drug is used in a religious setting. Twenty seminarians participated in a double-blind study, with half receiving 30 mg of psilocybin and half placebos, 90 minutes before attending a religious service. Tape recordings of the subjects' experiences were made immediately after the 2½-hour service, which was held in a chapel. Within a week a questionnaire was completed, followed by a similar one six months later. The first was directed at determining the magnitude and type of change that occurred during the experiment; the later one at assessing the durability of the change. Leary later summarized the outcome of the Good Friday study by saying,

> The results clearly support the hypothesis that, with adequate preparation and in an environment which is supportive and religiously meaningful, subjects report mystical experiences significantly more than placebo controls.[26]

The search for beneficial psychological effects of hallucinogens continues to a limited extent, with psilocybin replacing LSD. In addition to the study on creativity, one report suggests that psilocybin is useful in the treatment of obsessive-compulsive disorder.[27]

With access to some spores of the mushroom and proper growing conditions, one can cultivate *Psilocybe* in a closet. As a consequence of illegal production in the United States, the use of this mushroom has continued, with sporadic outbursts of availability. Although occasionally a major mushroom producer is

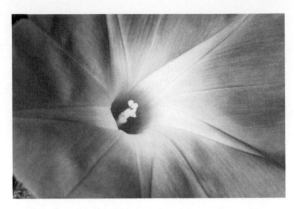

Although morning glory seeds were used as religious plants in Mexico before Columbus came to America, the seeds of most types of morning glories available in the United States have little or no hallucinogenic action.

discovered, most of the production seems to be on a local, amateur basis. Young people might obtain a few "shrooms" to consume at a party, usually in small quantities and in combination with alcoholic beverages. Under such circumstances it is difficult to tell how much of an effect is produced by the mushrooms and how much by the social situation and the alcohol.

Morning Glories and Hawaiian Baby Woodroses Of the psychoactive agents used freely in Mexico in the 16th century, *ololiuqui,* seeds of the morning glory plant *Rivea corymbosa,* perhaps had the greatest religious significance. These seeds tie America to Europe even today. When Albert Hofmann analyzed the seeds of the morning glory, he found several active alkaloids as well as *d*-lysergic acid amide, which is about one-tenth as active as LSD. The presence of *d*-lysergic acid amide is quite amazing (to botany majors) because before this discovery in 1960, lysergic acid had been found only in much more primitive groups of plants, such as the ergot fungus.[28]

The recreational use of seeds from *Argyreia nervosa,* commonly known as Hawaiian baby woodrose has also been reported.[29] These seeds contain higher levels of *d*-lysergic acid amide than morning glories. However,

Taking Sides

Can Ibogaine Cure Drug Dependence?

Ibogaine is a less well-known indole drug that comes from the African shrub *Tabernanthe iboga*. The drug has been used by the local natives as a stimulant at lower doses and a hallucinogen at higher doses. Animal experiments have demonstrated a short-term effect of reducing the self-administration of opioids or of cocaine, although the finding is not consistent. Also, there have been claims that humans who use ibogaine lose their craving for whatever drug they have been dependent upon. This has led to proposals to carry out full-scale testing of ibogaine as a possible treatment for dependence. However, these suggestions have been met by a great deal of skepticism from people with long experience in treating dependence, who are used to periodic claims of a miracle cure. Also, there has been considerable reluctance on the part of the federal drug-abuse research agency, NIDA, to promote a large-scale human study of ibogaine. This might be due partly to the drug's reputation as a hallucinogen and due partly to reports of neurotoxicity when high doses were given to animals. Researchers continue to be interested in the possible antidependence properties of both ibogaine and some less toxic chemical relatives.[30]

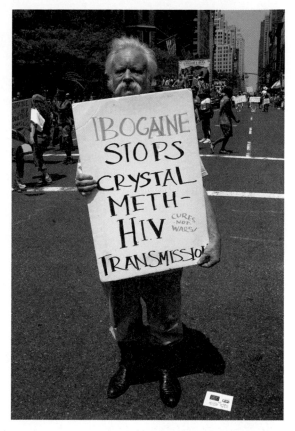

Some people have claimed that the indole drug ibogaine can reduce cravings for cocaine, opioids, and other drugs.

recreational use of these seeds often has adverse effects, probably because the fuzzy outer coating contains toxic cyanogenic glycosides (which can make one sick).

DMT Dimethyltryptamine (DMT) has never been widely used in the United States, although it has a long, if not noble, history. On a worldwide basis, DMT is one of the most important naturally occurring hallucinogenic compounds, and it occurs in many plants. DMT is the active agent in Cohoba snuff, which is used by some South American and Caribbean Indians in hunting rituals. Although DMT was synthesized in the 1930s, its discovery as the active ingredient in cohoba first led

to human examination of its psychoactive properties in 1956.

DMT is normally ineffective when taken orally and is usually snuffed, smoked, or taken by injection. The effective intramuscular dose is about 1 mg/kg body weight. Intravenously, hallucinogenic effects are seen within two minutes after doses of 0.2 mg/kg or more and last for less than 30 minutes. The freebase form of DMT can be smoked by adding the crystals to some type of plant, and 20 to 40 mg is the usual dose. The effect is brief, no matter how it is used. Well-controlled human studies have demonstrated that DMT is unique among classic hallucinogens in that tolerance does not develop to its psychological effects.[31]

Ayahuasca The word *ayahuasca* is from the Quechuan language of the Amazon region, and it means "vine of the soul." The term is used both for the vine *Banisteriopsis caapi* and for the medicinal/divinatory brew made from it. The brew is a traditional South American preparation most commonly combining the *Banisteriopsis* vine, which contains harmaline, with leaves of *Psychotria viridis,* which contains DMT. DMT is normally broken down quickly in the body by the enzyme monoamine oxidase (MAO). This means that, when DMT is taken orally, it is not usually effective. However, harmaline inhibits MAO (see Chapter 8 for a description of MAO inhibitors as antidepressants). Thus, neither plant alone has psychoactive properties, but together they are used by South American tribes as a psychoactive religious sacrament.[32] Doesn't it make you wonder how this combination was discovered before knowledge existed about these chemicals and how they work? Curiosity seekers from North America and Europe have been traveling to the Amazon to experience the effects of ayahuasca, often describing dramatic psychological effects.

Other Tryptamines There have been reports of a couple of "new" hallucinogenic drugs on the rave scene: 5-methoxy DIPT (known as "foxy methoxy") and alpha-methyltryptamine (AMT). Both may be taken orally. As of 2004, these substances were not specifically listed as federal controlled substances, but they are chemical analogues of DMT, so sellers can still be prosecuted.

Catechol Hallucinogens

The second group of phantastica, although having psychological effects quite similar to those of the indole types, is based on a different structure, that of the catechol nucleus. That nucleus forms the basic structure of the catecholamine neurotransmitters, norepinephrine and dopamine. Figure 14.2 shows the catechol structure and the structures of some catechol

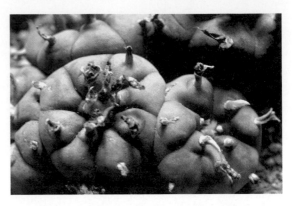

Only the top of the peyote cactus appears above ground, but the entire plant is psychoactive.

hallucinogens. Look for the catechol nucleus in each of the hallucinogens, and then compare these structures with the structure of the amphetamines and other stimulants shown in Chapter 6.

Mescaline Peyote (from the Aztec *peyotl*) is a small, spineless, carrot-shaped cactus, *Lophophora williamsii* Lemaire, which grows wild in the Rio Grande Valley and southward. It is mostly subterranean, and only the grayish-green pincushion-like top appears above ground. In pre-Columbian times the Aztec, Huichol, and other Mexican Indians ate the plant ceremonially either in the dried or green state, producing psychological effects lasting an entire day.

Only the part of the cactus that is above ground is easily edible, but the entire plant is psychoactive. This upper portion, or crown, is sliced into disks, which dry and are known as "mescal buttons." These slices of the peyote cactus remain psychoactive indefinitely and are the source of the drug between the yearly harvests. The Indians' journey in November and December to harvest the peyote is an elaborate ceremony, sometimes taking almost a month and a half. When the mescal buttons are to be used, they are soaked in the mouth until soft, then formed by hand into a bolus and swallowed.

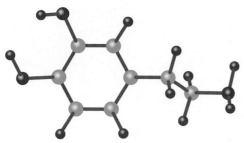

The basic catecholamine structure (dopamine)

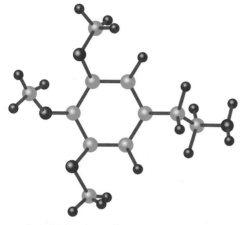

3, 4, 5 trimethoxyphenylethylamine (mescaline)

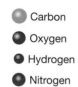

- 🔘 Carbon
- ⚫ Oxygen
- ⚫ Hydrogen
- ⚫ Nitrogen

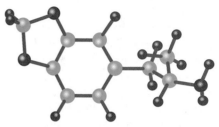

2', 5' dimethoxy –4' – methylamphetamine (DOM)

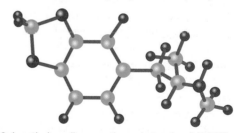

3, 4 methylenedioxy amphetamine (MDA)

3,4 methylenedioxy methamphetamine (MDMA)

Figure 14.2   Catechol Hallucinogens

Mescal buttons should not be confused with mescal beans—or with mescal liquor, which is distilled from the fermentation of the agave cactus and is the starting point for making tequila. Mescal buttons are slices of the peyote cactus and contain **mescaline** as the primary active agent. Mescal beans, however, are dark red seeds from the shrub *Sophora secundiflora.* These seeds, formerly the basis of a vision-seeking cult, contain a highly toxic alkaloid, cytisine, the effects of which resemble those of nicotine, causing nausea, convulsions, hallucinations, and occasionally death from respiratory failure. The mescal bean has a long history, and there is some evidence that use of the bean diminished and ceased when the safer peyote

peyote (pay *oh* tee): a type of hallucinogenic cactus.
mescaline (*mess* ka lin): the active chemical in the peyote cactus.

became available in the southwestern United States. In the transition from a mescal bean to a mescal button cult, some tribes experienced a period in which a mixture of peyote and mescal seeds was concocted and drunk. These factors contributed to considerable confusion in the early (and some recent) literature.[28]

Although there was evidence that the use of peyote had moved north into the United States as early as 1760, it was not until the late 19th century that a peyote cult was widely established among the Indians of the plains. From that time to the present, Indian missionaries have spread the peyote religion to almost a quarter of a million Indians, some as far north as Canada. The *Native American Church* of the United States was first chartered in Oklahoma in 1918 and is an amalgamation of Christianity and traditional beliefs and practices of the Native Americans, with peyote use incorporated into its ceremonies.

Peyotism continues to be an important religious practice among the Indians of the United States between the Rocky Mountains and the Mississippi. As in all religions, a variety of rituals has developed surrounding the use of peyote in religious ceremonies. Peyote is also used in other ways because the Indians attribute spiritual power to the peyote plant. As such, peyote is believed to be helpful, along with prayers and modern medicines, in curing illnesses. It is also worn as an amulet, much as some Christians wear a Saint Christopher's medal, to protect the wearer from harm.

For many years the use of peyote as a sacrament by the Native American Church was protected by the constitutional guarantee of freedom of religion. That protection had inspired Timothy Leary to attempt a similar exclusion for LSD in his newly founded 1960s League of Spiritual Discovery. However, in 1990 the Supreme Court ruled that the State of Oregon could prosecute its citizens for using peyote, and the freedom of religion argument was not allowed. A large group of religious and civil liberties organizations asked the court to reconsider its decision, but it declined to do so.

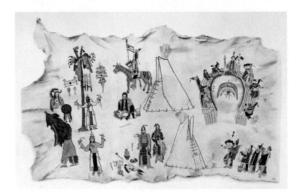

Peyotism remains an important religious practice among Indians in certain areas of the United States. This painting from the early twentieth century includes scenes of peyote cult practices.

The two defendants in the case were American Indians and members of the Native American Church. Federal law and many state laws specifically exclude sacramental peyote use, and the court pointed out that Oregon could exclude such use, too. Other states have not moved to outlaw religious use of peyote.

San Pedro Cactus Another mescaline-containing cactus, *Trichocereus pachanoi,* whose common name is the San Pedro cactus, is native to the Andes Mountains of Peru and Ecuador and has been used for thousands of years as a religious sacrament.[33] The San Pedro is a large, multibranched cactus, often growing to heights of 10 to 15 feet. Its mescaline content is less than that of peyote, and its recreational use more often results in adverse side effects than in the desired hallucinogenic experience.

Discovery and Early Research on Mescaline Near the end of the 19th century, Arthur Heffter isolated several alkaloids from peyote and showed that mescaline was the primary agent for the visual effect induced by peyote. Mescaline was synthesized in 1918, and most experiments on the psychoactive and/or behavioral effects since then have used synthesized mescaline. More than 30 psychoactive alkaloids have now been identified in peyote, but mescaline does seem to be the agent responsible for the vivid colors and other visual effects. The fact that mescaline is not equivalent to peyote is not always made clear in the literature.

One of the early investigators of the effects of peyote was Dr. Weir Mitchell, who used an extract of peyote and who reported, in part:

> The display which for an enchanted two hours followed was such as I find it hopeless to describe in language which shall convey to others the beauty and splendor of what I saw. Stars, delicate floating films of color, then an abrupt rush of countless points of white light swept across the field of view, as if the unseen millions of the Milky Way were to flow in a sparkling river before my eyes . . . zigzag lines of very bright colors . . . the wonderful loveliness of swelling clouds of more vivid colors gone before I could name them.[34]

Another early experimenter was Havelock Ellis. Interestingly, he took his peyote on Good Friday in 1897, 65 years before the Good Friday experiment with psilocybin. His experience is described in detail in a 1902 article titled "Mescal: A Study of a Divine Plant" in *Popular Science Monthly,* but a brief quotation gives the essence of the experience:

> On the whole, if I had to describe the visions in one word, I should say that they were living arabesques. There was generally a certain incomplete tendency to symmetry, the effect being somewhat as if the underlying mechanism consisted of a large number of polished facets acting as mirrors. It constantly happened that the same image was repeated over a large part of the field, though this holds good mainly of the forms, for in the colors there would still remain all sorts of delicious varieties. Thus at a moment when uniformly jewelled flowers seemed to be springing up and extending all over the field of vision, the flowers still showed every variety of delicate tone and tint.[35]

Not every individual wants every educational opportunity. William James, surprisingly, was one who did not. He wrote to his brother Henry: "I ate one but three days ago, was violently sick for twenty-four hours, and had no other symptoms whatever except that and the Katzenjammer the following day. I will take the visions on trust." Even Dr. Weir Mitchell, who had the effect previously recorded, said, "These shows are expensive. . . . The experience, however, was worth one such headache and indigestion but was not worth a second."

Even if you get by without too much nausea and physical discomfort, which the Indians also report, all might not go well. Huxley, whose 1954 *The Doors of Perception.*[36] made him a guru in this area, admitted, "Along with the happily transfigured majority of mescaline takers there is a minority that finds in the drug only hell and purgatory." It is reported that natives sometimes wished for bad trips when taking this or other plants. By meeting their personal demons, they hoped to conquer them and remove problems from their lives.

Pharmacology of Mescaline Mescaline is readily absorbed if taken orally, but it only very poorly passes the blood-brain barrier (which explains the high doses required). There is a maximal concentration of the drug in the brain after 30 to 120 minutes. About half of it is removed from the body in six hours, and there is evidence that some mescaline persists in the brain for up to 10 hours. Similar to the indole hallucinogens, the effects obtained with low doses, about 3 mg/kg body weight, are primarily euphoric, whereas doses in the range of 5 mg/kg give rise to a full set of hallucinations. Most of the mescaline is excreted unchanged in the urine, and the metabolites identified thus far are not psychoactive.

A dose that is psychoeffective in humans causes pupil dilation, pulse rate and blood pressure increases, and an elevation in body temperature. All of these effects are similar to those induced by LSD, psilocybin, and most other alkaloid hallucinogens. There are other signs of central stimulation, such as EEG arousal, after mescaline intake. In rats the LD_{50} is about 370 mg/kg body weight, 10 to 30 times the dose that causes behavioral effects. Death results from convulsions and respiratory arrest.

Tolerance develops more slowly to mescaline than to LSD, and there is cross-tolerance between them. As with LSD, mescaline intoxication can be blocked with chlorpromazine.

Although mescaline and the other catechol hallucinogens have a structure that resembles the catecholamine neurotransmitters, they act indirectly on the serotonin 2A receptor.

Amphetamine Derivatives A large group of synthetic hallucinogens is chemically related to the amphetamines. However, most of these drugs have little amphetamine-like stimulant activity. Thanks to certain chemical substitutions on the ring part of the catechol nucleus, these drugs are more mescaline-like (review Figure 14.2).

DOM (STP) DOM is 2,5-dimethoxy-4-methylamphetamine. In the 1960s and 1970s, DOM was called STP, and street talk was that the initials stood for serenity, tranquility, and peace. Its actions and effects are highly similar to those of mescaline and LSD, with a total dose of 1 to 3 mg yielding euphoria and 3 to 5 mg a six- to eight-hour hallucinogenic period. This makes DOM about a hundred times as potent as mescaline but only one-thirtieth as potent as LSD.

MDA and Others In addition to DOM, many other amphetamine derivatives have been synthesized and shown to have hallucinogenic properties. Most of these have effects very similar to those of DOM and mescaline, as well as LSD and the indole types. There is some indication that one type of derivative, MDA (review Figure 14.2), has effects that are subjectively somewhat different. MDA, which is somewhat more potent than mescaline, has seen some recreational use through illicit manufacture. Because of the variety of possible hallucinogenic amphetamine derivatives and because most of these chemicals are not specifically listed as controlled substances, illicit drug makers were drawn to this group of chemicals in the production of various designer drugs to be sold on the street as hallucinogens.

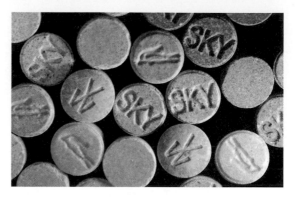

Some evidence suggests that Ecstasy may be neurotoxic, affecting serotonin neurons in the brain.

MDMA One of the amphetamine derivatives received special attention in July 1984 when the DEA first proposed scheduling it. MDMA is similar in structure to MDA but is apparently quite different from the other hallucinogens. Rats trained to discriminate DOM from saline did show some generalization from the DOM stimulus to MDA but not to MDMA. Furthermore, there is no cross-tolerance between MDA and MDMA. Although there had been some use of MDMA on the streets (it is called "Ecstasy" or "XTC"), a number of psychiatrists came forth who had been quietly using MDMA, a drug that, although not approved by the FDA, was not illegal. These psychiatrists testified against the scheduling of MDMA, insisting that it was not a true hallucinogen and that it had a special ability to promote empathy, thus aiding the psychoanalytic process.[37]

There is some evidence supporting this claim of increased empathy: In one study, 100 people completed detailed questionnaires describing the effects of their previous use of MDMA.[38] Although such retrospective reports are less reliable than reports obtained during or immediately after the experience, a remarkably common report (90 percent of the individuals) was that they experienced a heightened sense of "closeness" with other people. Other common effects were an increased heart rate, dry mouth, grinding of the teeth, profuse sweating, and other autonomic effects. Although several

Mind / Body Connection

Living in the Flow

During the 1960s, the spirit of kinship with a peer group helped fuel the spread of LSD. More recently, the feeling of making intense emotional connections seems to have helped spread a "rave" subculture in the United States and elsewhere. This scene, known for its all-night dance parties featuring techno tunes and the drug Ecstasy, has had a dedicated following since the early 1990s. It's not, however, just about the music or the drugs, according to those in the rave community. It's about being in the moment, having a brief conversation with a stranger who affects you, having an emotional internal experience.

What really makes people glad to be alive? What are the inner experiences that make life worthwhile? It's easier to talk about dancing than it is to describe a moment of mystical union with the universe. Joy can find us and lift us in moments of ordinary connection, though, and the opening we feel to life is not unlike that experienced through a spiritual quest or mystical practice. The elation comes when we know we belong—to another, to ourselves, to the mystery that is larger than ourselves.

In our society, celebrations and relaxation often involve moving away from the emotion, numbing ourselves with alcohol or drugs. Dance and music are exceptions to this, but too often we are simply spectators in our lives. Sometimes we discount the small joys in daily living. Sometimes we spoil the good by focusing on the less than perfect or seemingly incompatible. Perhaps we don't want to be let down, so we anticipate disappointment rather than expect success and happiness.

Can you think of a time when joy came unexpectedly and caught you off guard? Maybe it was a sudden realization that made you smile. Perhaps it was something you didn't even know you were looking for. Chances are it was a moment when you felt so alive that, ironically, you forgot yourself. Mihaly Csikszentmihalyi, a University of Chicago psychology professor who has devoted his life's work to studying what makes people happy, satisfied, and fulfilled, describes "flow" as a state of consciousness so focused that you are totally absorbed in an activity and lose track of time. It is a state of complete engagement with life in which you feel strong, alert, in effortless control, unself-conscious, and at the peak of your abilities. Examples of when you might experience flow include after completing a hard task, when feeling the wind in your hair during a walk on the beach, during yoga or sex, and when seeing your child respond to your smile for the first time.

What activities usually make you feel happy and completely engaged? During the next week, be aware of and record what activities give you this feeling of deep enjoyment. Then try to build some of these activities into your daily routine to improve the spiritual and emotional quality of your life.

people reported that objects seemed more "luminescent," very few reported actual visual hallucinations.

The bad news is that this otherwise fairly benign drug might cause brain damage. Several laboratories have reported that rats given MDMA injections show a selective destruction of serotonin neurons in their brains. Then a similar effect was reported in monkeys at only two to three times the normal human dose, and this led many observers to conclude that similar brain damage could occur in human MDMA users. It should be stressed that this effect is not caused by LSD, mescaline, psilocybin, or most other drugs. Although the evidence from the animal studies on MDMA is strong enough to be taken seriously, the evidence of long-term neurotoxic effects of MDMA use in humans is inconclusive.[39] The serotonin reuptake inhibitor fluoxetine (Prozac) (see Chapter 8) blocks the neurotoxicity in rats but does not appear to block the psychoactive effect in humans, and some human users have used fluoxetine with MDMA to reduce the chances of brain damage.[40] Although MDMA has been listed as a Schedule I controlled substance since 1988, it continues to be studied as a potential psychotherapeutic agent. It is once again ironic but by now no longer surprising—following the listing of MDMA (Ecstasy) as a Schedule I controlled substance, and the attendant publicity about its dangers, it appears to have become more popular than ever among young users at "raves."

2-CB and 2-C-T7 It's happened before and it will happen again: As federal and state agencies work to limit access to one drug, another arrives to fill the gap. In this case, two drugs have arrived to share the rave scene with MDMA: 4-bromo-2,5-dimethoxyphenethylamine (known as 2-CB) and 4-propylthio-2, 5-dimethoxyphenethylamine (2-C-T7). As phenylethylamines, both are chemical cousins to the amphetamine series of hallucinogens. Along with the recently popularized tryptamine derivatives MTA and "foxy methoxy" (see page 348), a confusing array of chemicals is being made available to "ravers," who may find themselves trying unknown amounts of unfamiliar drugs more often than they'd like.

Deliriants

If the indole and catechol hallucinogens are grouped together as "phantastica" with all having similar effects, and acting primarily through the serotonin 2A receptor, then how do we classify all the remaining hallucinogens? We have chosen the term *deliriants,* implying that the drugs to follow have somewhat more of a tendency to produce mental confusion and a loss of touch with reality. The drugs we describe next represent a variety of effects and act through different brain mechanisms, so it is perhaps better to think of each type by itself rather than as belonging to a group with common effects.

PCP

In the 1950s, Parke, Davis & Company investigated a series of drugs in the search for an efficient intravenous anesthetic. On the basis of animal studies, the company selected 1-(1-phenylcyclohexyl) piperidine hydrochloride (PCP, generic name *phencyclidine*) for testing in humans. The studies on monkeys had indicated that **PCP** was a good analgesic but did not produce good muscle relaxation or sleep. Instead, the animals showed a sort of "dissociation" from what was happening: "During the operation the animal had its eyes open and looked about unconcernedly." In 1958, the first report was published on the use of PCP (Sernyl) for surgical anesthesia in humans. Sernyl produced good analgesia without depressing blood circulation or respiration and did not produce irregularities in heartbeat. Loss of sensation occurred within two or three minutes of beginning the intravenous infusion, after about 10 mg of the drug had been delivered. The patients later had no memory of the procedure, did not remember being spoken to, and remembered no pain. Compared with existing anesthetics, which tend to depress both respiration and circulation through general depression of the CNS, this type of "dissociative" anesthetic seemed to be quite safe. However, the psychological reactions to the drug were unpredictable.

During administration of the drug a few patients became very excited, and a different anesthetic had to be used. Several patients were "unmanageable" as they emerged from the anesthetic, exhibiting severely manic behavior. This and later reports indicated that many people given anesthetic doses of Sernyl reported changes in body perception and hallucinations, and about 15 percent of the patients experienced a "prolonged confusional psychosis," lasting up to four days after the drug was given. This period of confusion was characterized by feelings of unreality, depersonalization, persecution, depression, and intense anxiety.

News of this new hallucinogen soon reached Dr. Luby, a psychiatrist, who began testing it in both normal and schizophrenic subjects.[41] All the subjects reported changes in perception of their own bodies, with one normal subject saying, "my arm feels like a twenty-mile pole with a pin at the end." Another said, "I am a small . . . not human . . . just a block of something in a great big laboratory." There were a number of reports of floating, flying, dizziness, and alternate contraction and expansion of body size. All subjects also showed a thought disorder. Some made up new words, uttered strings of unrelated words, or repeated words or simple phrases. Also, all became increasingly drowsy and apathetic. At times a subject would appear to be asleep but when asked a direct question would respond. When asked, "Can you hear me?" subjects often responded, "No." The majority became either angry or uncooperative. Many of the normal subjects said they felt as if they were drunk from alcohol. All subjects displayed diminished pain, touch, and position sense, and all showed nystagmus (rapid oscillations of the eyes) and a slapping, ataxic walk. Luby and his colleagues felt that PCP was different from LSD or mescaline in that there were few reports of intense visual experiences and many more reports of body image changes. The disorganized thinking, suspiciousness, and lack of cooperation made the PCP state resemble schizophrenia much more than the LSD state.

Thus, by 1960, PCP had been characterized as an excellent anesthetic for monkeys, a medically safe but psychologically troublesome anesthetic for humans, and a hallucinogen different from LSD and mescaline, with profound effects on body perception. Parke, Davis withdrew Sernyl as an investigational drug for humans in 1965 and in 1967 licensed another company to sell Sernylan as an animal anesthetic. It was particularly used with primates, in both research laboratories and zoos. Also, because of its rapid action and wide safety margin, Sernylan was used in syringe bullets to immobilize stray, wild, or dangerous zoo animals. Because of the popular term *tranquilizer gun* for this use, PCP became popularly, and inaccurately, known as an animal "tranquilizer."

Other PCP-like Drugs: Ketamine, Dextromethorphan, and Nitrous Oxide Even though Sernyl was never marketed for human use, a related chemical from the same series was marketed as a dissociative anesthetic. Ketamine hydrochloride (Ketalar) has been in continued human use for more than 30 years. A related veterinary product is also available. Although ketamine has more depressant effects than PCP and fewer prolonged reactions, clinical reports indicate that emergence reactions occur in about 12 percent of patients. These reactions include hallucinations and delirium, sometimes accompanied by confusion and irrational behavior. In 1999, widespread reports of ketamine abuse and its notoriety as a party drug (called Special K, or K) caused the Department of Health and Human Services to recommend adding ketamine to the list of Schedule III controlled substances.

Like PCP and ketamine, two more common substances are also capable of causing dissociative effects, perhaps by blocking NMDA-type glutamate receptors in the brain. Nitrous oxide (laughing gas, Chapter 7) and dextromethorphan, an over-the-counter cough suppressant (Chapter 12) can, at very high doses, produce dissociative-type hallucinations similar to those produced by PCP. Unfortunately, at these doses there is also evidence of pathological changes to neurons in the cerebral cortex of animals. Recently, it was reported that the combination of nitrous oxide and ketamine, sometimes used for general anesthesia, produces synergistic neurotoxic effects in animals.[42]

Recreational Use of PCP In late 1967, workers at the Haight-Ashbury Medical Clinic obtained samples of a substance being distributed as the "Peace Pill." The drug was analyzed and determined to be PCP, and its identity and dangers were publicized in the community in December 1967. By the next year, it was reported that this drug had enjoyed only brief popularity and then disappeared. It appeared briefly in New

> **PCP:** phencyclidine; originally developed as an anesthetic; has hallucinogenic properties.

York in 1968 as "hog" and at other times as "trank." Into the early 1970s, PCP was apparently regarded as pretty much a "garbage" drug by street people. In the early 1970s, PCP crystals were sometimes sprinkled onto oregano, parsley, or alfalfa and sold to unsuspecting youngsters as marijuana. In this form, it became known as **angel dust.** Because PCP can be made inexpensively and relatively easily by amateur chemists, when it is available it usually doesn't cost much. Eventually, the rapid and potent effects of angel dust made it a desired substance in its own right. Joints made with PCP sometimes contained marijuana, sometimes another plant substance, and were known as "killer joints" or "sherms" (because they hit the user like a Sherman tank). In the late 1970s, PCP use was the most common cause of drug-induced visits to hospital emergency rooms in many communities, and in some neighborhoods young users could be seen "moonwalking" down the street (taking very high, careful, and slow steps) on any Saturday night.

Some users develop a profound psychological dependence on PCP, despite its unpredictability and the behavioral impairment it produces. One user reported:

> Immediately after smoking the Dust I started experiencing the effects. All my troubles seemed to go away. I felt a little drunk and had some trouble walking around the apartment. Objects appeared either very far away or very close and I couldn't really judge distance at all. . . . I liked being apart from things, and felt outside my body for most of the trip. That was fun. Before I smoked I had been troubled about some exams coming up and felt I wasn't really prepared. . . . All that anxiety vanished with the Dust. . . . I felt at peace. It was a good feeling. . . . I want to be there always.[43]

That individual was unusually descriptive about the experience. Most often, a PCP user doesn't say much that makes sense while the drug is having its effects, and later the user doesn't remember much of what happened.

The dependence-producing properties of PCP have also been studied in monkeys, which will press a lever to obtain access to the drug.[44] This is in contrast to LSD and other hallucinogens, which do not support animal self-administration and do not produce psychological dependence in most users.

Because some PCP users have been reported to behave violently, there is a question as to whether PCP tends to promote violence directly or whether violence is a side effect of the suspicion and anesthesia produced by the drug. Most users do not report feeling violent and feel so uncoordinated that they can't imagine starting a fight. However, police who have tried to arrest PCP users have had trouble subduing them because many of the commonly used arrest techniques rely on restraining holds that result in pain if the arrestee resists. Because the PCP user is anesthetized, these restraint techniques are less effective. Manual restraint by more than one officer might be required to arrest some PCP users, although one might question how different this is from the problem of arresting a violent drunk who is "feeling no pain."

That PCP users might not feel pain has resulted in some gruesome legends about users biting or cutting off their own fingers and so forth. Like earlier stories about LSD users blinding themselves by staring at the sun, these legends cannot be substantiated and most likely have not really occurred. One oft-repeated story probably falls into the category of police folklore. Every cop knows for a fact the story about the PCP user who was so violent, had such superhuman strength, and was so insensitive to pain that he was shot 28 times (or a similar large number of times) before he fell. Although everyone "knows" that this happened, no one can tell you exactly when or where. One might dismiss such folklore as harmless, unless it contributes to events such as the shooting, six times at close range, of an unarmed, naked, 35-year-old biochemist who was trying to climb the street sign outside his laboratory. This story really did happen, on August 4, 1977, during the height of the PCP epidemic. The lethal shots were fired by a Los Angeles police officer. The coroner's office reported that the victim's blood did contain traces of a drug similar to PCP.[45] Several years later, Los Angeles police officers involved in the widely publicized videotaped beating of Rodney King said during their trial that they used such force because they believed King might have been "dusted"—under the influence of PCP.

The mechanism of PCP's action on the brain was a mystery for several years, because PCP alters many neurotransmitter systems but does not appear to act directly on any of them. In 1979, it was reported that a specific receptor for PCP was present in the brain, and in 1981 the identity between the receptor and another that had previously been considered a subtype of opiate receptor was reported. The drug cyclazocine, which has some opiate activity and has also been reported to produce hallucinations, binds well to this "sigma" receptor, but morphine, naloxone, and other opiates do not. Thus, the sigma receptor is probably better characterized as being selective for PCP, ketamine, and other similar drugs rather than as a type of opiate receptor. The presence of the sigma receptor implies that some endogenous substance should bind to it, but more than 20 years of research has not yet determined what that might be or what the normal functions are for this receptor. Several drugs have been developed that bind to the sigma receptor, but none has reached the market.[46]

Anticholinergic Hallucinogens

The potato family contains all the naturally occurring agents to be discussed in this section. Three of the genera—*Atropa, Hyoscyamus,* and *Mandragora*—have a single species of importance and were primarily restricted to Europe. The fourth genus, *Datura,* is worldwide and has many species containing the active agents.

The family of plants in which all these genera are found is *Solanaceae,* "herbs of consolation," and three pharmacologically active alkaloids are responsible for the effects of these plants. *Atropine,* which is *dl*-hyoscyamine, scopolamine, or *l*-hyoscine, and l-hyoscyamine are all potent central and peripheral cholinergic blocking agents. These drugs occupy the acetylcholine receptor site but do not activate it; thus, their effect is primarily to block muscarinic cholinergic neurons, including the parasympathetic system.

These agents have potent peripheral and central effects, and some of the psychological responses to these drugs are probably a reaction to peripheral changes. These alkaloids block the production of mucus in the nose and throat. They also prevent salivation, so the mouth becomes uncommonly dry, and perspiration stops. Temperature can increase to fever levels (109°F has been reported in infants with atropine poisoning), and heart rate can show a 50-beat-per-minute increase with atropine. Even at moderate doses these chemicals cause considerable dilation of the pupils of the eyes, with a resulting inability to focus on nearby objects. With large enough doses, a behavioral pattern develops that resembles toxic psychosis; there is delirium, mental confusion, loss of attention, drowsiness, and loss of memory for recent events. These two characteristics—a clouding of consciousness and no memory for the period of intoxication—plus the absence of vivid sensory effects separate these drugs from the indole and catechol hallucinogens. The anticholinergics are the original *deliriants.*

Belladonna

Atropine, which was isolated in 1831, is the active ingredient in the deadly nightshade, *Atropa belladonna.* The name of the plant reflects two of its major uses in the Middle Ages and before. The genus name reflects its use as a poison. Deadly nightshade was one of the plants used extensively by both professional and amateur poisoners; 14 of its berries contain enough of the alkaloid to cause death.

Belladonna, the species name, meaning "beautiful woman," comes from the use of the extract of this plant to dilate the pupils of the

angel dust: the street name for PCP sprinkled on plant material.

eyes. Interestingly, ancient Roman and Egyptian women knew something that science did not learn until more recently. In the 1950s, it was demonstrated, by using pairs of photographs identical except for the amount of pupil dilation, that most people judge the girl with the more dilated eyes to be prettier.

Of more interest here than pretty girls or poisoned men is the sensation of flying reported by some users of belladonna. The origin of this story goes back at least to the Middle Ages in Europe, and in particular to descriptions of witches and witchcraft. Every early society for which we have any history has a tradition of people with special knowledge of useful plants. In Europe, the people who were consulted for their special arcane knowledge of plant potions were most often women, and their traditions are kept alive in our modern concept of "witches." Among the rich folklore about witches are several accounts from the 1400s describing "flying ointments" (e.g., *The Book of the Sacred Magic of Abremelin the Mage,* 1458), and one ingredient often included in these ointments was deadly nightshade. The notion is that this ointment was spread upon the body and/or on a stick, or "staffe," which was straddled. This is certainly the origin of our notion that witches flew about on broomsticks, though in many accounts it seems that the sticks were used more as phallic symbols and were perhaps ridden in a different manner. What is actually known about witches and witchcraft of this era is confused considerably by what was written about witches by Catholic priests during the Inquisition.

During the Middle Ages, all such pagan rituals were considered to be heresy, and practitioners were tortured and killed. Admissions by witches that they "flew" long distances to celebrate Black Mass were extracted during torture and were likely to have reflected the beliefs of the inquisitors more than the history of the person being tortured. Some incredibly lurid accounts of the practices of witches associated drugs, sex, and human sacrifice. Similar lurid accounts linking other drugs (marijuana, LSD, cocaine) to sexual abandon and criminal

violence have appeared during more recent years, also promoted by those protecting the established order. The facts are usually not so exciting. Anticholinergics can make people feel lightheaded, and in conjunction with the power of suggestion one might get the *sensation* of floating, or flying, but it's not a realistic way to get from New York to Chicago.

Mandrake

The *mandrake* plant (*Mandragora officinarum*) contains all three alkaloids. Although many drugs can be traced to the Bible, it is particularly important to do so with mandrake because its close association with love and lovemaking has persisted from Genesis to recent times:

> In the time of wheat-harvest Reuben went out and found some mandrakes in the open country and brought them to his mother Leah. Then Rachel asked Leah for some of her son's mandrakes, but Leah said, "Is it so small a thing to have taken away my husband, that you should take my son's mandrakes as well?" But Rachel said, "Very well, let him sleep with you tonight in exchange for your son's mandrakes." So when Jacob came in from the country in the evening, Leah went out to meet him and said, "You are to sleep with me tonight; I have hired you with my son's mandrakes." That night he slept with her.[47]

The mandrake root is forked and, if you have a vivid imagination, resembles a human body. The root contains the psychoactive agents and was endowed with all sorts of magical and medical properties. The association with the human form is alluded to in Shakespeare's Juliet's farewell speech: "And shrieks like mandrakes torn out of the earth, That living mortals hearing them run mad."

Henbane

Compared with deadly nightshade and mandrake, *Hyoscyamus niger* has had a most uninteresting life. This is strange, because it is pharmacologically quite active and contains both scopolamine and *l*-hyoscyamine. Other plants of this genus contain effective levels of the alkaloids, but it is *Hyoscyamus niger* that appears throughout history as *henbane,* a highly poisonous substance and truly the bane of hens, as well as other animals.

Pliny in AD 60 said, "For this is certainly known, that, if one takes it in drink more than four leaves, it will put him beside himself." Shakespeare's Hamlet's father must have had more than four leaves because it was henbane that was used to poison him.

Datura

The distribution of the many *Datura* species is worldwide, but they all contain the three alkaloids under discussion—atropine, scopolamine, and hyoscyamine—in varying amounts. Almost as extensive as the distribution are its uses and its history. Although it is not clear when the Chinese first used *Datura metel* as a medicine to treat colds and nervous disorders, the plant was important enough to become associated with Buddha:

> The Chinese valued this drug far back into ancient times. A comparatively recent Chinese medical text, published in 1590, reported that "when Buddha preaches a sermon, the heavens bedew the petals of this plant with rain drops."[48]

Halfway around the world 2,500 years before the Chinese text, virgins sat in the temple to Apollo in Delphi and, probably under the influence of *Datura,* mumbled sounds that holy men interpreted as predictions that always came true. Engraved on the temple at Delphi were the words "Know thyself."

Datura is associated with the worship of Shiva in India, where it has long been recognized as an ingredient in love potions and has been known as "deceiver" and "foolmaker." In Asia the practice of mixing the crushed seeds of *Datura metel* in tobacco, cannabis, and food persists even today.

The ever-busy chronicler Hernandez mentioned the use of *Datura inoxia* (loco weed) by the Aztecs, and the use of various *Datura* species by Indians of the United States Southwest for magical and religious purposes is well substantiated.[26] One interesting use of *Datura stramonium,* which is native and grows wild in the eastern United States, was devised by the Algonquin Indians. They used the plant to solve the problem of the adolescent search for identity:

> The youths are confined for long periods, given " . . . no other substance but the infusion or decoction of some poisonous, intoxicating roots . . . " and "they became stark, staring mad, in which raving condition they were kept eighteen or twenty days." These poor creatures drink so much of that water of Lethe that they perfectly lose the remembrance of all former things, even of their parents, their treasure, and their language. When the doctors find that they have drunk sufficiently of the wysoccan . . . they gradually restore them to their senses again. . . . Thus they unlive their former lives and commence men by forgetting that they ever have been boys.[48]

The same plant is now called Jamestown weed, or jimsonweed, as a result of an incident in the 17th century. This was recorded for history in the book *The History and Present State of Virginia,* published first in 1705 by Robert Beverly.[49]

> The *James-Town* Weed (which resembles the Thorny Apple of *Peru,* and I take to be the Plant so call'd) is supposed to be one of the greatest Coolers in the World. This being an early Plant, was gather'd very young for a boil'd Salad, by some of the Soldiers sent thither, to pacifie the Troubles of *Bacon;* and some of them eat plentifully of it, the Effect of which was a very pleasant Comedy; for they turn'd natural Fools upon it for several Days.

Although there has been some recent abuse of jimsonweed, the unpleasant and dangerous side effects of this plant limit its recreational use.

Synthetic Anticholinergics

Anticholinergic drugs were once used to treat Parkinson's disease (before the introduction of *L*-dopa) and are still widely used to treat the pseudoparkinsonism produced by antipsychotic drugs (see Chapter 8). Particularly in older people there is concern about inadvertently producing an "anticholinergic syndrome," characterized by excessive dry mouth, elevated temperature, delusions, and hallucinations. Anticholinergic drugs such as trihexyphenidyl (Artane) and benztropine (Cogentin) have only rarely been abused for their delirium-producing properties.

Amanita Muscaria

The *Amanita muscaria* mushroom is also called "fly agaric," probably because of what it does to flies. It doesn't kill them, but when they suck its juice, it puts them into a stupor for two to three hours. It is one of the common poisonous mushrooms found in forests in many parts of the world. The older literature suggests that eating 5 to 10 *Amanita* mushrooms results in severe effects of intoxication, such as muscular twitching, leading to twitches of limbs and raving drunkenness, with agitation and vivid hallucinations. Later follow many hours of partial paralysis with sleep and dreams.

When the ancient Aryan invaders swept down from the north into India 3,500 years ago, they took soma, itself considered a deity. The cult of Soma ruled India's religion and culture for many years—the poems of the Rig Veda celebrate the sacramental use of this substance. It has only been within the past 30 years that scholars have discovered and agreed on the identity of soma as *Amanita*.[1]

The suggestion has been made that the ambrosia ("food of the gods") mentioned in the secret rites of the god Dionysius in Greece was a solution of the *Amanita* mushroom. And based on paintings representing the "tree of life" found in ancient European cave paintings, it has been suggested that *Amanita muscaria* use formed a basis for the cult that originated about 2,000 years ago and today calls itself Christianity.[50]

Until the Russians introduced them to alcohol, many of the isolated nomadic tribes of Siberia had no intoxicant but *Amanita:*

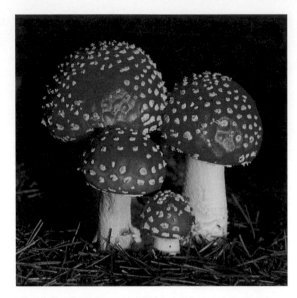

The red- and white-speckled mushroom *Amanita muscaria* played a major role in the early history of Indo-European and Central American religions.

> Use of the Amanita mushroom by Siberian tribes continues today largely free from social control of any sort. Use of the drug has a Shamanist aspect, and forms the basis for orgiastic communal indulgences. Since the drug can induce murderous rages in addition to more moderate hallucinogenic experiences, serious injuries frequently result.[51]

In the frozen northland, these mushrooms are expensive; sometimes several reindeer are exchanged for an effective number of the mushrooms. During the long winter months they might be worth the price. While the mushrooms themselves are not reusable (once eaten, they're gone), the hallucinogen is excreted unchanged in the urine. When the effect begins to wear off, "midway in the party the cry of 'pass the pot' goes out."[52] The active ingredient can be reused four or five times in this way.

There is evidence that *Amanita* was also used as a holy plant by several tribal groups in the Americas, ranging from Alaska and the Great Lakes to Mexico and Central America. In several of the legends, its origin is associated with thunder and lightning.[1]

Drugs in Depth

Toad-Licking: An Urban Legend

In the late 1980s, a story was going around about a substance called *bufotenin,* an indole that looks as if it might be hallucinogenic and was originally identified in the skins of toads (genus *Bufo*). In one version of the story, hippies living in the hills of Northern California were chasing toads through the woods and licking them to get high: California was said to have listed one species of toad as a controlled substance. In another version, it was the infamous cane toad of Australia, said to be licked or ingested both by aborigines and by Australian hippies.

It's a great story, seemingly plausible enough, and certainly colorful enough to repeat. It found its way into drug-abuse lectures and at least one textbook, and the Australian version was passed along as fact by *USA Today* in 1988. The idea even became the plot for one episode of the television program "LA Law." The only problem is that the story wasn't true.

Bufotenin was studied experimentally in the 1950s, during the heyday of research on hallucinogens as models of schizophrenia. Probably it was studied because it was found in *Amanita* mushrooms, and they were known to have been used as hallucinogens. However, when bufotenin was given to "volunteer" prison inmates (by injection, not licking) it was found to be a not very potent hallucinogen. It may have been toxic in other ways because the experimental subjects became quite cyanotic (meaning they turned blue, although the researcher in charge says it was more of a deep purple). That basically ended human research with bufotenin. It can't be proved that nobody ever licked a toad in California, but there is no documented evidence for this as a regular practice of any group at any time, nor is there any documented evidence that hallucinatory effects can be achieved in this way.

This legend could have tragic consequences, in that toads do have a variety of toxins in their skins that protect them from being eaten by predators. If a person actually were to eat toad skins or somehow obtain and use pure bufotenin, he or she could become quite ill or even die. One Australian youth is reported to have died after eating cane toad eggs.

This story is such a graphically gross one that it didn't want to go away, despite a small story debunking the myth published in *Scientific American* in 1990. Even after that came out, a Georgia legislator referred to "the extreme danger of cane-toad licking becoming the designer drug of choice." A warning was published in the *British Journal of Psychiatry* (November 1990) that "the Australian cane toad is popularly kept as a pet in the US, and licked by its owners for the resulting hallucinatory effects," with the note that two English toads also have the potential to be used in this way. The legend may be explained with a related truth (not uncommon). It was reported that the Sonoran desert toad, *Bufo alvarius,* secretes large amounts of 5-methoxy DMT, which is a potent hallucinogen, in its venom. Although the venom is toxic when eaten, the substance can be smoked to obtain the psychoactive effect. The authors speculated that anthropologists had long ago mistakenly concluded that the more common toad *Bufo marinus* was the one being referred to in their interviews with the native people of the region and depicted in pre-Columbian art of Central America.[53]

Two pieces of advice: Don't lick strange toads, and be especially cautious about believing any weird story you hear that involves hallucinogenic drugs, unless there is documented evidence (who, what, when, where, why, how, and how much?). The "mystical" nature of these substances has, no doubt, inspired more untrue legends than about any other type of drug.

For many years the active agent in this mushroom was thought to be *muscarine* (for which the muscarinic cholinergic receptors were named). This substance activates the same type of acetylcholine receptor that is blocked by the anticholinergics. However, pharmacological studies with other cholinergic agonists did not produce similar psychoactive effects. Next, attention focused on *bufotenin,* an indole that is found in high concentrations in the skins of toads (see the Drugs in Depth). However, the hallucinogenic properties of bufotenin have been in doubt, and *Amanita* species contain only small amounts of it. In the mid-1960s, meaningful amounts of two chemicals were found: ibotenic acid and muscimol.

The effects of *Amanita* ingestion are not similar to those of other hallucinogens, and that helped confuse the picture with regard to the mechanism. Muscimol can act as an agonist at GABA receptors, which are inhibitory and found throughout the CNS. Muscimol is more potent than ibotenic acid, and drying of the mushroom, which is usually done by those who use it, promotes the transformation of ibotenic acid to muscimol. Muscimol has been given to humans, resulting in confusion, disorientation in time and place, sensory disturbances, muscle twitching, weariness, fatigue, and sleep.[28]

Amanita muscaria and other related poisonous mushrooms are found in North America, and they are a particularly dangerous type of plant with which to experiment.

Salvia Divinorum

This member of the mint family is known by its botanical name, which is translated as "diviner's sage." It has been used for centuries by the Mazatec people of Oaxaca, Mexico, in religious ceremonies, and more recently some young people in Mexico have smoked it as a substitute for marijuana. The traditional methods of using the plant include chewing the leaves, drinking a tea made from the crushed leaves, or smoking the dried leaves. The resulting hallucinatory effect is reported to last for up to an hour.[54] People in the United States and in Europe have cultivated the plant for the past several years and use it as a legal hallucinogen. *Salvia* is not currently listed as a controlled substance in the United States.

The plant was identified in 1962 by Wasson and Hoffman, and the active agent, salvinorin A, was identified in 1982. Salvinorin A is nearly as potent as LSD, in that an effective human dose may be as little as 200 µg (micrograms) when smoked. It was reported in 1994 that salvinorin A binds selectively to the kappa opioid receptor, where it acts as an agonist. Thus, this drug represents a newly discovered type of chemical structure and a unique pharmacological effect, which is stimulating research to develop new, related compounds.[54]

Meanwhile, it will be interesting to see what happens to the legal status of *Salvia* and of salvinorin A. That will no doubt be influenced by whether there are highly publicized examples of abuse.

Summary

- Hallucinogenic plants have been used for many centuries, not only as medicines but for spiritual and recreational purposes as well.

- LSD, a synthetic hallucinogen, alters perceptual processes and enhances emotionality, so that the real world is seen differently and is responded to with great emotion.

- Other chemicals that contain the indole nucleus, such as psilocybin (from the Mexican mushroom), have effects similar to those of LSD.

- Mescaline, from the peyote cactus, and synthetic derivatives of the amphetamines represent the catechol hallucinogens. They have psychological effects quite similar to those of the indole types.

- MDMA is the only catechol hallucinogen that appears likely to be capable of producing permanent brain damage in its users.

- PCP, or angel dust, produces more changes in body perception and fewer visual effects than LSD.

- Anticholinergics are found in many plants throughout the world and have been used not only recreationally, medically, and spiritually but also as poisons.

Review Questions

1. What are the distinctions among phantastica, deliriants, psychedelics, psychotomimetics, entheogens, and hallucinogens?
2. What is the precise relationship between ergotism and LSD?
3. Why was LSD used in psychoanalysis in the 1950s and 1960s? How does this relate to its proposed use by the Army and the CIA?
4. Describe the dependence potential of LSD in terms of tolerance, physical dependence, and psychological dependence.
5. What is the diagnostic term for *flashbacks*?
6. What is the active agent in the "magic mushrooms" of Mexico, and is it an indole or a catechol?
7. Besides the psychological effects, what other effects are reliably produced by peyote?
8. Contrast MDMA and PCP in terms of how they appear to make people feel about being close to others.
9. Which of the hallucinogenic plants was most associated with witchcraft?
10. Describe what is actually known about bufotenin and the "toad-licking" phenomenon.
11. Which hallucinogen acts as an agonist at kappa opiate receptors?

References

1. Schultes, R.E., A. Hofmann. *Plants of the Gods.* New York: McGraw-Hill, 1979.
2. Caporael, L.R. "Ergotism: The Satan Loosed in Salem." *Science* 192 (1976), pp. 21–26.
3. Gottlieb, J., N.P. Spanos. "Ergotism and the Salem Village Witch Trials." *Science* 194 (1976), pp. 1390–94.
4. Hofmann, A. "Psychotomimetic Agents." In A. Burger, editor. *Drugs affecting the central nervous system* (Vol. 2). New York: Marcel Dekker, 1968.
5. Segal, J., editor. *Research in the Service of Mental Health, Research on Drug Abuse.* National Institute on Mental Health, Pub. No. (ADM) 75-236, U.S. Department of Health, Education, and Welfare. Washington, DC: U.S. Government Printing Office, 1975.
6. Johnston, L. "Ford Signs Grant of $750,000 in LSD Death in CIA Test." *The New York Times,* October 14, 1976, p. C43.
7. Treaster, J.B. "Mind-Drug Test a Federal Project for Almost 25 Years." *The New York Times,* August 11, 1975, p. M42.
8. "CIA Considered Big LSD Purchase." *Washington Star,* August 4, 1975. See also Knight, M. "LSD Creator Says Army Sought Drug." *The New York Times,* August 1, 1975.
9. Taylor, J.R., & W. N. Johnson. *Use of Volunteers in Chemical Agent Research.* Inspector General Report No. DAIGIN 21-75, Washington, DC: U.S. Department of Army, March 10, 1976.
10. Weil, A.T. "The Strange Case of the Harvard Drug Scandal." *Look,* November 5, 1963, pp. 38–48.
11. Blumenthal, R. "Leary Drug Cult Stirs Millbrook." *The New York Times,* June 14, 1967, p. 49.
12. "Celebration #1." *New Yorker* 42 (1966), p. 43.
13. Council on Mental Health and Committee on Alcoholism and Drug Dependence. "Dependence on LSD and Other Hallucinogenic Drugs." *JAMA* 202 (1967), pp. 141–44.
14. Leary and Liddy, Debating Specialists. *The New York Times,* September 3, 1981, p. B26.
15. Appel, J.B., & J.A. Rosecrans. "Behavioral Pharmacology of Hallucinogens in Animals: Conditioning Studies." In B.L. Jacobs, editor. *Hallucinogens: Neurochemical, Behavioral and Clinical Perspectives.* New York: Raven Press, 1984.
16. Julien, R.M. *A Primer of Drug Action,* 10th ed. New York: Worth, 2005.
17. Siegel, R.K. "The Natural History of Hallucinogens." In B.L. Jacobs, editor. *Hallucinogens: Neurochemical, Behavioral and Clinical Perspectives.* New York: Raven Press, 1984.
18. Krippner, S. "Psychedelic Experience and the Language Process." *Journal of Psychedelic Drugs* 3, no. 1 (1970), pp. 41–51.
19. Levine, J., & A.M. Ludwig. "The LSD Controversy." *Comprehensive Psychiatry* 5, no. 5 (1964), pp. 318–19.
20. Forsch, W.A., E.S. Robbins, and M. Stern. "Untoward Reactions to Lysergic Acid Diethylamide (LSD) Resulting in Hospitalization." *New England Journal of Medicine* 273 (1965), pp. 1235–39.
21. Halpern, J.H., and others. "Hallucinogen Persisting Perceptual Disorder: What Do We Know after 50 Years?" *Drug & Alcohol Dependence* 69 (2003), pp. 109–19.
22. Zegans, L.S., J.C. Pollard, and D. Brown. "The Effects of LSD-25 on Creativity and Tolerance to Regression." *Archives of General Psychiatry* 16 (1967), pp. 740–49.
23. Spitzer, M., and others. "Increased Activation of Indirect Semantic Associations Under Psilocybin." *Biological Psychiatry* 39 (1996), pp. 1055–57.
24. Hollister, L.E., J. Shelton, and G. Krieger. "A Controlled Comparison of Lysergic Acid Diethylamide (LSD) and Dextroamphetamine in Alcoholics." *American Journal of Psychiatry* 125 (1969), pp. 1352–57.
25. NIMH Research on LSD. "Extramural Programs Fiscal Year 1948 to Present." Prepared September 1, 1975.
26. Leary, T. "The Religious Experience: Its Production and Interpretation." *Journal of Psychedelic Drugs* 1, no. 2 (1967–1968), pp. 3–23.
27. Delgado, P.L., & F.A. Moreno. "Hallucinogens, Serotonin, and Obsessive-Compulsive Disorder." *Journal of Psychoactive Drugs,* 30 (1998), pp. 359–66.
28. Schultes, R.E., & A. Hofmann. *The Botany and Chemistry of Hallucinogens.* Springfield, IL: Charles C. Thomas, 1980.

29. Al-Assmar, S.E. "The Seeds of the Hawaiian Baby Woodrose Are a Powerful Hallucinogen [letter]." *Archives of Internal Medicine* 159 (1999), p. 2090.

30. Glick, S.D., and others. "18-Methoxycoronaridine (18-MC) and Ibogaine: Comparison of Antiaddictive Efficacy, Toxicity, and Mechanisms of Action." *Annals of the New York Academy of Sciences* 914 (2000), pp. 369–86.

31. Strassman, R.J., and others. "Differential Tolerance to Biological and Subjective Effects of Four Closely-Spaced Doses of N,N-dimethyltryptamine in Humans." *Biological Psychiatry* 39 (1996), pp. 784–95.

32. Grob, C.S., and others. "Human Psychopharmacology of Hoasca, a Plant Hallucinogen Used in Ritual Context in Brazil." *Journal of Nervous and Mental Disease* 184 (1996), pp. 86–94.

33. Dobkin de Rios, M., & M. Cardenas. "Plant Hallucinogens, Shamanism, and Nazca Ceramics." *Journal of Ethnopharmacology* 2 (1980), pp. 233–46.

34. De Ropp, R.S. *Drugs and the Mind.* New York: Grove Press, 1957.

35. Ellis, H. "Mescal: A Study of a Divine Plant." *Popular Science Monthly* 61 (1902), pp. 59, 65.

36. Huxley, A. *The Doors of Perception.* New York: Harper & Row, 1954.

37. MDMA. "Compound Raises Medical, Legal Issues." *Brain/Mind Bulletin,* April 15, 1985.

38. Peroutka, S.J., and others. "Subjective Effects of 3,4-methylenedioxymethamphetamine in Recreational Users." *Neuropsychopharmacology* 1 (1988), pp. 273–77.

39. Curran, H.V. "Is MDMA ("Ecstasy") Neurotoxic in Humans? An Overview of Evidence and of Methodological Problems in Research." *Neuropsychobiology* 42 (2000), pp. 34–41.

40. McGann, U.D., & G.A. Ricuarte. "Reinforcing Subjective Effects of 3,4-methylenedioxymethamphetamine ("Ecstasy") May Be Separable from its Neurotoxic Actions: Clinical Evidence." *Journal of Clinical Psychopharmacology* 13 (1993), p. 214.

41. Luby, E., and others. "Study of a New Schizophrenomimetic Drug—Sernyl." *American Medical Association Archive of Neurological Psychiatry* 81 (1959), pp. 113–19.

42. Jevtovic-Todorovic, V., and others. "Ketamine Potentiates Cerebrocortical Damage Induced by the Common Anaesthetic Agent Nitrous Oxide in Adult Rats." *British Journal of Pharmacology* 130 (2000), pp. 1692–98.

43. Siegel, R.K. "Phencyclidine and Ketamine Intoxication: A Study of Four Populations of Recreational Users." In R.C. Petersen, R.C. Stillman, editors. *Phencyclidine (PCP) Abuse: An Appraisal.* (NIDA Research Monograph No. 21). Washington, DC: U.S. Department of Health and Human Services, 1978.

44. Cosgrove, K.P., & M.E. Carroll. "Differential Effects of Bremazocine on Oral Phencyclidine (PCP) Self-Administration in Male and Female Rhesus Monkeys." *Experimental & Clinical Psychopharmacology* 12 (2004), pp. 111–17.

45. Overend, W. "PCP: Death in the 'Dust.'" *Los Angeles Times,* September 26, 1977.

46. Guitart, X., and others. "Sigma Receptors: Biology and Therapeutic Potential." *Psychopharmacology* 174 (2004), pp. 301–19.

47. Genesis 30:14–16. *The New English Bible.* Oxford University Press and Cambridge University Press, 1970.

48. Schultes, R.E. "The Plant Kingdom and Hallucinogens (Part III)." *Bulletin on Narcotics* 22, no. 1 (1970), pp. 43–46.

49. Beverly, R. *The History and Present State of Virginia, 1705.* Chapel Hill: University of North Carolina Press, 1947.

50. Allegro, J.M. *The Sacred Mushroom and the Cross.* New York: Doubleday, 1970.

51. Wasson, R.G. "Fly Agaric and Man." In D.H. Efron, editor. *Ethnopharmacologic Search for Psychoactive Drugs.* Washington, DC: National Institute of Mental Health, 1967. See also Wasson, R.G. *Soma, Divine Mushroom of Immortality.* New York: Harcourt Brace Jovanovich, 1971.

52. "Hallucinogens." *Columbia Law Review* 68, no. 3 (1968), pp. 521–60.

53. Weil, A.T., & W. Davis. "*Bufo Alvarius:* A Potent Hallucinogen of Animal Origin." *Journal of Ethnopharmacology* 41 (1994), pp. 1–8.

54. Sheffler, D.J., B.L. Roth, and A. Salvinorin. "The 'Magic Mint' Hallucinogen Finds a Molecular Target in the Kappa Opioid Receptor." *Trends in Pharmacological Sciences* 24 (2003), pp. 107–09.

Check Yourself

Match the plants on the left with the appropriate hallucinogenic chemical on the right:

ayahuasca

peyote

sacred mushrooms (from Mexico)

morning glories

belladonna

Amanita

mescaline

muscimol

d-lysergic acid amide

atropine

DMT and harmaline

psilocybin

15

Marijuana

Objectives

When you have finished this chapter, you should be able to:

- Describe the relationship among marijuana, cannabis, and THC and discuss different preparations of cannabis.

- Describe how Europeans became exposed to the psychological effects of cannabis.

- Explain how marijuana was described in the years leading up to the 1937 Marijuana Tax Act.

- Discuss the legal status of marijuana in the U.S. since 1937, including current debates.

- Draw parallels among the various scientific and medical studies on marijuana.

- Describe the type of receptor THC acts on in the brain and compare the time course of smoked vs. oral THC.

- List the two most consistent physiological effects of marijuana.

- Discuss evidence for the abuse potential of marijuana and influences on the psychological effects of marijuana.

- Describe the effects of marijuana use on driving ability, the lungs, sperm motility, and the immune system.

- Describe the range of evidence relating to whether marijuana smoking leads to brain damage in humans.

Marijuana has meant so many things to so many people over the years that it is hard to describe it from a single perspective. The matter of classifying marijuana among the other psychoactive drugs is so complex that we, like most authors, avoid the issue by setting it off by itself. Marijuana can produce some sedative-like effects, some pain relief, and, in large doses, hallucinogenic effects. Thus, many of its users treat it as a depressant; it has been called a narcotic (for both pharmacological, as well as political, reasons); and it is often included among descriptions of hallucinogenic plants. However, the effects it produces when used as most people use it are sufficiently different from those of other psychoactive drugs to justify its consideration as a unique substance.

Cannabis, the Plant

Marijuana (or *marihuana;* either spelling is correct) is a preparation of leafy material from the ***Cannabis*** plant that is smoked. The question

Online Learning Center Resources

www.mhhe.com/ksir12e

Visit our Online Learning Center (OLC) for access to these study aids and additional resources.

- Learning objectives
- Glossary flashcards
- Web activities and links
- Self-scoring chapter quiz
- Audio chapter summaries

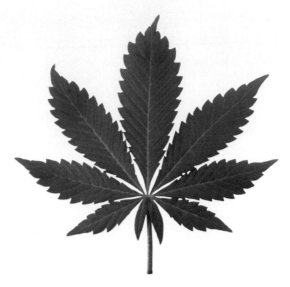

A leaf of the *Cannabis* (marijuana) plant.

is which *Cannabis* plant, because there is still botanical debate over whether there is one, three, or more species of *Cannabis.* In previous years, this issue spurred legal arguments because the laws mentioned only *Cannabis sativa.* Does that include all marijuana or not? The evidence is strong that there are three separate species. *Cannabis sativa* originated in Asia but now grows worldwide and primarily has been used for its fibers, from which hemp rope is made. This is the species that grows as a weed in the United States and Canada. *Cannabis indica* is grown for its psychoactive resins and is cultivated in many areas of the world, including selected planters and backyards of the United States. The third species, *Cannabis ruderalis,* grows primarily in Russia and not at all in America. The plant Linnaeus named *C. sativa* in 1753 is what is still known as *C. sativa.*[1]

George Washington grew *C. sativa* at Mount Vernon, most likely not to get high but to make rope and possibly for medicinal uses. From his fields and many others like it, *C. sativa* spread across the nation, growing spontaneously.

C. sativa that is cultivated for use as hemp grows as a lanky plant up to 18 feet high. *C. indica* plants cultivated for their psychoactive effects are more compact and usually only two or three feet tall. The psychoactive potency results from an interaction between genetics and environmental conditions. Plants of different species grown under identical conditions produce different amounts of psychoactive

material, and the same plants vary in potency from year to year, depending on the amount of sunshine, warm weather, and moisture.

Preparations from *Cannabis*

The primary psychoactive agent, delta-9-tetrahydrocannabinol **(THC),** is concentrated in the resin of *Cannabis;* most of the resin is in the flowering tops, less is in the leaves, and there is little in the fibrous stalks. The psychoactive potency of a *Cannabis* preparation depends on the amount of resin present and therefore varies, depending on the part of the plant used.[1] India has produced three traditional *Cannabis* preparations, each of which corresponds roughly to preparations available in the United States. The most potent of these is called *charas* in India, and it consists of pure resin that has been carefully removed from the surface of leaves and stems. **Hashish,** or hasheesh, is a substance widely known around the world and in its purest form is pure resin, like charas. It may be less pure, depending on how carefully the resin has been separated from the plant material. Hashish is rare in the

Drugs in the Media

Medical Marijuana in the News

Probably no single psychoactive drug topic has received more publicity in the past few years than the issue of medical marijuana, which has been placed as a referendum on the ballot in at least eight states. Each time, there are stories about the plight of people with AIDS who say they need marijuana to stimulate their appetites. And each time there are stories reflecting the views of local police and federal drug-control officials who say that medical marijuana is just an excuse for people who want to grow and use an illegal substance. Here is a sampling of a few days' headlines that reveal the complexity of the issues raised when these laws are considered and then passed:

"Push for medical marijuana raises many questions," by Jim Tiffin, *Gallup Independent,* January 23, 2006. SANTA FE—As the New Mexico State Legislature considers whether to pass legislation making the use of marijuana legal for certain medical conditions, there are some questions that need to be answered.

"Radio Station Pulls Medical Marijuana PSA After Complaints," Associated Press, February 24, 2006. RAWLINS, Wyo.—A pair of local radio stations has pulled a set of public service announcements advocating medical marijuana use after receiving complaints from the police chief and others.

"Legislation Allowing Medical Marijuana Advances to Senate," Associated Press, March 1, 2006. SPRINGFIELD, Ill.—Although an Illinois law has allowed the use of marijuana as medicine since 1978, the statute has sat on the books unused. Now a Chicago lawmaker has won the chance to take a practical medical marijuana bill to the Senate for a floor vote for the first time in three decades.

"Senate Committee OKs Bill to Allow Medical Marijuana Use," by Conrad Defiebre, *Minneapolis Star Tribune,* March 17, 2006. MINNEAPOLIS—A bill to legalize marijuana for medical use in Minnesota cleared the Senate Judiciary Committee on Thursday, advancing it another step in a long and uncertain journey toward possible enactment.

"State Asks Court to Toss SD County Medical Marijuana Suit," by Gig Conaughton, *North County Times,* March 21, 2006. NORTH COUNTY—State officials formally asked judges to throw out San Diego County's precedent-setting lawsuit seeking to overturn California's 10-year-old medical marijuana law, saying that the only controversy over the law was in the minds of county supervisors.

Judging from the small but increasing number of states that permit seriously ill patients to grow and use marijuana under medical supervision (California took the lead in 1996), the issue isn't going away any time soon. And this is separate from the issue of general legalization. Currently, marijuana maintains a slot alongside heroin and methamphetamine as a "drug of concern" in its listing on the federal Drug Enforcement Administration's Web site.

The average American so far seems uninterested in a serious national debate on the use of marijuana. The mere mention of legalizing any illegal drug means political suicide for any politician willing to broach the subject. A notable exception is former New Mexico Governor Gary Johnson, a Republican. An outspoken advocate for legalizing pot while in office, Johnson is also a triathlete who maintained steady popularity ratings in his state. Although most U.S. citizens may not be ready to embrace his stance, we will certainly be seeing more arguments in the media for legalizing medical marijuana use.

United States, constituting less than 1 percent of all confiscated marijuana samples in the past 10 years. The average THC content of hashish has ranged from 3 to 7 percent with rare samples as high as about 20 percent.

The second most potent preparation is traditionally called *ganja* in India, and it consists

Cannabis (can a biss): the genus of plant known as marijuana.

THC: delta-9-tetrahydrocannabinol, the most active chemical in marijuana.

hashish (hash *eesh* or *hash* eesh): concentrated resin from the *Cannabis* plant.

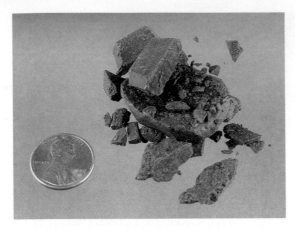

Hashish, concentrated resin from the *Cannabis* plant, is relatively rare in the United States.

of the dried flowering tops of plants with pistillate flowers (female plants). The male plants are removed from the fields before the female plants can become pollinated and put their energy into seed production. This increases the potency of the female plants and produces high-grade marijuana known as **sinsemilla** (from the Spanish *sin semilla,* "without seeds"). The average THC content of sinsemilla samples from the United States also varies widely, ranging from 7 to 12 percent.

The weakest form in India is *bhang,* which is made by using the entire remainder of the plant after the top has been picked, then drying it and grinding it into a powder. The powder can then be mixed into drinks or candies.[1] This type of preparation is rare in the United States, but it is similar to low-grade marijuana, which consists of the leaves of a plant, perhaps even a *sativa* plant found growing as a weed. Some of this low-grade marijuana contains less than 1 percent THC.

Manually scraping exuded resin off the plant to make hashish is a tedious process, and a more efficient method of separating the resin from plants has been known for many years. The plants are boiled in alcohol, then the solids filtered out and the liquid evaporated down to a thick, dark substance once known medically as "red oil of cannabis" and now referred to as

hash oil. Again, this product varies widely in its potency but can contain more than 50 percent THC. Until fairly recently, both the medical and the psychological effects of *Cannabis* preparations were variable. All the traditional methods could do was produce relatively pure plant resin, but that resin could vary considerably in its THC content.

If we consider only the marijuana available for smoking in the United States, we can see that it can vary widely in potency from a low-grade product containing less than 1 percent THC to a high-grade sinsemilla containing 9 percent or more THC. The usual range of potency for marijuana seems to be 2 to 5 percent, however. Since the early 1980s, repeated reports have stated that the marijuana available on the streets today is "10 times" more potent than the marijuana of the 1960s. The political message behind this is that the marijuana of the 1960s may have been relatively harmless, but the current marijuana is more dangerous. In fact, the entire range of these traditional preparations has been known, and scientific, literary, and medical descriptions of the wide range of effects have been based on this entire range of potencies, for 150 years. But it is true that U.S. marijuana growers are becoming more sophisticated and producing more sinsemilla. According to the Drug Enforcement Administration, the proportion of confiscated marijuana samples containing more than 9 percent THC has increased from 3 percent of the samples in 1992 to 15 percent of the samples in 2001.[2]

History
Early History

The earliest reference to *Cannabis* is in a pharmacy book written in 2737 BC by Chinese emperor Shen Nung. Referring to the euphoriant effects of *Cannabis,* he called it the "Liberator of Sin." He recommended it for some medical uses, including "female weakness, gout, rheumatism, malaria, beriberi, constipation and absent-mindedness." Social use of the plant had spread to the Muslim world and North Africa by AD 1000. In this period in the eastern Mediterranean area, a legend developed around a religious cult that committed murder for political reasons. The cult was called "hashishiyya," from which our word *assassin* developed. In 1299, Marco Polo told the story he had heard of this group and its leader. It was a marvelous tale and had all the ingredients necessary for a tale to survive through the ages: intrigue, murder, sex, the use of drugs, and mysterious lands. The story of this group and its activities was told in many ways over the years, and Boccaccio's *Decameron* contained one story based on it. Stories of this cult, combined with the frequent reference to the power and wonderment of hashish in *The Arabian Nights,* were widely circulated in Europe over the years.

The 19th Century: Romantic Literature and the New Science of Psychology

At the start of the 19th century, world commerce was expanding. New and exciting reports from the world travelers of the 17th and 18th centuries introduced new cultures and new ideas to Europe. Asia and the Middle East had yielded exotic spices, as well as the stimulants coffee and tea. Europe was ready for another new sensation, and got it. The returning veteran, as usual, gets part of the blame for introducing what Europe was ready to receive:

> Napoleon's campaign to Egypt at the beginning of the nineteenth century increased the Romantic's acquaintance with hashish and caused them to associate it with the Near East. . . . Napoleon was forced to give an order forbidding all French soldiers to indulge in hashish. Some of the soldiers brought the habit to France, however, as did many other Frenchmen who worked for the government or traveled in the Near East.[3]

By the 1830s and 1840s, everyone who was anyone was using, thinking about using, or decrying the use of mind-tickling agents such as opium and hashish. One of the earliest (1844) popular accounts of the use of hashish

is in *The Count of Monte Cristo* by Alexander Dumas. The story includes a reference to the Assassins tale and contains statements about the characteristics of the drug that still sound contemporary. During the 1840s, a group of artists and writers gathered monthly at the Hotel Pimodan in Paris's Latin Quarter to use drugs. This group became famous because one of the participants, Gautier, wrote a book, *Le Club de Hachischins,* that described their activities. From this group have come some of the best literary descriptions of hashish intoxication. These French Romantics, like the Impressionist painters of a later period, were searching for new experiences, new sources of creativity from within, and new ways of seeing the world outside. A few of the regulars were well-known writers, including Baudelaire, Gautier, and Dumas.

Baudelaire used hashish and was an astute observer of its effects in himself and in others. In his book *Artificial Paradises,* he echoed what Dumas had written about the kind of effect to expect from hashish:

> The intoxication will be nothing but one immense dream, thanks to intensity of color and the rapidity of conceptions; but it will always preserve the particular tonality of the individual. . . . The dream will certainly reflect its dreamer. He is only the same man grown larger . . . sophisticate and ingenu . . . will find nothing miraculous, absolutely nothing but the natural to an extreme.[4]

As the end of the 19th century approached, the use of psychoactive drugs increased, but the hashish experience held little interest for the dweller in middle America.

"Marijuana, Assassin of Youth"

At the beginning of the 20th century, public interest in *Cannabis* and its use was not very

---

sinsemilla (sin se *mee* ya): "without seeds"; a method of growing more potent marijuana.

widespread. In the early 1920s, a few references in the mass media reported the use by Mexican-Americans of something the newspapers called marijuana, but public concern was not aroused. In 1926, however, a series of articles associating marijuana and crime appeared in a New Orleans newspaper. As a result, the public began to take an interest in this "new" drug.

The U.S. commissioner of narcotics, Harry Anslinger, said that in 1931 the Bureau of Narcotics' file on marijuana was less than two inches thick. The same year, the Treasury Department stated:

> A great deal of public interest has been aroused by the newspaper articles appearing from time to time on the evils of the abuse of marijuana, or Indian hemp. This publicity tends to magnify the extent of the evil and lends color to an inference that there is an alarming spread of the improper use of the drug, whereas the actual increase in such use may not have been inordinately large.[5]

Even so, by 1935, 36 states had laws regulating the use, sale, and/or possession of marijuana. By the end of 1936, all 48 states had similar laws. The Federal Bureau of Narcotics also changed its tune. In 1937, at congressional hearings, Anslinger stated, "Traffic in marihuana is increasing to such an extent that it has come to be the cause for the greatest national concern."[6] From 1931 to 1937, the use of marijuana had spread throughout the country, but there is no evidence that there was extensive use in most communities. The primary motivation for the congressional hearings on marijuana came not because of the use of marijuana as an inebriant or a euphoriant but because of reports by police and in the popular literature stating, "Most crimes of violence are laid to users of marihuana."[7]

Scientific American reported in March 1936:

> Marijuana produces a wide variety of symptoms in the user, including hilarity, swooning, and sexual excitement. Combined with intoxicants, it often makes the smoker vicious, with a desire to fight and kill.[8]

And *Popular Science Monthly* in May 1936 contained a lengthy article with such statements as this:

> The Chief of Philadelphia County detectives declared that whenever any particularly horrible crime was committed—and especially one pointing to perversion—his officers searched first in marijuana dens and questioned marijuana smokers for suspects.[9]

It hardly seemed necessary for readers to be told that marijuana had arrived as "the foremost menace to life, health, and morals in the list of drugs used in America."[9]

In this period the association was repeatedly made between crime, particularly violent and/or perverted crime, and marijuana use. A typical report follows:

> In Los Angeles, Calif., a youth was walking along a downtown street after inhaling a marijuana cigarette. For many addicts, merely a portion of a "reefer" is enough to induce intoxication. Suddenly, for no reason, he decided that someone had threatened to kill him and that his life at that very moment was in danger. Wildly he looked about him. The only person in sight was an aged boot-black. Drug-crazed nerve centers conjured the innocent old shoe-shiner into a destroying monster. Mad with fright, the addict hurried to his room and got a gun. He killed the old man, and then, later, babbled his grief over what had been wanton, uncontrolled murder.
>
> "I thought someone was after me," he said. "That's the only reason I did it. I had never seen the old fellow before. Something just told me to kill him!"
>
> That's marijuana![10]

However, not all articles condemned marijuana as the precipitator of violent crimes. An article in *The Literary Digest* reported that the chief psychiatrist at Bellevue Hospital in New York City had reviewed the cases of more than 2,200 criminals convicted of felonies. Referring to marijuana, he said, "None of the assault cases could be said to have been committed under the drug's influence. Of the sexual crimes, there was none due to marihuana intoxication. It is quite probable that alcohol is more responsible as an agent for crime than is marihuana."[11]

There was very poor documentation of the relationship between marijuana and crime, which in the 1930s was stated as if it had been proved. A thorough review of Commissioner Anslinger's writings on marijuana concluded:

> In the works of Mr. Anslinger, there are either no references or references to volumes which my assistants and I have checked and which, in our checking, we find to be based upon much hearsay and little or no experimentation. We found a mythology in which later writers cite the authority of earlier writers, who also had little evidence. We have found, by and large, what can most charitably be described as a pyramid of prejudice, with each level of the structure built upon the shaky foundations of earlier distortions.[12]

Examples of this "pyramid of prejudice" abound, but here's one way it worked: One of Mr. Anslinger's Treasury agents would testify before Congress and relate one of the outrageous stories of marijuana-induced violence. Next, the testimony would be referred to in an editorial in a medical journal, such as the *Journal of the American Medical Association (JAMA)*. Then Anslinger or one of his people would write a magazine article, citing the prestigious *JAMA* as the source of the information.

With such poor evidence supporting the relationship between marijuana use and crime, it seems strange that the true story was never told. There are probably several reasons. One was the Great Depression, which made everyone acutely sensitive to, and wary of, any new and particularly foreign influences. The fact that it was lower-class Mexican-Americans and African-Americans who were associated with use of the drug made the drug doubly dangerous to the white middle class.

Another contributing factor probably was the regular reference in associating marijuana and crime to the murdering cult of Assassins as suggestive of the characteristics of the drug. The 1936 *Popular Science Monthly* reference to the Assassins is the most concise:

The origin of the word "assassin" has two explanations, but either demonstrates the menace of Indian hemp. According to one version, members of a band of Persian terrorists committed their worst atrocities while under the influence of hashish. In the other version, Saracens who opposed the Crusaders were said to employ the services of hashish addicts to secure secret murderers of the leaders of the Crusades. In both versions, the murderers were known as "haschischin," "hashshash" or "hashishi" and from those terms comes the modern and ominous "assassin."[9]

In none of the original stories and legends were the murders committed by individuals under the influence of hashish; rather, hashish may have been part of the reward for carrying out various crimes. No matter. As the 1930s rolled on, fear of marijuana users and of marijuana itself increased, as did state marijuana-control laws. In the mid-1930s, the Narcotics Bureau acted to support federal legislation, and in the spring of 1937 congressional hearings were held.

The Marijuana Tax Act of 1937

Passage of the Marijuana Tax Act was a foregone conclusion. Few witnesses testified other than law enforcement officers. People dealing in birdseed had the act modified so they could import sterilized *Cannabis* seed for use in their product. An official of the American Medical Association (AMA) testified on his own behalf, not representing the AMA, against the bill. His reasons for opposing the bill were multiple. Primarily, he thought the state antimarijuana laws were adequate and that the social-menace case against *Cannabis* had not been proved. It might be that most other medical doctors didn't associate the old remedies based on *Cannabis* with this new, foreign-sounding drug marijuana. The bill was passed in August and became effective on October 1, 1937.

The general characteristics of the law followed the regulation-by-taxation theme of the Harrison Act of 1914. The federal law did not outlaw *Cannabis* or its preparations; it just taxed the grower, distributor, seller, and buyer and made it, administratively, almost impossible for anyone to have anything to do with *Cannabis.* In addition, the Bureau of Narcotics prepared a uniform law that many states adopted. The uniform law on marijuana specifically named *C. sativa* as the species of plant whose leafy material is illegal. In later years, the defense in some court cases argued that the material confiscated by the police had come from *C. indica* and thus was not illegal. In the usual specimens obtained by police or presented in court, all distinguishing characteristics between species are either not present or are obliterated by drying and crushing. Because the cannabinoids are present in all species, there is no way of telling what species most confiscated marijuana belongs to. The current federal and uniform laws refer only to *Cannabis.*

The state laws made possession and use of *Cannabis* illegal per se. In May 1969, 32 years later, the U.S. Supreme Court declared the Marijuana Tax Act unconstitutional and overturned the conviction of Timothy Leary because there was

> in the Federal anti-marijuana law—a section that requires the suspect to pay a tax on the drug, thus incriminating himself, in violation of the Fifth Amendment: and a section that assumes (rather than requiring proof) that a person with foreign-grown marijuana in his possession knows it is smuggled.[13]

After the Marijuana Tax Act

Passage of the Marijuana Tax Act had an amazing effect. Almost immediately there was a sharp reduction in the reports of heinous crimes committed under the influence of marijuana. The price of the merchandise increased rapidly (the war came along, too), so that five years after passage of the act the cost of a marijuana cigarette—a reefer—had increased 6 to 12 times and cost about a dollar.

The year after the law was enacted, 1938, Mayor Fiorello LaGuardia of New York City remembered what no one else wanted to recall. What he recalled were two army studies on marijuana use by soldiers in the Panama Canal Zone around 1930. Both reports had found marijuana to be innocuous and had said that its reputation as a troublemaker "was due to its association with alcohol which was always found the prime agent."[14] Mayor LaGuardia asked the New York Academy of Medicine to study marijuana, its use, its effects, and the necessity for control. The report, issued in 1944, was intensive and extensive and a very good study for its time. Following is only a part of the report's summary:[15]

> It was found that marihuana in an effective dose impairs intellectual functioning in general. . . .
>
> Marihuana does not change the basic personality structure of the individual. It induces a feeling of self-confidence, but this expressed in thought rather than in performance. There is, in fact, evidence of a diminution in physical activity. . . .
>
> Those who have been smoking marihuana for a period of years showed no mental or physical deterioration which may be attributed to the drug.[15]

This 1944 report, which was completed by a very reputable committee of the New York Academy of Medicine, brought a violent reaction. The AMA stated in a 1945 editorial:

> For many years medical scientists have considered cannabis a dangerous drug. Nevertheless, a book called "Marihuana Problems" by New York City Mayor's Committee on Marihuana submits an analysis of seventeen doctors of tests on 77 prisoners and, on this narrow and thoroughly unscientific foundation, draws sweeping and inadequate conclusions which minimize the harmfulness of marijuana. Already the book has done harm. One investigator has described some tearful parents who brought their 16 year old son to a physician after he had been detected in the act of smoking marihuana. A noticeable mental deterioration had been evident for some time even to their lay minds. The boy said he had read an account of the LaGuardia Committee report and that this was his justification for using marihuana.[16]

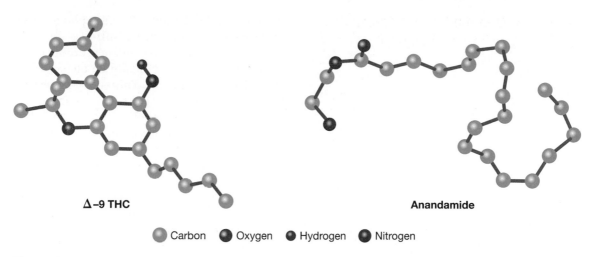

Δ–9 THC   **Anandamide**

● Carbon   ● Oxygen   ● Hydrogen   ● Nitrogen

Figure 15.1   Delta-9 THC, The Most Active Substance Found in *Cannabis,* and Anandamide, Isolated from Brain Tissue

As in all such reports and reactions to reports, there is little dispute over the facts, only over the interpretation. The LaGuardia Report is in substantial agreement with the Indian Hemp Commission Report of the 1890s, the Panama Canal Zone reports of the 1930s, and the comprehensive reports in the 1970s by the governments of New Zealand, Canada, Great Britain, and the United States, in addition to the 1981 report to the World Health Organization and the 1982 report by the National Academy of Science to the Congress of the United States, so it is likely that the conclusions of the LaGuardia Report were and are for the most part valid.

The 1950s and 1960s were a unique period in the history of marijuana. There was a hiatus in scientific research on *Cannabis,* but experimentation in the streets increased. With the arrival of the "psychedelic 60s," the popular press emphasized the more sensational hallucinogens. Marijuana, however, became the most common symbol of youthful rejection of authority and identification with a new era of personal freedom. According to the annual high school senior survey and the NIDA household survey (see Chapter 1), marijuana apparently peaked in popularity in the United States around 1980.

During the 1980s and early 1990s, marijuana use became much less popular than it had been in the 1970s, but the mid-1990s saw the beginning of a significant rise in the number of young people using marijuana.

Pharmacology
Cannabinoid Chemicals

The chemistry of *Cannabis* is quite complex, and the isolation and extraction of the active ingredient are difficult even today. The active agent in *Cannabis* is unique among psychoactive plant materials in that it contains no nitrogen and thus is not an alkaloid.

There are more than 400 chemicals in marijuana, but only 66 of them are unique to the *Cannabis* plant—these are called cannabinoids. One of them, delta-9-tetrahydrocannabinol (THC), was isolated and synthesized in 1964 and is clearly the most pharmacologically active. Structures of some of these chemicals are shown in Figure 15.1. The major active metabolite in the body of THC is 11-hydroxy-delta-9-THC.

The relationship of THC to *Cannabis* is probably more similar to the relationship of nicotine to tobacco than of alcohol to beer, wine, or distilled spirits. Alcohol is the only behaviorally active agent in alcoholic beverages, but there might be several active agents in *Cannabis.*

Absorption, Distribution, and Elimination

When smoked, THC is rapidly absorbed into the blood and distributed first to the brain, then redistributed to the rest of the body, so that within 30 minutes much is gone from the brain. The peak psychological and cardiovascular effects occur together, usually within 5 to 10 minutes. The THC remaining in the blood has a half-life of about 19 hours, but metabolites (of which there are at least 45), primarily 11-hydroxy-delta-9-THC, are formed in the liver and have a half-life of 50 hours. After one week, 25 to 30 percent of the THC and its metabolites might still remain in the body. Complete elimination of a large dose of THC and its metabolites might take two or three weeks. THC taken orally is slowly absorbed, and the liver transforms it to 11-hydroxy-delta-9-THC; therefore, much less THC reaches the brain after oral ingestion, and it takes much longer for it to have psychological and cardiovascular effects. The peak effects following oral ingestion usually occur at about 90 minutes.

The high lipid solubility of THC means that it (like its metabolites) is selectively taken up and stored in fatty tissue to be released slowly. Excretion is primarily through the feces. All of this has two important implications: (1) there is no easy way to monitor (in urine or blood) THC/metabolite levels and relate them to behavioral and/or physiological effects, as can be done with alcohol, and (2) the long-lasting, steady, low concentration of THC and its metabolites on the brain and other organs might have effects not yet determined.

Mechanism of Action

Scientists searched for years for a key to help them unlock the mystery of marijuana's action on the central nervous system. The identification and purification of THC was a necessary step. A significant breakthrough was made by researchers in 1988 who developed a technique to identify and measure highly specific and selective binding sites for THC and related compounds in rat brains. One result was the

development and testing of more potent marijuana analogues. Another result was the 1992 discovery of a natural substance produced in the body that has marijuana-like effects when administered to animals. This endogenous substance (see Figure 15.1) is called **anandamide** (*ananda* is sanskrit for "bliss").[17]

THC and other cannabinoids are known to bind to two receptors, designated CB1 and CB2.[18] There are substantial differences in the structures of these two receptors and their anatomical distribution in the body. CB2 receptors are found mainly outside the brain in immune cells, suggesting that cannabinoids may play a role in the modulation of the immune response. CB1 receptors are found throughout the body, but primarily in the brain. These receptors are much more abundant than receptors for morphine and heroin,[16] suggesting that the potential actions of cannabinoids are widespread. The locations of CB1 receptors in the brain also may provide some clues about their functions. For example, the highest density of CB1 receptors has been found in cells of the basal ganglia; its primary components include the caudate nucleus, putamen, and globus pallidus. Cells of the basal ganglia are involved in coordinating body movements. Other regions that also contain a larger number of CB1 receptors include the: *cerebellum,* which coordinates fine body movements; *hippocampus,* which is involved in aspects of memory storage; *cerebral cortex,* which regulates the integration of higher cognitive functions; and *nucleus accumbens,* which is involved in reward.

A number of drugs have been developed in an effort to more selectively act on these receptors. Rimonabant, a selective CB1 receptor antagonist, is being tested in Phase III clinical trials and has shown some promise both in reducing food intake and in assisting people trying to stop smoking tobacco cigarettes. However, there are concerns about reports of psychological depression among some of the research participants, plus general uneasiness that rimonabant is the first drug that blocks these

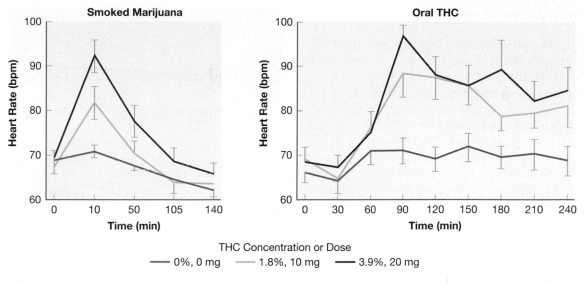

Figure 15.2   The Time Course for Heart Rate after Smoking Marijuana (left) and Ingesting Oral THC (right)

receptors. Since we don't yet know what all the normal functions are for anandamide's actions on CB1 receptors, there could be unexpected side effects that will appear only after rimonabant (trade name Accomplia) is marketed and large numbers of people begin to use it.[19]

Physiological Effects

One of the most consistent acute physiological effects of both smoked marijuana and oral THC is an increase in heart rate. Figure 15.2 shows that both smoked marijuana and oral THC increased the heart rate of marijuana smokers in a dose-dependent fashion (i.e., larger THC doses produced larger heart rate elevations).[20, 21] While the peak effects produced by smoking marijuana containing 4 percent THC are similar to 20 mg oral THC, the drug's time course of action is different. Peak heart-rate elevations produced by smoked marijuana occurred within 10 minutes and returned to baseline levels after about 90 minutes, whereas peak heart-rate elevations produced by oral THC did not occur until 90 minutes following ingestion and remained elevated for at least four hours after drug administration. The effect of

cannabis-based drugs on blood pressure is more variable, with some studies reporting slight increases and others reporting no effect. Concern has been raised that smoking marijuana might have permanent deleterious effects on the cardiovascular system, but there is no evidence to indicate that marijuana-related cardiovascular effects are associated with serious health problems for most young, healthy users.[22] Patients with hypertension, cerebrovascular disease, and coronary atherosclerosis, however, should probably avoid smoking marijuana or ingesting THC because of the drug's effects on heart rate. Other consistent acute effects of smoked marijuana are reddening of the eyes and dryness of the mouth and throat. Except for bronchodilation, acute exposure to marijuana has little effect on breathing as measured by conventional pulmonary tests. Heavy marijuana smoking over a much longer period could lead to clinically significant and less readily reversible impairment of pulmonary function.

anandamide (an *and* a mide): a chemical isolated from brain tissue that has marijuana-like properties.

Behavioral Effects

While physiological effects produced by cannabis-based drugs provide important information, the behavior of most interest for the assessment of abuse potential is drug taking. Until recently, cannabinoids were not shown to maintain self-administration in laboratory animals, suggesting that the abuse potential of cannabis-based drugs was minimal. This seemed inconsistent with epidemiological data showing that marijuana is the most widely used illicit drug in the world[23] and that more Americans sought treatment for marijuana abuse and dependence than for any other illicit substance.[24] Findings from recent studies, however, demonstrate clearly that rats and squirrel monkeys will consistently self-administer cannabinoids.[25] The success of recent attempts to obtain reliable self-administration in laboratory animals has been attributed to intravenously injecting THC doses more rapidly than had been previously tried.

Several laboratory studies have shown that marijuana produces robust self-administration by human marijuana smokers, and that marijuana self-administration is related to the THC content of the cigarettes. That is, marijuana cigarettes containing a higher concentration of THC are preferred to those containing a lower THC concentration.[26] These findings not only confirm the abuse potential of smoked marijuana, but they also suggest that THC administered alone (e.g., oral administration of THC capsules) might have abuse potential. In a recent study, experienced marijuana smokers were given repeated opportunities to self-administer oral THC capsules or to receive $2. They selected the money on more occasions than the capsules, despite the fact that oral THC produces marijuana-like effects on many measures, including ratings of euphoria. This study suggests that oral THC does *not* have high abuse potential.[21]

Some have argued that before novice marijuana smokers are able to experience marijuana-associated positive subjective effects (e.g., euphoria, stoned), they must go through a process by which they learn to recognize and

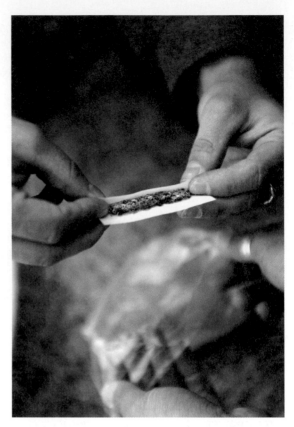

Experienced marijuana smokers report euphoria, "high," hunger, and mellowness after smoking; the magnitude of the effects depends on the THC concentration.

interpret the psychoactive effects produced by smoked marijuana.[27] While this position remains open for debate, the subjective effects on experienced marijuana smokers have been well characterized. In general, experienced smokers report increased ratings of euphoria, "high," mellowness, hunger, and stimulation after smoking marijuana. These effects peak within 5 to 10 minutes and last for about two hours; they are usually THC concentration-dependent (i.e., the magnitude of effects is increased with increasing THC concentrations). Subjective effects reported by infrequent smokers are similar but more intense because these individuals are less tolerant to marijuana-associated effects. Also, at higher

THC concentrations some infrequent smokers may report negative effects such as mild paranoia and hallucination. As seen with heart rate, peak subjective effects of oral THC are similar to those produced by smoked marijuana except that the time course of the effects is different. Peak subjective effects occur about 90 minutes following oral ingestion and can last for several hours. An important factor in determining whether a drug is likely to be abused is the rapidity of the onset of its effects. The more rapidly a drug's effects are experienced, the more likely it will be abused. This might be why the abuse potential of oral THC is limited.

While an earlier study demonstrated that relatively less-experienced marijuana smokers reported being intoxicated after smoking a placebo cigarette, more recent studies demonstrate that regular marijuana smokers are not so readily duped. Placebo cigarettes were made by extracting the THC and other cannabinoids from marijuana—the cigarettes looked and smelled like regular marijuana cigarettes. In these studies, participants "sampled" marijuana cigarettes (containing placebo or different THC concentrations) and alternative reinforcers (e.g., money or snack food), and subsequently were given an option to choose. Participants selected cigarettes containing THC on more than 75 percent of choice opportunities compared to only about 40 percent when placebo cigarettes were available.[28] Furthermore, subjective effects produced by the placebo cigarette were identical to baseline levels, whereas subjective effects produced by cigarettes containing THC were significantly elevated.

The effect of marijuana on cognitive performance has received a great deal of attention in the popular press and the scientific literature for many years with little resolution. Unfortunately, many discussions on this topic add to the confusion because they fail to differentiate between the direct (acute) effects and long-term (chronic) effects of marijuana. They also fail to consider the marijuana use history of the user. Following acute administration of smoked marijuana to infrequent marijuana smokers, cognitive performance is disrupted temporarily in several domains: The amount of time that is required to complete cognitive tasks is increased (*slowed cognitive processing*); performance on immediate recall tasks is decreased (*impaired short-term memory*); premature responding is increased (*impaired inhibitory control*); performance on tracking tasks is decreased (*loss of sustained concentration or vigilance*); and performance on tasks requiring participants to reproduce computer-generated patterns is disrupted (*impaired visuospatial processing*). The acute effects of marijuana on the performance of frequent smokers are less dramatic, leading some to hypothesize that regular marijuana smokers are tolerant to many marijuana-related cognitive effects.[20] Some negative cognitive effects, however, have been reported. For example, slowing of cognitive performance is a consistent finding, even in regular users. This effect may have significant behavioral consequences under circumstances requiring complex operations that must be accomplished in a limited time frame, such as certain workplace tasks and the operation of machinery and automobiles.

It is also difficult to make definitive statements about *long-term* cognitive effects of marijuana use because of divergent findings and interpretations. More general conclusions, however, are possible. Based on the available evidence, it appears that following a sufficient period of abstinence (greater than one month), regular marijuana use produces minimal effects on cognition as measured by standard neuropsychological tests.[29] The reader is cautioned, though, because as the number of better controlled studies increase, the current conclusions about the long-term effects of marijuana on cognition may change.

We've all heard about someone smoking marijuana and then getting a case of the "munchies," a marked increase in food intake. Data from a large number of studies clearly demonstrate that marijuana and oral THC significantly increase total daily caloric intake. These findings provided the basis for at least one clinical use of cannabis-based drugs—appetite stimulation (see "Medical Uses of Cannabis"). A related question that has received less scientific attention is: Why aren't most chronic marijuana users overweight? Some have speculated that tolerance develops to the food intake-enhancing effect of cannabis-based drugs, but no empirical data support this view. The bottom line is that the average weight of chronic marijuana users is not known because there have been no studies addressing this issue. Thus, the average chronic marijuana user may indeed be overweight.

Another consistent behavioral effect of marijuana is on verbal behavior (talking). Stimulant drugs such as amphetamines, have been shown to increase verbal interactions, as have moderate doses of alcohol. Marijuana appears to be different. Several researchers have reported that while nonverbal social interactions are increased following marijuana smoking, verbal exchanges are dramatically decreased.[30]

Medical Uses of *Cannabis*

Cannabis has never attained the medical status of opium, but the first report of medical use was by Shen Nung in 2737 BC. About 2,900 years after the Shen Nung report, another Chinese physician, Hoa-tho (AD 200) recommended *Cannabis* resin mixed with wine as a surgical anesthetic. Although *Cannabis* preparations were used extensively in medicine in India and after about AD 900 in the Near East, almost nothing about it appeared in European medical journals until the 1800s.

Early reports in Europe, such as de Sacy's 1809 article titled "Intoxicating Preparations Made with Cannabis," awakened more interest among the writers and artists of the period than among physicians. In 1839, however, a lengthy article, "On the Preparations of the Indian Hemp, or Gunjah," was published by a British physician working in India.[31] He reviewed the use of *Cannabis* in Indian medicine and reported on his own work with animals, which

suggested that *Cannabis* preparations were quite safe. Having shown *Cannabis* to be non-toxic, he used it clinically and found it to be an effective anticonvulsant and muscle relaxant, as well as a valuable drug for the relief of the pain of rheumatism.

In 1860, the Ohio State Medical Society's Committee on *C. indica* reported its successful use in the treatment of stomach pain, chronic cough, and gonorrhea. One physician felt he had to "assign to the Indian hemp a place among the so-called hypnotic medicines next to opium."[32]

One difficulty that has always plagued the scientific, medical, and social use of *Cannabis* is the variability of the product. An 1898 brochure reviewed the assay and standardization techniques used with many of the common plant drugs and stated: "In Cannabis Indica we have a drug of great importance and one which of all materia medica is undoubtedly the most variable."[33] Four years later, Parke, Davis,[34] using new standardization procedures, claimed that "each lot sent out upon the market by us is of full potency and to be relied upon." The company listed a variety of *Cannabis* products available for medical use, including "a Chocolate Coated Tablet Extract Indian Cannabis 1/4 grain."

Passage of the Marijuana Tax Act of 1937 resulted in all 28 of the legal *Cannabis* preparations being withdrawn from the market, and in 1941 *Cannabis* was dropped from *The National Formulary and The U.S. Pharmacopoeia.* The decline in the medical use of *Cannabis* occurred long before 1937, and the law did not eliminate an actively used therapeutic agent. Four factors, however, contributed to the declining prescription rate of this plant. One was the development of new and better drugs for most illnesses. Second was the variability of the available medicinal preparations of *Cannabis,* which was repeatedly mentioned in the 1937 hearings.[6] Third, the active ingredient is very insoluble in water and thus not amenable to injectable preparations. Last, taken orally it has an unusually long (one- to two-hour) latency to onset of action.

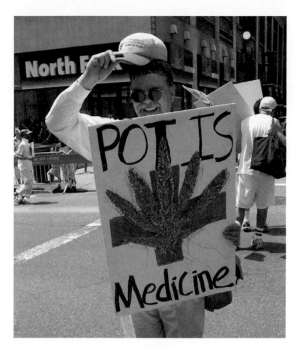

The potential medical benefits of marijuana is an issue with a long and controversial history.

With the recent renewed interest in marijuana as a social drug has come some reevaluation of the implications of some of the older therapeutic reports. Scientists have looked again at some of the most interesting reported therapeutic effects of *Cannabis.* One is its anticonvulsant activity. A 1949 report found it effective in some cases in which phenytoin (Dilantin), the anticonvulsant of choice both then and now, was ineffective.[35] The fact that both Queen Victoria's physician and Sir William Osler, as well as others, found *Cannabis* to be very effective against tension and migraine headaches also caused some interest.

A 1972 report showed that marijuana smoking was effective in reducing the fluid pressure of the eye in a glaucoma patient.[36] That report became a cause célèbre in 1975, when a glaucoma patient was arrested for growing marijuana plants on his back porch for medical purposes. Fifteen months later, this man (1) saw the charges against him dropped,

(2) had his physician certify that the only way for him to avoid blindness was to smoke five joints a day, and (3) had these marijuana joints legally supplied to him by the United States government.[37] This began a very limited program in which the National Institute on Drug Abuse (NIDA) provided medical-grade marijuana cigarettes to patients with the FDA's approval of a "compassionate use" protocol.

A second possible important medical use was reported in 1975. Medication containing THC, the active ingredient in marijuana, was the only kind that was effective in reducing the severe nausea caused by certain drugs used to treat cancer. A 1982 report from the National Academy of Sciences stated:

> Cannabis and its derivatives have shown promise in the treatment of a variety of disorders. The evidence is most impressive in glaucoma . . . ; in asthma . . . ; and in the nausea and vomiting of cancer chemotherapy . . . and might also be useful in seizures, spasticity, and other nervous system disorders.[38]

On the other hand, Dr. Gabriel Nahas, a medical researcher and prominent foe of medical marijuana, felt that

> for each of these uses, there are other modern drugs with greater bioavailability, specificity, and effectiveness. . . . Reproducible absorption, consistent and predictable pharmacological effects may not be achieved. . . . It appears that it will not become a useful therapeutic agent.[39]

In 1985, the FDA licensed a small drug company, Unimed, Inc., to begin producing a capsule containing THC for sale to cancer chemotherapy patients who are experiencing nausea. The drug is referred to by the generic name **dronabinol** and the brand name **Marinol.** Dronabinol has helped cancer chemotherapy patients gain weight, and in 1993 the FDA also

dronabinol (dro *nab* i noll): the generic name for prescription THC in oil in a gelatin capsule.
Marinol (*mare* i noll): the brand name for dronabinol.

approved its use for stimulating appetite in AIDS patients.

The National Organization for the Reform of Marijuana Laws (NORML) wants marijuana cigarettes themselves approved, under the theory that the dose can be better controlled and smoking is therefore safer. Its position received some support from the DEA's chief administrative law judge in 1988, who recommended that the DEA move marijuana from Schedule I to Schedule II, so that physicians could use it to treat the nausea produced by cancer chemotherapy and to relieve suffering in cases of multiple sclerosis. He called natural marijuana "one of the safest therapeutically active substances known to man."[40] The DEA finally decided in 1992 that there was insufficient evidence to justify rescheduling marijuana to Schedule II, so it will remain officially "without medical usefulness"; part of the DEA's reasoning was that, because "pure" THC was now available by prescription, there was no justification for providing the raw plant material to be smoked. Also in 1992, apparently in response to a number of "compassionate use" requests from AIDS patients seeking improved appetites, the FDA terminated the process of reviewing any new compassionate use protocols for marijuana cigarettes.[41]

The question of medical usefulness for marijuana seemed to some to have been taken away from federal agencies and put in the hands of the public when, in November 1996, both Arizona and California voters passed ballot initiatives allowing physicians to recommend marijuana for serious illnesses and allowing patients to possess and use marijuana if their physicians recommend it. There was still no legal way for patients to purchase marijuana, of course, and no legal growers or distributors. More than half the states had previously passed laws allowing medicinal use of marijuana, so in a sense this was not new. However, those previous laws had passed in the 1970s, when decriminalization and even legalization of marijuana were being debated openly. Also, many of those older laws allowed marijuana to be used only as part of an approved research effort, not for individual patients. As of 2004, 11 states had some form of legislation allowing a patient, with a physician's authorization (or prescription), to use marijuana for medical purposes (see Taking Sides).

In 1997, in response to public pressure to allow the medical use of marijuana, the White House Office of National Drug Control Policy funded another study by the Institute of Medicine (IOM) of the National Academy of Sciences to perform a comprehensive review of the scientific evidence for potential benefits and risks of using marijuana as a medicine. The resulting 1999 report has been pointed to by proponents of medical marijuana as supporting the idea that marijuana is a relatively safe and effective medicine for patients suffering from chronic conditions, such as AIDS wasting syndrome or chronic pain. However, the report also recommends more research on cannabinoid biology, additional clinical studies on marijuana and synthetic cannabinoids, and the development of an effective inhaler to solve the problem of poor oral absorption of THC. In the meantime, the panel recommended that the compassionate use of smoked marijuana cigarettes be allowed for no more than six months for patients with debilitating, intractable pain or vomiting, when the following conditions are met:

- The failure of approved medications to provide relief has been documented.
- The symptoms can reasonably be expected to be relieved by rapid-onset cannabinoid drugs.
- Such treatment is administered under medical supervision in a manner that allows for the assessment of treatment effectiveness.
- An oversight strategy is in place to approve or reject requests within 24 hours after a physician seeks permission to provide marijuana to a patient for a specified use.

The entire report can be found on the Internet at books.nap.edu/catalog/9586.html.

Taking Sides

Should Medical Patients Have Access to Marijuana?

At least eleven states have passed ballot initiatives allowing patients to use marijuana on the advice of their physicians. Passage of these initiatives has fueled public interest in this topic. The best-demonstrated effects of marijuana (and of THC) are the reduction of the nausea caused by chemotherapy for cancer and the stimulation of appetite, which might benefit AIDS patients. With such serious illnesses involved, many feel that the compassionate thing is to allow marijuana to be used if it might help, since the risk of dependence seems to be a rather small issue in such cases. In fact, "*Cannabis* buyers clubs" sprang up in many large cities—most notably, San Francisco—and patients who had notes from the physicians could purchase from them. These clubs were illegal, but local law enforcement agencies for the most part left them alone, not wanting to arrest seriously ill patients. Of course, because the clubs were illegal and informally operated, there was no guarantee that everyone purchasing marijuana was, in fact, seriously ill.

Following the passage of the first ballot initiatives, the U.S. government in December 1996 announced that it would move to revoke the DEA registration of any physician who advised a patient to use illegal drugs. This caused some to wonder about violations of the tradition of privileged communications between doctors and patients, and so far the legality of all of this is open to question. In early 1998, the U.S. Justice Department announced plans to shut down all *Cannabis* buyers clubs in California.

In September 2000, the U.S. District Court in San Francisco issued an injunction permanently barring the government from revoking a physician's license to prescribe medicine "merely because the doctor recommends medical marijuana to a patient based on a sincere medical judgement." The court also prevented the government from initiating an investigation of a doctor's other prescribing practices solely because he or she had recommended marijuana.

In November 2000, at the White House's request, the U.S. Supreme Court issued an emergency ban (by a vote of seven to one) on the distribution of marijuana for medical purposes. The court struck down the U.S. Court of Appeals ruling in San Francisco, which would have made "medical necessity" a defense against violation of federal drug statutes. The court voted 8–0 against such defenses in May 2001. In November 2004, the Supreme Court heard arguments in *Raich v Ashcroft*, a case brought on behalf of Angel Raich, a California patient, and others. They asserted that because the marijuana was provided to Ms. Raich free, the transactions did not constitute "commerce." And, since the growing, transfer, and use of the marijuana were all done within California, the federal government could not assert jurisdiction based on its ability to regulate interstate commerce. In June 2005, the U.S. Supreme Court disagreed ruling that federal law enforcement personnel could prosecute patients for possessing marijuana even if their physicians recommended marijuana use for a serious illness. Despite this ruling, the medical marijuana issue is far from being resolved. In fact, in January 2006, Rhode Island became the eleventh state to legalize the medical use of marijuana.

Do you think medical necessity is a compelling argument for the use of marijuana? Why or why not?

Causes for Concern

Abuse and Dependence

The evidence now suggests that if high levels of marijuana are used regularly over a sustained period, tolerance can develop to many marijuana-related effects, including the cognitive-impairing, physiological, and subjective effects.

However, tolerance may not develop uniformly across each of these variables. For example, it has been demonstrated that heavy marijuana smokers exhibit minimal cognitive impairment following acute marijuana smoking, while showing dramatic heart rate increases and reporting significant levels of euphoria. These findings suggest that tolerance may develop more readily to marijuana-related cognitive effects than to heart rate responses and subjective effects.[20]

Relative to other drugs of abuse, many people perceive marijuana to be an innocuous drug with limited abuse potential. People have made comparisons between marijuana abuse and abuse of other drugs such as crack cocaine. However, the social consequences associated with marijuana use and those associated with crack cocaine use are dissimilar, making one-to-one comparisons imperfect. Research showing that THC and marijuana produce robust self-administration in laboratory animals and in human research participants clearly demonstrates that the drug has some abuse potential. In addition, of the 7.1 million Americans classified with dependence on or abuse of illicit drugs in 2001, 4.3 million were dependent on or abused marijuana.[24] Although this number represents a relatively small fraction of current marijuana users (less than 30 percent), it shows that a significant number of marijuana smokers do suffer ill effects from using the drug.

Can regular marijuana use produce a withdrawal syndrome? According to the DSM-IV-TR (the standard diagnostic instrument), the answer is no. The DSM-IV-TR does not recognize a diagnosis of cannabis withdrawal. Data from a variety of human laboratory and clinical studies, however, demonstrate that an abstinence syndrome can be observed following abrupt cessation of several days of smoked marijuana administration[42] or oral Δ^9-THC administration.[43] Cannabinoid withdrawal is not life threatening, but symptoms can be unpleasant. Marijuana withdrawal syndrome in humans may include negative mood states (e.g., anxiety, restlessness, depression, and irritability), disrupted sleep, decreased food intake, and in some cases, aggressive behavior.[44] These symptoms have been reported to begin 1 day after cannabinoid cessation and persist from 4 to 12 days, depending on an individual's level of marijuana dependence. Clearly, the majority of marijuana users do not experience withdrawal symptoms nor do they meet DSM-IV-TR criteria for cannabis-use disorders. But these findings indicate that regular marijuana use may not be as innocuous as previously perceived.

Toxicity Potential

Acute Physiological Effects The acute physiological effects of marijuana, primarily an increase in heart rate, have not been thought to be a threat to health. However, as the marijuana-using population ages, there is concern that individuals with high blood pressure, heart disease, or hardening of the arteries might be harmed by smoking marijuana.[37] The lethal dose of THC has not been extensively studied in animals, and no human deaths have been reported from "overdoses" of *Cannabis*.

Driving Ability A large number of studies have investigated the effects of marijuana on driving performance, but the findings have been inconsistent. Some studies have reported marijuana-related driving impairments, while others have not. Traditionally, two types of studies have been conducted: (1) *epidemiological:* These studies determine whether marijuana use is over-represented among drivers involved in automobile accidents; and (2) *laboratory:* These studies determine the direct effects of marijuana on skills related to driving performance. Findings from the majority of the epidemiological studies show little evidence that drivers who use marijuana alone are more likely to be involved in an accident than non-drug-using drivers. But data from laboratory studies of computer-controlled driving simulators indicate that marijuana produces significant impairments.[36] Most of the laboratory studies have employed relatively infrequent marijuana users as participants, a group that would be expected to show marked impairments. Because tolerance can develop to many of the cognitive-impairing effects of marijuana, further laboratory studies should include heavy marijuana smokers.

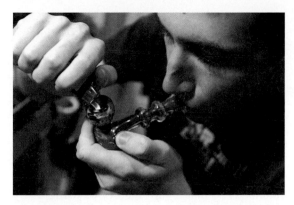

Inhaling marijuana smoke.

Panic Reactions The other major behavioral problem associated with acute marijuana intoxication is the panic reaction. Much like many of the bad trips with hallucinogens, the reaction is usually fear of loss of control and fear that things will not return to normal. This reaction is more common among less-experienced marijuana users. Even Baudelaire understood this and advised his readers to surround themselves with friends and a pleasant environment before using hashish. Although many people do seek emergency medical treatment for marijuana-induced panic and are sometimes given sedatives or tranquilizers, the best treatment is probably "talking down," or reminding the person of who and where they are, that the reaction is temporary, and that everything will be all right.

Chronic Lung Exposure There has been a great deal of concern about the possible long-term effects of chronic marijuana use. A couple of physiological concerns merit attention. One is the effect on lung function and the concern about lung cancer. Experiments have shown that chronic, daily smoking of marijuana impairs air flow in and out of the lungs.[45] It is hard to tell yet whether years of such an effect results in permanent, major obstructive lung disease in the same way that smoking tobacco cigarettes does. Also, no direct evidence links marijuana smoking to lung cancer in humans. Remember that it took many years of cigarette smoking by millions of Americans before the links between tobacco and lung cancer and other lung diseases were shown.

Marijuana smoke has been compared with tobacco smoke.[37] Some of the constituents differ (there is no nicotine in marijuana smoke and no THC in tobacco), but many of the dangerous components are found in both. Total tar levels, carbon monoxide, hydrogen cyanide, and nitrosamines are found in similar amounts (except for tobacco-specific nitrosamines, which are carcinogens). Another potent carcinogen, *benzopyrene*, is found in greater amounts in marijuana than in tobacco. Everyone suspects that marijuana smoking will eventually be shown to cause cancer, but how much of a problem this will be compared with tobacco is hard to say. On the one hand, few marijuana smokers smoke 20 marijuana cigarettes every day, whereas tobacco smokers regularly smoke this much. On the other hand, the marijuana cigarette is not filtered and the user generally gets as much concentrated smoke as possible as far down in the lungs as possible and holds it there. So, while some wait and see when the data will come out, others are participating in the experiment.

Reproductive Effects Another area of concern is reproductive effects in both men and women. Heavy marijuana smoking can decrease testosterone levels in men, although the levels are still within the normal range and the significance of those decreases is not known. Diminished sperm counts and abnormal sperm structure in heavy marijuana users has been reported, perhaps because anandamide plays a role in normal sperm function.[46] A number of studies have reported either lower birth weight or shorter length at birth for infants whose mothers smoked marijuana during pregnancy, but because so many of the women also smoked tobacco or drank alcohol, it is not possible to determine the exact contribution of marijuana to these effects. It is, of course, wise to avoid the use of all drugs during pregnancy.

The Immune System Effects There have also been reports that marijuana smoking impairs some measures of the functioning of the immune system.[47] Animal studies have found that THC injections can reduce immunity to infection, but at doses well above those obtainable by smoking marijuana. Some human studies of marijuana smokers have suggested reduced immunity, but most have not. If the effect were real, it could result in marijuana smokers' being more susceptible to infections, cancer, and other diseases, such as genital herpes. One might suspect that such problems would eventually be reflected in the overall death rate of marijuana users. However, a report examining 10 years of mortality data for more than 65,000 people found no relationship between marijuana use and overall death rates.[48]

Amotivational Syndrome Since 1971, when some psychiatric case reports were published identifying an *amotivational* syndrome in marijuana smokers, concern has been expressed about the effect of regular marijuana use on behavior and motivation. A number of experiments and correlational studies have been aimed at answering this question. There does seem to be evidence for this diminished motivation, impaired ability to learn, and school and family problems in some adolescents who are chronic, heavy marijuana smokers. If they stop smoking and remain in counseling, the condition improves.[49] This probably implies a constant state of intoxication rather than a long-lasting change in brain function or personality.

Insanity The connection between marijuana use and insanity was one of the main arguments for outlawing the drug in the 1930s, and the notion still remains that marijuana can cause a type of psychosis. There have been reports of psychotic "breakdowns" occurring with rare frequency after marijuana has been smoked, but the causal relationship is in question. The psy-

chotic episodes are generally self-limiting and seem to occur in individuals with a history of psychiatric problems.[49]

Brain Damage For about 30 years, it has been speculated that amotivational or prolonged psychotic reactions could reflect an underlying damage to brain tissue produced by marijuana. For example, a 1972 report from England indicated that two individuals who demonstrated cerebral atrophy had a history of smoking marijuana. They also had a history of using many other illicit drugs, plus other medical problems, but it was suggested that the brain damage might have been caused by the marijuana. Several experiments have since been done, and all have failed to find a relationship between marijuana smoking and cerebral atrophy.

Most other incomplete or poorly controlled reports from animal research of potential brain damage have been dismissed as inconclusive. However, two experiments on rats, one appearing in 1987 and the other in 1988, gave stronger evidence that THC causes permanent changes in the structure of neurons in the hippocampus. One of the reports related these changes to a persistent deficit in the rats' performance on a radial arm maze. The doses used were in the range of what a very heavy marijuana smoker might obtain, and the treatment was given to the rats every day for 90 days. It's not clear what the implications might be for human beings smoking less heavily and only occasionally.

Ironically, some of the nonpsychoactive ingredients in marijuana, including cannabidiol, have been shown to have powerful antioxidant properties that protect brain cells from the toxic effects of other chemicals.[50] This effect was strong enough that the NIMH filed a patent in 1988 entitled "Cannabinoids as Antioxidants and Neuroprotectants."

Emotion has played an obvious and influential role. Scientists on both sides have become crusaders for their cause. Some individuals seem to think it is their professional duty to seek out and publicize every potential evil associated with marijuana, even if no strong scientific evidence supports their views. Others seem to automatically question the negative reports and look for ways to discredit them. We can predict that the emotion, the premature announcements of new scary findings, the repeating of long discredited stories, and the conflicting reports will continue.

Marijuana and American Society

Our patterns of drug use are but one facet of our evolving society. Drug use affects and is affected by other social trends, including a couple of significant themes from the 1980s.

One trend was the increased emphasis on physical health. Jogging, working out, dieting, drinking less alcohol and caffeine, and smoking less all were reflections of our national concern over shaping up. The health trend obviously worked against marijuana use: How many people who wouldn't smoke tobacco felt good about inhaling marijuana smoke? Second, the 1980s saw a move toward social and political conservatism, which worked against such counterculture behavior as marijuana smoking. And, of course, drug use tends to be faddish. If marijuana was the fashionable drug of the 1970s, then it couldn't be the fashionable drug of the 1980s. However, in the 1990s the drug came back into fashion, at least somewhat.

Data from the yearly survey of high school seniors shows the trends most clearly. After peaking in 1978–1979, the number of high school seniors who had ever smoked marijuana dropped from just over 60 percent to 32 percent in 1992, then rebounded to 45 percent by the class of 2005. Equally dramatic were the trends in daily use, which went from 11 percent in 1978 to 2 percent in 1992 and back to 6 percent by 2005.[51] The earlier decreases in marijuana use went along with a steady increase in the belief among these students that "people risk harming themselves if they smoke marijuana regularly." Whereas just over one-third of the high school seniors agreed with

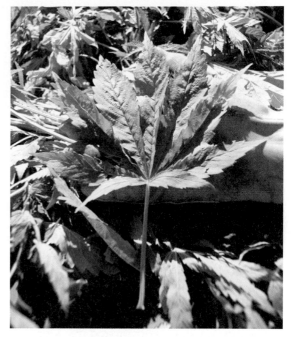

Federal and state laws and penalties related to marijuana possession tend to reflect other social trends, becoming more severe in periods of social and political conservatism.

that statement in 1978, more than three-fourths agreed in 1992. Fads being what they are, this downward trend in marijuana use had to end sometime, and the turnaround was seen in the high school senior class of 1992. Significant increases in marijuana use in the 1992–2005 period were accompanied by decreased estimates of risk (see Chapter 1).

Although marijuana is not used by most Americans, it is still remarkable how many people have used and continue to use a substance that shouldn't exist at all in our society, according to the Controlled Substances Act and the DEA. That a large fraction of the society continues to violate the laws regarding marijuana is a matter for concern. It is easy to look back and wish that the 1937 Marijuana Tax Act had never happened. Marijuana use was spreading slowly across the United States and, with any luck, it might have become acculturated. Society would have adapted to marijuana and adapted marijuana to society. Soon it would have become part of society: Perhaps most people would never have used it regularly; of those who did use it, most would have known how to use it; some, of course, would have abused it. It has happened before with coffee, tea, tobacco, and alcohol.

The 1937 law prevented all that. It didn't affect most Americans a great deal until the 1960s, when a large number of young people began experimenting with drugs. Marijuana, more than anything else, convinced many young people that the government had been lying to them about drugs. They had been told that marijuana would make them insane, enslave them in drug dependence, and lead to violence and perverted sexual acts. Their experience told them that marijuana was pretty innocuous, compared with those stories, and it became an important symbol: Smoking marijuana struck a blow for truth and freedom. The problem was that laws existed that allowed young people to be sent to jail for 20 years for striking this blow, and that didn't sit well with some people. Voice was given to the millions of marijuana users in 1970 when a young Washington lawyer established the National Organization for the Reform of Marijuana Laws (NORML) with a grant from the Playboy Foundation. As the founder of NORML put it, "The only people working for reform then were freaks who wanted to turn on the world, an approach that was obviously doomed to failure. I wanted an effective, middle-class approach, not pro-grass but antijail."

Also, in 1970 the Comprehensive Drug Abuse Prevention and Control Act of 1970 established the Commission on Marijuana and Drug Abuse. Its 1972 report recommended that federal and state laws be changed so that private possession of small amounts of marijuana for personal use, and casual distribution of small amounts without monetary profit, would no longer be offenses. The year 1972 was a turning point in the fight to decriminalize marijuana. In June the American Medical Association came out in favor of dropping penalties for possession

of "insignificant amounts" of marijuana and noted that "there is no evidence supporting the idea that marijuana leads to violence, aggressive behavior, or crime." In August the American Bar Association called for the reduction of criminal penalties for possession, and a year later the organization recommended decriminalization. Both traditional liberals and conservatives could support the idea, not to declare marijuana legal but to make possession of marijuana a civil offense, punishable only by a fine.

In October 1973, Oregon abolished criminal penalties for marijuana use, substituting civil fines of up to $100. Marijuana offenders were given citations that are processed similar to traffic tickets. Did marijuana use increase in Oregon as a result of the decriminalization? Yes. By leaps and bounds? No. From the fall of 1974, a year after decriminalization, to the fall of 1977, the percentage of adults over 18 who had ever used marijuana went from 19 percent to 25 percent. Current users went from 9 percent to 10 percent over the same period. However, marijuana use was increasing toward its 1978 to 1979 peak all over the country at the same time. Possession of a small amount of marijuana was made only a civil offense by eight other states: Maine, Colorado, California, Ohio, Minnesota, Mississippi, New York, and North Carolina. In Alaska, private possession of up to four ounces of marijuana was not illegal. Changing marijuana possession from a felony to a misdemeanor saved money on court costs, juries, and jails. The state of California enjoyed an estimated average annual savings of more than $95 million between 1976 and 1985 as a result of its citation plan for marijuana possession.[52]

At the federal level, action picked up in 1977. In January, Rosalynn Carter joined her husband, the president, in calling for the decriminalization of marijuana and revealed that their oldest son had been discharged from the Navy for smoking marijuana. Bills to decriminalize marijuana possession were introduced into both houses of Congress, and in August President Carter sent a message to Congress in which he asked them to abolish all federal criminal penalties for the possession of small amounts of marijuana.

In the late 1970s, de facto decriminalization had already occurred in many areas of the country. Law enforcement agencies in many of the larger U.S. cities had stopped arresting marijuana users and did not search out those with small amounts for personal use.

When the Reagan administration came into office in 1981, any hope of federal decriminalization was gone, replaced by a "get tough" attitude toward all illegal drugs. Marijuana was no exception. In addition to increased efforts to intercept marijuana shipments from abroad, a nationwide effort was launched to combat the cultivation of marijuana plants. More than 100 million plants were tugged out of the ground in 1987 by state, local, and federal law enforcement teams.[53] Add to that the zero tolerance seizures of boats, cars, and planes containing even traces of marijuana and the 1988 legislation putting extra pressure on the user (e.g., $10,000 fines at the federal level; see Chapter 3), and we can see that the pendulum had definitely swung back. The states began to follow suit: In 1989, Oregon raised its civil penalty for possession from a $100 maximum to a $500 minimum. In 1990, Alaska voters approved the recriminalization of marijuana possession, making it a misdemeanor punishable by a jail term and up to a $1,000 fine. In 1993, an Alaska Court of Appeals ruled that individuals did have the right to possess up to four ounces of marijuana for personal use. An initiative in 2004 that would have removed criminal penalties for marijuana possession and allowed its regulated (and taxed) sale in Alaska, failed to pass.

Summary

- *Cannabis* has a rich history relating both to its medicinal use and to its recreational uses.
- Marijuana became famous as the "Assassin of Youth" in the 1930s and was outlawed in 1937.

- *Cannabis* contains many active chemicals, but the most active is delta-9-THC.
- THC is absorbed rapidly by smoking but slowly and incompletely when taken by mouth.
- THC has a long half-life of elimination, and its metabolites can be found in the body for up to several weeks after THC enters the body.
- Selective THC receptors exist in brain tissue, leading to the discovery of a naturally occurring brain cannabinoid, anandamide.
- Marijuana causes an increase in the heart rate and reddening of the eyes as its main physiological effects.
- Psychologically, THC has some sedative properties, produces some analgesia, and at high doses can produce hallucinations.
- Marijuana is useful in the treatment of glaucoma, the reduction of nausea in patients undergoing cancer chemotherapy, and the increase of appetite in AIDS patients. A legal form of THC is available by prescription.
- Although strong dependence is not common, it does occur in some individuals.
- Marijuana can impair driving skills, but it is not clear that smoking marijuana leads to an increased frequency of accidents.
- Most experts agree that chronic smoking of marijuana impairs lung function somewhat and probably increases the risk of lung cancer.

Review Questions

1. What are the major differences between *C. sativa* and *C. indica*?
2. How are hashish and sinsemilla produced?
3. When and where was the earliest recorded medical use of cannabis?
4. Why were Harry Anslinger's writings on marijuana referred to as a "pyramid of prejudice"?

5. What were the general conclusions of the 1944 LaGuardia Commission?

6. What is meant by "cannabinoid," and about how many are there in *Cannabis?* What is the cannabinoid found in brain tissue?

7. How is the action of THC in the brain terminated after about 30 minutes, when the half-life of metabolism is much longer than that?

8. What are the two most consistent physiological effects of smoking marijuana?

9. What two medical uses have been approved by the FDA for dronabinol?

10. What evidence suggests that marijuana use might interfere with reproduction?

References

1. Schultes, R.E., & A. Hofmann. *The Botany and Chemistry of Hallucinogens.* Springfield, IL: Charles C Thomas, 1980.

2. National Drug Intelligence Center. *Intelligence Brief: National Drug Threat Assessment, Marijuana Update.* Washington, DC: U.S. Department of Justice Document No. 2002-J0403-002, 2002.

3. Mickel, E.J. *The Artificial Paradises in French Literature.* Chapel Hill: University of North Carolina Press, 1969.

4. Baudelaire, C.P. *Artificial Paradises; on Hashish and Wine as Means of Expanding Individuality.* Translated by Ellen Fox. New York: Herder & Herder, 1971.

5. Musto, D.F. *The American Disease: Origins of Narcotic Control,* 3rd ed. New York: Oxford, 1999, p. 221.

6. *Taxation of Marihuana, Hearings before the Committee on Ways and Means, House of Representatives, Seventy-fifth Congress, First Session, on HR 6385, April 27–30 and May 4, 1937.* Washington, DC: U.S. Government Printing Office.

7. Parry, A. "The Menace of Marihuana." *American Mercury* 36 (1935), pp. 487–88.

8. "Marihuana Menaces Youth." *Scientific American* 154 (1936), p. 151.

9. Wolf, W. "Uncle Sam Fights a New Drug Menace . . . Marijuana." *Popular Science Monthly* 128 (1936), p. 14.

10. Anslinger, H.J., & C.R. Cooper. "Marijuana: Assassin of Youth." *The American Magazine* 124 (1937), pp. 19, 153.

11. "Facts and Fancies about Marihuana." *Literary Digest* 122 (1936), pp. 7–8.

12. Whitlock, L. "Review: Marijuana." *Crime and Delinquency Literature* 2, no. 3 (1970), p. 367.

13. Fort, J. "Pot: A Rational Approach." *Playboy,* October 1969, pp. 131, 154.

14. "The Marihuana Bugaboo." *Military Surgeon* 93 (1943), p. 95.

15. "Mayor LaGuardia's Committee on Marijuana." In D. Solomon, editor. *The Marihuana Papers.* New York: New American Library, 1966.

16. "Marijuana Problems." *JAMA* 127 (1945), p. 1129.

17. DiMarzo, V., and others. "Formation and Inactivation of Endogenous Cannabinoid Anandamide in Central Neurons." *Nature* 372 (1994), p. 686.

18. Sim, L.I., and others. "Differences in G-protein Activation by Mu- and Delta-opioid, and Cannabinoid, Receptors in Rat Striatum." *European Journal of Pharmacology* 307 (1996), pp. 97–105.

19. Fogoros, R.N. "Rimonabant Still Impressive, But . . . ." *About Heart Disease,* November 16, 2004. Retrieved from http://heartdisease.about.com/od/dietandobesity/a/rimonabant5.htm.

20. Hart, C.L., and others. "Effects of Acute Smoked Marijuana on Complex Cognitive Performance." *Neuropsychopharmacology* 25 (2001), pp. 757–65.

21. Hart, C.L., and others. "Reinforcing effects of oral Δ^9-THC in male marijuanna smokers in a laboratory choice procedure." *Psychopharmacology,* 181 (2005) pp. 237–243.

22. Jones, R.T. "Cardiovascular System Effects of Marijuana." *Journal of Clinical Pharmacology* 42, no. 11 (2002), pp. 585–635.

23. Anthony, J.C., & J. Helzer. "Epidemiology of Drug Dependence." In M.T. Tsuang and others, eds. *Textbook in Psychiatric Epidemiology.* New York: John Wiley & Sons, 1995, pp. 361–406.

24. Substance Abuse and Mental Health Services Administration. *Overview of Findings from the 2002 National Survey on Drug Use and Health.* (NHSDA Series H-21, DHS Publication No. SMA 03-3774.) Rockville, MD: Office of Applied Studies, 2003.

25. Justinova, Z., and others. "Self-Administration of Delta9-tetrahydrocannabinol (THC) by Drug Naive Squirrel Monkeys." *Psychopharmacology* 169 (2003), pp. 135–40.

26. Kelly, T.H., and others. "Effects of D^9-THC on Marijuana Smoking, Dose Choice, and Verbal Report of Drug Liking." *Journal of the Experimental Analysis of Behavior* 61 (1994), pp. 203–11.

27. Becker, H.S. "Becoming a Marijuana User." *American Journal of Sociology* 59 (1953), pp. 235–43.

28. Ward, A.S., and others. "The Effects of a Monetary Alternative on Marijuana Self-administration." *Behavioural Pharmacology* 8 (1997), pp. 275–86.

29. Pope, H.G., and others. "Neuropsychological Performance in Long-Term Cannabis Users." *Archives of General Psychiatry* 58 (2001), pp. 909–15.

30. Foltin, R.W., & M.W. Fischman. "Effects of Smoked Marijuana on Human Social Behavior in Small Groups." *Pharmacology, Biochemistry, and Behavior* 30 (1988), pp. 539–41.

31. O'Shaughnessy, W.B. "On the Preparations of the Indian Hemp, or Gunja." *Transactions of the Physical and Medical Society of Bengal,* 1838–1840, pp. 71–102, 1842, pp. 421–61.

32. Mikuriya, T.H. "Marijuana in Medicine: Past, Present and Future." *California Medicine* 110 (1969), pp. 34–40.

33. *Standardization of Drug Extracts,* promotional brochure. Detroit: Parke, Davis & Co., 1898.

34. Letter to EP Delabarre, 9 Arlington Ave., Providence, RI, from Parke, Davis & Co., Manufacturing Department, Main Laboratories, Detroit, Superintendent's Office, Control Department, March 10, 1902.

35. Davis, J.P., & H.H. Ramsey. "Antiepileptic Action of Marihuana-active Substances." *Federation Proceedings* 8 (1949), pp. 284–85.

36. Ramaekers, J.G., and others. "Dose-related Risk of Motor Vehicle Crashes after Cannabis Use." *Drug and Alcohol Dependence* 73 (2004), pp. 109–19.

37. "Medical Therapy, Legalization Issues Debated at Marijuana Reform Conference." *National Drug Reporter* 7, no. 1 (1977), pp. 3–5.

38. Institute of Medicine, National Academy of Sciences. *Marijuana and Health.* Washington, DC: National Academy Press, 1982.

39. Nahas, G.G. "The Medical Use of Cannabis." In G.G. Nahas, ed. *Marijuana in Science and Medicine.* New York: Raven Press, 1984.

40. Conlan, M.F. "Top Drug Cop Weighs Use of Marijuana as an Rx Drug." *Drug Topics,* December 12, 1988.

41. Karel, R. "Hopes of Many Long-Term Sufferers Dashed as FDA Ends Medical Marijuana Program." *Psychiatric News,* May 1, 1992.

42. Budney, A.J., and others. "Marijuana Abstinence Effects in Marijuana Smokers Maintained in Their Home Environment." *Archives of General Psychiatry* 58 (2001), pp. 917–24.

43. Haney, M., and others. "Abstinence Symptoms Following Oral THC Administration to Humans." *Psychopharmacology* 141 (1999), pp. 385–94.

44. Kouri, E.M., and others. "Changes in Aggressive Behavior During Withdrawal from Long-term Marijuana Use." *Psychopharmacology* 43 (1999), pp. 302–08.

45. Tashkin, D.P. "Airway Effects of Marijuana, Cocaine and Other Inhaled Illicit Agents." *Current Opinion in Pulmonary Medicine* 7 (2001), pp. 43–61.

46. Schuel, H., and others. "Evidence That Anandamide-signalling Regulates Human Sperm Functions Required for Fertilization." *Molecular Reproduction and Development* 63 (2002), pp. 376–87.

47. Shay, A.H., and others. "Impairment of Antimicrobial Activity and Nitric Oxide Production in Alveolar Macrophages from Smokers of Marijuana and Cocaine." *Journal of Infectious Diseases* 187 (2003), pp. 700–04.

48. Sidney, S., J.E. Beck, G.D. Friedman. "Marijuana Use and Mortality." *American Journal of Public Health* 87 (1997), pp. 585–90.

49. Smith, D.E., R.B. Seymour. "Clinical Perspectives on the Toxicology of Marijuana: 1967–1981." In *Marijuana and Youth: Clinical Observations on Motivation and Learning.* Washington, DC: U.S. Department of Health and Human Services, U.S. Government Printing Office, 1982.

50. Hampson, A.J., and others. "Neuroprotective Antioxidants from Marijuana." *Annals of the New York Academy of Sciences* 899 (2000), pp. 274–82.

51. Johnston, L.D., P.M. O'Malley, J.G. Bachman, and J.E. Schulenberg. "Monitoring the Future national results on adolescent drug use: Overview of Key Findings, 2005. (NIH Publication No. 06-5882). Bethesda, MD: National Institute on Drug Abuse, 2006.

52. Aldrich, M.R., & T. Mikuriya. "Savings in California Marijuana Law Enforcement Costs Attributable to the Moscone Act of 1976—a Summary." *Journal of Psychoactive Drugs* 20 (1988), pp. 75–81.

53. Drug Enforcement Administration, *1987 Domestic Cannabis Eradication/Suppression Program Final Report.* Washington, DC: US Department of Justice, 1987.

Check Yourself

Short-term Memory

One of the most consistent findings about the effects of marijuana is that it impairs short-term memory. To learn more about short-term memory and get an idea of the types of tests that are used to measure it, go to the following Web site, which has an interactive test for short-term memory: faculty.washington.edu/chudler/stm0.html. You can use this chart to record your responses.

Trial #	The letters I remember are
1	
2	
3	
4	
5	
6	

16 Performance-Enhancing Drugs

Objectives

When you have finished this chapter, you should be able to:

- **Relate historical uses of performance-enhancing drugs by athletes.**

- **Describe the history of use of stimulants to enhance performance.**

- **Describe the development and current state of drug testing in sports.**

- **Explain why the BALCO scandal received so much publicity.**

- **Describe the performance-enhancing effects and primary dangers of stimulant drugs.**

- **Distinguish between androgenic and anabolic effects of testosterone and other related steroid hormones.**

- **Describe the desired effects and undesirable side-effects of steroids in men, women, and adolescents.**

- **Explain the effects of human growth hormone as well as its dangers.**

- **Explain the effects of creatine.**

- **Discuss the usefulness of dietary supplements in relation to their label claims.**

Why is there so much concern over drug use by athletes? Why not focus on drug use by clarinet players or muffler repair people? There are several answers to this question, and together they demonstrate the special reasons to be concerned about drug use in sport. First, well-known athletes are seen as role models for young people, portraying youth, strength, and health. When a famous athlete is reported to be using steroids or some other illicit substance, there is concern that impressionable young people will see drug use in a more positive light. Corporate sponsors pay these athletes to endorse their products, from shoes to breakfast cereal, based on this presumed influence over young consumers.

Second, some of the drugs used by athletes are intended to give the user an advantage over the competition, an advantage that is clearly viewed as being unfair. This is inconsistent with our tradition of fair play in sports, and widespread cheating of any kind tends to diminish a sport and public interest in it. Professional wrestling, which is widely viewed as being rigged or staged, is enjoyed more as a form of comic entertainment than as an athletic contest. Most professional and amateur athletes guard their honor carefully, and the use of performance-enhancing drugs is seen as a threat to that honor.

Online Learning Center Resources

www.mhhe.com/ksir12e

Visit our Online Learning Center (OLC) for access to these study aids and additional resources.

- Learning objectives
- Glossary flashcards
- Web activities and links
- Self-scoring chapter quiz
- Audio chapter summaries

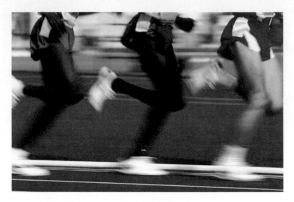

One of the major concerns over the use of performance-enhancing drugs is that they violate the tradition of fair play in sports.

Third, there is a concern that both the famous and the not-so-famous athletes who use drugs are endangering their health and perhaps their lives for the sake of a temporary burst of power or speed. Athletes should be aware of the risks associated with the use of these drugs. Because these drugs are often obtained illicitly, we can assume that the providers of the drugs do not present a balanced cost/benefit analysis to the potential user but, instead, probably maximize any possible benefit and minimize the dangers.

Historical Use of Drugs in Athletics

Ancient Times

Although we tend to think of drug use by athletes as a recent phenomenon, the use of chemicals to enhance performance might be as old as sport itself. As with many early drugs, some of these concoctions seemed to make sense at the time but probably had only placebo value. We no longer think that the powdered hooves of an ass will make our feet fly as fast as that animal's, but perhaps it was a belief in that powder that helped the ancient Egyptian competitor's self-confidence. Also, if all the others are using it, why take chances?

The early Greek Olympians used various herbs and mushrooms that might have had some pharmacological actions as stimulants,

and Aztec athletes used a cactus-based stimulant resembling strychnine. Athletic competitions probably developed in tribal societies as a means of training and preparing for war or for hunting, and various psychoactive plants were used by tribal peoples during battles and hunts, so it is not surprising that the drugs were also used in athletic contests from the beginning.

Early Use of Stimulants

During the 1800s and early 1900s, three types of stimulants were reported to be in use by athletes. *Strychnine,* which became famous as a rat poison, can at low doses act as a central nervous system stimulant. However, if the dose is too high, seizure activity will be produced in the brain. The resulting convulsions can paralyze respiration, leading to death. At least some boxers were reported to have used strychnine tablets. This might have made them more aggressive and kept them from tiring very quickly, but it was a dangerous way to do it. We'll never know how many of those rugged heroes were killed in this way, but there must have been a few. Thomas Hicks won the marathon in the 1904 St. Louis Olympics, then collapsed and had to be revived. His race was partly fueled by a mixture of brandy and strychnine.[1] Although the availability of amphetamines later made highly dangerous drugs such as strychnine less

Drugs in the Media

Banned Substances and How to Avoid Them

Television and other news from the 2004 Olympic Games in Athens, Greece, reported several instances of athletes being disqualified for using banned substances. In some cases, the disqualification was not contested, but in others the athletes thought they had been disqualified unfairly because they had taken something prescribed for them or something that they were not aware had been banned. The following list, from an article in *Technique* magazine by Jack Swarbick, lawyer for USA Gymnastics, includes tips for athletes on how to avoid the problem. Even if you aren't an Olympic competitor, these tips should give you an idea of how complex and difficult this problem can be.

1. Be familiar with the banned substances list of the governing body (International Olympic Committee or NCAA). This means knowing not only what drugs are on the list but also the types of medications or even foods in which those drugs are often found.
2. Make certain that others who ought to know, such as the athlete's parents, physician, and school nurse, are also familiar with the banned substances list.
3. Know what medications you are using. Athletes should consult with the governing body regarding the potential for any medications to contain elements of banned substances and should be

careful to list all medications when completing the screening form as part of the drug-testing program.
4. At competitions, drink only out of containers that were sealed when you got them, and once you have begun drinking out of a container do not leave it unattended. Several sports have implemented fairly rigorous security measures for the handling of coolers and water bottles.
5. When you are required to produce a urine sample as part of the drug-testing procedures, never surrender possession of the sample or leave it unattended until after you have sealed it inside the shipping canister provided by the officials.
6. If there are any irregularities in the process by which you give a urine sample and place that sample in the sealed container (e.g., a cracked beaker, a spilled sample, or unauthorized individuals on-site), immediately bring those irregularities to the attention of the drug-control administrator on-site.
7. If you are informed that you have tested positive for a banned substance (and you dispute that result), you will be invited to witness the testing of the second half (i.e., the "B sample") of your urine sample. Attend the test of the B sample, take with you an individual qualified to evaluate the process, and consider videotaping the test.

attractive, some evidence indicates the occasional use of strychnine continued at the level of world competition into the 1960s.

Cocaine was also available in the 1800s, at first in the form of Mariani's Coca Wine (used by the French cycling team), which was referred to in some advertisements as "wine for athletes."[2] When pure cocaine became available, athletes quickly adopted this more potent form. Many athletes used coffee as a mild stimulant, and some added pure *caffeine* to their coffee or took caffeine tablets. There were numerous reports of the suspected doping of swimmers, cyclists, boxers, runners,

and other athletes during this period. Then, as now, some of the suspicions were raised by the losers, who might or might not have had any evidence of doping. Our use of the word *dope* for illicit drugs is derived from a Dutch word used in South Africa to refer to a cheap brandy, which was sometimes given to racing dogs or horses to slow them down. From this came the term for doping horses and then people, more often in an effort to improve rather than impair performance. Dogs and horses received all the substances used by humans, including coca wine and cocaine, before the days of testing for drugs.

Amphetamines

It isn't clear when athletes first started using amphetamines for their stimulant effects, but it was probably not long after the drugs were introduced in the 1930s. Amphetamines were widely used throughout the world during World War II, and in the 1940s and 1950s there were reports of the use of these pep pills by professional soccer players in England and Italy. Boxers and cyclists also relied on this new synthetic energy source. More potent than caffeine, longer-lasting than cocaine, and safer than strychnine, it seemed for a while to be the ideal **ergogenic** (energy-producing) drug for both training and competition.

In 1952, the presence of syringes and broken ampules in the speed-skating locker room at the Oslo Winter Olympics was an indication of amphetamines' presence in international competition. There were other reports from the 1952 summer games in Helsinki and the 1956 Melbourne Olympics. Several deaths during this period were attributed to overdoses of amphetamines or other drugs. By the time of the 1960 Rome games, amphetamine use had spread around the world and to most sports. On opening day a Danish cyclist died during time trials. An autopsy revealed that his death resulting from "sunstroke" was aided by the presence of amphetamines, which reduce blood flow to the skin, making it more difficult for the body to cool itself. Three other cyclists collapsed that day, and two were hospitalized.[1] This and other examples of amphetamine abuse led to investigations and to antidoping laws in France and Belgium. Other nations, including the United States, seemed less concerned.

International Drug Testing

Some sports, especially cycling, began to test competitors for drugs on a sporadic basis. Throughout the 1960s, some athletes refused to submit to tests or failed tests and were disqualified. These early testing efforts were not enough to prevent the death of cyclist Tommy Simpson, an ex-world champion, who died during the 1967 *Tour de France*. His death was seen on television, and weeks later it was reported that his body contained two types of amphetamines and that drugs had been found in his luggage. This caused the International Olympic Committee in 1968 to establish rules requiring the disqualification of any competitor who refuses to take a drug test or who is found guilty of using banned drugs. Beginning with fewer than 700 urine tests at the 1968 Mexico City Olympics, each subsequent international competition has had more testing, more disqualifications, and more controversy.

American Football

Most Americans did not seem to be very concerned about drug use by athletes until reports surfaced in the late 1960s and early 1970s that professional football players were using amphetamines during games. Before that, people might not have been very concerned about it even if they had known. Remember from Chapter 6 that the amphetamines underwent a major status change in the United States during the 1960s. For years an increasing number of Americans had used amphetamines to keep them awake, to provide extra energy, or to lose weight. They were seen by most people as legal, harmless pep pills. It was in that context that the physicians for professional football teams ordered large quantities of the drugs as a routine part of their supplies, and trainers dispensed them liberally.

At the end of the 1960s, amphetamines were widely considered to be drugs of abuse, dangerous drugs that could lead to violent behavior. In this context, revelations that many professionals were playing high made for sensational headlines. Several National Football League (NFL) players sued their teams for injuries received while playing under the influence of drugs, and the NFL officially banned the distribution of amphetamines by team physicians and trainers in 1971. Although the drugs were no longer condoned by the league, the NFL did little at that time to enforce the

Mind/Body Connection

Promoting Overall Fitness

A sharp rise in the use of illegal anabolic steroids by teenage girls, which some attribute to "reverse anorexia," has health authorities worried. This new interest in steroids among girls, experts say, reflects their desire to excel in high school sports, as well as a gradual change in fashion, attitude, and peer pressure away from a preoccupation with thinness. The desired style is to look more healthy and somewhat muscular, leading some girls to a compulsion for fitness and larger muscles. In pursuit of sports stardom or the perfect body, they expose themselves to the same severe health risks as boys taking steroids, but with the added complications of unwanted masculinizing effects.[3]

Young girls are not the only ones who may succumb to an "addiction to the mirror." Researchers at Harvard Medical School's McLean Hospital recently completed a study of 32 women bodybuilders, 17 of whom showed signs of an emotional disorder called "body dysmorphism," or the excessive preoccupation with a trait or traits of the body viewed as defective or ugly, whether they are or not. The researchers found that several of the women studied were so dependent on working out that they cut off close personal relationships and job opportunities to do so.[3]

Although these cases take building a better body to an unhealthy extreme, most of us would agree that overall body fitness helps us feel better, mentally and physically. Even a modest increase in our daily activity level can be rewarding, reducing stress, decreasing susceptibility to illness, and providing more energy to keep up the pace of school, family activities, and work. And an increase in physical well-being often goes hand in hand with the emotional benefits of good health.

How can we increase self-esteem in young athletes and educate them about the long-term benefits of avoiding steroid use? Unless young people are taught to know that it's not right to try to win at all costs or to try to look good at all costs, they won't listen when they hear that steroids put their lives at risk. A program called Atlas, supported by the National Institute on Drug Abuse, is aimed at reducing steroid use among young male athletes by getting them to teach one another about the problems. After the program was instituted at 31 high schools in Oregon and Washington—involving 3,200 male athletes—the number of male students who reported having used steroids within the past year was cut by 50 percent. A similar program for girls is under development.[3]

An additional deterrent is for role models to take a public stance against steroid use, as was done in the campaign kicked off by a group of former Olympians from a variety of sports. Gold medal winners Jim Ryan, Edwin Moses, Frank Shorter, Donna de Varona, John Nabor, and Bruce Baumgartner have made the point that it's possible to achieve athletic success through hard work, personal sacrifice, and determination.

---

ban, except to request copies of each team's orders for medical supplies. Athletes who wanted amphetamines still obtained and used them, often through a legal prescription from their own physicians. The attitude seemed to be that, if the players wanted to use pep pills and obtained them on their own, that was their business, but team physicians and trainers shouldn't be using medications to push the athletes beyond their normal endurance. The current NFL policy, of course, restricts all use of amphetamines, as well as many other drugs, no matter where they are obtained.

Steroids

During and after World War II, it was found that malnourished people could gain weight and build themselves up more rapidly if they were given the male hormone testosterone. The Soviets were the first to put this hormone to use on a wide scale to build up their athletes. An American team physician at the 1956

> **ergogenic (er go *gen* ic):** producing work or energy; a general term for performance enhancement.

Olympics reported that the Soviet athletes were using straight testosterone, sometimes in excessive doses and with unfortunate side effects. Testosterone helps both men and women become more muscular, but its masculinizing effects on women and enlargement of the prostate gland in men are definite drawbacks. The American physician at the 1956 Olympics returned to the United States and helped develop and test **anabolic** steroids, which were quickly adopted by American weight lifters and bodybuilders.[4]

American and British athletes in events such as discus and shotput were the first to acknowledge publicly that they had used steroids, and there was evidence that steroid use was widespread during the 1960s in most track and field events. These drugs were not officially banned, nor were they tested for in international competition until the early 1970s, mainly because a sensitive urine test was not available until then. Of the 2,000 urine samples taken during the 1976 Olympics, fewer than 300 were tested for the presence of steroids, and 8 of those were positive.[1] The first international athletes to be found guilty of taking steroids were a Bulgarian discus thrower, a Romanian shotputter, a Polish discus thrower, and weight lifters from several countries. By that time, individual Western athletes might have chosen to use steroids, but some of the Eastern European countries seemed to have adopted their use almost as a matter of official policy. When the East German swimming coach was asked during the 1976 Olympics why so many of their women swimmers had deep voices, the answer was, "We have come here to swim, not sing."[5]

The BALCO Scandal

For years, rumors had circulated around professional baseball that certain players were using steroids, but Major League Baseball did not test for them. When Barry Bonds came into the 2001 season looking bigger and stronger, and went on to hit a record 79 home runs, some speculated that he might have used steroids, but the rumors were always denied. In 2002, former player Ken Caminiti admitted to using steroids and claimed that "half" the Major League players were doing so. Major League Baseball did institute a limited testing program that was generally considered to be too weak to have much effect.

In June 2003, an unidentified track coach delivered to the U.S. Anti-Doping Agency a syringe containing an "undetectable" steroid, naming the source as Victor Conte, founder of BALCO Laboratories. Analysis determined that the syringe contained tetrahydrogestrinone (THG), a steroid previously unknown to the agency that did not show up in agency tests. The BALCO investigation led to a raid on the laboratory and the discovery of other steroids and human-growth hormone.[6] Conte testified before a grand jury in San Francisco after being given immunity from prosecution and named a long list of Olympic and professional athletes who had been his clients, including Barry Bonds and many other professional baseball players. As of this writing, the fallout from all this is not clear, but President George W. Bush issued a statement in December 2004 stating that Major League Baseball and the players' union should take strong steps to clear up the problem of performance-enhancing drugs in baseball.

The Battle over Testing

During the 1980s, public revelations of drug use by athletes became common and cocaine was often mentioned. Professional basketball, baseball, and football players in the United States were being sent into treatment centers for cocaine dependence, and several either dropped out or were kicked out of professional sports. Most amateur and professional sports organizations adopted longer and more complicated lists of banned substances and rules providing for more and more participants to be tested. For example, in 1986, the National Collegiate Athletic Association (NCAA) adopted a list of more than 3,000 brand-name drugs containing banned substances. All participants are to be tested during the championship contest and after all postseason football games. In many events around the world, all contestants must now be subjected to urine tests as a matter of routine.

Because of both the expense and the inconvenience, some have questioned the wisdom of trying to test every athlete for everything. Despite the enormous expense to which sports organizations have gone, the use of steroids, stimulants, and other performance-enhancing substances seems to be as great as ever. Both the extent of testing and the ingenuity of athletes trying to beat the tests continue to escalate. The BALCO scandal demonstrates that chemists will keep coming up with new ways to help the athletes avoid detection.

Stimulants as Performance Enhancers

The first question to be answered about the use of a drug to increase energy or otherwise enhance athletic performance is, Does it work? We might not worry so much about unfair competition if we didn't feel that the use of a drug would really help the person using it. Also, if we could prove that these drugs were ineffective, then we could presumably convince young people not to take the risk of using drugs because there would be no gain to be had. But experiments can never prove that a drug has no effect—you might have done a hundred experiments and not used the right dose or the right test (peak output? endurance? accuracy?). The possibility always exists that someone will come along later with the right combination to demonstrate a beneficial effect. Therefore, be wary when someone tries to use scientific evidence to argue that a drug doesn't work, has no effect, is not toxic, or is otherwise inactive.

We've had a pretty good idea of the effectiveness of the amphetamines since 1959, when Smith and Beecher published the results

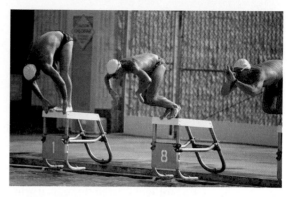

Stimulants have been shown to improve endurance.

of a double-blind study comparing amphetamines and placebos in runners, swimmers, and weight throwers.[7] They concluded that most of the athletes performed better under amphetamines, but the improvement was small (a few percentage points' improvement). Several studies have reported no differences or very small differences in performance, and some medical experts in the 1960s wanted to argue that amphetamines were essentially ineffective and there was no reason for people to use them. An excellent 1981 review of the existing literature put it all into perspective. Pointing out that it had been taking athletes an average of about seven years for each 1 percent improvement in the world record speed for the mile run, if amphetamines produced even a 1 percent improvement they could make an important difference at that level of competition. The study concluded that there is an amphetamine margin. It is usually small, amounting to a few percent under most circumstances. But even when that tiny, it can spell the difference between a gold medal and sixth place.[8]

Whether amphetamines or other stimulants increase physical ability (provide pep or energy) or produce their actions only through

anabolic (an a _ball_ ick): promoting constructive metabolism; building tissue.

effects on the brain is an interesting question, which might not be answerable. Surely a person who feels more confident will train harder, compete with a winning attitude, try harder, and keep trying longer. With amphetamines, improvements have been seen both in events requiring brief, explosive power (shotput) and in events requiring endurance, such as distance running. In laboratory studies, increases have been found in isometric strength and in work output during endurance testing on a stationary bicycle (the subjects rode longer under amphetamine conditions). This endurance improvement could be due to the masking of fatigue effects, allowing a person to compete to utter exhaustion.

Caffeine has also been shown to improve endurance performance under laboratory conditions. In one experiment, 330 mg of caffeine (approximately equivalent to three cups of brewed coffee) increased the length of a stationary bicycle ride by almost 20 percent. In another experiment, when subjects rode for two hours, their total energy output was 7 percent higher after 500 mg caffeine than in the control condition.[9] The effectiveness of caffeine might depend on other factors: For example, one study reported no benefit from caffeine when athletes ran long distances (12 miles) in hot, humid conditions.[10] Small amounts of caffeine are acceptable in most sports, but a urine level above 12 micrograms/mL will lead to disqualification in many competitions. The doses needed to produce large performance increases produce much higher levels than that, but there could still be a slight improvement even at legal levels.

Apparently no controlled laboratory or field experiments have tested the performance-enhancing capabilities of cocaine, but especially during the 1980s many athletes believed in its power. Cocaine's stimulant properties are generally similar to those of the amphetamines, so we can assume that cocaine would be effective under some circumstances. Given cocaine's shorter duration of action, it would not be expected to improve endurance over a several-hour period as well as either amphetamines or caffeine.

For years, athletes had another readily available stimulant in the form of ephedrine, either as a drug or in the form of ephedra extract. Ephedra (ma huang) was introduced in Chapter 6 as the herbal source of ephedrine, and it was the ephedrine molecule that was modified in the 1920s to produce amphetamine. When Olympic and NCAA officials developed lists of banned substances, ephedrine soon made its way onto the lists (except for people whose physicians said they suffered from asthma—ephedrine relaxes bronchial passages and is an ingredient in asthma medications). Professional sports organizations were at first less concerned about ephedrine, but eventually the National Football League also banned it. Major League Baseball did not, and baseball players used it to provide extra energy, or in some cases to reduce weight, since ephedra was also found in many weight-control dietary supplements (Chapter 12). In 2003, Baltimore Orioles pitcher Steve Bechler died after collapsing during practice—his temperature rose to 108 degrees in the hospital before his death, which was attributed to heat stroke due to the ingestion of "significant amounts" of ephedrine from a dietary supplement.[11] This widely publicized death finally gave the FDA enough political backing to go along with the years of evidence it had been accumulating, leading to the 2004 ban on ephedra and ephedrine in dietary supplements.

With all these and several other CNS stimulants banned by most sports associations, some athletes have continued to use them during training, to allow them to run, ride, or swim harder. They then do not use the drug for several days before the competition or during the competition, hoping that traces of the substance will not appear in the urine test. This might make sense, but no one knows whether training under one drug condition has an effect on competition under another condition. Also, overexertion under the influence of a fatigue-masking drug might be most dangerous during training, leading to muscle injury, a fall or another accident, or heat exhaustion.

Athletes and others who use amphetamines or cocaine regularly run the risk of developing a dependence on the drug, developing paranoid or violent behavior patterns, and suffering from the loss of energy and psychological depression that occur as the drugs wear off (see Chapter 6).

Steroids

The male sex hormone testosterone has two major types of effects on the developing man. **Androgenic** effects are masculinizing actions: Initial growth of the penis and other male sex glands, deepening of the voice, and increased facial hair are examples. This steroid hormone also has anabolic effects. These include increased muscle mass, increases in the size of various internal organs, control of the distribution of body fat, increased protein synthesis, and increased calcium in the bones. In the 1950s, drug companies began to synthesize various steroids that have fewer of the androgenic effects and more of the anabolic effects than testosterone. These are referred to as *anabolic steroids,* although none of them is entirely free of some masculinizing effect.

Whether or not these drugs are effective in improving athletic performance has been controversial: For many years the medical position was that they were not, whereas the lore around the locker room was that they would make anyone bigger, stronger, and more masculine-looking. A lot of people must have had more faith in the locker-room lore than in the official word. The 1989 *Physician's Desk Reference* contained the following statement in boldface type: **"Anabolic Steroids Have Not Been Shown to Enhance Athletic Ability."** Try telling that to any current major league baseball player, sports writer, or fan. That disclaimer is no longer required by the FDA.

There is no doubt that testosterone has a tremendous effect on muscle mass and strength during puberty, and experiments on castrated animals clearly show the muscle-developing ability of the synthetic anabolics.[12] What is not

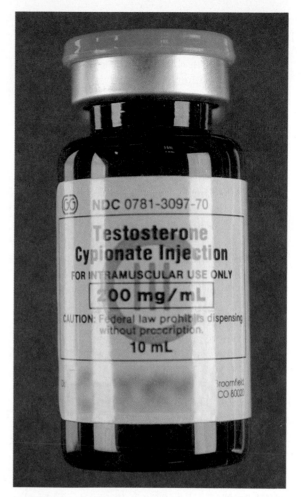

Testosterone, a male sex hormone, is sometimes abused by athletes for its protein-building (anabolic) effect.

so clear is the effect of adding additional anabolic stimulation to adolescent or adult males who already have normal circulating levels of testosterone.

Laboratory research on healthy men who are engaged in weight training and are maintained on a proper diet has often found that anabolic steroids produce small increases in lean muscle

androgenic (an drow *gen* ick): masculinizing.

mass and sometimes small increases in muscular strength. There is no evidence for an overall increase in aerobic capacity or endurance in those studies. However, it might never be possible to conduct experiments demonstrating the effectiveness of the high doses used by some athletes. Many athletes report that they take 10 or more times the dose of a steroid that has been tested and recommended for treatment of a deficiency disorder.[13] It is also common for athletes to take more than one steroid at a time (both an oral and an injectable form, for example). This practice is known as "stacking." To expose research subjects to such massive doses would clearly be unethical.

Another impediment to doing careful research on this topic is that these steroids produce detectable psychological effects. When double-blind experiments have been attempted, almost always the subjects have known when they were on steroids, thus destroying the blind control.[14] This is important because steroid users report that they feel they can lift more or work harder when they are on the steroids. This may be due to CNS effects of the steroids leading to a stimulant-like feeling of energy and loss of fatigue or to increased aggressiveness expressed as more aggressive training. There is a further possibility of what is known as an *active placebo effect,* with a belief in the power of steroids, enhanced by the clear sensation that the drug is doing something because one can "feel" it. Until recently, many of the scientists studying steroid hormones believed that their main effects were psychological, combined with a "bloating" effect on the muscle, in which the muscle retains more fluids, is larger, weighs more, but has no more physical strength.[1]

Psychological Effects of Steroids

The reported psychological effects of steroids, including a stimulant-like high and increased aggressiveness, might be beneficial for increasing the amount of work done during training and for increasing the intensity of effort during competition. However, there are also concerns that these psychological effects might produce great problems, especially at high doses. One concern is that a psychological dependence seems to develop in some users, who feel great when they are on the steroids but become depressed when they are off them. Many users take the drugs in cycles, and their mood swings can interfere with their social relationships and other life functions.

There has been a great deal of discussion about "roid rage," a kind of manic rage that has been reported by some steroid users.[15] We should be careful about attributing instances of violence to a drug on the basis of uncontrolled retrospective reports, especially when the perpetrator of a violent crime might be looking for an excuse.[16] However, there are a sufficient number of reports of violent feelings and actions among steroid users for us to be concerned and to await further research. Says Dr. William Taylor, a leading authority on anabolic steroids, "I've seen total personality changes. A passive, low-key guy goes on steroids for muscle enhancement, and the next thing you know, he's being arrested for assault or disorderly conduct."[17]

Adverse Effects on the Body

There are many concerns about the effects of steroid use on the body. In young users who have not attained their full height, steroids can cause premature closing of the growth plates of the long bones, thus limiting their adult height. For all users the risk of peliosis hepatitis (bloody cysts in the liver) and the changes in blood lipids possibly leading to atherosclerosis, high blood pressure, and heart disease are potentially serious concerns. Acne and baldness are reported, as are atrophy of the testes and breast enlargement in men using anabolic steroids.

There are also considerations for women who use anabolic steroids. Because women usually have only trace amounts of testosterone produced by the adrenals, the addition of even relatively small doses of anabolic steroids can

Drugs in Depth

Nutritional Ergogenic Aids

If athletes can't get or refuse to use pharmacological aids in athletic competition, most believe that certain foods or nutritional supplements are a "natural" way to enhance their performance. Following is a very abbreviated description of a more complete review of this topic.[18]

Amino acids are the natural building blocks of the protein required to build muscle, and one certainly requires a basic minimum intake. There is some evidence that very active people can benefit from a somewhat increased intake of dietary protein, slightly above the recommended daily allowances, but there is no demonstrated need to purchase expensive amino acid supplements to achieve this. Marketers of these "muscle-building" dietary supplements walk a fine line by avoiding making specific claims on the product labels, so they do not fall under the FDA's rules for demonstrating effectiveness. Usually nearby posters or pamphlets link amino acids to the idea of muscle growth. These supplements are probably of little or no value to an athlete who is receiving proper nutrition.

Carbohydrates are burned as fuels, especially during prolonged aerobic exercise. Carbohydrates taken two to four hours before an endurance performance lasting for more than an hour may enhance the performance by maintaining blood glucose levels and preventing the depletion of muscle stores of glycogen. Carbohydrate loading before marathon runs consists of resting for the last day or two while ingesting extra carbohydrates, increasing both muscle and liver stores of carbohydrates. In either case, there is not much evidence to support the value of carbohydrate supplements for athletic performances lasting less than an hour.

Fats, in experiments with fat supplements, have not been found to be a useful ergogenic aid.

Vitamins, especially the water-soluble B vitamins, are necessary for normal utilization of food energy.

Deficiencies in these vitamins, such as might result when a wrestler is dieting to meet a weight limit, can clearly impair physical performance. However, once the necessary minimum amount is available for metabolic purposes, further supplements are of no value. Many experiments have been done with supplements of C, E, and B-complex vitamins or with multivitamin supplements, the so-called vitamin B_{15}, and with bee pollen, and there is no evidence for enhanced performance or faster recovery after workouts. Again, these supplements are probably of no value to an athlete who is receiving proper nutrition.

Minerals, in the form of various mineral supplements, are widely used by athletes. Once again, most are probably not needed or useful, but there may be some exceptions. Electrolyte drinks are designed to replace both fluids and electrolytes, such as sodium and chloride that are lost in sweat. Actually, sweat contains a lower concentration of these electrolytes than does blood, so it is more important to replace the fluids than the electrolytes under most circumstances. Sodium supplementation may be useful for those engaged in ultraendurance events, such as 100-mile runs.

Iron supplements are helpful in athletes who are iron-deficient, as may occur especially in female distance runners. However, if iron status is normal, there is probably no value in iron supplements.

The jury is still out on whether "buffering" the blood pH with sodium bicarbonate (baking soda) enhances performance in anaerobic events, such as 400- to 800-meter runs. Some studies indicate improvements, whereas others do not.

Water is needed by endurance athletes to keep their body temperatures down, especially in a warm environment. Drinking water both before and during prolonged exercise can deter dehydration and improve performance. Visit the Online Learning Center for links to more information on supplements.

have dramatic effects, in terms of both muscle growth and masculinization. Some of the side effects, such as mild acne, decreased breast size, and fluid retention, are reversible. The enlargement of the clitoris might be reversible if steroid use is stopped soon after it is noticed. Other effects, such as increased facial hair and deepening of the voice, might be irreversible.[14]

Taking Sides

Has Creatine Killed Wrestlers?

In 1997, three wrestlers died while in training, and traces of creatine were found in one of the young men. Sensational news articles followed, in which the death was linked to creatine use. However, a look at what this athlete had done might indicate a different explanation.[20] Jeff Reese, the 21-year-old wrestler who was found to have elevated levels of creatine in his blood, had worked out for two hours in a 92-degree gym wearing a rubber suit, in an attempt to lose 12 pounds in a single day. The other two wrestlers were undertaking similar extreme measures when they died, and there is no evidence they were using creatine. Clearly, we cannot say that creatine caused Reese's death. With thousands of creatine users, the risk of acute toxicity appears to be small. What we don't yet know is the effect of chronic use for months or years. Although creatine is considered a dietary supplement, it is being used in a druglike manner: a pure chemical taken in doses well above normal physiological ranges. No matter how safe creatine appears to be now, we should be cautious about long-term use until more is known.

For more on this topic, visit the Online Learning Center.

Regulation

As we found in Chapter 2, when a drug produces dependence, violent behavior, and toxic side effects, society may feel justified in trying to restrict the drug's availability. In 1988, congressional hearings were held on the notion of placing anabolic steroids on the list of controlled substances. Evidence was presented that a large black market had developed for these drugs, amounting to perhaps $100 million per year. In addition, there was concern that adolescent boys, many of whom were not athletic at all, had begun to use steroids in the belief that they would quickly become more muscular and "macho" looking. As part of the Omnibus Crime Control Act of 1990, anabolic steroids became listed as a Schedule III controlled substance, requiring more record-keeping and limited prescription refills.[19]

Other Hormonal Manipulations

Whereas the anabolic steroids have been in wide use, other treatments have been experimented with on a more limited basis. Female sex hormones have been used to feminize men, so that they could compete in women's events. The women's gold medal sprinter in the 1964 Olympics was shown by chromosome testing to have been a man, and he had to return the medal. Hormone receptor–blocking drugs have probably been used to delay puberty in female gymnasts. In women, puberty shifts the center of gravity lower in the body and changes body proportions in ways that adversely affect performance in some gymnastic events. Smaller women appear to be more graceful, spin faster on the uneven bars, and generally have the advantage, which is why top female gymnasts are usually in their teens. However, the Soviets were suspected of tampering with nature: Their top three international gymnasts in 1978 were all 17 or 18 years old, but the following were their heights and weights: 53 inches, 63 pounds; 60 inches, 90 pounds; and 57 inches, 79 pounds.

We have certainly not seen the end of growth-promoting hormonal treatments. **Human growth hormone,** which is released from the pituitary gland, can potentially increase the height and weight of an individual to gigantic proportions, especially if administered during childhood and adolescence. In rare instances, the excessive production of this hormone creates giants well over 7 feet tall. These giants usually die at an early age because their internal organs continue to grow. However, administration of a few doses of this hormone at the right time might produce a more controlled increase in body size. Likewise, the growth-hormone-releasing hormone, and some of the cellular intermediary hormones by which growth hormone exerts its effects, might work to enhance growth. It is not currently possible to test for the presence of these substances. Despite the possible dangers, the lure of an otherwise capable basketball player growing a couple of inches taller or of a football player being 30 pounds heavier has no doubt caused many young athletes to experiment with these substances. Experiments in which growth hormone was given to men found no increase in muscle protein synthesis or in strength.[21] The 1990 legislation that placed anabolic steroids on the list of controlled substances also made it a crime to distribute human growth hormone for nonmedical purposes.

Beta-2 Agonists

At the beginning of the 1992 Olympics, the leader of the British team was disqualified because of the detection of a new drug. Clenbuterol was developed as a treatment for asthma and is a relative of several other bronchodilators that are found in prescription inhalers. These drugs have sympathomimetic effects on the bronchi of the lungs but are designed to be more specific than older sympathomimetics, such as ephedrine or the amphetamines (see Chapter 6). Their specificity comes from a selective stimulation of the beta-2 subtype of adrenergic receptors. Research with cows had revealed an increase in muscle mass, and speculation was beginning that this might represent a new type of nonsteroidal anabolic agent. Apparently someone in Great Britain was keeping an eye on the animal research literature and decided to try the anabolic actions on at least one Olympic athlete. Presumably it was hoped that such a new drug would not be tested for, but the Olympic officials were also well informed and ready, at least for clenbuterol. More recent human studies have shown some increases in strength of selected muscle types with clenbuterol or a similar drug, but there is no evidence that beta-2 agonists improve athletic performance.[22]

Creatine

One widely used substance among bodybuilders has been creatine, a natural substance found in meat and fish. This legal product is sold as a food supplement. There is clear evidence that creatine helps regenerate ATP, which provides the energy for muscle contractions. Users of creatine tend to gain some weight, some of which is water weight. There is considerable evidence that the use of creatine can improve strength and short-term speed in sprinting. However, studies of longer-distance running, cycling, and swimming often find no effect, and in one case a significant slowing was reported, probably due to weight gain.[4]

Getting "Cut"

If getting "cut," "ripped," and "shredded" sounds like something you'd want to avoid, then you're probably not into bodybuilding. These terms refer to the appearance of someone who is both muscular and lean. Because amateur wrestlers compete in weight classes and they need to be strong, they have always had the problem of eating well to build strength and train hard, but then needing to "cut" weight before the weigh-ins for matches. Jockeys have had a similar problem. Over the years, some of these athletes have engaged in fairly extreme methods to achieve short-term weight reduction, such as purging, taking diuretic drugs to lose water weight, and exercising in a heated environment or wearing nonporous clothing to maximize sweating (see Taking Sides). The entire

human growth hormone: a pituitary hormone responsible for some types of giantism.

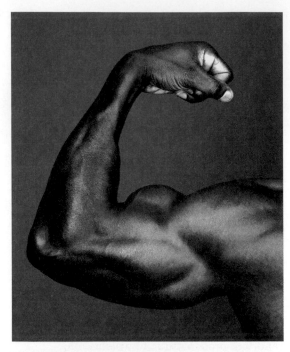

Bodybuilders and other athletes have used steroids or other supplements to develop a lean, strong, muscular body—to become "cut" or "ripped."

list of weight-control drugs mentioned in Chapters 6 and 12 have been used as well, ranging from amphetamine to ephedrine to caffeine.

Increasingly, bodybuilders are seeking the look of someone who is both strong and lean, with lots of muscle definition. That appearance is referred to as looking "cut," probably derived from the idea of cutting weight or cutting fat, but perhaps also carrying the connotation of "sculpted." A more extreme version of looking cut is looking "ripped," or sometimes "shredded." These are the men and women whose every muscle fiber and vein can be seen through the skin, perhaps with a body fat percentage down to an unhealthy 6 to 9 percent (14 to 20 percent is considered ideal for a healthy male). They also are using drugs and nutritional supplements to help achieve this appearance. Steroids increase muscle mass, but they don't produce this kind of lean definition. A brisk market has developed in dietary supplements

containing the word *ripped* in their name, such as "Ripped Fuel" and "Ripped Fast." For many years these products relied mainly on ephedra as the main active ingredient. Once ephedra was banned, these profitable products did not go away, they simply changed their formulas and kept making the same claims about being "fat burners" and promising incredible results. They contain a bewildering variety of plant extracts, many of which contain caffeine in unknown amounts (e.g., guarana extract, green tea extract, and coffee bean extract).

Remember that these dietary supplements do not have to be demonstrated to be effective, and the beneficial claims have not been evaluated by the FDA (or anyone else). If an included ingredient should turn out to be dangerous, it might take a long time for this to come to the attention of the FDA, and it would then take a long time for the agency to build a case to remove the ingredient from the market (it took 10 years for ephedra). No such product has ever been shown to actually be a "fat burner," so it's unlikely that these are either. If you buy them, the closest you'll get to being "ripped" as a result is probably feeling "ripped off" when the magic pill doesn't deliver what you hoped.

Summary

- Performance-enhancing drugs have been used by athletes throughout history.

- Athletic use of stimulants appears to have increased and spread to most sports with the use of amphetamines during the 1950s and 1960s.

- Amphetamines and caffeine have both been shown to increase work output and to mask the effects of fatigue.

- Some athletes continue to use stimulants for training, despite the dangers of injury and overexertion.

- Anabolic steroids are capable of increasing muscle mass and probably strength, although it has been difficult to separate the psychological stimulant-like effect of these drugs from the physical effects on the muscles themselves.

- Anabolic steroids can also produce a variety of dangerous and sometimes irreversible side effects.

- It is difficult to do ethical and well-controlled research on the effects of steroids.

- Misuse of human growth hormone and related substances might be the next problem to arise.

- Creatine is a legally available nutritional supplement that can increase strength but might slow distance runners because of resultant weight gain.

Review Questions

1. What was the first type of stimulant drug reported to be used by boxers and other athletes in the 1800s?
2. What was the first type of drug known to be widely used in international competition and that led to the first Olympic urine-testing programs?
3. When and in what country were the selective anabolic steroids first developed?
4. Do amphetamines and caffeine actually enhance athletic performance? If so, how much?
5. How was ephedrine used by athletes, and what happened to it?
6. What muscle effect do we know for certain that anabolic steroids can produce in healthy men?
7. What is meant by "roid rage," and what double-blind studies have been done on this phenomenon?
8. What specific effect of anabolic steroids might be of concern to young users? to females?
9. Why do "pituitary giants" often die at an early age?
10. How does creatine increase strength?

References

1. Donohue, T., & N. Johnson. *Foul Play: Drug Abuse in Sports.* Oxford, England: Basil Blackwell, 1986.
2. Asken, M.J. *Dying to Win: The Athlete's Guide to Safe and Unsafe Drugs in Sports.* Washington, DC: Acropolis, 1988.
3. Noble, H.B. "Steroid Use by Teen-age Girls Is Rising, *The New York Times,* June 1, 1999.
4. Eichner, E.R. "Ergogenic Aids: What Athletes Are Using—and Why." *Physician and Sportsmedicine* 25 (1997), pp. 70–83.
5. Goldman, B. *Death in the Locker Room.* South Bend, IN: Icarus Press, 1984.
6. Fainaru-Wada, M., & L. Williams. "Sports and Drugs: How the Doping Scandal Unfolded. Fallout from BALCO Probe Could Taint Olympics, Pro Sports." *San Francisco Chronicle,* December 21, 2003.
7. Smith, G.M., & H.K. Beecher. "Amphetamine Sulfate and Athletic Performance." *JAMA* 170 (1959), pp. 542–57.
8. Laties, V.G., & B. Weiss. "The Amphetamine Margin in Sports." *Federation Proceedings* 40 (1981), pp. 2689–92.
9. Noble, B.J. *Physiology of Exercise and Sport.* St Louis: Mosby, 1986.
10. Cohen, B.S., and others. "Effects of Caffeine Ingestion on Endurance Racing in Heat and Humidity." *European Journal of Applied Physiology* 73 (1996), pp. 358–63.
11. Bodley, H. "Medical Examiner: Ephedra a Factor in Bechler Death." *USA Today,* March 13, 2003.
12. Williams, M.H. *Ergogenic Aids in Sports.* Champaign, IL: Human Kinetics, 1983.
13. Marshall, E. "The Drug of Champions." *Science* 242 (1983), pp. 183–84.
14. Taylor, W.N. *Hormonal Manipulation: a New Era of Monstrous Athletes.* Jefferson, NC: McFarland & Co., 1985.
15. Pope, H.G., & D.L. Katz. "Affective and Psychotic Symptoms Associated with Anabolic Steroid Use." *American Journal of Psychiatry* 145 (1988), pp. 487–90.
16. Lubell, A. "Does Steroid Abuse Cause—or Excuse—Violence? *Physician and Sportsmedicine* 17 (1989), pp. 176–85.
17. Fultz, O. "'Roid Rage." *American Health* 10 (1991), p. 60.
18. Burke, L., and others. "Supplements and Sports Foods." *Clinical Sports Nutrition,* 3rd ed. Edited by L. Burke and V. Deakin. Sydney: McGraw-Hill, 2006, pp. 485–579. Available at http://www.ais.org.au/nutrition/documents/16Complete.pdf
19. Nightingale, S.L. "Anabolic Steroids as Controlled Substances." *JAMA* 265 (1991), p. 1229.
20. Persky, A.M., & G.A. Brazeau. Clinical Pharmacology of the Dietary Supplement Creatine Monohydrate." *Pharmacology Review* 53 (2001), p. 161.
21. Yarasheski, K.E., and others. "Short-term Growth Hormone Treatment Does Not Increase Muscle Protein Synthesis in Experienced Weight Lifters." *Journal of Applied Physiology* 74 (1993), pp. 3073–76.
22. Spann, S. "Effect of Clenbuterol on Athletic Performance." *Annals of Pharmacotherapy* 29 (1995), p. 75.

Check Yourself

How Would You Run the Race?

Imagine that you have gone out for the track team. You compete in the 3,000-meter races and have been training hard for the past two years. It seems as though you have worked as hard as you could every day, yet it's clear that your times have gotten as fast as they're going to get. The conference championships are tomorrow. Your parents have traveled 300 miles to see you run, and lots of your friends will be there, cheering you on. You know your own times, and you know the competition, and, although you expect a close race for the top three spots, you figure to come in fourth. You yourself have never used any type of stimulant drug, but you have heard rumors that several of the fastest runners take amphetamines before the race, and you suspect that it is true. Your conference has not yet adopted a drug-screening program for track, however, so there's no way to know for sure.

Under these circumstances, what would you do if

1. Someone you don't know very well but who you heard is a drug dealer offers you some "speed" just for the race?
2. A friend of yours has some prescription diet pills that contain amphetamines, and the friend offers you one?
3. You are offered some cocaine to snort right before the race?
4. You are offered an OTC asthma pill that contains ephedrine?
5. You are offered coffee or tea?

Or would you rather not take artificial stimulants at all, come in fourth, and know you did your best and ran a clean race?

Prevention and Treatment

This final section on prevention and treatment comes at the end of the book for a reason. Now that you're more familiar with the wide spectrum of substances that people can abuse, and also with the wide variety of forms of substance abuse and dependence, we are better able to talk about what we're trying to prevent, and what we're trying to treat. Because many of the medication-based treatments depend on specific interactions with the targeted substances of abuse, you now should understand how those medications have been developed and used.

17 Preventing Substance Abuse
What kinds of prevention programs have been tested in the schools, and which ones seem to be effective? What can parents and communities do?

18 Treating Substance Abuse and Dependence
What are the differences among the various approaches to treating alcoholism, opioid dependence, cocaine use, and others? How well do these programs work?

Preventing Substance Abuse

Objectives

After you have studied this chapter, you should be able to:

- **Distinguish between education and propaganda programs based on their goals and approaches.**

- **Describe two systems for classifying prevention programs: one based on stages of involvement, the other based on target populations defined by risk for drug use.**

- **Describe the historical shifts in substance abuse prevention programs from the knowledge-attitudes-behavior model to affective education to anti-drug norms.**

- **Explain how the social influence model for smoking prevention led to the development of DARE and similar programs.**

- **Describe the outcome of research on DARE's effectiveness and how DARE America has responded.**

- **List some examples of effective prevention programs that have been adopted as model programs by SAMHSA.**

- **Give some examples of peer, family, and community approaches to prevention.**

- **Describe the most consistent feature of workplace prevention programs.**

Why can't we *do* something to keep young people from ruining their lives with drugs? As our society seeks to prevent drug abuse by limiting the availability of such drugs as heroin and cocaine, we are forced to recognize several other facts. First, as long as there is a sizable market for these substances, there will be people to supply them. Thus, only if we can teach people not to want the drugs can we attack the source of the problem. Second, these substances will never disappear, so we should try to teach people to live in a world that includes them. Third, our society has accepted the continued existence of tobacco and alcohol, yet some people are harmed by them. Can we teach people to coexist with both legal and illegal substances and to live in such a way that their lives and health are not impaired by them?

Defining Goals and Evaluating Outcomes

Think about the process you are engaged in while reading and studying this book. The text is aimed at teaching its readers about drugs: their effects, how they are used, and how they

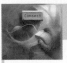

Online Learning Center Resources

www.mhhe.com/ksir12e

Visit our Online Learning Center (OLC) for access to these study aids and additional resources.

- Learning objectives
- Glossary flashcards
- Web activities and links
- Self-scoring chapter quiz
- Audio chapter summaries

relate to society. The goal of the authors is *education*. A person who understands all this information about all these drugs will perhaps be better prepared to make decisions about personal drug use, more able to understand drug use by others, and better prepared to participate in social decisions about drug use and abuse. We hope that a person who knew all this would be in a position to act more rationally, neither glorifying a drug and expecting miraculous changes from using it nor condemning it as the essence of evil. But our ultimate goal is not to change the readers' behavior in a particular direction. For example, the chapter on alcohol, although pointing out the dangers of its use and the problems it can cause, does not attempt to influence readers to avoid all alcohol use. The success of this book is measured by how much a person knows about alcohol, tobacco, or marijuana, not by whether he or she is convinced never to drink or smoke.

On the other hand, a tradition exists, going back to the "demon rum" programs of the late 1800s, of presenting negative information about alcohol and other drugs in the public schools with the clear goal of *prevention* of use. Some of these early programs presented information that was so clearly one-sided that they could have been classified as propaganda rather than education. We would not measure the success of such a program by how much objective information the students gained about the pharmacology of cocaine, for example. A more appropriate

index might be how many of the students did subsequently experiment with the drugs against which the program was aimed. Until the early 1970s, it was simply assumed that these programs would have the desired effect, and few attempts were made to evaluate them.

Types of Prevention

The goals and methods of a prevention program also depend on the drug-using status of those served by the program. The programs designed to prevent young people from starting smoking might be different from those used to try to prevent relapse in smokers who have quit, for example. Until recently, drug-abuse prevention programs have been classified according to a public health model:

- **Primary prevention** programs are those aimed mainly at young people who have not yet tried the substances in question or who may have tried tobacco or alcohol a few times. As discussed in the section "Defining Goals and Evaluating Outcomes," such programs might encourage abstinence from specific drugs or might have the broader goal of teaching people how to view drugs and the potential influences of drugs on their lives, emotions, and social relationships. Because those programs are presented to people with little personal experience with drugs, they might be expected to be especially effective. But, there is the danger of introducing large numbers of children to information about drugs that they might otherwise never have heard of, thus arousing their curiosity.

- **Secondary prevention** programs can be thought of as designed for people who have tried the drug in question or a variety of other substances. The goals of such programs are usually the prevention of the use of other, more dangerous substances and the prevention of the development of more dangerous forms of use of the substances they are already experimenting with. We

Drugs in the Media

Prime-Time Drug-Prevention Programming

In late 1997, the U.S. Congress approved the expenditure of $1 billion over a five-year period for anti-drug advertising on television networks. This was a lot of revenue for the networks, but the catch was that they had to broadcast the messages at half the normal market price. After industry protests, the White House Office of National Drug Control Policy struck deals to discharge networks from the half-cost advertising time requirements if they would incorporate drug-abuse prevention messages into the content of television shows. For example, the program *"E.R.,"* about a hospital emergency room, has included several episodes dramatizing the consequences of illicit drug use. The agreement was brought to light in early 2000 by the online newsmagazine salon.com, which raised concerns about hidden government "propaganda."

See if you can get a few people to keep an eye out for such integrated anti-drug content for one week. Did you find some obvious examples? Have you been aware of this type of integrated content before? What is the danger involved in having the federal government influence the content of television programming in this subtle way?

might describe the clientele here as more "sophisticated" substance users who have not suffered seriously from their drug experiences and who are not obvious candidates for treatment. Many college students fall into this category, and programs aimed at encouraging responsible use of alcohol among college students are good examples of this stage of prevention.

- **Tertiary prevention,** in our scheme, is relapse prevention, or follow-up programs. For alcoholics or cocaine or heroin addicts, treatment programs are the first order of priority. However, once a person has been treated or has stopped the substance use without assistance, we enter another stage of prevention.

The Institute of Medicine has proposed a new classification of the "continuum of care," which includes prevention, treatment, and maintenance.[1] Prevention efforts are categorized according to the intended target population, but the targets are not defined only by prior drug use:

- **Universal prevention** programs are designed for delivery to an entire population—for example, all schoolchildren or an entire community.

- **Selective prevention** strategies are designed for groups within the general population that are deemed to be at high risk—for example, students who are not doing well academically or the poorest neighborhoods in a community.

- **Indicated prevention** strategies are targeted at individuals who show signs of developing problems, such as a child who began smoking cigarettes at a young age or an adult arrested for a first offense of driving under the influence of alcohol.

Prevention Programs in the Schools

The Knowledge-Attitudes-Behavior Model

After the increase in the use of illicit drugs by young middle-class people in the 1960s, there was a general sense that society was not doing an adequate job of drug education, and most school systems increased their efforts. However, there was confusion over the methods to be used. Traditional anti-drug programs had relied heavily on representatives of the local police, who went into schools and told a few horror stories, describing the legal trouble due anyone who got caught with illicit drugs.

Targeting Prevention

Preventing Inhalant Abuse

The abuse by children of spray paints and other products containing solvents appears to have increased somewhat in recent years (see Chapter 7). Several characteristics of this type of abuse make it an interesting problem for prevention workers. First, the variety of available products and their ready availability in stores, the home, and even in schools make preventing access to the inhalants an impossibility. Second, most of the kids who use these substances probably know it's unhealthy and dangerous to do so, so further information of that sort may not add much in the way of preventing their use. Third, this use is very "faddish"—a group of eighth-graders in one school might start inhaling cleaning fluid; a group of sixth-graders in another neighborhood might be into gold paint (in distinct preference to black, yellow, or white).

Given these characteristics, where does a school-based prevention education program begin to attack the problem? Does it focus on a particular product and try to talk kids out of using gold paint? Does it talk about a whole variety of products and thereby perhaps introduce the kids to new things they hadn't thought of? One videotape (*Inhalants: Kids in Danger, Adults in the Dark*) took the approach of attempting to inform parents and teachers of the varieties of paints, perfumes, solvents, and other spray products used by abusers and to inform them of some of the subterfuges used by some of the kids (carrying a small cologne vial to school, spraying paint into empty soft drink cans, etc.). However, this video is *not* meant to be shown to children, because it describes exactly what to do and how to do it. Probably the best idea in prevention classes is to reinforce to children in general terms the dangers of inhalants without describing a particular substance or method of use.

Sometimes the officers showed what the drugs looked like or demonstrated the smell of burning marijuana, so that the kids would know what to avoid. Sometimes, especially in larger cities, a former user described how easy it was to get "hooked," the horrible life of the junkie, and the horror of withdrawal symptoms. The 1960s saw more of that, plus the production of a large number of scary anti-drug films.

Teachers and counselors knew little about these substances, and many teachers attended courses taught by experts. Some of the experts were enforcement-oriented and presented the traditional scare-tactics information, whereas others were pharmacologists who presented the "dry facts" about the classification and effects of various drugs. The teachers then brought many of these facts into their classrooms. It was later pointed out that the programs of this era were based on an assumed model: that providing information about drugs would increase the students' *knowledge* of drugs and their effects, that this increased knowledge would lead to changes in *attitudes* about drug use, and that these changed attitudes would be reflected in decreased drug-using *behavior*.[2]

In the early 1970s, this model began to be questioned. A 1971 study indicated that students who had more knowledge about drugs tended to have a more positive attitude toward drug use.[3] Of course, it may have been that pro-drug students were more interested in learning about drugs, so this was not an actual assessment of the value of drug education programs. A 1973 report by the same group indicated that four different types of drug education programs were equally effective in producing increased knowledge about drugs and equally ineffective in altering attitudes or behavior.[4] Nationwide, drug use had increased even with the greater emphasis on drug education. Concern arose about the possibility that drug education may even have contributed to increased drug use. Before the 1960s, the use of marijuana and LSD was rare among school-age youngsters. Most of them didn't know much about these things, had given them little thought, and had probably never considered using them. Telling them over and over not to use drugs was a bit like telling a young boy not to put beans in his nose. He probably hadn't thought of it before, and your warning gives him the idea. These concerns led the federal government in 1973 to stop supporting the production of drug-abuse films and educational materials until it could determine what kinds of approaches would be effective.

The question of effectiveness depended greatly on the goals of the program. Did we want all students *never to experiment* with cigarettes, alcohol, marijuana, or other drugs? Or did we want students to be prepared to *make rational decisions* about drugs? For example, a 1976 report indicated that students in drug education programs did increase their use of drugs over the two years after the program, but they were less likely to show drastic escalation of the amount or type of drug use over that period, when compared with a control group.[5] Perhaps by giving the students information about drugs, we make them more likely to try them, but we also make them more aware of the dangers of excessive use. For a time in the 1970s, it seemed as though teaching students to make rational decisions about their own drug use with the goal of reducing the overall harm produced by misuse and abuse could be a possible goal of prevention programs.

Affective Education

Educators have been talking for several years about education as including both a "cognitive domain" and an "*affective* domain," the domain of emotions and attitudes. One reason that young people might use psychoactive drugs is to produce certain feelings: of excitement, of relaxation, of power, of being in control. Or perhaps a child might not really want to take drugs but does so after being influenced by others. Helping children know their own feelings and express them, helping them achieve altered emotional states without drugs, and teaching

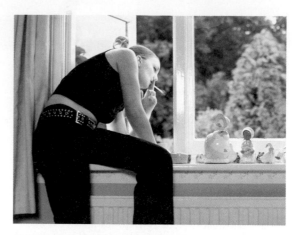

Helping young people learn to deal with emotions in healthy ways and giving them successful experiences may reduce their rates of smoking, drinking, and drug use.

them to feel valued, accepted, and wanted are all presumed to be ways of reducing drug use.

Values Clarification The values clarification approach makes the assumption that what is lacking in drug-using adolescents is not factual information about drugs but, rather, the ability to make appropriate decisions based on that information.[6] Perhaps drug use should not be "flagged" for the students by having special curricula designed just for drugs but, instead, emphasis should be placed on teaching generic decision-making skills. Teaching students to analyze and clarify their own values in life is accomplished by having them discuss their reactions to various situations that pose moral and ethical dilemmas. Groups of parents or other citizens who are concerned about drug abuse sometimes have great difficulty understanding and accepting these approaches because they do not take a direct anti-drug approach. In the 1970s, when these programs were developed, it seemed important that the schools not try to impose a particular set of values but, rather, allow for differences in religion, family background, and so on. For this reason, the programs were often said to be *value-free*. To many parents, the purpose of **values clarification** training is not

Table 17.1 Some Suggested Alternatives to Drug Use		
Level of Experience	**Motives**	**Possible Alternatives**
Physical	Relaxation	Relaxation exercises
	Increased energy	Athletics, dancing
Sensory	Stimulation Magnify senses	Skydiving Sensory awareness training
Interpersonal	Gain acceptance	Learn about social 'norms', finding a group that "fits"
Spiritual/ mystical	Develop spiritual insight	Meditation

immediately clear, and teaching young children to decide moral issues for themselves may run contrary to the particular set of values the parents want their children to learn.

Alternatives to Drugs Along with values clarification, another aspect of affective education involves the teaching of **alternatives** to drug use (Table 17.1). Under the assumption that students might take drugs for the experience, for the altered states of consciousness that a drug might produce, students are taught so-called natural highs, or altered states, that can be produced through relaxation exercises, meditation, vigorous exercise, or an exciting sport. Students are encouraged to try these things and to focus on the psychological changes that occur. These alternatives should be discussed with some degree of sensitivity to the audience; for example, it would make little sense to suggest to many inner-city 13-year-olds that expensive activities as scuba diving and snow skiing would be good alternatives to drugs.

Personal and Social Skills Several studies indicate that adolescents who smoke, drink, or use marijuana also get lower grades and are less involved in organized sports or school clubs. One view of this is that students might take up substance use in response to personal or social failure. Therefore, teaching students how to communicate with others and giving them success experiences is another component of affective education approaches. For example, one exercise that has been used is having the students operate a school store. This is done as a group effort with frequent group meetings. The involved students are expected to develop a sense of social and personal competence without using drugs. Another approach is to have older students tutor younger students, which is designed to give the older students a sense of competence. An experiment carried out in Napa, California, combined these approaches with a drug education course, small-group discussions led by teachers, and classroom management techniques designed to teach discipline and communication skills and to enhance the students' self-concepts.[7] Although a small effect on alcohol, marijuana, and cigarette use was found among the girls, the effects were gone by the one-year follow-up.

Anti-drug Norms

A 1984 review of prevention studies concluded that

> (1) most substance abuse prevention programs have not contained adequate evaluation components; (2) increased knowledge has virtually no impact on substance abuse or on intentions to smoke, drink, or use drugs; (3) affective education approaches appear to be experiential in their orientation and to place too little emphasis

values clarification: teaching students to recognize and express their own feelings and beliefs.
alternatives: alternative nondrug activities, such as relaxation or dancing.

Taking Sides

Are "Alternatives to Drugs" Really Alternatives?

As one part of many drug education programs, students are taught that they can produce natural highs—that is, altered states of consciousness similar to those produced by drugs, but without using drugs.

One such alternative that has been mentioned in these programs is skydiving. Obviously an activity of that sort has all the glamour, danger, and excitement most of us would want. Maybe if the kids could do this whenever they wanted, they wouldn't want to try cocaine or marijuana. But let's examine this as an alternative for a bunch of junior high school kids. First, there's the matter of cost and availability. How realistic is it to think that most of these kids would have access to skydiving? Second, there's the issue of convenience. Even if you were a rich kid, with your own airplane, parachute, and pilot, it's unlikely that you'd be able to go skydiving every afternoon after school. Drugs and alcohol may not provide the best highs in the world, but often they are easy to get and use, compared with activities, such as skydiving.

Maybe skydiving isn't a *practical* alternative to drugs for a lot of people. Still, it seems more wholesome and desirable. Let's become social philosophers and ask ourselves why the image of a person skydiving is more positive than the image of a person snorting cocaine. After all, skydiving doesn't make any obvious contributions to society. Let's play devil's advocate and propose that skydiving is not preferable to taking cocaine. Either way, the person is engaged in dangerous, expensive, self-indulgent activity. Contrast skydiving with cocaine, and see if you can answer for yourself why skydiving has a more positive image than cocaine use. You may have to talk about this with several people before you get a consistent feeling for why our society respects one of these activities so much more than the other. What about skiing? bungee-cord jumping?

on the acquisition of skills necessary to increase personal and social competence, particularly those skills needed to enable students to resist the various interpersonal pressures to begin using drugs; and (4) few studies have demonstrated any degree of success in terms of actual substance abuse prevention.[8]

This last point is not entirely a criticism of the programs themselves but reflects the difficulty of demonstrating statistically significant changes in behavior over a period of time after the programs.

Refusal Skills In response to the third point, that affective education approaches were too general and experiential, the next efforts at preventing drug use focused on teaching students to recognize peer pressure to use drugs and on teaching specific ways to respond to such pressures without using drugs. This is sometimes referred to as psychological inoculation. In addition to the focus on substance use, "refusal skills" and "pressure resistance" strategies are taught in a broader context of self-assertion and social skills training. The first successful application of this technique was a film in which young actors acted out situations in which one person was being pressured to smoke cigarettes. The film then demonstrated effective ways of responding to the pressure gracefully without smoking. After the film, students discuss alternative strategies and practice the coping techniques presented in the film. This approach has been demonstrated to be successful in reducing cigarette smoking in adolescent populations. It has been adapted for use with groups of various ages and for a wider variety of drugs and other behaviors, and students are taught from kindergarten on to "just say no" when someone is trying to get them to do something they know is wrong.

Drug-Free Schools In 1986 the federal government launched a massive program to support "drug-free schools and communities." Among other things, the government provided millions of dollars' worth of direct aid to local school districts to implement or enhance drug-prevention activities. Along with this, the Department of Education produced a small book called *What Works: Schools Without Drugs,*[9] which made specific recommendations for schools to follow. This book did not recommend a specific curriculum; its most significant feature was the emphasis on factors other than curriculum, such as school policies on drug and alcohol use. It suggested policies regarding locker searches, suspension, and expulsion of students. The purpose was not so much to take a punitive approach to alcohol or drug use as to point out through example and official policy that the school and community were opposed to drug and alcohol use by minors. Following this general drug-free lead, schools adopted "tobacco-free" policies, stating that not only the students but also teachers and other staff people were not to use tobacco products at school or on school-sponsored trips or activities.

According to this approach, the curriculum should include teaching about the laws against drugs, as well as about the school policies. In other words, as opposed to the 1970s values clarification approach of teaching students how to make responsible decisions for themselves, this approach wants to make it clear to the students that the society at large, the community in which they live, and the school in which they study have already made the decision not to condone drug use or underage alcohol use. This seems to be part of a more general educational trend away from "value-free" schools toward teaching values that are generally accepted in our society. For schools to be eligible for federal Drug-Free Schools funding, they must certify that their program teaches that "illicit drug use is wrong and harmful."

Development of the Social Influence Model

Some of the most sophisticated prevention research in recent years has been focused directly on cigarette smoking in adolescents. This problem has two major advantages over other types of drug use, as far as prevention research is concerned. First, a large enough fraction of adolescents do smoke cigarettes so that measurable behavior change is possible in a group of reasonable size. In contrast, one would have to perform an intervention with tens of thousands of people before significant alterations in the proportion of heroin users would be statistically evident. Second, the health consequences of smoking are so clear with respect to cancer and heart disease that there is a fairly good consensus over goals: We'd like to prevent adolescents from becoming smokers. One research advantage is the relatively simple verification available for self-reported use of tobacco: Saliva samples can be measured for cotinine, a nicotine metabolite.

Virtually all the various approaches to drug-abuse prevention have been tried with smoking behavior; in fact, Evans's 1976 smoking prevention paper introduced the use of the psychological inoculation approach based on the **social influence model.**[10] Out of all this research, certain consistencies appear. The most important of these is that it *is* possible to design smoking prevention programs that are effective in reducing the number of adolescents who begin smoking. Some practical lessons about the components of those programs have also emerged.[11] For example, presenting information about the delayed consequences of smoking (possible lung cancer many years later) is relatively ineffective. Information about the immediate physiological effects (increased heart rate, shortness of breath) is included instead. Some of the most important key elements that were shown to be effective were the following:

- *Training refusal skills* (for example, eight ways to say no). This was originally based on films demonstrating the kinds of social pressures that peers might use to encourage smoking and modeling a variety of appropriate responses. Then the students

social influence model: a prevention model adopted from successful smoking programs.

engage in role-playing exercises in which they practice these refusal skills. By using such techniques as changing the subject or having a good excuse handy, students learn to refuse to "cooperate" without being negative. When all else fails, however, they are taught to be assertive and insist on their right to refuse.

- *Public commitment.* Researchers found that having each child stand before his or her peers and promise not to start smoking and sign a pledge not to smoke are effective prevention techniques.

- *Countering advertising.* Students are shown examples of cigarette advertising, and then the "hidden messages" are discussed (young, attractive, healthy, active models are typically used; cigarette smoking might be associated with dating or with sports). Then the logical inconsistencies between these hidden messages and the actual effects of cigarette smoking (e.g., bad breath, yellow teeth, shortness of breath) are pointed out. The purpose of this is to "inoculate" the children against cigarette advertising by teaching them to question its messages.

- *Normative education.* Adolescents tend to overestimate the proportion of their peers who smoke. Presenting factual information about the smoking practices of adolescents provides students with a more realistic picture of the true social norms regarding smoking and reduces the "everybody is doing it" attitude. When possible, statistics on smoking from the specific school or community should be used in presenting this information.

- *Use of teen leaders.* Presenting dry facts about the actual proportion of smokers should ideally be reinforced by example. If you're presenting the program to junior high students, it's one thing to *say* that fewer than one-fifth of the high school students in that community smoke, but it's another to bring a few high school students into the room and have them discuss the

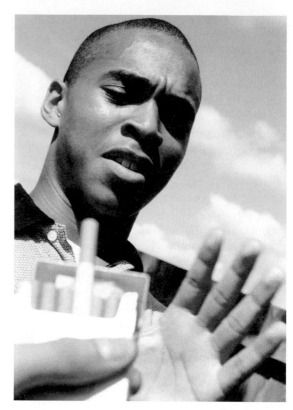

Training in refusal skills, including role-playing exercises, is a key component of the social influence model.

fact that neither they nor their friends smoke, their attitudes about smokers, and ways they have dealt with others' attempts to get them to smoke.

Possible improvements to those approaches are offered by the *cognitive developmental* approach to smoking behavior. McCarthy criticized the social influence/social skills training model for assuming that all students should be taught social skills or refusal skills without regard to whether they need such training.[12] The model "is that of a defenseless teenager who, for lack of general social skills or refusal skills, passively accedes to social pressures to smoke." Alternative models have been proposed in which the individual makes active, conscious decisions in preparation for trying cigarettes, trying smoking and becoming an occasional or regular user. The decision-making processes, and thus the appropriate prevention strategy, might be different at each of these "stages of cognitive development" as a smoker. Furthermore, smokers who begin smoking very young behave differently than smokers who begin as older adolescents (e.g., those who start young show more unanimity in selecting the most popular brand). Unfortunately, adolescents continue to initiate smoking every year, and the risk and protective factors reviewed in Chapter 1 have more influence on smoking behavior (and on alcohol and other drug use) than any information or education programs yet devised.[13]

DARE

Perhaps the most amazing educational phenomenon in a long time had fairly modest beginnings in 1983 as a joint project of the Los Angeles police department and school district. Those who are familiar with the Drug Abuse Resistance Education **(DARE)** program will have recognized its components described under the social influence model of smoking cessation. The difference here is that the educational program with DARE is delivered by police officers, originally in fifth- and sixth-grade classrooms. By basing the curriculum on sound educational research, by maintaining strict training standards for the officers who were to present the curriculum, and by encouraging the classroom teacher to participate, some of the old barriers to having nonteachers responsible for curriculum were overcome. The officers are in uniform, and they use interactive techniques as described for the social influence model. Most of the components are there: refusal skills, teen leaders, and a public commitment not to use illicit drugs. In addition, some of the affective education components are included: self-esteem building, alternatives to drug use, and decision making. The component on consequences of drug abuse is, no doubt, enhanced by the presence of a uniformed officer who can serve as an information source and symbol for

Drugs in Depth

How Much Do You Know About DARE?

1. Almost everyone in the United State has heard of DARE. What do the letters stand for?
2. One component of DARE is practicing how to refuse using drugs. Do you know the origin of DARE's eight ways to say no?
3. DARE has been implemented in more schools than any other substance-abuse prevention program. Does research on its effectiveness show that it's one of the best at preventing drug abuse?
4. Besides school-based programs, what other kinds of substance-abuse prevention programs have been developed?
5. The Institute of Medicine has a relatively new way of categorizing prevention programs into various types. Do you know what factor is used to differentiate among the types?

Answers
1. Drug Abuse Resistance Education
2. This and most components of DARE were adopted from smoking prevention programs developed in the 1970s.
3. Research on the effectiveness of DARE has not demonstrated a strong impact on preventing drug use. Other programs described in this chapter appear to be more effective.
4. Parent, family, and community programs and public media campaigns have also been developed to prevent drug abuse.
5. The target population (the entire population, at-risk populations, and individuals with early signs of problems).

concerns over gang activity and violence and can discuss arrest and incarceration. The 17-week program is capped by a commencement assembly at which certificates are awarded.

DARE: Drug Abuse Resistance Education, the most popular prevention program in schools.

This program happened to be in place at just the right time, both financially and politically. With the assistance of drug-free schools money and with nationwide enthusiasm for new drug-prevention activities in the 1980s, the program spread rapidly across the United States. By the early 1990s, DARE programs were found in every state.

This program was accepted quickly by many schools, and endorsed enthusiastically by educators, students, parents, and police participants, even though its effectiveness in preventing drug use was not evaluated extensively until 1994.

In 1994, two important, large-scale studies of the effects of DARE were reported. One was based on a longitudinal study in rural, suburban, and urban schools in Illinois, comparing students exposed to DARE with students who were not.[14] Although the program had some effects on reported self-esteem, there was no evidence for long-term reductions in self-reported use of drugs. The other report was based on a review of eight smaller outcome evaluations of DARE, selected from 18 evaluations based on whether the reports had a control group, a pretest-posttest design, and reliable outcome measures.[15] The overall impact of these eight programs was to increase drug knowledge and knowledge about social skills, but the effects on drug use were marginal at best. There was a very small but statistically significant reduction of tobacco use and no reliable effect on alcohol or marijuana use.

A more recent review of all the experimental studies on DARE published in peer-reviewed journals found an average effect size that was small and not statistically significant. The authors reported that their results supported previous conclusions about the ineffectiveness of DARE.[16] The repeated failures to demonstrate a significant impact of the DARE program on drug use remain a dilemma in light of its widespread popularity. Communities have not abandoned the program. Instead, DARE America has developed additional programs, including DARE + PLUS (Play and Learn Under Supervision) as an extension to the elementary program, and curriculum for middle school and high school DARE programs designed to follow up with these older adolescents. We cannot yet evaluate the effectiveness of these additional programs.

Programs That Work

Several school-based drug-use prevention programs have been modeled after the successful social influence model and have components similar to those of DARE. A few of these programs have been demonstrated to have beneficial effects on actual drug use:

Project ALERT was first tested in 30 junior high schools in California and Oregon.[17] The program targeted cigarette smoking, alcohol use, and marijuana use. Before the program, each student was surveyed and classified as a nonuser, an experimenter, or a user for each of the three substances. The curriculum was taught either by health educators or by educators with the assistance of trained teen leaders. Control schools simply continued whatever health or drug curriculum they had been using. The program was delivered in the seventh grade, and follow-up surveys were done 3, 12, and 15 months later. Three "booster" lessons were given in the eighth grade.

The program surprisingly had no measurable effect on initiation of smoking by nonusers. However, those who were cigarette experimenters before the program began were more likely to quit or to maintain low rates of smoking than the control group. The group with teen leader support showed the largest reduction: 50 percent fewer students were weekly smokers at the 15-month follow-up.

The experimental groups drank less alcohol soon after the program was presented, for previous alcohol nonusers, experimenters, and users. However, this effect diminished over time and disappeared by the end of the study.

The most consistent results were in reducing initiation of marijuana smoking and reducing levels of marijuana smoking. For

Drugs in Depth

Effective Prevention Programs

The Center for Substance Abuse Prevention (CSAP), a branch of the Substance Abuse and Mental Health Administration in the U.S. Department of Health and Human Services, has been studying research on effective prevention programs. It has developed a list of model programs. Some of the programs on this partial list are described within this chapter, and more information on the others can be obtained from the SAMHSA Web site. Also, as new programs are approved, they are being added to the list, so for the most current list, check on the Web at www.prevention.samhsa.gov.

Model Programs
- Across Ages
- Athletes Training and Learning to Avoid Steroids (ATLAS)
- Child Development Project
- Communities Mobilizing for Change on Alcohol
- Creating Lasting Family Connections
- Dare to Be You
- Families and Schools Together
- Keep a Clear Mind
- Life Skills Training
- Project ALERT
- Project Northland
- Project Towards No Tobacco Use
- Reconnecting Youth
- Residential Student Assistance Program
- Safe Dates
- SMART Team
- Strengthening Families Program
- Too Good for Drugs

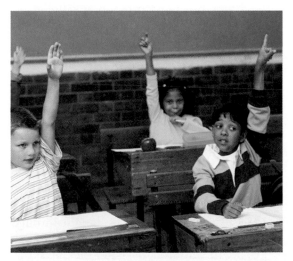

School-based drug-use prevention programs have been shown to reduce initiation and levels of drug use.

example, among those who were not marijuana users at the beginning, about 12 percent of the control-group students had begun using marijuana by the 15-month follow-up. In the treatment groups, only 8 percent began using during that time period, representing a one-third decrease in initiation to marijuana use.

Another program, the Life Skills Training program, has been subjected to several tests and has shown long-term positive results. This three-year program is based on the social influence model and teaches resistance skills, normative education, and media influences. Self-management skills and general social skills are also included. One study of this program found significantly lower use of marijuana, alcohol, and tobacco after six years. A subsequent application of this program among ethnic minority youth (Latino and African American) in New York City found reduced use on a two-year follow-up.[18]

Peers, Parents, and the Community

Our nation's public schools clearly are the most convenient conduit for attempts to achieve widespread social changes among young people, and that is why most efforts at drug-abuse prevention have been carried out there. However, peers, parents, and the community at large also exert powerful social influences on young people. Because these groups are less accessible than the schools, fewer prevention programs have been based on using parent and community influences. Nevertheless, important efforts have been made in all these areas.

Peer Programs

Most peer programs have occurred in the school setting, but some have used youth-oriented community service programs (such as YMCA, YWCA, and recreation centers) or have focused on "street" youth by using them in group community service projects.

- *Peer influence* approaches start with the assumption that the opinions of an adolescent's peers are significant influences on the adolescent's behavior. Often using an adult group facilitator/coordinator, the program's emphasis is on open discussion among a group of children or adolescents. These discussions might focus on drugs, with the peer group discussing dangers and alternatives, or they might simply have the more general goal of building positive group cohesiveness, a sense of belonging, and communication skills.

- *Peer participation* programs often focus on groups of youth in high-risk areas. The idea here is that young people participate in making important decisions and in doing significant work, either as "peers" with co-operating adults or in programs managed almost entirely by the youth themselves. Sometimes participants are paid for community service work, in other cases they engage in money-making businesses, and sometimes they provide youth-oriented information services. These groups almost never focus on drug use in any significant way; rather, the idea is to help people become participating members of society.

The benefits of these "extracurricular" peer approaches are measurable in terms of acquired skills, improved academic success, higher self-esteem, and a more positive attitude toward peers and school. As to whether they alter drug use significantly, the data either are not available or are inconclusive for the most part.

Parent and Family Programs

The various programs that have worked with parents have been described as taking at least one of four approaches.[19] Most of the programs include more than one of these approaches.

- *Informational* programs provide parents with basic information about alcohol and drugs, as well as information about their use and effects. Although the parents often want to know simply what to look for, how to tell if their child is using drugs, and what the consequences of drug abuse are, the best programs provide additional information. One important piece of information is the actual extent of the use of various types of drugs among young people. Another goal might be to make parents aware of their own alcohol and drug use to gain a broader perspective of the issue. A basic rationale is that well-informed parents will be able to teach appropriate attitudes about drugs, beginning when their child is young, and will be better able to recognize potential problems relating to drug or alcohol use.

- *Parenting skills* might be taught through practical training programs. Communication with children, decision-making skills, how to set goals and limits, and when and how to say no to your child can be learned in the abstract and then practiced in role-playing exercises. One risk factor for adolescent drug and alcohol use is poor family relationships, and improving family interaction and strengthening communication can help prevent alcohol and drug abuse.

- *Parent support groups* can be important adjuncts to skills training or in planning community efforts. Groups of parents meet regularly to discuss problem solving, parenting skills, their perceptions of the problem, actions to be taken, and so on.

- *Family interaction* approaches call for families to work as a unit to examine, discuss, and confront issues relating to alcohol and drug use. Other exercises might include more general problem solving or response to emergencies. Not only do these programs attempt to improve family communication, but also the parents are placed in the roles of teacher of drug facts and coordinator of family action, thus strengthening their knowledge and skills.

One selective prevention program, called the Strengthening Families program, targets children of parents who are substance abusers. This program has been successfully implemented several times within diverse populations. It has three major goals: improving parenting skills, increasing children's skills (such as communication skills, refusal skills, awareness of feelings, and emotion expression skills), and improving family relationships (decreasing conflict, improving communication, increasing parent-child time together, and increasing the planning and organizational skills of the family). Children and parents attend evening sessions weekly for 14 weeks to learn and practice these skills. Evaluations of this program indicate that it reduces tobacco and alcohol use in the children as well as reduces substance abuse and other problems in the parents.[20]

Community Programs

Two basic reasons exist for organizing prevention programs at the community level. The first is that a coordinated approach using schools, parent and peer groups, civic organizations, police, newspapers, radio, and television can have a much greater impact than an isolated

Mind / Body Connection

Integrating Treatment and Prevention with Pregnancy Services

Does your community provide needed services and compassionate support for pregnant women who use alcohol and drugs? An emerging consensus views alcohol, tobacco, and other drug use during pregnancy as a community problem. During this period when women anticipate major life change, prevention initiatives can enhance their motivation to have a healthy baby. And, for women with substance-abuse problems, pregnancy provides a similarly strong motivation to seek help.

Fear of blame, legal intervention, and loss of child custody prevent many women from getting help. To counteract these barriers to services, prevention initiatives should promote services that are safe and confidential. Services should be not only physically accessible but also culturally accessible. Efforts that recognize the importance of relationships to women can call on the support of family members and others for alcohol-free and other drug-free pregnancies. Prevention strategies that combine information with options for change have shown promising results in reducing drug use during pregnancy.

Find out if women in your area have access to an integrated system of alcohol, tobacco, and other drug treatment and maternal and child health care. An example is the Women's and Infants Clinic at Boston City Hospital, which since 1989 has provided pediatric care, child development services, and drug-abuse treatment services in an integrated service system.

program that occurs only in the school, for example. Another reason is that drug-abuse prevention and drug education are controversial and emotional topics. Parents might question the need for or the methods used in drug education programs in the schools. Jealousy and mistrust about approaches can separate schools, police, church, and parent groups. A program that starts by involving all these groups in the planning stages is more likely to

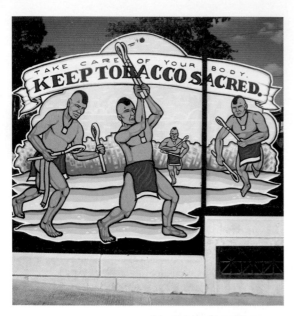

Community-based programs work best when they have widespread community support. This anti-tobacco mural is tied to the values of a local community and focuses on the traditional sacred origins of tobacco use among Native Americans.

receive widespread community support. Clearly, the spread of the DARE program in the schools is based partly on the fact that it demonstrates and encourages cooperation between the police and the schools, as well as encourages parental involvement.

Community-based programs can bring other resources to bear. For example, the city council and local businesses can be involved in sponsoring alcohol-free parties, developing recreational facilities, and arranging field trips so that, when the school-based program talks about alternatives, the alternatives are available. The public media can be enlisted not only to publicize public meetings and programs but also to present drug- and alcohol-related information that reinforces what is learned in the other programs.

Communities Mobilizing for Change on Alcohol is one of SAMHSA's model prevention programs (see page 425). The program works for change in alcohol ordinances in the community and alcohol policies of schools, universities, and civic organizations. It encourages parents, faith organizations, the police, city government, and all businesses and organizations within the community to promote the idea of limiting alcohol availability for 13-to-18-year-olds. The program was studied in 15 communities over a five-year period and resulted in decreased alcohol sales to minors, decreases in friends providing alcohol to minors, and decreases in self-reported drinking in the targeted age group.

Prevention in the Workplace

As a part of its efforts to reduce the demand for drugs, the federal government has encouraged private employers, especially those who do business with the government, to adopt policies to prevent drug use by their employees. The most consistent feature of these programs is random urine screens. In 1989, rules went into effect requiring all companies and organizations that obtain grants or contracts from the federal government to adopt a "drug-free workplace" plan. The exact nature of the plan is up to the company, but guidelines were produced by the Department of Labor. Modeled after the Education Department's *What Works* book, the Labor Department's is called *What Works: Workplaces Without Drugs*.[21] At a minimum, the Labor Department expects employers to state clearly that drug use on the job is unacceptable and to notify employees of the consequences of violating company policy regarding drug use. The ultimate goal is not to catch drug users and fire them but to prevent drug use by making it clear that it is not condoned.

What Should We Be Doing?

By now you have picked up some ideas for things to do to reduce drug use, as well as some things to avoid doing. But the answer as to what needs to be done in a particular situation depends on the motivations for doing it. Most states require drug- and alcohol-abuse prevention education as part of a health curriculum, for example. If that is the primary motive for doing something, and if there doesn't seem to be a particular problem with substance abuse in the schools, then the best thing would be to adopt one of the modern school-based programs that have been developed for this purpose, to make sure the teachers and other participants are properly trained in it, and to go ahead. In selecting from among the curricula, a sensible, balanced approach that combines some factual information with social skills training, perhaps integrated into the more general themes of health, personal values, and decision making, would be appropriate. The ones mentioned in the section "Programs That Work" fit this general description, and each deserves a careful look. Above all, avoid sensational scare stories, preachy approaches from the teacher to the student, and untrained personnel developing their own curricula. Another good thing to avoid is the inadvertent demonstration of how to do things you don't want students to do.

If, on the other hand, there is a public outcry about the "epidemic" of drugs and alcohol abuse in the community, speakers have inflamed passions, and there is a widespread fervor to do something about it, this presents both a danger and an opportunity. The danger is that this passionate group might attack and undermine the efforts already being made in the schools, substituting scary, preachy, negative approaches, which can have negative consequences. The opportunity lies in the possibility that this energy can be organized into a community planning effort, out of which could develop cooperation, increased parent understanding, a focus on family communication, interest in the lives of the community's young people, and increased recreational and creative opportunities.

The key to making this happen is convincing the aroused citizenry of the possibly negative consequences of doing what seems obvious and selling them on the idea of studying what needs to be done. A good place to start is by visiting the Web site of the Center for Substance Abuse Prevention (www.samhsa.gov/csap). This agency produces updated materials for groups interested in developing drug- and alcohol-abuse prevention programs, provides technical assistance and training to communities interested in developing programs, and offers Community Partnership Grants. (A list of CSAP model programs was shown in the Drugs in Depth on page 425.)

Summary

- We can distinguish between education programs with the goal of imparting knowledge and prevention programs aimed at modifying drug-using behavior.

- Most of the research over the past 30 years has failed to demonstrate that prevention programs can produce clear, meaningful, long-lasting effects on drug-using behavior.

- The affective education programs of the 1970s have been criticized for being too value-free.

- Based on the success of the social influence model in reducing cigarette smoking, a variety of school-based prevention programs have used the same techniques with illicit drugs.

- The DARE program has been adopted rapidly and widely, despite research showing limited impact on drug-using behavior.

- Current school-based approaches use refusal skills, countering advertising, public commitments, and teen leaders. Several of these programs have been demonstrated to be effective.

- Other nonschool programs are peer-based through after-school groups or activities, parent-based through parent and family training, or community-based.

Review Questions

1. What is the distinction between secondary and tertiary prevention?
2. What is the knowledge-attitudes-behavior model, and what information first called it into question?
3. Explain what is meant by "value-free" values clarification programs, and why they fell out of favor in the 1980s.
4. When the Drug-Free Schools programs began in 1986, the emphasis shifted away from curriculum to what?
5. What were the five successful components of the social influence model for smoking prevention?
6. In Project ALERT, what was the impact of using teen leaders to assist the instructors?
7. What distinguishes DARE from other similar programs based on the social influence model?
8. What do ALERT and Life Skills Training have in common, besides their effectiveness?
9. What are some of the "parenting" skills that might be taught and practiced in a prevention program?
10. What is the most common component of "drug-free workplace" plans?

References

1. National Institute on Drug Abuse. *Drug Abuse Prevention for the General Population*. Washington, DC: U.S. Department of Health and Human Services, 1997.
2. Goodstadt, M.S. "School-based Drug Education in North America: What Is Wrong? What Can Be Done?" *Journal of School Health* 56 (1986), pp. 278–81.
3. Swisher, J.D., and others. "Drug Education: Pushing or Preventing?" *Peabody Journal of Education* 49 (1971), pp. 68–75.
4. Swisher, J.D., and others. "A Comparison of Four Approaches to Drug Abuse Prevention at the College Level." *Journal of College Student Personnel* 14 (1973), pp. 231–35.
5. Blum, R.H., E. Blum, and E. Garfield. *Drug Education: Results and Recommendations*. Lexington, MA: D.C. Heath, 1976.
6. Swisher, J.D. "Prevention Issues." In R.I. DuPont, A. Goldstein, J. O'Donnell, eds. *Handbook on Drug Abuse.*
   Washington, DC: NIDA, U.S. Government Printing Office, 1979.
7. Schaps, E., and others. *The Napa Drug Abuse Prevention Project: Research Findings*. Washington, DC: DHHS Publication No. (ADM) 84-1339, U.S. Government Printing Office, 1984.
8. "Prevention Research." In *Drug Abuse and Drug Abuse Research*. Washington, DC: DHHS Publication No. (ADM) 85-1372, U.S. Government Printing Office, 1984.
9. U.S. Department of Education. *What Works: Schools without Drugs*. Washington, DC: 1987.
10. Evans, R.I. "Smoking in Children: Developing a Social Psychological Strategy of Deterrence." *Preventive Medicine* 5 (1976), pp. 122–27.
11. Flay, B.R. "What We Know About the Social Influences Approach to Smoking Prevention: Review and Recommendations." In C.S. Bell, R. Battjes, eds. *Prevention Research: Deterring Drug Abuse Among Children and Adolescents*. Washington, DC: NIDA Research Monograph 63, DHHS Publication No. (ADM) 85-1334, U.S. Government Printing Office, 1985.
12. McCarthy, W.J. "The Cognitive Developmental Model and Other Alternatives to the Social Skills Deficit Model of Smoking Onset." In C.S. Bell, R. Battjes, eds. *Prevention Research: Deterring Drug Abuse Among Children and Adolescents*. Washington, DC: NIDA Research Monograph 63, DHHS Publication No. (ADM) 85-1334, U.S. Government Printing Office, 1985.
13. Albaum, G., and others. "Smoking Behavior, Information Sources, and Consumption Value of Teenagers: Implications for Public Policy and Other Intervention Failures." *Journal of Consumer Affairs* 36 (2002), pp. 50–76.
14. Ennett, S.T., and others. "Long-term Evaluation of Drug Abuse Resistance Education." *Addictive Behaviors* 19 (1994), p. 113.
15. Ennett, S.T., and others. "How Effective Is Drug Abuse Resistance Education? A Meta-analysis of Project DARE Outcome Evaluations." *American Journal of Public Health* 84 (1994), p. 1394.
16. West, S.L., & K.K. O'Neal. "Project D.A.R.E. Outcome Effectiveness Revisited." *American Journal of Public Health,* 94 (2004), pp. 1027–30.
17. Ellickson, P.L., & R.M. Bell. "Drug Prevention in Junior High: A Multi-site Longitudinal Test." *Science* 247 (1990), pp. 1299–1305.
18. Botvin, G.J., & S.P. Schinke. "Effectiveness of Culturally Focused and Generic Skills Training Approaches to Alcohol and Drug Abuse Prevention Among Minority Adolescents: Two-Year Follow-up Results." *Psychology of Addictive Behaviors* 9 (1995), p. 183.
19. "Parent Education." In *Prevention Plus: Involving Schools, Parents, and the Community in Alcohol and Drug Education*. Washington, DC: DHHS Publication No. (ADM) 84-1256, U.S. Government Printing Office, 1984.
20. National Institute on Drug Abuse. *Drug Abuse Prevention for At-risk Groups*. Washington, DC: U.S. Department of Health and Human Services, 1997.
21. U.S. Department of Labor. *What Works: Workplaces Without Drugs*. Washington, DC: 1989.

Check Yourself

If you are a parent, think about your own family for a moment. Several of the risk and protective factors mentioned in Chapter 2 are related to family, and some of the effective prevention strategies target family activities. Consider the following questions (they can be answered either from the perspective of a child or a parent).

1. Is the interaction between the parent(s) and child generally positive?
2. Do the parents provide attention and praise to the child?
3. Is discipline consistent and usually effective and never involves physical punishment?
4. Is the child able to communicate his or her feelings to the parent(s)?
5. Does the child feel comfortable discussing rules and consequences, especially when it comes to the use of substances or other inappropriate behavior?
6. Does the family spend time together doing things every week?
7. Is the family capable of planning and organizing family activities?

If the answer to most of these questions is yes, then your family is probably functioning pretty well. If the answer to most of them is no, then think about what steps you can take to change this situation. That might include scheduling some time with a family therapist or counselor.

18

Treating Substance Abuse and Dependence

Objectives

After you have studied this chapter, you should be able to:

- Discuss different types of treatment goals for substance abuse and how those goals relate to one's belief about the nature of substance abuse.

- Describe the influence of Alcoholics Anonymous on substance abuse treatment programs for alcohol and for other substances.

- Explain how motivational interviewing is used in conjunction with the notion of stages of change to better prepare people for treatment.

- List the benefits and limitations of using contingency management to maintain abstinence.

- Explain why drugs are sometimes used during the initial detoxification phase of treatment.

- Discuss the three drugs that are available for use in treating alcohol dependence.

- Describe the various forms of nicotine-replacement therapies and the use of Zyban in nicotine dependence treatment.

- Explain both antagonist and substitution treatment for opioid dependence and list the most commonly used medication for substitution.

- Describe the status of development of medications for treating cocaine dependence and cannabis dependence.

- Explain why, despite the well-known failure rates in substance abuse treatment, the book still concludes that these treatments are effective.

Every year, hundreds of thousands of Americans undergo treatment for substance abuse and dependence. The word *treatment* conjures up images of hospitals, nurses, and physicians, but traditional medical approaches form only a small part of the overall treatment picture. As we will see, the variety of treatment approaches reflects the variety of substance abuse problems, as well as the variety of theories about substance abuse. The various treatment approaches are often used in combination.

Behavioral/ Psychosocial Treatments

Many early theories of substance dependence were based primarily on studying alcohol-dependent individuals, so it should come as no surprise that the history of behavioral/ psychosocial treatment approaches also began with the treatment of alcohol dependence.

Online Learning Center Resources

www.mhhe.com/ksir12e

Visit our Online Learning Center (OLC) for access to these study aids and additional resources.

- Learning objectives
- Glossary flashcards
- Web activities and links
- Self-scoring chapter quiz
- Audio chapter summaries

However, most behavioral/psychosocial treatment programs today are not designed for a particular substance, but treat a variety of types of substance dependence. Below, we present some behavioral/psychosocial treatment approaches often used in helping individuals deal with their substance abuse problems.

Defining Treatment Goals

The particular theoretical view one has of substance abuse influences not only the treatment approaches one is likely to take but also the goals of treatment. For example, if one accepts the increasingly predominant view of alcohol dependence as a biological disease, which someone either "has" or does not have and which has an inevitable progression to more and more drinking, then the only acceptable treatment goal is total **abstinence.** Other experts view alcohol dependence as representing one end of a continuum of drinking, with no clear dividing line. For some of these theorists, a possible beneficial outcome of treatment is **controlled** social **drinking.** Likewise, if one views opioid dependence as inherently evil, undermining the physical and mental health of its victims (a common view until fairly recently), then abstinence from opioids is the only acceptable goal. Americans seem to have accepted dependence on the legal opioid methadone as preferable to heroin dependence, so the goal has changed from eliminating

opioid use to eliminating heroin use. The case with cigarette smoking is similar; some programs have focused on cutting down on smoking, whereas most programs aim for complete abstinence.

When we look for indicators of a treatment program's success, if we find that some people are still using, but using less, should we claim any benefit? Or should we assume, as some do, that any decreases will be temporary and that, unless the person quits entirely, there has been no real improvement? Although the answer depends on your goals, the DSM-IV-TR can provide a useful guide for answering this question. Researchers have begun to estimate the cost savings resulting from increased employment and decreased crime after treatment, and to compare these savings with the cost of treatment itself, to develop a cost/benefit analysis of the effectiveness of treatment.

Alcoholics Anonymous

The formation of **Alcoholics Anonymous** (AA) in 1935 can now be seen as an important milestone in treatment. This group, which has total abstinence as a goal, has given support to the disease model of alcohol dependence. One of the basic tenets of this group is that the "alcoholic" is biologically different from others and therefore can never safely drink any alcohol. Central to this disease model is the idea that the disease takes away the person's control of his or her own drinking behavior and therefore removes the blame for the problem. AA members are quick to point out that removing blame for the disease does not remove responsibility for dealing with it. By analogy, we would not blame diabetics for being diabetic, but we do expect diabetics to control their diets, take their medication, and so on. Thus, the alcohol-dependent person is seen as having the responsibility for managing the disease on a day-by-day basis but need not feel guilty about being different. The major approach used by AA has been group support and a buddy system. The members of AA help each other

Drugs in the Media

Hollywood Knows, and Shows, Hard Truth About Drugs

Hollywood stars and the talented creators in their orbit are hardly immune to the effects of substance abuse and dependence. The list of people who have battled drug-, drink-, and smoking-related problems includes some of the most famous names in show business: Robert Downey, Jr.; Drew Barrymore; Matthew Perry; Melanie Griffith; and others.

Many actors, directors, producers, and writers have recognized the media's responsibility to make others aware of how substance abuse destroys families, careers, health, and lives. These numerous luminaries attend the annual PRISM Awards, which honor creative achievement in accurate depictions of drug, alcohol, and tobacco use and dependence. The awards spotlight films, TV shows, comic books, community service efforts, and individual volunteerism, as well as special honors. They are presented jointly by the Entertainment Industries Council, the National Institute on Drug Abuse, and the Robert Wood Johnson Foundation, the nation's largest philanthropic organization dedicated exclusively to health and health care.

For decades Hollywood actors' personal nightmares with drugs have been kept under wraps by an industry mentality that tried to protect star and box-office receipts from scandal. And, often on the screen, smoking, alcohol, and drugs have been portrayed as glamorous, fun, or cool. Many stars now realize they can use the power of their celebrity to help millions in their struggles against drugs. By giving an accurate depiction of the dangers of these substances, they believe they can prevent many others from taking that first step down a precarious path. To see recent PRISM Award honorees and video clips, go to www.prismawards.com.

Companion efforts to assist the creative community and complement the PRISM Awards include the publication of special drug abuse, alcohol, and tobacco volumes of "Spotlight on Depiction of Health and Social Issues," a resource encyclopedia; a technical assistance program called "First Draft"; and "PRISM Generation Next," a program to take the responsive depiction process to students enrolled in television and film schools.

Do you think the film industry can make a big impact on children and the general public by showing them the negative effects of drugs? Would hearing that a movie or TV show had received a PRISM award make you more interested in viewing it?

---

through difficult periods and encourage each other in their sobriety.

Although AA has been described as a loose affiliation of local groups, each with its own character, they have in common adherence to a method. Nevertheless, formal evaluations of the success of AA have been few and have not been very positive. For example, studies of court-ordered referrals to AA or to other types of interventions have not shown AA to be more effective. However, AA was developed by and for people who have made a personal decision to stop drinking and who want to affiliate with others who have made that decision, and it might not be the most appropriate approach for individuals who are coerced into attending meetings as an alternative to jail. More appro-

priate (and more difficult and expensive) evaluations of AA should be done to determine which types of drinkers are most likely to benefit from this organization's program.

This point is particularly important because many treatment programs, such as the Betty Ford Center, Hazelden, and Phoenix House, rely mostly on the 12-step model of AA

abstinence: no alcohol or drug use at all.
controlled drinking: the idea that alcohol abusers may be able to drink under control.
Alcoholics Anonymous: a worldwide organization of self-help groups based on alcoholics helping each other achieve and maintain sobriety.

DSM-IV-TR

Psychiatric Diagnosis of Substance Disorders

Diagnostic Criteria for Substance Dependence

A maladaptive pattern of substance use, leading to clinically significant impairment or distress, as manifested by three (or more) of the following, occurring at any time in the same 12-month period:

1. Tolerance, as defined by either of the following:
   a. A need for markedly increased amounts of the substance to achieve intoxication or desired effect
   b. Markedly diminished effect with continued use of the same amount of the substance
2. Withdrawal, as manifested by either of the following:
   a. The characteristic withdrawal syndrome for the substance
   b. The same (or a closely related) substance is taken to relieve or avoid withdrawal symptoms
3. The substance is often taken in larger amounts or over a longer period than was intended.
4. There is a persistent desire or unsuccessful efforts to cut down or control substance use.
5. A great deal of time is spent in activities necessary to obtain the substance.

6. Important social, occupational, or recreational activities are given up or reduced because of substance use.
7. The substance use is continued despite knowledge of having a persistent or recurrent physical or psychological problem that is likely to have been caused or exacerbated by the substance.

Diagnostic Criteria for Substance Abuse

A. A maladaptive pattern of substance use leading to clinically significant impairment or distress, as manifested by one (or more) of the following, occurring within a 12-month period:
   1. Recurrent substance use resulting in failure to fulfill major role obligations at work, school, or home.
   2. Recurrent substance use in situations in which it is physically hazardous.
   3. Recurrent substance-related legal problems.
   4. Continued substance use despite having persistent or recurrent social or interpersonal problems caused or exacerbated by the effects of the substance.
B. The symptoms have never met the criteria for substance dependence for this class of substance.

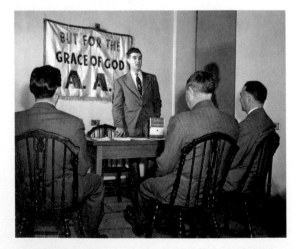

The major approach of Alcoholics Anonymous, founded in 1935, is group support and a buddy system.

(see Drugs in Depth). Moreover, a wide variety of other self-help groups, including Cocaine Anonymous (CA), Narcotics Anonymous (NA), and Gamblers Anonymous (GA), have modeled the AA treatment approach.

Motivational Enhancement Therapy

For many years, the predominant theories on why people seek treatment for substance abuse were based on the anecdotal experiences of alcohol-dependent individuals. According to the conventional wisdom, most substance abusers use the defense mechanism of *denial* and are obstinately unwilling to admit either that their substance use is unusual or that it has serious consequences for themselves or others. In this context, only when the abuser

Drugs in Depth

The 12 Steps of Alcoholics Anonymous

1. We admitted we were powerless over alcohol—that our lives had become unmanageable.
2. Came to believe that a Power greater than ourselves could restore us to sanity.
3. Made a decision to turn our will and our lives over to the care of God *as we understood Him*.
4. Made a searching and fearless moral inventory of ourselves.
5. Admitted to God, to ourselves, and to another human being the exact nature of our wrongs.
6. Were entirely ready to have God remove all these defects of character.
7. Humbly asked Him to remove our shortcomings.
8. Made a list of all persons we had harmed and became willing to make amends to them all.
9. Made direct amends to such people wherever possible, except when to do so would injure them or others.
10. Continued to take moral inventory and when we were wrong promptly admitted it.
11. Sought through prayer and meditation to improve our conscious contact with God *as we understood Him*, praying only for knowledge of His will for us and the power to carry that out.
12. Having had a spiritual awakening as the result of these steps, we tried to carry this message to alcoholics, and to practice these principles in all our affairs.

Source: The Twelve Steps are reprinted with permission of Alcoholics Anonymous World Services, Inc. Permission to reprint the Twelve Steps does not mean that AA has reviewed or approved the contents of this publication, nor that AA agrees with the views expressed herein. AA is a program of recovery from alcoholism *only*—use of the Twelve Steps in connection with programs and activities which are patterned after AA, but which address other problems, or in any other non-AA context, does not imply otherwise.

"hits bottom"—that is, suffers sufficient consequences that the reality of the problem finally sinks in—will he or she be ready to seek help. The obvious problem with this perspective is that grave consequences (e.g., death) may occur before the abuser's perception of "hitting bottom."

One relatively new treatment approach, motivational enhancement therapy, attempts to shift the focus away from denial and toward motivation to change.[1] The idea is that targeting the abuser's degree of motivation to quit substance use could enhance the effectiveness of treatment. Hence, ambivalent or less ready substance abusers should first receive *motivational interviewing*. During this nonconfrontational process, an assessment of the substance-using behavior and its consequences is completed to determine the abuser's current **stage of change** because, according to this view, to help someone move from one stage to another through motivational interviewing, you need to know where he or she is in the decision-making process. In the *precontemplation* stage, the individual does not recognize that a problem exists. In the *contemplation* stage, the individual believes that a problem might exist and gives some consideration to the possibility of changing her or his behavior. In the *preparation* stage, the individual decides to change and makes plans to do so. In the *action* stage, the individual takes active steps toward change, such as entering treatment. Finally, the *maintenance* stage involves activities intended to maintain the change. The motivational interviewer attempts to help the client focus on the concerns and problem behavior but does not directly tell the client what to do. Ideally, if the therapist knows which stage of change the

stages of change: a model for decision making consisting of precontemplation, contemplation, preparation, action, and maintenance.

client is in, the discussion can be guided appropriately to help move the client to the next stage. Although this approach has been demonstrated to decrease substance use,[2] it is probably best conceptualized as a preparation for other therapies rather than as a stand-alone treatment.

Contingency Management

A behavioral approach to treating substance abuse that has received substantial attention in recent years is *contingency management.* This approach has produced consistent reductions in substance-using behaviors among diverse substance-abusing populations.[3] In this approach, individuals receive immediate rewards (e.g., vouchers redeemable for goods or services) for providing drug-free urine samples, and the value of the rewards is increased with consecutive drug-free urine samples. However, rewards are withheld if the client's urine sample is positive for an illicit drug. In addition to receiving rewards, clients participate in counseling sessions weekly, where they learn a variety of skills to help them minimize substance use. A weakness of contingency management is the cost of the rewards, which could preclude the use of this procedure by small, less well-funded treatment programs.

Relapse Prevention

Another behavioral strategy is called relapse prevention, an approach that uses cognitive-therapy techniques with behavioral-skills training. Individuals learn to identify and change behaviors that may lead to continued drug use, such as going out to bars or associating with users. Relapse prevention has been shown to be more effective at decreasing substance use than most standard psychotherapies, and the beneficial effects persist for as long as a year following treatment).[4] This approach is criticized for placing greater demands on the patients compared to other substance abuse treatments, and it may be particularly challenging for individuals who have cognitive limitations.[5]

Targeting Prevention

Avoiding Relapse

One important type of substance-abuse prevention involves those who have been in treatment and are trying to avoid relapsing, or going back to their previously abusive behavior. Think about the messages these people receive each day from public media (such as television, movies, newspapers, and the Web) and from other individuals. Which of these messages support relapse prevention and which tend to encourage relapse? Have a conversation with a friend, relative, or classmate who has been in treatment for substance abuse and has had to deal with the problem of relapse prevention. Ask what was helpful for him or her and what made it more difficult to avoid substance abuse.

Pharmacotherapies (Medication Treatments)

Substance abuse and dependence is increasingly viewed as a "brain disease," much like, for example, Parkinson's disease. But the overwhelming majority of individuals who use substances do not become dependent, whereas virtually all of the individuals who lose greater than 80 percent of nigrostriatal dopamine neurons will exhibit symptoms of Parkinson's disease. Nevertheless, an intense amount of research efforts have focused on developing medications to treat substance abuse and dependence. The rationale is that as we increase our understanding of brain mechanisms mediating substance abuse, we should be better able to use medications to target these mechanisms, thereby blocking the reinforcing effects of drugs of abuse (i.e., the "magic bullet approach"). Despite the enthusiasm accompanying medication development efforts, most experts do not believe that pharmacotherapies alone will cure a chronic, relapsing disorder such as substance abuse, in part, because the problem of substance abuse is expressed behaviorally. Thus, a major hope is that pharmacotherapies will provide a window of opportunity by relieving withdrawal symptoms, for example, so that behavioral/psychosocial treatments can be used. Below we describe some medications that have been used to help substance abusers deal with withdrawal symptoms and maintain abstinence. The focus of our discussion will be limited to alcohol, nicotine, the opioids, cocaine, and cannabis. These substances were selected for their public health importance and because a large amount of research has been conducted regarding their use.

Detoxification and Maintenance Phase

Pharmacological interventions are typically initiated at two different phases of the dependence cycle: detoxification and maintenance. Detoxification can be viewed as an *initial and immediate goal* during which medications are administered to alleviate unpleasant withdrawal symptoms that may appear following abrupt cessation of drug use (e.g., the nicotine patch and nicotine gum have been used to treat individuals experiencing cigarette smoking abstinence symptoms). Medications used in the detoxification phase are also sometimes used in the maintenance phase (e.g., nicotine replacement medications). Thus, the distinction between a detoxification medication and a maintenance medication is sometimes less clear.

Maintenance on pharmacological agents can be viewed as a *longer-term strategy* used to help the dependent individual avoid relapsing to the abused drug. Three major maintenance strategies are used. First, *agonist or substitution therapy* is used to induce cross-tolerance to the abused drug. Methadone, a long-acting μ-opioid agonist, for heroin dependence, and nicotine replacement medications for tobacco dependence have been used as agonist maintenance treatments to prevent relapse and cravings in individuals attempting to maintain abstinence. Agonist maintenance agents typically have safer routes of administration and/or

diminished psychoactive effects. Second, *antagonist therapy* is used to produce extinction by preventing the user from experiencing the reinforcing effects of the abused drug (e.g., the opioid antagonist naltrexone, which selectively blocks opioid effects). Finally, *punishment therapy* is used to produce an aversive reaction following ingestion of the abused drug. Disulfiram (Antabuse) for the treatment of alcohol dependence is an example of punishment therapy. Disulfiram inhibits aldehyde dehydrogenase, a major enzyme involved in alcohol metabolism, which, in the presence of alcohol, can produce unpleasant symptoms including headache, vomiting, and breathing difficulties.

Alcohol

Pharmacotherapies have become increasingly important in the treatment of alcohol dependence, in part, because of the serious nature of the acute alcohol withdrawal syndrome. This syndrome is typically characterized by tremors, tachycardia (rapid heartbeat), hypertension, perfuse sweating, insomnia, hallucinations, and seizures. Medical risks associated with the alcohol withdrawal process often require an inpatient medical setting. During detoxification, two of the central tasks for the clinician are to reduce autonomic hyperactivity and to prevent the development of seizures. For several reasons, administration of a benzodiazepine during alcohol detoxification is the standard treatment approach. There is a high degree of cross-tolerance between alcohol and the benzodiazepines. Because benzodiazepines can serve as substitutes for alcohol and generally have longer half-lives than alcohol, the withdrawal process can be safely completed. Benzodiazepines, by potentiating the inhibitory actions of GABA on the central nervous system, significantly decrease the risk of seizures during detoxification. In addition, the increased autonomic arousal that occurs during alcohol withdrawal is similar to the initiation of the "stress response" (i.e., increased heart rate, blood pressure, respiration, and anxiety). This suggests the mechanisms that mediate the stress response may also play a role in alcohol withdrawal symptoms. Because it is well documented that increased GABAergic transmission markedly diminishes the stress response,[6] it is not surprising that benzodiazepines are also effective in attenuating the autonomic hyperactivity that accompanies alcohol withdrawal symptoms. Some clinicians might be wary about the potential for abuse associated with the use of some rapid-acting benzodiazepines (e.g., alprazolam), particularly in alcohol-abusing populations.[7] Thus, benzodiazepines with a slower onset of action such as clonazepam or oxazepam may be more suitable in this population.

Three medications have received Food and Drug Administration (FDA) approval for the treatment of alcohol abuse and dependence: disulfiram (Antabuse), naltrexone, and acamprosate (calcium acetylhomotaurinate). All of these medications are used during the maintenance phase, although the length of use could vary. Typically, these medications are used for weeks or months, but indefinite maintenance for years is unusual with these approaches. Nearly a half century ago it was discovered that ingestion of disulfiram in the presence of alcohol resulted in an unpleasant reaction, including facial flushing, accelerated pulse, throbbing headache, nausea, and vomiting.[8] As stated above, these symptoms occur as a result of the increased amount of acetaldehyde in the body following inhibition of aldehyde dehydrogenase by disulfiram. Since this initial observation, several studies have assessed disulfiram as a pharmacotherapeutic option in treating alcohol-use disorders. In general, disulfiram has not been shown to be effective in achieving abstinence or delaying relapse; most individuals simply do not take the medication.

Naltrexone was developed as an opioid antagonist and has been used in the treatment of opioid dependence. In the early 1990s, data from two large studies of naltrexone for the treatment of alcohol dependence showed that the medication substantially reduced days of alcohol drinking per week, the rate of relapse among those who drank, and alcohol craving.[9] The precise mechanism of action for naltrexone-related reductions in alcohol drinking is not fully understood, but it has been suggested that the medication blocks opioid receptors, thereby preventing the release of alcohol-induced dopamine, which in turn blocks the reinforcing effects of alcohol.[10] Although great fanfare accompanied the approval of naltrexone and many alcohol-dependent individuals were treated with this medication, it has not had a big impact on overall treatment success.

The latest medication to receive approval for the treatment of alcohol-use disorders is acamprosate, a compound that bears a structural resemblance to GABA. Acamprosate exerts at least two actions that have been proposed to be important for its clinical utility in treating alcohol dependence: normalizing basal GABA concentrations, which are proposed to be disrupted in alcohol-dependent individuals, and blocking the glutamate increases observed during alcohol withdrawal.[11] In several studies, acamprosate has been shown to be effective in decreasing alcohol relapse. But, because the medication only recently received FDA approval, the impact of its availability on treating alcohol-use disorder in broader clinical populations has yet to be determined.

Nicotine

More than 98 percent of tobacco users are cigarette smokers. Despite the declining social acceptability and rates of cigarette smoking, a substantial proportion of individuals remain dependent. Tobacco smoke contains as many as 4,000 chemical constituents, but nicotine is thought to be the primary component responsible for the maintenance of continued use. When most smokers attempt to quit, they experience withdrawal symptoms, such as anxiety, depression, dysphoria, irritability, decreased concentration, insomnia, increased food intake, and cigarette craving. Pharmacotherapies have been used primarily to attenuate these symptoms. Five nicotine-replacement therapies have received FDA-approval for treating nicotine dependence: transdermal nicotine patch, nicotine gum, nicotine nasal spray, nicotine vapor inhaler, and nicotine lozenge. Before initiating nicotine-replacement treatments, smokers are advised to discontinue the use of other nicotine-containing products because of concerns about nicotine toxicity that might result from concurrent use of nicotine-containing products (e.g., cigarettes in combination with the nicotine patch). All of these treatments have been demonstrated to increase quit rates in controlled clinical studies.[12] These studies have been conducted under fairly strict conditions, with a prescribed quitting period, several visits to the clinic to assess progress, and the usual trappings of a clinical research study, often including the collection of saliva or other samples to detect tobacco use. That's a far cry from buying nicotine gum at the corner store, with no plan for quitting, no follow-up interviews, and no monitoring. Thus, it is not surprising that the average person might have great difficulties quitting even with the aid of nicotine-replacement medications.

In 1997, the FDA approved bupropion (Zyban), the first non-nicotine pharmacotherapy for smoking cessation. Bupropion is also used in the treatment of depression, where it is referred to as Wellbutrin. Although the neurochemical mechanisms that underlie bupropion's therapeutic effects have yet to be definitively determined, the mechanism of action most commonly attributed to bupropion is inhibition of dopamine and norepinephrine reuptake and, to a lesser extent, blockade of acetylcholine receptors.[13] Unlike nicotine-replacement therapies, there is no absolute requirement for the smoker to abstain from the

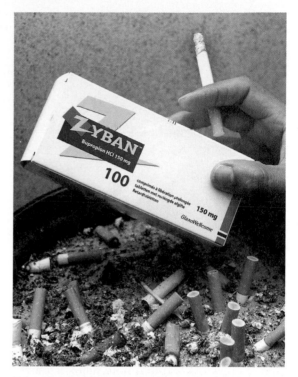

Zyban (bupropion) was the first non-nicotine pharmacotherapy for smoking cessation. The drug, also used to treat depression, appears to gradually reduce cravings for cigarettes.

use of nicotine-containing products. Bupropion has been shown to gradually decrease cigarette craving and use in some clinical trials. Because nicotine-replacement medications and bupropion have been demonstrated to decrease cigarette smoking when administered alone, it has been suggested that greater treatment success might be achieved if the two strategies were combined. Unfortunately, data from a recent investigation indicated that the addition of bupropion treatment to nicotine-replacement therapy did not significantly increase smoking cessation rates.[14]

Opioids

Historically, anticholinergic drugs, such as belladonna, were used in the treatment of opioid

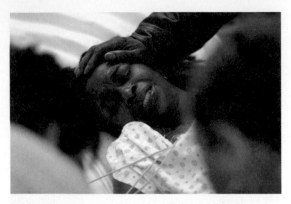

Drug withdrawal can have unpleasant and potentially dangerous symptoms. Drugs may be administered to reduce withdrawal symptoms.

dependence.[15] The idea was that anticholinergics would produce a state of delirium for several days, after which the dependent person would emerge cured of dependence without remembering the dreadful experience of the withdrawal process. A more recent version of this approach is "rapid opioid detoxification." Opioid-dependent individuals are anesthetized and, while unconscious, are given an opioid antagonist, so that withdrawal will occur while they are unconscious. After 24 hours the patient is released and enters a period of counseling, combined with continued opioid antagonist treatment. This procedure has been vehemently criticized because it increases the risk of problems during the withdrawal process and because aftercare (behavioral/psychosocial treatment) is often deemphasized.

Although opioid withdrawal is not life threatening, symptoms such as nausea, vomiting, diarrhea, aches, and pain can be unpleasant. Medications are administered to minimize discomfort. Methadone (Dolophine), an opioid analgesic developed in Germany during World War II, is commonly used in this capacity. It has a long duration of action, which means that it needs to be taken less frequently to prevent withdrawal symptoms. Another medication that has been shown to decrease opioid withdrawal symptoms is buprenorphine, a partial opioid agonist. Buprenorphine has a relatively large margin of safety and a low overdose potential. In addition, it has a long duration of action and blocks the effects of other opioid agonists such as heroin. As a result of these features, both methadone and buprenorphine are FDA-approved opioid-dependence medications. These medications are not only used during detoxification, but they are also used during maintenance. Methadone maintenance, the most common form of treatment for opioid dependence, may continue for months or years. The duration of buprenorphine maintenance might be similar, but because the medication has only recently received approval, this is not yet known.

One major concern in the treatment of opioid dependence is opioid-induced overdose, which could lead to a coma and eventual death via respiratory depression. Because the short-acting opioid antagonist naloxone has a greater affinity for brain opioid receptors than do most opioid agonists, including heroin, it is often used for treating opioid overdose. Following its administration, naloxone displaces the opioid agonist from the receptors, and thereby rapidly reverses the overdose. This observation led to speculations about the use of opioid antagonists in treating opioid dependence. That is, if a user takes heroin, for example, while being maintained on an opioid antagonist, the effects of heroin would not be felt. This rationale provided the basis for the approval of the long-acting opioid antagonist naltrexone for treating opioid dependence. Although naltrexone therapy has been shown to be effective in the treatment of opioid dependence, this therapy appears to be appropriate for only highly motivated individuals because most opioid abusers enrolled in naltrexone therapy prematurely discontinue treatment. To circumvent compliance problems, a new depot formulation of naltrexone, which requires one administration per month, is being studied as a potential opioid-dependence treatment medication. Initial findings are encouraging, as depot naltrexone has been demonstrated to block heroin-related effects for up to six weeks.[16] An interesting problem arises if a patient on naltrexone is involved in an accident and requires some pain relief. Current practice is to give high doses of hydromorphone (Dilaudid) to overcome the antagonism. This should be done only in a hospital and with extreme caution.

Cocaine

Although a cocaine withdrawal syndrome has been difficult to demonstrate in humans under controlled laboratory conditions, this syndrome has been described in clinical settings. Cocaine withdrawal is characterized by self-reports of depression, nervousness, dysphoria, **anhedonia,** fatigue, irritability, sleep and activity disturbances, and craving for cocaine.[17] Since risk of relapse may be greatest during the initial withdrawal period, it has been hypothesized that a withdrawal syndrome may underlie vulnerability.[18] The behavioral and mood changes that accompany cocaine withdrawal are thought to correlate with neurochemical changes. Specifically, although acute administration of cocaine increases the activity of dopamine, norepinephrine, and serotonin, chronic administration may produce an opposite effect.[19] During withdrawal from cocaine, monoaminergic activity is thought to be hyporesponsive (reduced activity); it has been suggested that reduced dopaminergic activity underlies anhedonia and craving,[20] whereas reduced serotoninergic activity underlies dysphoria, negative affect, and impulsivity.[21] Because administration of cocaine increases the activity of these neurotransmitters[22] and transiently improves mood,[23] it has been proposed that medications that increase dopaminergic and/or serotoninergic activity may be useful in treating withdrawal symptoms and thereby prevent relapse. Although numerous medications (e.g., several antidepressants) have been evaluated according to this theory, none has been found to be useful in treating cocaine withdrawal symptoms or dependence. Regarding potential cocaine maintenance medications, the situation is similar—many have been studied, but few have shown promise. Currently, there are no approved pharmacotherapies for cocaine dependence.

Cannabis

While most users of cannabis consume the drug infrequently without apparent negative consequences, a small proportion experience problems related to frequent cannabis use. An estimated one in 11 cannabis users will become dependent:[24] Rates of cannabis dependence in several developed countries (e.g., Australia, North America, South Africa) have increased substantially over the past decade[25] as well as the number of individuals seeking treatment.[26] Many individuals seeking treatment for cannabis dependence reported experiencing withdrawal symptoms and that these symptoms made it more difficult to maintain abstinence.[27] As a result, efforts to develop medication for cannabis dependence have primarily focused on relieving withdrawal symptoms. Cannabis withdrawal is characterized by symptoms of irritability, anxiety, sleep disruptions, and aches.[28] A growing number of medications have been tested for efficacy in relieving these symptoms, but only one has been demonstrated to be effective—oral Δ^9-THC. The primary reason for evaluating the effects of oral Δ^9-THC on cannabis withdrawal was based on the idea of substituting a longer-acting pharmacologically equivalent drug for the abused substance, stabilizing the individual on that drug, and then gradually withdrawing the substituted drug, thus decreasing the likelihood of precipitating abstinence symptoms. It was recently demonstrated that oral Δ^9-THC markedly reduced symptoms associated with cannabis abstinence including self-reported ratings of cannabis craving, anxiety, misery,

anhedonia [an hee *doe'* nee ya]: lack of emotional response; especially an inability to experience joy or pleasure.

Mind / Body Connection

The Nature of Dependence

Is drug dependence strictly a matter of neurotransmitters and neural adaptation, as seems increasingly to be the accepted viewpoint, or will it ultimately be impossible to understand such a complex set of behaviors by reducing the problem to its biochemical correlates? This has been a huge and ongoing debate among proponents of the various views of drug dependence, but currently the research funding and most of the information seen in the popular media favor biological approaches to understanding these problems. This chapter's focus on drug treatments for substance dependence seems to be based on an implied acceptance that some biochemical imbalance is at the heart of people who are seemingly unable to exert control over their own drug-using behavior.

However, many, including proponents of the Alcoholics Anonymous philosophy, believe that substance dependence is a "spiritual" disorder—essentially that an individual human is not recognizing the need to draw upon either God or some other source of spiritual strength to help win the struggle with the bottle or needle or pill. For these people, drug treatments, especially of the substitution/maintenance type, are often seen as a crutch that does not address the individual's basic problem and cannot therefore be of much long-term benefit.

To others, substance abuse and dependence can be approached through behavioral techniques such as contingency management or through a variety of psychosocial approaches such as group therapy. For them, medication might be seen as a temporary aid in assisting the person to "reprogram" his or her thinking, routines, and social interactions, but it is ultimately these changes in relationships, attitudes, and activities that are the key to longer-term success.

How do you feel about the evidence showing that former heroin users can often be maintained for years on methadone, a legal substitute, while they attend school, work, and otherwise enjoy more productive and less dangerous lives than if they had continued to use heroin?

---

and sleep disturbance.[29] The medication also reversed the withdrawal-associated psychomotor performance decrements as well as the anorexia and weight loss associated with cannabis withdrawal. These results indicate that moderate doses of oral Δ^9-THC might be beneficial in the treatment of cannabis dependence.[30] To date, no medications are approved for the treatment of cannabis dependence.

Treatment: The Big Picture in the United States

In each state, the agency that has primary responsibility for public funding of substance abuse treatment programs submits annual reports to the U.S. Substance Abuse and Mental Health Services Administration (SAMHSA). Between 1993 and 2003, the data from more than 1.3 million admissions each year for substance abuse were compiled into the *Treatment Episode Data Set*.[31] In 2003, four substances accounted for about 90 percent of these admissions: alcohol (42 percent), opioids (18 percent), marijuana (16 percent), and cocaine (14 percent). Of those who reported opioids as their primary drug of abuse, 84 percent were heroin users, and 72 percent of those who reported cocaine as the primary drug were crack cocaine smokers. The average age of those admitted with marijuana as the primary drug was 23 years of age. In 2003, 61 percent of the substance-abuse clients were treated as outpatients, 22 percent as hospital inpatients (detoxification), and 17 percent in a residential setting. These data suggest that the bulk of our substance-abuse treatment should focus on developing more effective interventions for alcohol, opioid, marijuana, and cocaine abuse that can be delivered on an outpatient basis. As reviewed previously, most recent research efforts to develop pharmacotherapies to treat substance abuse have been aimed at decreasing the use of these substances (and nicotine). But, without effective outpatient behavioral/psychosocial interventions, the overall success of pharmacotherapies alone to treat substance abuse is likely to be unimpressive. This is because substance abusers may show poor medication compliance, even on medications that have been demonstrated to be effective at decreasing substance use (e.g., disulfiram for alcohol dependence and naltrexone for opioid dependence). Moreover, substance abusers often present with additional mental disorders and multiple other functional impairments. Thus, behavioral/psychosocial treatments are needed to address these issues so that overall treatment success is enhanced.

Is Treatment Effective?

There is a widespread belief that substance-abuse treatment is often ineffective. We've all heard of well-known athletes who have been in treatment programs and later are found to be using illegal drugs, and we might know an alcohol abuser who went into treatment and later began drinking again. Treatment doesn't work for every client every time, especially if our expectation is that one treatment exposure will eliminate the use of the substance for the rest of the person's life. Substance dependence is often a chronic illness that shares many characteristics with other chronic illnesses such as diabetes, hypertension, and asthma. There are no reliable "cures," and all of these conditions may require continuing care throughout the patient's life.

An important question is whether substance-abuse treatment programs have any beneficial effect—and, if they do, are their effects worth the cost? A report from the Institute of Medicine addressed these questions by studying heroin abusers.[31] The report concluded (1) methadone maintenance pays for itself (in reduced crime and increased employment) during the time it is administered, and

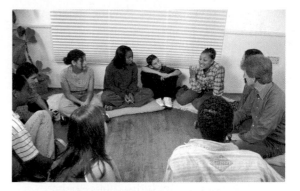

Drug treatment doesn't work for every person every time, but overall, treatment does reduce drug use, reduce associated criminal activity, and increase employment. By continuing to participate in outpatient drug rehabilitation meetings, these teens increase the likelihood that their substance-abuse treatment will be a success over the long term.

posttreatment effects are an economic bonus; (2) although therapeutic communities cost more than methadone maintenance, they result in better status after treatment; and (3) outpatient drug-free programs attract more clients without a criminal background and therefore do not reduce criminal activity as much as the other two approaches; they are inexpensive, however, and do produce a net benefit because of increased employment. In addition, a report by the California Department of Alcohol and Drug Programs concluded that, on average, seven dollars are saved for every dollar invested in the treatment of alcohol and other drug abuse.[32] Alcohol and other drug use was reduced by about two-fifths after treatment; treatment for crack cocaine, powder cocaine, and methamphetamine use was equally effective as for alcohol; and criminal activity declined by about two-thirds after treatment.

One report reviewed 53 studies of the effectiveness of substance-abuse treatments for adolescents. Overall, most of the treated adolescents had significant reductions in substance use and problems in other life areas in the year following treatment, and an average of 32 percent remained abstinent at the end of a year. Successful program completion, involvement in outpatient therapy, and the inclusion of the family therapy as one treatment component all appeared to predict success.[33]

Overall, substance abuse treatment does work. It saves lives, saves money, and is, therefore, a worthwhile investment.

Summary

- Treatment for substance abuse and dependence may include both behavioral/psychosocial approaches and the use of various medications.

- Many of today's psychosocial treatment programs are heavily influenced by the philosophy developed by Alcoholics Anonymous. These are often referred to as 12-step programs.

- Motivational interviewing is usually used in conjunction with stages of change theory, to help move people from one stage to another in the process of quitting.

- Medications are often used to ease withdrawal during detoxification. Maintaining abstinence may be assisted by either agonist substitution or by antagonist treatment.

- Antabuse (disulfiram) interferes with alcohol metabolism to produce illness if the patient uses alcohol. Naltrexone and acamprosate are also available to assist in preventing relapse.

- Zyban (bupropion) may be used alone or in combination with various forms of nicotine-replacement therapy to aid smoking cessation.

- Methadone is the drug most commonly used to treat opioid dependence, although buprenorphine is now also available for use in substitution/maintenance treatment. Naltrexone blocks the effects of any opioids the user might take, but it has not been as effective as methadone in helping people to abstain from heroin or other abused opioids. Rapid opioid detoxifica-

tion is a short-term method to avoid experiencing withdrawal symptoms.

- Despite many attempts, no medication has yet been developed specifically for treatment of cocaine dependence.

- Cannabis withdrawal symptoms can be relieved by the use of oral THC, which shows promise as a treatment for cannabis dependence.

- Overall, substance-abuse treatment programs are considered to be effective because they do help many people to abstain, sometimes only for a few months, but often for many years. The benefits far exceed the cost of providing the programs.

Review Questions

1. List at least 8 of the 12 steps of Alcoholics Anonymous.
2. What are the four "stages of change" listed in the text?
3. Describe the kinds of contingencies used in contingency management: What happens if the client has several "clean" urine samples in a row? What happens if the client fails one of the urine sample tests?
4. Give one example for each: agonist/substitution therapy, antagonist therapy, and punishment therapy.
5. What drugs are typically used to reduce withdrawal symptoms during alcohol detoxification?
6. Compare and contrast the use of disulfiram (Antabuse) versus either naltrexone or acamprosate for alcohol dependence.
7. List four of the five types of available nicotine replacement therapy.
8. How are methadone and buprenorphine similar to each other and different from naltrexone as treatments for opioid dependence?
9. The effort to develop drugs to treat cocaine dependence has targeted which neurotransmitter systems?

10. How big a problem is cannabis dependence, and what seems to be the most promising drug treatment currently being studied?

References

1. Rollnick, S., & W.R. Miller. "What Is Motivational Interviewing?" *Behavioural and Cognitive Psychotherapy* 23 (1995), pp. 325–34.
2. Polcin, D.L., G.P. Galloway, J. Palmer, and W. Mains. "The Case for High-Dose Motivational Enhancement Therapy." *Substance Use and Misuse* 39 (2004), pp. 331–43.
3. Higgins, S.T., S.H. Heil, and J.P. Lussier. "Clinical Implications of Reinforcement as a Determinant of Substance Use Disorders. *Annual Review of Psychology* 55 (2004), pp. 431–61.
4. Carroll, K.M., B.J. Rounsaville, C. Nich, L.T. Gordon, P.W. Wirtz, and F. Gawin. "One-year Follow-up of Psychotherapy and Pharmacotherapy for Cocaine Dependence. Delayed Emergence of Psychotherapy Effects." *Archives of General Psychiatry* 51 (1994), pp. 989–97.
5. Aharonovich, E., E. Nunes, and D. Hasin. "Cognitive Impairment, Retention and Abstinence Among Cocaine Abusers in Cognitive-behavioral Treatment." *Drug and Alcohol Dependence* 71 (2003), pp. 207–11.
6. Chrousos, G.P., & P.W. Gold. "The Concepts of Stress and Stress System Disorders: Overview of Physical and Behavioral Homeostasis." *JAMA* 267 (1992), pp. 1244–52.
7. Woods, J.H., J.L. Katz, and G. Winger. "Benzodiazepines: Use, Abuse, and Consequences." *Pharmacology Review* 44 (1992), pp. 151–347.
8. Hald, J., E. Jacobsen, and V. Larsen. "The Sensitizing Effect of Tetraethylthiuram Disulfide (Antabuse) to Ethyl Alcohol." *Acta Pharmocologica et Toxicologica* 4 (1948), pp. 285–96.
9. O'Malley, S.S., A.J. Jaffe, and G. Chang, et al. "Naltrexone and Coping Skills Therapy for Alcohol Dependence: A Controlled Study." *Archives of General Psychiatry* 49 (1992), pp. 894–98; and Volpicelli, J., C. O'Brien, and A. Alterman, et al. "Naltrexone in the Treatment of Alcohol Dependence." *Archives of General Psychiatry* 49 (1992), pp. 867–80.
10. Sinclair, J.D. "Evidence About the Use of Naltrexone and for Different Ways of Using It in the Treatment of Alcoholism." *Alcohol* 36 (2001), pp. 2–10.
11. Dahchour, A., & P. De Witte. "Ethanol and Amino Acids in the Central Nervous System: Assessment of the Pharmacological Actions of Acamprosate." *Progress in Neurobiology* 60 (2000), pp. 343–62.
12. George, T.P., & S.S. O'Malley. "Current Pharmacological Treatments for Nicotine Dependence. *Trends in Pharmacological Sciences* 25 (2004), pp. 42–48.
13. Ascher, J.A., J.O. Cole, J. Colin, J.P. Feighner, R.M. Ferris, H.C. Fibiger, R.N. Golden, P. Martin, W.Z. Potter, E. Richelson, and F. Sluser. "Bupropion: A Review of Its Mechanism of Antidepressant Activity." *Journal of Clinical Psychiatry* 56 (1995), pp. 395–401; and Slemmer, J.E., B.R. Martin, and M.I. Damaj. "Bupropion Is a Nicotinic Antagonist." *Journal of Pharmacology Experimental Therapies* 295 (2000), pp. 321–27.
14. Simon, J.A., C. Duncan, T.P. Carmody, and E.S. Hudes. "Bupropion for Smoking Cessation: A Randomized Trial." *Archives of Internal Medicine* 164 (2004), pp. 1797–1803.
15. Latimer, D., & J. Goldberg. *Flowers in the Blood: The Story of Opium.* New York: Arno Press, 1981.
16. Comer, S.D., E.D. Collins, H.D. Kleber, E.S. Nuwayser, J.H. Kerrigan, and M.W. Fischman. "Depot Naltrexone: Long-lasting Antagonism of the Effects of Heroin in Humans." *Psychopharmacology* 159 (2002), pp. 351–60.
17. Gawin, F.H., & H.D. Kleber, "Abstinence Symptomatology and Psychiatric Diagnosis in Cocaine Abusers. Clinical Observations." *Archives of General Psychiatry* 43 (1986), pp. 107–13.
18. Kampman, K.M., J.R. Volpicelli, F. Mulvaney, M. Rukstalis, A.I. Alterman, H. Pettinati, R.M. Weinrieb, and C.P. O'Brien. "Cocaine Withdrawal Severity and Urine Toxicology Results from Treatment Entry Predict Outcome in Medication Trials for Cocaine Dependence." *Addictive Behaviors* 27 (2002), pp. 251–60.
19. Woolverton, W.L., & K.M. Johnson. "Neurobiology of Cocaine Abuse." *Trends in Pharmacological Sciences* 13 (1992), pp. 193–200.
20. Rothman, R.B., B.E. Blough, and M.H. Baumann. "Appetite Suppressants as Agonist Substitution Therapies for Stimulant Dependence." *Annals of the New York Academy of Sciences* 965 (2002), pp. 109–26; and Weiss, F., A. Markou, M.T. Lorang, and G.F. Koob. "Basal Extracellular Dopamine Levels in the Nucleus Accumbens Are Decreased During Cocaine Withdrawal After Unlimited-access Self-administration." *Brain Research* 593 (1992), pp. 314–18.
21. Baumann, M.H., K.M. Becketts, and R.B. Rothman. "Evidence for Alterations in Presynaptic Serotonergic Function During Withdrawal from Chronic Cocaine in Rats." *European Journal of Pharmacology* 282 (1995), pp. 87–93.
22. Andrews, C.M., & I. Lucki. "Effects of Cocaine on Extracellular Dopamine and Serotonin Levels in the Nucleus Accumbens." *Psychopharmacology* 155 (2001), pp. 221–29.
23. Fischman, M.W., C.R. Schuster, J. Javaid, Y. Hatano, and J. Davis. "Acute Tolerance Development to the Cardiovascular and Subjective Effects of Cocaine." *Journal of Pharmacology and Experimental Therapeutics* 235 (1985), pp. 677–82.
24. Anthony, J.C., L.A. Warner, and R.C. Kessler. "Comparative Epidemiology of Dependence on Tobacco, Alcohol, Controlled Substances, and Inhalants: Basic Findings from the National Comorbidity Survey." *Experimental and Clinical Psychopharmacology* 2 (1994), pp. 244–68.
25. Bhana, A., C.D. Parry, B. Myers, A. Pluddemann, N.K. Morojele, and A.J. Flisher. "The South African Community Epidemiology Network on Drug Use (SACENDU) Project, Phases 1–8—Cannabis and Mandrax." *South African Medical Journal* 92 (2002), pp. 542–47; and Substance Abuse and Mental Health Services Administration (SAMHSA). *Overview of Findings from the 2002 National Survey on Drug Use and Health* (NHSDA Series H-21, DHHS Publication No. SMA 03-3774). Rockville, MD: Office of Applied Studies, 2003.
26. *Treatment Episode Data Set (TEDS)* 1996–1999. National Admissions to Substance Abuse Treatment Services. Rockville, MD: U.S. Department of Health and Human Services, Substance Abuse and Mental Health Services Administration, 2001.

27. Stephens, R.S., T.F. Babor, R. Kadden, M. Miller. "The Marijuana Treatment Project: Rationale, Design and Participant Characteristics." *Addiction* 97, Supplement 1 (2002), pp. 109–24.

28. Budney, A.J., J.R. Hughes, B.A. Moore, and R. Vandrey. "Review of the Validity and Significance of Cannabis Withdrawal Syndrome." *American Journal of Psychiatry* 161 (2004), pp. 1967–77.

29. Haney, M., C.L. Hart, S.K. Vosburg, J. Nasser, A. Bennett, C. Zubaran, and R.W. Foltin. "Marijuana Withdrawal in Humans: Effects of Oral THC or Divalproex." *Neuropsychopharmacology* 29 (2004), pp. 158–70.

30. Lichtman, A.H., J. Fisher, and B.R. Martin. "Precipitated Cannabinoid Withdrawal Is Reversed by Delta(9)-tetrahydrocannabinol or Clonidine." *Pharmacology, Biochemistry and Behavior* 69 (2001), pp. 181–88.

31. *Treatment Episode Data Set (TEDS)* 1993–2003. SAMHSA Office of Applied Studies. Rockville, MD: U.S. Department of Health and Human Services, November 2005.

32. Lewis, D.C. "More Evidence That Treatment Works." *The Brown University Digest of Addiction Theory and Application* 13 (1994), p. 12.

33. Williams, R.J., & S.Y. Chang. "A Comprehensive and Comparative Review of Adolescent Substance Abuse Treatment Outcome." *Clinical Psychology, Science and Practice* 7 (2000), pp. 138–66.

Appendix A Drug Names

A

Abilify (aripiprazole): a typical antipsychotic.

acamprosate (Campral): treatment for alcohol dependence.

acetaminophen: OTC analgesic. Similar to aspirin in its effects.

acetophenazine: Tindal. Antipsychotic.

acetylsalicylic acid: aspirin. OTC analgesic.

alprazolam: Xanax. Benzodiazepine sedative.

Amanita muscaria: hallucinogenic mushroom.

Ambien: zolpidem. Non-benzodiazepine sedative-hypnotic.

amitriptyline: Elavil, Endep. Tricyclic antidepressant.

amobarbital: Amytal. Barbiturate sedative-hypnotic.

amoxapine: Asendin. Tricyclic antidepressant.

amphetamine: Benzedrine. CNS stimulant and sympathomimetic.

Amytal: amobarbital. Barbiturate sedative-hypnotic.

Anavar: oxandrolone. Anabolic steroid.

angel dust: street name for PCP.

Antabuse: disulfiram. Alters metabolism of alcohol; used to treat alcohol dependence.

aprobarbital: Alurate. Barbiturate sedative-hypnotic.

Artane: trihexyphenidyl. Anticholinergic used to control extrapyramidal symptoms.

Asendin: amoxapine. Tricyclic antidepressant.

aspirin: acetylsalicylic acid. OTC analgesic.

Ativan: lorazepam. Benzodiazepine sedative.

atropine: anticholinergic.

Aventyl: nortriptyline. Tricyclic antidepressant.

ayahuasca: a combination of two plants, one of which contains DMT. Hallucinogen.

B

belladonna: poisonous anticholinergic plant.

Benzedrine: amphetamine. CNS stimulant and sympathomimetic. Brand name no longer used.

benzodiazepines: class of sedative-hypnotics that includes diazepam (Valium).

benztropine: Cogentin. Anticholinergic used to control extrapyramidal symptoms.

black tar: a type of illicit heroin.

bromide: group of salts with sedative properties.

buprenorphine (Subutex): opioid used as a maintenance treatment for heroin users.

bupropion: Wellbutrin. Atypical antidepressant. Also Zyban, to reduce craving during tobacco cessation.

butabarbital: Butisol. Barbiturate sedative-hypnotic.

Butisol: butabarbital. Barbiturate sedative-hypnotic.

C

caffeine: mild stimulant found in coffee and in OTC preparations.

cannabis: the marijuana plant.

carbamazepine: Tegretol. Anticonvulsant also used as a mood stabilizer in bipolar disorder.

Catapres: clonidine. Antihypertensive drug shown to reduce narcotic withdrawal symptoms.

Celexa: citalopram. Atypical antidepressant.

chloral hydrate: Noctec. Nonbarbiturate sedative-hypnotic.

chlordiazepoxide: Librium. Benzodiazepine sedative.

chlorpheniramine maleate: OTC antihistamine.

chlorpromazine: Thorazine. Antipsychotic.

chlorprothixene: Taractan. Antipsychotic.

Cibalith: lithium citrate. Salt used in treating mania and bipolar affective disorders.

Citalopram: Celexa. Atypical antidepressant.

clenbuterol: an alpha-2 adrenergic agonist developed to treat asthma, but used by athletes to build muscle.

clonidine: Catapres. Antihyperintensive drug shown to reduce narcotic withdrawal symptoms.

clorazepate: Tranxene. Benzodiazepine sedative.

clozapine: Clozaril. Atypical antipsychotic.

Clozaril: clozapine. Atypical antipsychotic.

cocaine: CNS stimulant and local anesthetic.

codeine: opioid analgesic found in opium.

Cogentin: benztropine. Anticholinergic used to control extrapyramidal symptoms.

Compazine: prochlorperazine. Antipsychotic.

creatine: natural substance found in meat and fish that might have anabolic properties and is used by athletes.

Cylert: pemoline. Stimulant used to treat ADD with hyperactivity.

D

Dalmane: flurazepam. Benzodiazepine hypnotic.

Darvon: propoxyphene. Opioid analgesic.

Datura: genus of plants, many of which are anticholinergic.

Demerol: meperidine. Opioid analgesic.

Depakene: valproic acid. Anticonvulsant also used as a mood stabilizer in bipolar disorder.

desipramine: Norpramin, Pertofrane. Tricyclic antidepressant.

Desoxyn: methamphetamine. CNS stimulant and sympathomimetic.

Desyrel: trazodone. Atypical antidepressant.

Dexedrine: dextroamphetamine. CNS stimulant and sympathomimetic.

dexfenfluramine: Redux. Appetite suppressant, removed from the market in 1997.

dextroamphetamine: Dexedrine. CNS stimulant and sympathomimetic.

dextromethorphan: OTC cough suppressant.

diazepam: Valium. Benzodiazepine sedative.

diethylpropion: Tenuate, Tepanil. Amphetamine-like appetite suppressant.

dihydrocodeine: opioid analgesic.

Dilaudid: hydromorphone. Opioid analgesic.

diphenhydramine: antihistamine.

disulfiram: Antabuse. Alters metabolism of alcohol; used to treat alcoholism.

DMT: dimethyltryptamine. Hallucinogen.

Dolophine: methadone. Opioid analgesic.

DOM: hallucinogen.

doxepin: Sinequan. Tricyclic antidepressant.

dronabinol: Marinol. Prescription form of delta-9-tetrahydrocannabinol.

E

Effexor: venlafaxine. Antidepressant (SSRI).

Elavil: amitriptyline. Tricyclic antidepressant.

Endep: amitriptyline. Tricyclic antidepressant.

endorphin: endogenous substance with effects similar to those of the opioid analgesics.

enkephalin: endogenous substance with effects similar to those of the opioid analgesics.

ephedrine: sympathomimetic used to treat asthma.

Equanil: meprobamate. Nonbarbiturate sedative-hypnotic.

Eskalith: lithium carbonate. Salt used in treating mania and bipolar affective disorders.

eszopiclone: Lunesta. Non-benzodiazepine sedative-hypnotic.

F

fenfluramine: Pondimin. Appetite suppressant, removed from the market in 1997.

fentanyl: Sublimaze. Potent synthetic analgesic.

flunitrazepam: Rohypnol. Benzodiazepine hypnotic, not sold in the U.S. Known as a "date-rape" drug.

fluoxetine: Prozac. Antidepressant (SSRI).

fluphenazine: Permitil, Prolixin. Antipsychotic.

flurazepam: Dalmane. Benzodiazepine hypnotic.

G

GEOdon: Ziprasidone. Atypical antipsychotic.

GHB: gamma hydroxybutyrate. CNS depressant, produced naturally in small amounts in the human brain. Has been used recreationally and, in combination with alcohol, has some reputation as a "date-rape" drug.

Ginkgo biloba: a dietary supplement believed by some to increase blood circulation.

H

Halcion: triazolam. Benzodiazepine hypnotic.

Haldol: haloperidol. Antipsychotic.

haloperidol: Haldol. Antipsychotic.

henbane: poisonous anticholinergic plant.

heroin: Diacetylmorphine Narcotic analgesic.

hydrocodone: Opioid analgesic.

hydromorphone: Dilaudid. Opioid analgesic.

I

ibogaine: hallucinogen, also proposed to reduce craving in drug addicts.

ibuprofen: analgesic and anti-inflammatory.

imipramine: Janimine, Tofranil. Tricyclic antidepressant.

isocarboxazid: Marplan. MAO inhibitor used as antidepressant.

J

Janimine: imipramine. Tricyclic antidepressant.

K

Ketalar: ketamine. Dissociative anesthetic.

ketamine: Ketalar. Dissociative anesthetic.

Klonopin: Clonazepam. Benzodiazepine sedative-hypnotic, also used as an anticonvulsant.

L

LAAM: L-alpha-acetyl-methadol. Long-lasting synthetic opioid used in maintenance treatment of narcotic addicts.

Lamictal: lamotrigine. Anticonvulsant also used as a mood stabilizer in bipolar disorder.

lamotrigine: Lamictal. Anticonvulsant also used as a mood stabilizer in bipolar disorder.

laudanum: tincture (alcohol solution) of opium.

Lexapro: escitalopram. Atypical antidepressant.

Librium: chlordiazepoxide. Benzodiazepine sedative.

Lithane: lithium carbonate.

lithium carbonate, lithium citrate: salts used in treating mania and bipolar affective disorders.

Lithobid: lithium carbonate.

lorazepam: Ativan. Benzodiazepine sedative.

Lortab: acetaminophen-hydrocodone combination, Analgesic.

loxapine: Loxitane. Antipsychotic.

Loxitane: loxapine. Antipsychotic.

LSD: lysergic acid diethylamide. Hallucinogen.

Ludiomil: maprotiline. Tricyclic antidepressant.

Luminal: phenobarbital. Barbiturate sedative-hypnotic.

Lunesta: eszopiclone. Non-benzodiazepine sedative-hypnotic.

M

mandrake: anticholinergic plant.

maprotiline: Ludiomil. Tricyclic antidepressant.

Marijuana: Common name for the cannabis plant and for its dried leaves.

Marinol: dronabinol. Prescription form of delta-9-tetrahydrocannabinol.

Marplan: isocarboxazid. MAO inhibitor used as antidepressant.

Mazanor: mazindol. Appetite suppressant.

mazinodol: Mazanor, Sanorex. Appetite suppressant.

MDA: hallucinogen.

MDMA: hallucinogen.

Mebaral: mephobarbital. Barbiturate sedative-hypnotic.

Mellaril: thioridazine. Antipsychotic.

meperidine: Demerol. Opioid analgesic.

mephobarbital: Mebaral. Barbiturate sedative-hypnotic.

meprobamate: Equanil, Miltown. Nonbarbiturate sedative-hypnotic.

mescaline: hallucinogen found in peyote cactus.

mesoridazine: Serentil. Antipsychotic.

methadone: Dolophine. Narcotic analgesic.

methamphetamine: Desoxyn, Methedrine. CNS stimulant and sympathomimetic.

methaqualone: Quaalude, Sopor. Nonbarbiturate sedative-hypnotic.

methylphenidate: Ritalin. Stimulant used to treat ADD with hyperactivity.

Metrazol: pentylenetetrazol. Convulsant formerly used in convulsive therapy.

Miltown: meprobamate. Nonbarbiturate sedative-hypnotic.

mirtazapine: Remeron. Atypical antidepressant.

Moban: molindone. Antipsychotic.

molindone: Moban. Antipsychotic.

morphine: opioid analgesic.

N

naloxone: Narcan. Opioid antagonist.

naltrexone: Trexan, reVIA. Opioid antagonist. Used in treating alcoholism.

Nardil: phenelzine. MAO inhibitor used as antidepressant.

Navane: thiothixene. Antipsychotic.

Nembutal: pentobarbital. Barbiturate sedative-hypnotic.

Norpramin: desipramine. Tricyclic antidepressant.

nortriptyline: Aventyl, Pamelor. Tricyclic antidepressant.

Novocain: Procaine. Local anesthetic.

Numorphan: oxymorphone. Opioid analgesic.

O

olanzepine: Zyprex. Atypical antipsychotic.

opium: opioid analgesic.

oxandrolone: Anavar. Anabolic steroid.

oxazepam: Serax. Benzodiazepine sedative.

oxycodone: Percodan. Opioid analgesic.

Oxycontin: continuous-release form of oxycodone.

oxymorphone: Numorphan. Opioid analgesic.

P

Pamelor: nortriptyline. Tricyclic antidepressant.

paraldehyde: nonbarbiturate sedative-hypnotic.

paregoric: tincture (alcohol solution) of opium.

Parnate: tranylcypromine. MAO inhibitor used as antidepressant.

paroxetine: Paxil. Antidepressant (SSRI).

Paxil: paroxetine. Antidepressant (SSRI).

PCP: phencyclidine, angel dust. Hallucinogen.

pemoline: Cylert. Stimulant used to treat ADD with hyperactivity.

pentazocine: Talwin. Opioid analgesic.

pentobarbital: Nembutal. Barbiturate sedative-hypnotic.

pentylenetetrazol: Metrazol. Convulsant formerly used in convulsive therapy.

Percodan: oxycodone. Opioid analgesic.

Permitil: fluphenazine. Antipsychotic.

perphenazine: Trilafon. Antipsychotic.

Pertofrane: desipramine. Tricyclic antidepressant.

peyote: cactus containing mescaline (hallucinogenic).

phencyclidine: PCP, angel dust. Hallucinogen.

phendimetrazine: amphetamine-like appetite suppressant.

phenelzine: Nardil. MAO inhibitor used as antidepressant.

phenmetrazine: Preludin. Amphetamine-like appetite suppressant.

phenobarbital: Luminal. Barbiturate sedative-hypnotic.

phentermine: Amphetamine-like appetite suppressant.

phenylpropanolamine (PPA): OTC appetite suppressant.

Pondimin: fenfluramine. Appetite suppressant, removed from the market in 1997.

Preludin: phenmetrazine. Amphetamine-like appetite suppressant.

prochlorperazine: Compazine. Antipsychotic.

Prolixin: fluphenazine. Antipsychotic.

propoxyphene: Darvon. Narcotic analgesic.

protriptyline: Vivactil. Tricyclic antidepressant.

Prozac: fluoxetine. Antidepressant (SSRI).

pseudoephedrine: OTC sympathomimetic.

psilocybin: hallucinogen from the Mexican psilocybe mushroom.

Q

Quaalude: methaqualone. Nonbarbiturate sedative-hypnotic.

R

Redux: dexfenfluramine. Appetite suppressant, removed from the market in 1997.

Remeron: mirtazapine. Atypical antidepressant.

Restoril: temazepam. Benzodiazepine hypnotic.

reVIA: naltrexone. Opioid antagonist used in treating alcohol dependence.

Risperdal: risperidone. Atypical antipsychotic.

risperidone: Risperdal. Atypical antipsychotic.

Ritalin: methylphenidate. Stimulant used to treat ADHD.

Rohypnol: flunitrazepam. Benzodiazepine hypnotic, not sold in the U.S., known as a "date-rape" drug.

S

Saint-John's-wort: a dietary supplement used by some to treat depression.

SAMe: S-adenosyl-L-methionine. Dietary supplement proposed as a possible treatment for depression.

Sanorex: mazindol. Appetite suppressant.

scopolamine: anticholinergic.

secobarbital: Seconal. Barbiturate sedative-hypnotic.

Seconal: secobarbital. Barbiturate sedative-hypnotic.

Serax: oxazepam. Benzodiazepine sedative.

Serentil: mesoridazine. Antipsychotic.

Sernyl: former brand name for PCP.

sertraline: Zoloft. Antidepressant (SSRI).

Sinequan: doxepin. Tricyclic antidepressant.

Sonata: zaleplon. Non-benzodiazepine sedative-hypnotic.

Sopor: methaqualone. Nonbarbiturate sedative-hypnotic.

Steroids: Various important hormones and their chemical derivatives. Usually refers to the anabolic steroids used by athletes and body builders.

stanozolol: Winstrol. Anabolic steroid.

Stelazine: trifluoperazine. Antipsychotic.

Sublimaze: fentanyl. Potent synthetic analgesic.

T

Talwin: pentazocine. Opioid analgesic.

Taractan: chlorprothixene. Antipsychotic.

Tegretol: carbamazepine. Anticonvulsant also used as a mood stabilizer in bipolar disorder.

temazepam: Restoril. Benzodiazepine hypnotic.

Tenuate: diethylpropion. Amphetamine-like appetite suppressant.

Tepanil: diethylpropion. Amphetamine-like appetite suppressant.

Teslac: testolactone. Anabolic steroid.

testolactone: Teslac. Anabolic steroid.

theophylline: mild stimulant found in tea; used to treat asthma.

thioridazine: Mellaril. Antipsychotic.

thiothixene: Navane. Antipsychotic.

Thorazine: chlorpromazine. Antipsychotic.

Tindal: acetophenazine. Antipsychotic.

TMA: indole hallucinogen.

Tofranil: imipramine. Tricyclic antidepressant.

Tranxene: clorazepate. Benzodiazepine sedative.

tranylcypromine: Parnate. MAO inhibitor used as an antidepressant.

trazodone: Desyrel. Atypical antidepressant.

Trexan: naltrexone. Opioid antagonist.

triazolam: Halcion. Benzodiazepine hypnotic.

trifluoperazine: Stelazine. Antipsychotic.

trihexyphenidyl: Artane. Anticholinergic used to control extrapyramidal symptoms.

Trilafon: perphenazine. Antipsychotic.

2-CB: catechol hallucinogen.

V

Valium: diazepam. Benzodiazepine sedative.

valproic acid: Depakene. Anticonvulsant also used as a mood stabilizer in bipolar disorder.

venlafaxine: Effexor. Antidepressant (SSRI).

Vesprin: triflupromazine. Antipsychotic.

Vicodin: Hydrocodone-acetaminophen combination. Analgesic.

Vivactil: protriptyline. Tricyclic antidepressant.

W

Wellbutrin: bupropion. Atypical antidepressant.

Winstrol: stanozolol. Anabolic steroid.

X

Xanax: alprazolam. Benzodiazepine sedative.

Z

zaleplon: Sonata. Non-benzodiazepine sedative-hypnotic.

Ziprasidone: Gedon. Atypical antipsychotic.

Zoloft: Sertraline. Antidepressant (SSRI).

Zyban: bupropion. To reduce craving during tobacco cessation.

zolpidem: Ambien. Non-benzodiazepine sedative-hypnotic.

Zyprexa: olanzepine. Atypical antipsychotic.

Appendix B

Resources for Information and Assistance

Federal Government Agencies

National Clearinghouse for Alcohol and Drug Information
Office of Substance Abuse Prevention (OSAP)
P.O. Box 2345
Rockville, MD 20852
(301) 468-2600
(800) 729-6686

Drugs & Crime Data Center
Bureau of Justice Statistics
1600 Research Blvd.
Rockville, MD 20850
(800) 666-3332

NIDA Cocaine Hot Line
(800) 662-HELP
Office on Smoking and Health
5600 Fishers Lane
Rockville, MD 20857
(301) 443-1575

Alcohol

Alcohol Research Information Service
1106 E. Oakland
Lansing, MI 48906
(517) 485-9900

Alcoholics Anonymous World Services
P.O. Box 459, Grand Central Station
New York, NY 10163
(212) 686-1100

American Council on Alcoholism
5024 Campbell Blvd., Suite H
Whitemarsh Business Center
Baltimore, MD 21236
(301) 529-9200

American Health and Temperance Society
6830 Eastern Ave., N.W.
Washington, DC 20012
(202) 722-6736

BACCHUS of the U.S.
(Boost Alcohol Consciousness Concerning the Health of University Students)
P.O. Box 10430
Denver, CO 80210
(303) 871-3068

Licensed Beverage Information Council
1250 I St., Suite 900
Washington, DC 20005
(202) 628-3544

MADD (Mothers Against Drunk Driving)
669 Airport Fwy., Suite 310
Hurst, TX 76053
(817) 268-6233

National Alcohol Hot Line
(800) ALCOHOL

National Council on Alcoholism
12 W. 21st St.
New York, NY 10010
(212) 206-6770

National Woman's Christian Temperance Union
1730 Chicago Ave.
Evanston, IL 60201
(312) 864-1396

RID (Remove Intoxicated Drivers)
P.O. Box 520
Schenectady, NY 12301
(518) 372-0034

Smoking

ASH (Action on Smoking and Health)
2013 H St., N.W.
Washington, DC 20006
(202) 659-4310

Smoking Control Advocacy Resource Center
1730 Rhode Island Ave., N.W.
Washington, DC 20036
(202) 659-8475

Tobacco Institute
1875 I St., N.W.
Washington, DC 20006
(202) 457-4800

Drugs

Alcohol and Drug Problems Association of
    North America
444 N. Capitol St., N.W., Suite 706
Washington, DC 20001
(202) 737-4340

American Council for Drug Education
204 Monroe St., Suite 110
Rockville, MD 20850
(301) 294-0600

Do It Now Foundation
Box 27568
Tempe, AZ 85285
(602) 257-0797

Drug Policy Foundation
4801 Massachusetts Ave., N.W., Suite 400
Washington, DC 20016-2087

Fair Oaks Hospital
19 Prospect St. Box 100
Summit, NJ 07901
(201) 552-7000
(800) COCAINE

Narcotic Educational Foundation of America
5055 Sunset Blvd.
Los Angeles, CA 90027
(213) 663-5171

National Drug Information Center of Families
    in Action, Inc.
2296 Henderson Mill Rd., Suite 204
Atlanta, GA 30345
(404) 934-6364

National Federation of Parents for a
    Drug-Free Youth
1423 N. Jefferson
Springfield, MO 65802-1988
(407) 836-3709

NIDA (National Institute on
    Drug Abuse)
5600 Fishers Lane
Rockville, MD 20857

NORML (National Organization for the Reform
    of Marijuana Laws)
2001 S. St., N.W., Suite 640
Washington, DC 20009
(202) 483-5500

PRIDE (Parent Resource Institute for Drug
    Education)
100 Edgewood Ave., Suite 1002
Atlanta, GA 30303
(800) 241-7946

Drug Information on the Internet

Much information, opinion, misinformation, and discussion about drugs is available on the Internet. It is possible to learn about the latest drug fads, to get involved in arguments about drug policy, and occasionally even to learn some solid facts by browsing on the Internet. But be warned that there is no quality control on many of these computer sites—they represent the ultimate in free expression! You're liable to find such things as a bogus recipe for making LSD from Foster's beer, warnings about water addiction, and other foolishness mixed in with potentially useful information, so take care. Links to some relevant Internet sites are found on the Online Learning Center.

Glossary

A

abstinence Refraining completely from the use of alcohol or another drug. Complete abstinence from alcohol means no drinking at all. Abstinence syndrome: see withdrawal syndrome.

abstinence violation effect The tendency of a person who has been abstaining (as from alcohol), and "slips," to go on and indulge fully, because the rule of abstinence has been broken.

acetaldehyde The chemical product of the first step in the liver's metabolism of alcohol. It is normally present only in small amounts because it is rapidly converted to acetic acid.

acetaminophen An aspirinlike analgesic and antipyretic.

acetylcholine Neurotransmitter found in the parasympathetic branch and in the cerebral cortex.

acetylsalicylic acid The chemical known as aspirin; an over-the-counter drug that relieves pain and reduces fever and inflammation.

action potential A brief electrical signal transmitted along a neuron's axon.

active metabolites Pharmacologically active chemicals formed when enzymes in the body act on a drug.

acute In general, "sharp." In medicine, "rapid." Referring to drugs, the short-term effects or effects of a single administration, as opposed to chronic, or long-term, effects of administration.

additive effects When the effects of two different drugs add up to produce a greater effect than either drug alone. As contrasted with antagonistic effects, in which one drug reduces the effect of another, or synergistic effects, in which one drug greatly amplifies the effect of another.

adenosine A chemical believed to be a neurotransmitter in the CNS, primarily at inhibitory receptors. Caffeine might act by antagonizing the normal action of adenosine on its receptors.

ADHD Attention deficit hyperactivity disorder, a learning disability. Terminology of the DSM-IV-TR.

affective education In general, education that focuses on emotional content or emotional reactions, in contrast to cognitive content. In drug education, one example is learning how to achieve certain "feelings" (of excitement or belonging to a group) without using drugs.

AIDS Acquired immunodeficiency syndrome, a disease in which the body's immune system breaks down, leading eventually to death. Because the disease is spread through the mixing of body fluids, it is more prevalent in intravenous drug users who share needles. The infectious agent is the human immunodeficiency virus (HIV).

alcohol Generally refers to grain alcohol, or ethanol, as opposed to other types of alcohol (for example, wood or isopropyl alcohol), which are too toxic to be drinkable.

alcohol abuse In the DSM-IV-TR, defined as a pattern of pathological alcohol use that causes impairment of social or occupational functioning. Compare with alcohol dependence.

alcohol dehydrogenase The enzyme that metabolizes almost all of the alcohol consumed by an individual. It is found primarily in the liver.

alcohol dependence In the DSM-IV-TR, alcohol dependence is considered a more serious disorder than alcohol abuse, in that dependence includes either tolerance or withdrawal symptoms.

alcoholic personality Personality traits, such as immaturity and dependency, that are frequently found in alcoholics in treatment. Many of these consistent traits might be a result of years of heavy drinking rather than a cause of alcoholism.

Alcoholics Anonymous (AA) A worldwide organization of self-help groups based on alcoholics helping each other achieve and maintain sobriety.

alcoholism The word has many definitions and therefore is not a precise term. Definitions might refer to pathological drinking behavior (e.g., remaining drunk for two days), to impaired functioning (e.g., frequently missing work), or to physical dependence. See also alcohol abuse and alcohol dependence.

alternatives (to drugs) Assuming that there are motives for drug use, such as the need to be accepted by a group, many prevention and treatment programs teach alternative methods for satisfying these motives; may include activities such as relaxation or dancing.

Alzheimer's disease A progressive neurological disease that occurs primarily in the elderly. It causes loss of memory and then progressively impairs more aspects of intellectual and social functioning. Large acetylcholine-containing neurons of the brain are damaged in this disease.

Amanita muscaria The fly agaric mushroom, widely used in ancient times for its hallucinogenic properties.

amotivational syndrome A hypothesized loss of motivation that has been attributed to chronic marijuana use.

amphetamine A synthetic CNS stimulant and sympathomimetic.

anabolic Promoting constructive metabolism; building tissue.

anabolic steroids Substances that increase anabolic (constructive) metabolism, one of the functions of male sex hormones. The result is increased muscle mass.

analgesic Pain-relieving. An analgesic drug produces a selective reduction of pain, whereas an *anesthetic* reduces all sensation.

anandamide A naturally occurring brain chemical with marijuana-like properties.

androgenic Masculinizing.

anesthetic Sense-deadening. An anesthetic drug reduces all sensation, whereas an *analgesic* drug reduces pain.

angel dust A street name for phencyclidine (PCP) when sprinkled on plant material.

anhedonia Lack of emotional response; especially an inability to experience joy or pleasure.

animism The belief that objects and plants contain spirits that move and direct them.

Antabuse Brand name for disulfiram, a drug that interferes with the normal metabolism of alcohol, so that a person who drinks alcohol after taking disulfiram will become quite ill. Antabuse interferes with the enzyme aldehyde dehydrogenase, so that there is a buildup of acetaldehyde, the first metabolic product of alcohol.

antecedents In the context of Chapter 1, behaviors or individual characteristics that can be measured before drug use and might therefore be somewhat predictive of drug use. These are not necessarily causes of the subsequent drug use.

anticonvulsant A drug that prevents or reduces epileptic seizures.

antidepressant A group of drugs used in treating depressive disorders. The MAO inhibitors, the tricyclics, and the SSRIs are the major examples.

antihistamines A group of drugs that act by antagonizing the actions of histamine at its receptors. Used in cold and sinus remedies and in OTC sedatives and sleep aids.

anti-inflammatory Reducing the local swelling, inflammation, and soreness caused by injury or infection. Aspirin has anti-inflammatory properties.

antipsychotics A group of drugs used to treat psychotic disorders, such as schizophrenia. Also called neuroleptics or major tranquilizers.

antipyretic Fever-reducing. Aspirin is a commonly used antipyretic.

antitussive Cough-reducing. Narcotics have this effect. OTC antitussives generally contain dextromethorphan.

anxiety disorders Mental disorders characterized by excessive worry, fears, avoidance, or a sense of impending danger. At pathological levels, these disorders can be debilitating.

anxiolytics Drugs, such as Valium, used in the treatment of anxiety disorders. Literally, "anxiety-dissolving."

aphrodisiac Any substance that is said to promote sexual desire.

aspirin Originally Bayer's brand name for acetylsalicylic acid, now a generic name for that chemical.

assassin The story is that this term for a hired killer is derived from a hashish-using cult, the hashshiyya.

ataxia Loss of coordinated movement; for example, the staggering gait of someone who has consumed a large amount of alcohol.

attention-deficit hyperactivity disorder A learning disability accompanied by hyperactivity. More common in male children. This *DSM-IV-TR* diagnostic category replaces *hyperkinetic syndrome* and *minimal brain dysfunction.*

autonomic nervous system The branch of the peripheral nervous system that regulates the visceral, or automatic ("involuntary") functions of the body, such as heart rate and intestinal motility.

In contrast to the *somatic,* or voluntary, nervous system.

axon A region of a neuron that extends from the cell body and is responsible for conducting the electrical signal to the presynaptic terminals.

B

BAC Blood alcohol concentration, also called blood alcohol level (BAL). The proportion of blood that consists of alcohol. For example, a person with a BAC of 0.10 percent has alcohol constituting one-tenth of 1 percent of the blood and is legally intoxicated in all states.

balanced placebo A research design in which alcohol is compared with a placebo beverage, and subjects either believe they are drinking alcohol or believe they are not.

barbiturate A major class of sedative-hypnotic drugs, including amobarbital and sodium pentothal.

basal ganglia A subcortical brain structure containing large numbers of dopamine synapses. Responsible for maintaining proper muscle tone as a part of the *extrapyramidal motor system.* Damage to the basal ganglia, as in Parkinson's disease, produces muscular rigidity and tremors.

behavioral tolerance Repeated use of a drug can lead to a diminished effect of the drug (tolerance). When the diminished effect occurs because the individual has learned to compensate for the effect of the drug, it is called behavioral tolerance. For example, a novice drinker might be unable to walk with a BAC of 0.20 percent, whereas someone who has practiced walking while intoxicated would be able to walk fairly well at the same BAC.

behavioral toxicity Refers to the fact that a drug can be toxic because it impairs behavior and amplifies the danger level of many activities. The effect of alcohol on driving is an example.

benzodiazepine The group of drugs that includes Valium (diazepam) and Librium (chlordiazepoxide). They are used as *anxiolytics* or *sedatives,* and some types are used as sleeping pills.

bhang A preparation of cannabis (marijuana) that consists of the whole plant, dried and powdered. The weakest of the forms commonly used in India.

binding The interaction between a molecule and a receptor for that molecule. Although the molecules float onto and off the receptor, there are chemical and electrical attractions between a specific molecule and its receptor, so that there is a much higher probability that the receptor will be occupied by its proper molecule than by other molecules.

biopsychosocial A theory or perspective that relies on the interaction of biological, individual psychological, and social variables.

bipolar disorder One of the major mood disorders. Periods of mania and periods of depression have occurred in the same individual. Also called *manic-depressive illness.*

blackout A period of time during which a person was behaving, but of which the person has no memory. The most common cause of this phenomenon is excessive alcohol consumption, and blackouts are considered to indicate pathological drinking.

black tar A type of illicit heroin usually imported from Mexico.

blood alcohol concentration A measure of the concentration of alcohol in the blood, expressed in grams per 100 ml (percentage).

blood-brain barrier Refers to the fact that many substances, including drugs, that can circulate freely in the blood do not readily enter the brain tissue. The major structural feature of this barrier is the tightly jointed epithelial cells lining blood capillaries in the brain. Drug molecules cannot pass between the cells but must instead go through their membranes. Small molecules and molecules that are lipid- (fat-) soluble cross the barrier easily. Obviously, all psychoactive drugs must be capable of crossing the blood-brain barrier.

brain stem The medulla oblongata, pons, and midbrain. Located between the spinal cord and the forebrain, and generally considered to contain the "oldest" (in an evolutionary sense) and most primitive control centers for such basic functions as breathing, swallowing, and so on.

brand name The name given to a drug by a particular manufacturer and licensed only to that manufacturer. For example, *Valium* is a brand name for diazepam. Other companies may sell diazepam, but Hoffman-LaRoche, Inc., owns the name *Valium.*

C

caffeinism Excessive use of caffeine.

Camellia sinesis The plant from which tea is made.

Cannabis Genus of plants known as marijuana or hemp. Includes *C. indica* and *C. sativa.*

carbon monoxide A poisonous gas found in cigarette smoke.

catheter A piece of plastic or rubber tubing that is inserted or implanted into a vein or other structure.

central nervous system Brain and spinal cord.

charas A preparation of cannabis, or marijuana, that is similar to hashish. The most potent form of marijuana commonly used in India.

chemical name For a drug, the name that is descriptive of its chemical structure. For example, the chemical name *sodium chloride* is associated with the *generic* name *table salt,* of which there may be several *brand* names, such as *Morton's.*

chipper An individual who uses heroin occasionally.

chlorpheniramine maleate A common over-the-counter antihistamine found in cold products.

chronic Occurring over time. Chronic drug use is long-term use; chronic drug effects are persistent effects produced by long-term use.

chronic obstructive lung disease A group of disorders that includes emphysema and chronic bronchitis. Cigarette smoking is a major cause of these disorders.

cirrhosis A serious, largely irreversible, and frequently deadly disease of the liver. Usually caused by chronic heavy alcohol use.

club drugs Drugs associated with use at all-night dance parties, known as "raves," held in dance clubs, abandoned warehouses, and increasingly in more traditional nightclubs as the rave-party generation moves into its 20s. The drugs most commonly included in this group include the hallucinogen MDMA and the depressants GHB and Rohypnol.

coca The plant *Erythroxylon coca*, from which cocaine is derived. Also refers to the leaves of this plant.

cocaethylene A potent stimulant formed when cocaine and alcohol are used together.

cocaine A CNS stimulant and local anesthetic; the primary active chemical in coca.

cocaine hydrochloride The most common form of pure cocaine; it is stable and water soluble.

coca paste A crude, smokable extract derived from the coca leaf in the process of making cocaine.

codeine A narcotic chemical present in opium.

comatose A state of unconsciousness from which the individual cannot be aroused.

congeners In general, members of the same group. With respect to alcohol, the term refers to other chemicals (alcohols and oils) that are produced in the process of making a particular alcoholic beverage.

controlled drinking The concept that individuals who have been drinking pathologically can be taught to drink in a controlled, nonpathological manner.

controlled substance A term coined for the 1970 federal law that revised previous laws regulating *narcotics and dangerous drugs*. Heroin and cocaine are examples of controlled substances.

correlate A variable that is statistically related to some other variable, such as drug use.

crack Street name for a smokable form of cocaine. Also called rock.

crank Street name for illicitly manufactured methamphetamine.

crystal meth Street term for a form of methamphetamine crystals, also called *ice.*

cumulative effects Drug effects that increase with repeated administrations, usually due to the buildup of the drug in the body.

CYP450 Cytochrome P450 refers to a group of enzymes found in the liver that are responsible for metabolizing foreign chemicals, including most drugs.

D

DARE Drug Abuse Resistance Education, the most popular prevention program in schools.

date-rape drug A substance given to someone without her knowledge to cause unconsciousness in order to have nonconsensual sex. Rohypnol and GHB have become known for such use. A 1996 U.S. law provides serious penalties for using drugs in this manner.

Datura A plant genus that includes many species used for their hallucinogenic properties. These plants contain anticholinergic chemicals.

DAWN Drug Abuse Warning Network, a federal government system for reporting drug-related medical emergencies and deaths.

DEA United States Drug Enforcement Administration, a branch of the Department of Justice.

delirium tremens Alcohol withdrawal symptoms, including tremors and hallucinations.

demand reduction Efforts to control drug use by reducing the demand for drugs, as opposed to efforts aimed at reducing the supply of drugs. Demand reduction efforts include education and prevention programs, as well as increased punishments for drug users.

dendrite Treelike region of a neuron that extends from the cell body and contains in its membrane receptors that recognize and respond to specific chemical signals.

depressant Any of a large group of drugs that generally slow activity in the CNS and at high doses induce sleep. Includes alcohol, the barbiturates, and other sedative-hypnotic drugs.

depression A major type of mood disorder.

detoxification The process of allowing the body to rid itself of a large amount of alcohol or another drug. Often the first step in a treatment program.

deviance Behavior that is different from established social norms and that social groups take steps to change.

dextromethorphan An over-the-counter cough control ingredient.

diagnosis The process of identifying the nature of an illness. A subject of great controversy for mental disorders.

distillation The process by which alcohol is separated from a weak alcohol solution to form more concentrated distilled spirits. The weak solution is heated, and the alcohol vapors are collected and condensed to a liquid form.

dopamine A neurotransmitter found in the basal ganglia and other regions of the brain.

dose-response curve A graph showing the relationship between the size of a drug dose and the size of the response (or the proportion of subjects showing the response).

double-blind procedure A type of experiment in which the patients and those evaluating them do not know which patients are receiving a placebo and which are receiving the test drug.

dronabinol The generic name for prescription THC in oil in a gelatin capsule.

drug Any substance, natural or artificial, other than food, that by its chemical nature alters structure or function in the living organism.

drug abuse The use of a drug in such a manner or in such amounts or in situations such that the drug use causes problems or greatly increases the chance of problems occurring.

drug dependence A state in which a person uses a drug so frequently and consistently that the individual appears to need the drug to function. This may take the form of *physical dependence,* or behavioral signs may predominate (e.g., unsuccessful attempts to stop or reduce drug use).

drug disposition tolerance The reduced effect of a drug, which can result from more rapid metabolism or excretion of the drug.

drug misuse The use of prescribed drugs in greater amounts than, or for purposes other than, those prescribed by a physician or dentist.

DSM-IV-TR *Diagnostic and Statistical Manual of Mental Disorders,* fourth edition text revised, published by the American Psychiatric Association. It has become a standard for naming and distinguishing among mental disorders.

E

Ecstasy Street name for the hallucinogen MDMA. Also called "XTC."

ECT Electroconvulsive therapy, or electroconvulsive shock treatment. A procedure in which an electrical current is passed through the head, resulting in an epileptic-like seizure. Although this treatment is now used infrequently, it is still considered to be the most effective and rapid treatment for severe depression.

ED_{50} The effective dose for half the subjects in a drug test.

effective dose The dose of a drug that produces a certain effect in some percentage of the subjects. For example, an ED_{50} produces the effect in 50 percent of the subjects. Note that the dose will depend on the effect that is monitored.

emphysema A chronic lung disease in which tissue deterioration results in increased air retention and reduced exchange of gases. The result is difficulty breathing and shortness of breath. An example of a *chronic obstructive lung disease,* often caused by smoking.

endorphins Morphine-like chemicals that occur naturally in the brains and pituitary glands of humans and other animals. There are several proper endorphins, and the term is also used generically to refer to both the endorphins and the enkephalins.

enkephalins Morphine-like chemicals that occur naturally in the brains and adrenal glands of humans and other animals. The enkephalins are smaller molecules than the endorphins.

enzyme A large, organic molecule that works to speed up or help along a specific chemical reaction. Enzymes are found in brain cells, where they are needed for most steps in the synthesis of neurotransmitter molecules. They are also found in the liver, where they are needed for the metabolism of many drug molecules.

ephedrine A drug derived from the Chinese medicinal herb *ma huang* and used to relieve breathing difficulty in asthma. A sympathomimetic from which amphetamine was derived.

epilepsy A disorder of the nervous system in which recurring periods of abnormal electrical activity in the brain produce temporary malfunction. There might or might not be loss of consciousness or uncontrolled motor movements (seizures).

ergogenic Energy-producing. Refers to drugs or other methods (e.g., blood doping) designed to enhance an athlete's performance.

ergotism A disease caused by eating grain infected with the ergot fungus. There are both psychological and physical manifestations.

F

FAS Fetal alcohol syndrome.

FDA United States Food and Drug Administration.

fen-phen A combination of two prescription weight-control medications, fenfluramine and phentermine. No longer prescribed due to concerns with toxicity to heart valves.

fermentation The process by which sugars are converted into grain alcohol through the action of yeasts.

fetal alcohol effect Individual developmental abnormalities associated with the mother's alcohol use during pregnancy.

fetal alcohol syndrome Facial and developmental abnormalities associated with the mother's alcohol use during pregnancy.

flashback An experience reported by some users of LSD in which portions of the LSD experience recur at a later time without the use of the drug.

fly agaric mushroom *Amanita muscaria,* a hallucinogenic mushroom that is also considered poisonous.

freebase In general, when a chemical salt is separated into its basic and acidic components, the basic component is referred to as the free base. Most psychoactive drugs are bases that normally exist in a salt form. Specifically, the salt cocaine hydrochloride can be chemically extracted to form the cocaine free base, which is volatile and can therefore be smoked.

functional disorder A mental disorder for which there is no known organic cause. Schizophrenia is a form of psychosis that is considered to be a functional disorder.

G

GABA An inhibitory neurotransmitter found in most brain regions; gamma-aminobutyric acid.

gamma hydroxybutyrate (GHB) CNS depressant, produced naturally in small amounts in the human brain; has been used recreationally and, in combination with alcohol, has some reputation as a date-rape drug; chemically related to GABA.

ganja A preparation of *cannabis* (marijuana) in which the most potent parts of the plant are used.

gateway substances Substances, such as alcohol, tobacco, and sometimes marijuana, that most users of illicit substances will have tried before their first use of cocaine, heroin, or other less widely used illicit drugs.

generic name For drugs, a name that specifies a particular chemical without being chemically descriptive or referring to a brand name. As an example, the *chemical name* sodium chloride is associated with the *generic name* table salt, of which there may be several *brand names,* such as Morton's.

glia Brain cells that provide firmness and structure to the brain, get nutrients into the system, eliminate waste, form myelin, and create the blood-brain barrier.

glutamate An excitatory neurotransmitter found in most brain regions.

GRAE "Generally recognized as effective"; a term defined by the FDA with reference to the ingredients found in OTC drugs (see also *GRAS*).

GRAHL "Generally recognized as honestly labeled" (see also *GRAE* and *GRAS*).

grain neutral spirits Ethyl alcohol distilled to a purity of 190 proof (95 percent).

grand mal An epileptic seizure that results in convulsive motor movements and loss of consciousness.

GRAS "Generally recognized as safe"; a term defined by the FDA with reference to food additives and the ingredients found in OTC drugs.

H

hallucinogen A drug, such as LSD or mescaline, that produces profound alterations in perception.

hashish A potent preparation of concentrated resin from the *Cannabis* plant.

hash oil A slang term for oil of cannabis, a liquid extract from the marijuana plant.

henbane A poisonous plant containing anticholinergic chemicals and sometimes used for its hallucinogenic properties. *Hyoscyamus niger*.

heroin Originally Bayer's name for diacetylmorphine, a potent narcotic analgesic synthesized from morphine.

HIV Human immunodeficiency virus. The infectious agent responsible for AIDS.

homeostasis A state of physiological balance maintained by various regulatory mechanisms; body functions such as blood pressure and temperature must be maintained within a certain range.

hooka A water pipe, often with more than one mouthpiece. Used to smoke tobacco or marijuana.

human growth hormone A pituitary hormone responsible for some types of giantism.

hyperactive Refers to a disorder characterized by short attention span and a high level of motor activity. The *DSM-IV-TR* term is *attention-deficit hyperactivity disorder*.

hypnotic Sleep-inducing. For drugs, refers to sleeping preparations.

hypodermic syringe A device to which a hollow needle can be attached, so that solutions can be injected through the skin.

hypothalamus A group of nuclei found at the base of the brain, just above the pituitary gland.

I

ibogaine A hallucinogen that has been shown to reduce self-administration of cocaine and morphine in rats and is proposed to reduce craving in drug addicts.

ibuprofen An aspirin-like analgesic and anti-inflammatory.

ice The street name for crystals of methamphetamine hydrochloride.

illicit drug A drug that is unlawful to possess or use.

IND Approval to conduct clinical investigations on a new drug, filed with the FDA after animal tests are complete.

indole A type of chemical structure. The neurotransmitter serotonin and the hallucinogen LSD both contain an indole nucleus.

inhalants Any of a variety of volatile solvents or other products that can be inhaled to produce intoxication.

insomnia Inability to sleep. The most common complaint is difficulty falling asleep. Often treated with a hypnotic drug.

intramuscular A type of injection in which the drug is administered into a muscle.

intravenous (IV) A type of injection in which the drug is administered into a vein.

L

laissez-faire A theory that government should not interfere with business or other activities.

LD_{50} The lethal dose for half the animals in a test.

lethal dose The dose of a drug that produces a lethal effect in some percentage of the animals on which it is tested. For example, LD_{50} is the dose that would kill 50 percent of the animals to which it was given.

leukoplakia A whitening and thickening of the mucous tissues of the mouth. The use of chewing tobacco is associated with an increase in leukoplakia, considered to be a "precancerous" tissue change.

limbic system A system of various brain structures that are involved in emotional responses.

lipid solubility The tendency of a chemical to dissolve in oils or fats, as opposed to in water.

lithium A highly reactive metallic element, atomic number 3. Its salts are used in the treatment of mania and *bipolar disorder*.

longitudinal study A study done over a period of time (months or years).

look-alikes Drugs sold legally, usually through the mail, that are made to look like controlled, prescription-only drugs. The most common types contain caffeine and resemble amphetamine capsules or tablets.

M

ma huang A Chinese herb containing ephedrine, which is a sympathomimetic drug from which amphetamine was derived.

major depression A serious mental disorder characterized by a depressed mood. A specific diagnostic term in the *DSM-IV-TR.*

malting The process of wetting a grain and allowing it to sprout, to maximize its sugar content before fermentation to produce an alcoholic beverage.

mandrake *Mandragora officinarum,* a plant having a branched root that contains anticholinergic chemicals. Now classed among the other anticholinergic hallucinogens, this plant was widely believed to have aphrodisiac properties.

marijuana Also spelled marihuana; dried leaves of the *Cannabis* plant.

Marinol The brand name for prescription THC in oil in a gelatin capsule.

MDMA Methylenedioxy methamphetamine, a catechol hallucinogen related to MDA. Called "Ecstasy" or "XTC" on the street.

medial forebrain bundle A group of neuron fibers that projects from the midbrain to the forebrain, passing near the hypothalamus. Now known to contain several chemically and anatomically distinct pathways, including dopamine and norepinephrine pathways.

medical model With reference to mental disorders, a model that assumes that abnormal behaviors are *symptoms* resulting from a *disease.*

mental illness A term that, to some theorists, implies acceptance of a medical model of mental disorders.

mescaline The active hallucinogenic chemical in the peyote cactus.

mesolimbic dopamine pathway A group of dopamine-containing neurons that have their cell bodies in the midbrain and their terminals in the forebrain, on various structures associated with the limbic system. Believed by some theorists to be important in explaining the therapeutic effects of antipsychotic medications. Also believed by some theorists to be important for many types of behavioral reinforcers.

metabolism (of drugs) The breakdown or inactivation of drug molecules by enzymes, often in the liver.

metabolite A product of enzyme action on a drug.

metabolize To break down or inactivate a neurotransmitter (or a drug) through enzymatic action.

methadone A long-lasting synthetic opioid; commonly used in the long-term treatment for opioid dependence.

methadone maintenance A program for treatment of narcotic addicts in which the synthetic drug methadone is provided to the addicts in an oral dosage form, so that they can maintain their addiction legally.

methylphenidate A stimulant used in treating ADHD; brand name Ritalin.

Mexican brown A form of heroin that first appeared on American streets in the mid-1970s. Because the heroin is made from the hydrochloride salt of morphine, it is brown in its pure form.

moist snuff A type of oral smokeless tobacco that is popular among young American men. A "pinch" of this finely chopped, moistened, flavored tobacco is held in the mouth, often between the lower lip and the gum.

monoamine oxidase (MAO) inhibitor A drug that acts by inhibiting the enzyme monoamine oxidase (MAO). Used as an antidepressant.

mood disorder Mental disorders characterized by depressed or manic symptoms.

morphine A narcotic; the primary active chemical in opium. Heroin is made from morphine

morphine A narcotic; the primary active chemical in opium. Heroin is made from morphine.

morphinism An older term used to describe dependence on the use of morphine.

motivational interviewing A technique for encouraging alcoholics or addicts to seek treatment by first assessing their degree of dependence and then discussing the assessment results. Direct confrontation is avoided.

N

naloxone An opioid antagonist used in treating alcoholism.

narcolepsy A form of sleep disorder characterized by bouts of muscular weakness and falling asleep suddenly and involuntarily. The most common treatment employs stimulant drugs such as amphetamine to maintain wakefulness during the day.

narcotic Opioid (in pharmacology terms), or a drug that is produced or sold illegally (in legal terms); in the United States, a "controlled substance."

narcotic antagonists Drugs that can block the actions of narcotics.

Native American Church A religious organization active among American Indians, in which the hallucinogenic peyote cactus is used in conjunction with Christian religious themes.

NDA In FDA procedures, a New Drug Application. This application, demonstrating both safety and effectiveness of a new drug in both animal and human experiments, must be submitted by a drug company to the FDA before a new drug can be marketed.

neuroleptic A general term for the antipsychotic drugs (also called *major tranquilizers*).

neuron Brain cell that analyzes and transmits information via chemical and electrical signals.

neurotransmitter A chemical messenger that is released by one neuron and that alters the electrical activity in another neuron; its effects are brief and local.

Nicotiana Any of several types of tobacco plant, including *N. tobacum* and *N. rustica*.

nicotine The chemical contained in tobacco that is responsible for its psychoactive effects and for tobacco dependence.

nigrostriatal dopamine pathway A group of dopamine-containing neurons that have their cell bodies in the *substantia nigra* of the midbrain and their terminals in the *corpus striatum* (basal ganglia), which is part of the extrapyramidal motor system. It is this pathway that deteriorates in Parkinson's disease and on which antipsychotic drugs act to produce side effects resembling Parkinson's disease.

nitrosamines A group of organic chemicals, many of which are highly carcinogenic. At least four are found only in tobacco, and these might account for much of the cancer-causing property of tobacco.

nonspecific effects Effects of a drug that are not changed by changing the chemical makeup of the drug. Also referred to as placebo effects.

norepinephrine A neurotransmitter that might be important for regulating waking and appetite.

NORML National Organization for the Reform of Marijuana Laws.

NSAIDs Nonsteroidal anti-inflammatory drugs, such as ibuprofen and naproxen.

nucleus basalis A group of large cell bodies found just below the basal ganglia and containing acetylcholine. These cells send terminations widely to the cerebral cortex. In Alzheimer's disease, there is a loss of these neurons and a reduction in the amount of acetylcholine in the cortex.

O

opioid One of a group of drugs similar to morphine, used medically primarily for their analgesic effects. Opioids include drugs derived from opium and synthetic drugs with opium-like effects.

opioid antagonist Any of several drugs that are capable of blocking the effects of opioids. Used in emergency medicine to treat overdose and in some addiction treatment programs to block the effect of any illicit opioid that might be taken. Nalorphine and naltrexone are examples.

opium A sticky raw substance obtained from the seed pods of the opium poppy and containing the narcotic chemicals morphine and codeine.

organic disorder For mental disorders, those with a known physical cause (e.g., psychosis caused by long-term alcohol use).

OTC Over-the-counter. OTC drugs are those drugs that can be purchased without a prescription.

P

Papaver somniferum The opium poppy.

paraphernalia In general, the equipment used in some activity. Drug paraphernalia include such items as syringes, pipes, scales, or mirrors.

parasympathetic The branch of the autonomic nervous system that has acetylcholine as its neurotransmitter and, for example, slows the heart rate and activates the intestine.

Parkinson's disease A degenerative disease of the extrapyramidal motor system, specifically involving damage to the nigrostriatal dopamine system. Early symptoms include muscular rigidity, tremors, a shuffling gait, and a masklike face. Occurs primarily in the elderly.

passive smoking The inhalation of tobacco smoke from the air by nonsmokers.

patent medicines Proprietary medicines. Originally referred to medicines that were, in fact, treated as inventions and patented in Great Britain. In America, the term came to refer to medicines sold directly to the public.

PCP Phenycyclidine; 1-(1-phenylcyclohexl) piperidine. A drug with hallucinogenic properties that was originallly developed as an anesthetic; it is not legally available for human use. This hallucinogen is often referred to as angel dust.

PDR *Physician's Desk Reference,* a book listing all prescription drugs and giving prescribing information about each. Updated yearly.

pekoe A grade of tea.

peptide A class of chemicals made up of sequences of amino acids. Enkephalins are small peptides containing only five amino acids, whereas large proteins may contain hundreds.

peyote A hallucinogenic cactus containing the chemical mescaline.

phantastica Hallucinogens that create a world of fantasy.

pharmacodynamic tolerance Reduced effectiveness of a drug resulting from altered nervous system sensitivity.

phenothiazines A group of chemicals that includes several antipsychotic medications.

phenylpropanolamine (PPA) Until 2000, an active ingredient in OTC weight-control products.

physical dependence Defined by the presence of a consistent set of symptoms when use of a drug is stopped. These withdrawal symptoms imply that homeostatic mechanisms of the body had made adjustments to counteract the drug's effects and without the drug the system is thrown out of balance.

placebo An inactive drug, often used in experiments to control for nonspecific effects of drug administration.

postsynaptic Refers to structures associated with the neural membrane on the receiving side of a synapse.

potency Measured by the amount of a drug is required to produce a given effect.

precursor Something that precedes something else. In biochemistry, a precursor molecule may be acted upon by an enzyme and changed into a different molecule. For example, the dietary amino acid tryptophan is the precursor for the neurotransmitter serotonin.

prodrugs Drugs that are administered in an inactive form and become effective after they are chemically modified in the body by enzymes.

Prohibition The period 1920–1933, during which the sale of alcoholic beverages was prohibited in the United States.

proof A measure of a beverage's alcohol content; twice the alcohol percentage.

proprietary A medicine that is marketed directly to the public. Also called *OTC, patent,* or *nonprescription* medicines.

prostaglandins Local hormones, some of which are synthesized in response to cell injury and are important for initiating pain signals. Aspirin and similar drugs inhibit the formation of prostaglandins.

protective factors Behaviors, attitudes, or situations that correlate with low rates of deviant behavior, including use of illicit drugs. Examples include commitment to school, religiosity, and having parents who communicate opposition to drug use.

protein binding The combining of drug molecules with blood proteins.

psilocybin The active hallucinogenic chemical in *Psilocybe* mushrooms.

psychedelic Another name for hallucinogenic drugs. Has a somewhat positive connotation of mind viewing or mind clearing.

psychoactive A term used to describe drugs that have their principal effect on the CNS.

psychological dependence Behavioral dependence, indicated by a high rate of drug use, craving for the drug, and a tendency to relapse after stopping use.

psychopharmacology Science that studies the behavioral effects of drugs.

psychosis A type of mental disorder characterized by a loss of contact with reality and by deterioration in social and intellectual functioning.

psychotomimetic Another name for hallucinogenic drugs. Has a negative connotation of mimicking psychosis.

Q

quid A piece of something to be chewed, such as a wad of chewing tobacco.

R

receptors Specialized cell structures that recognize and respond to signals from specific chemicals (neurotransmitters or drugs).

reinforcement The process of strengthening a behavioral tendency by presenting a stimulus contingent on the behavior. For example, the tendency to obtain and take a drug might be strengthened by the stimulus properties of the drug that occur after it is taken, thus leading to psychological dependence.

reuptake One process by which neurotransmitter chemicals are removed from synapses. The chemical is taken back up into the cell from which it was released.

Reye's syndrome A rare brain infection that occurs almost exclusively in children and adolescents. There is some evidence that it is more likely to occur in children who have been given aspirin during a bout of flu or chicken pox.

risk factors Behaviors, attitudes, or situations that correlate with, and might indicate the development of, a deviance-prone lifestyle that includes drug or alcohol abuse. Examples are early alcohol intoxication, absence from school, and perceived peer approval of drug use.

rock Another street name for *crack,* a smokable form of cocaine.

Rohypnol (flunitrazepam) A benzodiazepine hypnotic; not sold legally in the United States and known as the "date-rape drug."

S

safety margin Dose range between an acceptable level of effectiveness and the lowest toxic dose.

salicylate A class of chemicals that includes aspirin.

schizophrenia A chronic psychotic disorder for which the cause is unknown.

sedative A drug used to relax, tranquilize, or calm a person, reducing stress and excitement.

serotonin A neurotransmitter found in the raphe nuclei that might be important for impulsivity and depression.

shisha Sweetened, flavored tobacco for use in a hooka.

side effects Unintended drug effects that accompany the desired therapeutic effect.

sidestream smoke Smoke that comes from the ash of a cigarette or cigar.

sinsemilla A process for growing marijuana that is especially potent in its psychological effects because of a high THC content; from the Spanish for "without seeds."

smokeless tobacco Various forms of chewing tobacco and snuff.

social influence model A prevention model adapted from successful smoking-prevention programs.

somatic system The part of the nervous system that controls the voluntary, skeletal muscles, such as the large muscles of the arms and legs.

specific effects Those effects of a drug that depend on the amount and type of chemical contained in the drug.

speed A street term used at one time for cocaine, then for injectable amphetamine, and later for all types of amphetamine. Probably shortened from *speedball.*

SSRI Selective serotonin reuptake inhibitor; a class of antidepressants that includes Prozac.

stages of change Theoretical description of the cognitive stages through which an addict would go in moving from active use to treatment and abstinence: precontemplation, contemplation, preparation, action, and maintenance.

stimulant Any of a group of drugs that has the effect of reversing mental and physical fatigue.

subcutaneous Under the skin. A form of injection in which the needle penetrates through the skin (about 3/8 inch) but does not enter a muscle or vein.

sympathetic nervous system The branch of the autonomic nervous system that contains norepinephrine as its neurotransmitter and, for example, increases heart rate and blood pressure.

sympathomimetic Any drug that stimulates the sympathetic branch of the autonomic nervous system— for example, amphetamine.

symptom In medical terms, an abnormality that indicates a disease. When applied to abnormal behavior, seems to imply a medical model in which an unseen disease causes the abnormal behavior.

synesthesia A phenomenon in which the different senses become blended or mixed—for example, a sound is "seen." Might be reported by a person taking hallucinogens.

synthesis The formation of a chemical compound. For example, some neurotransmitter chemicals must be synthesized within the neuron by the action of enzymes on precursors.

T

tachyphylaxis A rapid form of tolerance in which a second dose of a drug has a smaller effect than a first dose taken only a short time before.

tar With regard to tobacco, a complex mixture of chemicals found in cigarette smoke. After water, gases, and nicotine are removed from the smoke, the remaining residue is considered to be tar.

tardive dyskinesia Movement disorders that appear after several weeks or months of treatment with antipsychotic drugs and that usually become worse if use of the drug is discontinued.

temperance With reference to alcohol, temperance originally meant avoiding hard liquor and consuming beer and wine in moderation. Eventually the temperance movement adopted complete abstinence as its goal and prohibition as the means.

tetrahydrocannabinol The most active of the many chemicals found in cannabis (marijuana).

THC Tetrahydrocannabinol.

theobromine A mild stimulant similar to caffeine and found in chocolate; a xanthine.

theophylline A mild stimulant similar to caffeine and found in tea; a xanthine.

therapeutic index (TI) Ratio of the lethal dose to the effective dose for half the animals in an experiment (LD_{50}/ED_{50}).

time course Timing of the onset, duration, and termination of a drug's effect in the body.

tolerance The reduced effectiveness of a drug after repeated administration.

toxic Poisonous, dangerous.

transporter Mechanism in the nerve terminal membrane responsible for removing neurotransmitter molecules from the synapse by taking them back into the neuron.

tricyclics A group of chemicals used in treating depression.

truth serum Any drugs used to "loosen the tongue," in association with either psychotherapy or interrogation. Although people might speak more freely after receiving some drugs, there is no guarantee that anything they say is true.

U

uptake The process by which a cell expends energy to concentrate certain chemicals within itself. For example, precursor substances to be synthesized into neurotransmitters must be taken up by the neuron.

V

values clarification A type of affective education that avoids reference to drugs but focuses on helping students recognize and express their own feelings and beliefs.

W

Wernicke-Korsakoff syndrome Chronic mental impairments produced by heavy alcohol use over a long period of time.

withdrawal syndrome The set of symptoms that occur reliably when someone stops taking a drug; also called *abstinence syndrome*.

X

xanthine The chemical class that includes caffeine, theobromine, and theophylline.

Photo Credits

Chapter 1
p. 3: Emma Lee/Life File/Getty Images; **p. 8:** Getty Images; **p. 9:** © Digital Vision/Getty Images; **p. 12:** McGraw-Hill Companies, Inc./Gary He, photographer; **p. 19:** © Brand X Pictures/PunchStock; **p. 21:** © BananaStock/ PunchStock

Chapter 2
p. 31: Dynamic Graphics/JupiterImages; **p. 32:** © Annie Griffiths Belt/Corbis; **p. 36:** McGraw-Hill Companies, Inc./Gary He, photographer; **p. 39:** The McGraw-Hill Companies, Inc./Jill Braaten, photographer; **p. 42:** © Mikael Karlsson

Chapter 3
p. 54 (*top*): Library of Congress Prints and Photographs Division (09335u); **p. 54** (*bottom*): Library of Congress Prints and Photographs Division (3C03376U); **p. 59:** PhotoLink/Getty Images; **p. 61:** © The McGraw-Hill Companies, Inc./Elite Images; **p. 74:** © Thorne Anderson/Corbis

Chapter 4
p. 97 (*left*): National Cancer Institute Visuals Online (Dr. Giovanni Dichiro, Neuroimaging Section, National Institute of Neurological Disorders and Stroke); **p. 97** (*right*): © Royalty-Free/Corbis

Chapter 5
p. 111, 113: © Royalty-Free/Corbis; **p. 114:** Doug Menuez/Getty Images

Chapter 6
p. 130: © Royalty-Free/Corbis; **p. 134:** McGraw-Hill Companies,

Inc./Gary He, photographer; **p. 137:** Spike Mafford/Getty Images; **p. 140:** Drug Enforcement Administration

Chapter 7
p. 158: Spike Mafford/Getty Images; **p. 183:** Jonnie Miles/Getty Images; **p. 164:** © Royalty-Free/Corbis; **p. 169:** © Michael Newman/PhotoEdit; **p. 170:** © Barbara Stitzer/PhotoEdit

Chapter 8
p. 177: The McGraw-Hill Companies, Inc./Lars A. Niki, photographer; **p. 184:** Mel Curtis/Getty Images; **p. 189:** Royalty-Free/Corbis

Chapter 9
p. 196: John A. Rizzo/Getty Images; **p. 198:** Andersen Ross/Getty Images; **p. 199:** Library of Congress Prints and Photographs Division (3g06495u); **p. 203:** National Photo Company Collection; Library of Congress Prints and Photographs Division (3b42859u); **p. 208:** © BananaStock/PunchStock; **p. 216:** Tomi/PhotoLink/Getty Images; **p. 220:** Ryan McVay/Getty Images; **p. 223:** Fletcher, C. D. M. and McKee, P. H. *An Atlas of Gross Pathology.* © 1987 Mosby-Wolfe Europe Limited, London, UK; **p. 224:** © David H. Wells/Corbis

Chapter 10
p. 237: Flora Torrance/Life File/Getty Images; **p. 240:** Library of Congress Prints and Photographs Division (3G04309U); **p. 241:** Library of Congress Prints and Photographs Division (3b04259); **p. 242:**

Dynamic Graphics/JupiterImages; **p. 244:** The McGraw-Hill Companies, Inc./Christopher Kerrigan, photographer; **p. 245:** Emma Lee/Life File/Getty Images; **p. 247:** Steve Mason/Getty Images; **p. 250:** © Royalty-Free/Corbis; **p. 251:** Getty Images; **p. 254:** McGraw-Hill Companies, Inc./Gary He, photographer; **p. 256:** Stockdisc/PunchStock

Chapter 11
p. 262: Ryan McVay/Getty Images; **p. 264** (*top*): C. Sherburne/PhotoLink/Getty Images; **p. 264** (*bottom*): B: Jules Frazier/Getty Images; **p. 265:** S. Meltzer/PhotoLink/Getty Images; **p. 266:** PhotoLink/Getty Images; **p. 267:** Library of Congress Prints and Photographs Division (3A25022U); **p. 268:** Spike Mafford/Getty Images; **p. 269:** L. Hobbs/PhotoLink/Getty Images; **p. 270:** © Royalty-Free/Corbis; **p. 271:** Library of Congress Prints and Photographs Division (3G12222U); **p. 273:** © McGraw-Hill Companies/Jill Braaten, photographer; **p. 276:** Stockbyte/PunchStock; **p. 278:** © Royalty-Free/Corbis

Chapter 12
p. 285: Don Farrall/Getty Images; **p. 289:** Mitch Hrdlicka/Getty Images; **p. 291, 295:** © Royalty-Free/Corbis; **p. 300:** McGraw-Hill Companies, Inc./Gary He, photographer

Chapter 13
p. 313: © Steven L. Raymer/Getty Images/National Geographic; **p. 314:** Drug Enforcement

Administration; **p. 319:** Don Farrall/Getty Images; **p. 328:** Photodisc Green/Doug Menuez

Chapter 14
p. 340: © Bettmann/Corbis; **p. 342:** Drug Enforcement Administration; **p. 346:** Alan Pappe/Getty Images; **p. 347:** The McGraw-Hill Companies: Inc./Lars A. Niki, photographer; **p. 348:** US Fish & Wildlife; **p. 350:** © Stapleton Collection/Corbis; **p. 352:** Drug Enforcement Administration; **p. 360:** Digital Vision/PunchStock

Chapter 15
p. 368: Brand X Pictures/PunchStock; **p. 370:**

Drug Enforcement Administration; **p. 378:** Doug Menuez/Getty Images; **p. 381:** The McGraw-Hill Companies, Inc./Lars A. Niki, photographer; **p. 385:** McGraw-Hill Companies, Inc./Gary He, photographer; **p. 387:** Getty Images

Chapter 16
p. 396: Karl Weatherly/Getty Images; **p. 401:** PhotoLink/Getty Images; **p. 403:** Drug Enforcement Administration; **p. 408:** Anthony Saint James/Getty Images

Chapter 17
p. 418: Imagesource/PictureQuest; **p. 422:** © Royalty-Free/Corbis; **p. 425:**

Stockbyte/PunchStock; **p. 428:** The McGraw-Hill Companies, Inc./John Flournoy, photographer

Chapter 18
p. 436: © Bettmann/Corbis; **p. 441:** © Robert Vanden Brugge/BELGA/epa/Corbis; **p. 442:** © Ed Kashi/Corbis; **p. 445:** © Mary Kate Denny/PhotoEdit

Index